Aphasiology

Aphasiology

ANDRÉ ROCH LECOURS
FRANÇOIS LHERMITTE
and
BONNIE BRYANS

with the collaboration of
André Ali-Chérif, Michèle Bergeron, Louise Bérubé, Mihai Ioan Botez, Rémi Bouchard, David Caplan, Louise Coderre, Guy A. Courtois, Caroline Cronk, Laurent Descarries, Gérard Dordain, John Dudley, Raymond Escourolle, Yves Joanette, Maurice-André Lacroix, Denise Lafond, Ginette Lavallée-Huynh, Andrée Lemay, Charles-Joseph Nasser, Jean-Luc Nespoulous, Mireille Olivier, Michel Paradis, Gilbert Pinard, Michel Poncet, Jacques Ponzio, Michèle Ramade-Poncet, Françoise Rouillon, Michèle Sébahoun-Balsamo, Cheryl Trépagnier, Marie Vanier

Preface by
JOHN C. MARSHALL

Baillière Tindall · London

Published by Baillière Tindall,
a division of Cassell Ltd,
1 St Anne's Road, Eastbourne, East Sussex BN21 3UN

Publication of this book was encouraged by a grant awarded in the context of France–Quebec Cooperation

Results from several investigations have been integrated into this text. Much of this research was made possible by Grant MA-4210 from the Conseil de la Recherche Médicale du Canada

First English edition 1983
ISBN 0-7020-1014-6

Typeset, printed and bound in Great Britain by
Butler & Tanner Ltd, Frome and London

British Library Cataloguing in Publication Data

Lecours, André Roch
Aphasiology.
1. Aphasia 2. Languages—Psychology
I. Title II. Lhermitte, François
III. Bryans, Bonnie IV. L'aphasie. English
616.85′52 RC425

ISBN 0-7020-1014-6

Contributors

André AL-Chérif, Médicin, Service de Neurologie et de Neuropsychologie, Hôpital de la Timone, Marseilles, France.

Michèle Bergeron, Professor Agrégé, Faculté de Médecine, Université de Montréal, Ecole d'Orthophonie et d'Audiologie, Montreal, Quebec, Canada.

Louise Bérubé, Psychologue, Service de Neurologie, Hôtel-Dieu, Montreal, Quebec, Canada.

Mihai Dan Botez, Professeur, Faculté de Médecine, Université de Montréal, Service de Neurologie, Hôtel-Dieu, Montreal, Quebec, Canada.

Rémi Bouchard, Service de Neurologie, Hôpital de l'Enfant-Jésus, Quebec, Quebec, Canada.

Bonnie Bryans, Associate Professor, School of Human Communication Disorders, Dalhousie University, Halifax, Nova Scotia, Canada.

David Caplan, Associate Professor, Faculty of Medicine, Temple University, Philadelphia, PA, USA.

Louise Coderre, Professeur Agrégé, Faculté de Médecine, Université de Montréal; Directrice de l'Ecole d'Orthophonie et d'Audiologie, Montreal, Quebec, Canada.

Guy A. Courtois, Professeur, Faculté de Médecine, Université de Montréal, Montreal, Quebec, Canada.

Caroline Cronk, Professeur Adjoint, Faculté de Médecine, Université de Montréal, Ecole d'Orthophonie et d'Audiologie, Montreal, Quebec, Canada.

Laurent Descarries, Professeur, Faculté de Médecine, Université de Montréal; Membre du Centre de Recherches en Sciences Neurologiques, Université de Montréal, Montreal, Quebec, Canada.

Gerard Dordain, Professeur Agrégé, Faculté de Médecine de Clermont-Ferrand, Service de Neurologie, Hôpital Fontmaure, Chamalières, France.

John Dudley, Professeur Agrégé, Faculté de Médecine, Université de Montréal, Ecole d'Orthophonie et d'Audiologie, Montreal, Quebec, Canada.

Raymond Escourolle, Professeur, Faculté de Médecine, Université de Paris VI; Chef, Service de Neuropathologie, Hôpital de la Salpêtrière, Paris, France.

Yves Joanette, Scholar, Conseil de la Recherch Médicale du Canada, Chercheur Adjoint, Faculté de Médecine, Université de Montréal; Laboratoire Théophile Alajouanine, Centre de Recherche, Centre Hospitalier Côte-des-Neiges, Montreal, Quebec, Canada.

Maurice-André Lacroix, Psychologue, Centre de Rééducation du Langage et de Recherche Neuropsychologique, Hôtel-Dieu, Montreal, Quebec, Canada.

Denise Lafond, Orthophoniste, Laboratoire Théophile Alajouanine, Centre de Recherche, Centre Hospitalier Côte-des-Neiges, Montreal, Quebec, Canada.

Ginette Lavallée-Huynh, Linguiste, Laboratoire Théophile Alajouanine, Centre de Recherche, Centre Hospitalier Côte-des-Neiges, Montreal, Quebec, Canada.

André Roch Lecours, Professeur, Faculté de Médecine, Université de Montréal; Directeur du Laboratoire Théophile Alajouanine, Centre de Recherche, Centre Hospitalier Côte-des-Neiges, Montreal, Quebec, Canada. Recipient of grant MT-4210 from the Conseil de la Recherche médicale du Canada.

Andrée Lemay, Orthophoniste, Laboratoire Théophile Alajouanine, Centre de Recherche, Centre Hospitalier Côte-des-Neiges, Montreal, Quebec, Canada.

François Lhermitte, Membre de l'Institut, Professeur à la Faculté de Médecine, Université de Paris VI; Directeur du Groupe de Recherches INSERM U-84; Chef de Service, Clinique de Neurologie et de Neuropsychologie, Hôpital de la Salpêtrière, Paris, France.

Charles-Joseph Nasser, Centre du Langage, Service de Neurologie et de Neuropsychologie, Hôpital de la Timone, Marseilles, France.

Jean-Luc Nespoulous, Professeur Agrégé, Département de Linguistique et Philologie, Université de Montréal; Co-directeur du Laboratoire Théophile Alajouanine, Centre de Recherche, Centre Hospitalier Côte-des-Neiges, Montreal, Quebec, Canada.

Mireille Olivier, Psychologue, Service de Neurologie, Hôtel-Dieu, Montreal, Quebec, Canada.

Michel Paradis, Associate Professor, Department of Linguistics, McGill University, Montreal, Quebec, Canada.

Gilbert Pinard, Professeur, Faculté de Médecine, Université de Sherbrooke, Département de Psychiatrie, CHU de Sherbrooke, Sherbrooke, Quebec, Canada.

Michel Poncet, Professeur Agrégé, CHU de Marseille-la-Timone; Directeur de Centre du Langage, Service de Neurologie et de Neuropsychologie, Hôpital de la Timone, Marseilles, France.

Jacques Ponzio, Centre du Langage, Service de Neurologie et Neuropsychologie, Hôpital de la Timone, Marseilles, France.

Michèle Ramade-Poncet, Centre du Langage, Service de Neurologie et Neuropsychologie, Hôpital de la Timone, Marseilles, France.

Françoise Rouillon, Orthophoniste.

Michèle Sébahoun-Balsamo, Psychologue, Centre du Langage, Service de Neurologie et de Neuropsychologie, Hôpital de la Timone, Marseilles, France.

Cheryl Trépagnier, Assistant Professor, Department of Linguistics, Boston University, Boston, MA, USA.

Marie Vanier, Psychologue, Laboratoire Théophile Alajouanine, Centre de Recherche, Centre Hospitalier Côte-des-Neiges, Montreal, Quebec, Canada.

Table of Contents

Preface

Of all our cognitive capacities there can be few that hold the intrinsic and practical significance of language. To imagine the emergence of human-like societies and sciences in a species *without* language strains credulity well past breaking point. Small wonder, then, that a professional concern with language should characterize not only poets and philologists but also philosophers and physicians.

It is, of course, the frailty of language that draws the physician's attention, for the skills that underlie linguistic communication are all too susceptible to trauma and disease. In the earliest extant medical records, Egyptian surgeons recorded their observations of language loss consequent upon head injury. 'The breath of an outside god or death', they argued, had entered the brains of their patients who henceforth became 'silent in sadness'[4]. And the practice of trepanning was instituted, presumably to encourage and facilitate the exit of the god's breath. Later, the physicians of the Hippocratic School knew that wounds to one side of the head frequently resulted in spasm or paralysis of the opposite side of the body; they furthermore observed the correlation of speechlessness with paralysis of the right arm and leg[5]. For us, the conjunction of these observations implies that language is a function not of the brain as a whole but rather of the left hemisphere. Yet as Benton and Joynt[3] point out, there is no evidence that this deduction was drawn by the writers of the Hippocratic Corpus, and two millennia were to pass before Paul Broca convinced the medical community that aphasia-provoking lesions had a 'singular predilection' for the left cerebral hemisphere.

Despite the antiquity of concern with the biology of language and its pathologies, real progress was slow and sporadic until the nineteenth century. All too often, understanding and care were blocked by inadequate techniques, imprecise description and closed ideologies. The unprepossessing appearance of the brain led Aristotle to regard it as a cold sponge whose primary function is to cool the blood. And when Shakespeare (1596) wrote, in *The Merchant of Venice*,

'Tell me where is fancie bred,
Or in the heart, or in the head?'

the inquiry was not wholly a flippant anacronism. Even when the 'lower' functions of animal sensation and motion could safely be regarded as dependent upon a material substrate, the idea that the brain is responsible for human thought and language remained anathema in many circles.

In this magnificent compendium of current knowledge, Professors Lecours and Lhermitte justly begin their brief historical survey with the work of Franz Joseph Gall (1758–1828). On anatomic, physiological and psychological grounds, Gall argued passionately that the brain is not a single organ but rather comprises as many distinct, independent (yet interacting) organs as there are primary mental powers. 'It was this theory', writes Hollander[9], 'which aroused the antagonism of three schools of thought. The theologians called it blasphemy, the introspective philosophers of the time called it materialism, and the current scientific opinion was committed to the belief that the brain acted as a whole and not in parts.' When the Emperor Francis I signed the order to ban Gall's lectures in Vienna in 1802, the prohibition noted that 'His Majesty entertains the apprehension that Gall's theory appears to lead to materialism, and consequently to militate against the first principle of morality and religion'[9]. Yet Gall's central claim, that the mind/brain is modular, has become the cornerstone of current neuroscience, and his localization of the neuronal substrate of 'articulate language' at the basal extremity of the third frontal convolution and the island of Reil was the initial impetus that led to modern clinico-pathological correlations between discrete lesion sites and (relatively) isolated behavioural impairments.

Since the time of Gall we have witnessed a veritable explosion of information about the relationship of brain to behaviour, with language studies at the leading edge. The modern clinician who aims to describe and treat the patient with aphasia, and to contribute further to the development of neurolinguistic theory, must have a firm grasp of neurology, anatomy, physiology, linguistics and cognitive psychology. The most solid virtue of the volume written by Lecours, Lhermitte and their many collaborators is that it provides exactly the comprehensive, multi-faceted survey of the field that will be of inestimable value to scholars at every degree of experience and knowledge. The student is provided with a lucid summary of the classical clinical taxonomy of the aphasias; this classification, originally devised by French, German and English neurologists in the second half of the nineteenth century, still provides the framework, although not the limits, of current work (Chapter 4). The authors show how to conduct a detailed, careful examination of the patient with aphasia, an examination that provides an overall picture of the patient's impaired and preserved skills and is a necessary prerequisite to the study of the unique features of each case (Chapters 15 and 16).

The varied aetiologies of aphasia are outlined; the diagnosis and prognosis of cerebrovascular accident, head trauma, tumour and many degenerative, metabolic and infective conditions are described in relation to their effects upon linguistic performance (Chapter 9). At a somewhat finer level, the neuroanatomy and neurophysiology of brain areas committed to language are awarded ample coverage and related to parameters that measure the physical development of the brain (Chapter 8). Moving up in scale, the complexities of hemispheric dominance for language in child and adult—a 'strange fact' as Broca noted—are clearly reported; the relationship of handedness to speech representation is described with regard to both the highly heterogeneous population of left-handers and the extremely atypical right-hander who manifests right-hemisphere dominance for language (Chapter 11).

These chapters form essential 'core' reading for any serious student of the aphasias. One must, however, admit that even the most conscientious student will occasionally (perhaps frequently) be bewildered by the lavish proliferation of technical terms that our field has generated. But, happily, it is here that the authors have been most helpful: in Chapter 2, they provide an extensive glossary of neurolinguistic terminology, and they furthermore illustrate each expression with copious examples drawn from both normal and pathological language. No longer will the student have any excuse for believing that the morpheme is part of the hippocampus! This exposition of terms for the description of language ensures that the student will come to Chapter 12—'The Interaction between Linguistics and Aphasiology'—with some appreciation of why explicit linguistic analyses of aphasic symptomatology are crucial to future advances. Chapter 12 then exemplifies some of the ways in which normative linguistic theory can contribute to a deeper understanding of aphasic breakdown.

The student who reads the primary literature on the aphasias is confronted with yet further perplexities. It sometimes seems that every neurologist, linguist and psychologist who has investigated the pathology of language wants to construct not only his own new theory but also needs to rephrase the results of his predecessors in his own new terminology. In Chapter 10, the authors review the contributions to the description and classification of the aphasias made by 16 major scholars from Baillarger and Jackson in the nineteenth century to such contemporary masters as Hécaen and Goodglass. Lecours and his colleagues are scrupulous in showing where these leading figures have made distinguished original contributions, how their work fits into the overall pattern of scientific progress in the understanding of language pathology and where their phraseology serves to obscure areas of common agreement.

In addition to their full coverage of all the central topics of aphasiology, Lecours and Lhermitte treat many issues that are given scant regard in most texts. Thus the varied forms of writing disorder are discussed (Chapter 3); the language syndromes of frontal lobe pathology are carefully analysed (Chapter 6); language patterns of 'functional' origin in psychotic and neurotic patients are compared and contrasted with typical aphasic manifestations consequent upon focal damage (Chapter 13); temporary lapses of language performance in 'normal' individuals (consequent upon fatigue, distraction, haste or stress) are outlined for the light they may throw upon analogous disturbance due to structural damage (Chapter 14); the possibility of well-preserved non-verbal reasoning and intelligence is reported in the context of severe language impairment (Chapter 19).

Two further topics at the forefront of current

concern are reviewed. For many years almost exclusive emphasis has been laid on the role of the *cortical* brain areas that subserve language. Recently, however, more and more data have accumulated to implicate thalamic structures in the mediation of linguistic performance. The anatomy of the thalamus and its cortical connections is summarized in Chapter 7, with the evidence from lesion studies and electrical stimulation that suggests thalamic involvement in many aspects of language skill. In Chapter 18, the nature of aphasias in bilingual and polyglot individuals is briefly but expertly discussed. Such cases were widely reported in the nineteenth century and their unique potential was well recognized. Interest lapsed somewhat this century but has now revived[1] as cross-language characteristics of aphasia assume greater theoretical significance. With respect to lesion-localization, the multilingual patient acts as his own control for these comparisons between languages.

The ultimate and most important goal of aphasiological inquiry is, of course, to help the aphasic patient recover effective language skills. We are all familiar with the frustration attendant upon attempting to communicate in a language that we know but dimly, a feeling that is perhaps a pale shadow of what the aphasic patient must suffer. And indeed, Elvin and Oldfield[7] have described a young man with a deep penetrating injury to the left temporal area who 'on becoming aware of his surroundings . . . thought that he must be in a foreign country as speech had no meaning.' How terrifying it must be suddenly to become a stranger in one's own language. In *Pale Fire*, Vladimir Nabokov attempts to capture the experience:

'She still could speak. She paused and groped
and found
What seemed at first a serviceable sound,
But from adjacent cells imposters took
The place of words she needed, and her look
Spelt imploration as she sought in vain
To reason with the monsters in her brain.'

What, then, of prognosis and remediation? The neurologist and neurosurgeon will treat the underlying proximate cause of the patient's condition (stroke, penetrating missile injury, space-occupying lesion or whatever); but what hope can we offer the patient by way of behavioural treatment for overt aphasic symptoms? Can therapies be devised that will speed rate of recovery and reduce the degree and scope of persisting impairment? Attempts to assess the efficacy of speech therapy for aphasia have usually been somewhat equivocal, despite the occasional report of good success[2]. It is often difficult to show that the 'technical' content of a remediation programme has an effect over and above any improvement due to the provision of thoughtful encouragement and psychological support[6]. The problems of constructing and assessing therapeutic procedures are described with great skill and insight in Chapter 17. Particular attention is paid to matching the therapy to the specific pattern of impaired and preserved functions in the individual patient, a constraint that further emphasizes the crucial importance of detailed clinical examination. Here, and throughout the volume, Lecours and his colleagues stress the fact that the aphasic patient's performance is not static but is rather subject to both quantitative and qualitative change. Multiple, longitudinal assessments are required to monitor the patient's progress and ensure that therapy remains attuned to the patient's evolving condition[12].

In short, Lecours and Lhermitte have produced a superb volume, a treasure house of acute clinical observation and wise council. But what of the future? In what directions does the work displayed here point us? As the authors note in their introduction, the study of aphasia stands 'at the cross-roads of several scientific disciplines'. Their text should, as they hope, be readily accessible to scholars in neurology, linguistics, psychology and speech pathology, disciplines that have all contributed to our current understanding of aphasic impairment. Yet these approaches have often seemed to offer independent facts that, whilst informative at their own level, are difficult to relate (except by fiat) to facts discovered at other levels of analysis (Marshall, 1980). Lecours and Lhermitte bring out the problem most clearly in their introductory discussion of the difference between lesion localization and function localization. The resolution of what Lecours and Lhermitte aptly call 'a psycho-physiological hiatus' is still as urgent now as when John Hughlings Jackson[10] first noted that 'to locate the damage which destroys speech and to locate speech are two different things'. Once we move beyond relatively elementary sensory and motor functions it is still very difficult (if not impossible) to see *why* particular symptoms should be consequent upon particularly placed lesions.

What we lack is an overall model of normal

language functioning in which the relevant mechanisms are explicated in sufficient detail that one could sensibly inquire into the fine structure of the neural substrate in which they are instantiated. If we could link (normative) functional representations with their anatomico-physiological realization in a *principled* fashion, we would be able to understand the effects of differentially-placed lesions in an explanatory rather than merely descriptive mode. In such a fashion we might eventually be able to see the truth of two seemingly incompatible propositions: that the organization of the mind/brain is modular *and* that it operates as a functionally unified whole. As Goldstein[8] phrased the issue, the problem is *not* 'where is a definite function or symptom localized?' but rather 'how does a definite lesion modify the function of the brain so that a definite symptom comes to the fore?'

Such questions are of more than theoretical interest, for we shall need serious answers about *functional* localization if we are to understand the nature and limits of cerebral plasticity and its implications for language recovery and re-training. Lecours and Lhermitte (in the 'Introduction') note that 'very little is known about the biological mechanisms underlying recovery of language'; it is clear that the evaluation of the various possible mechanisms that they outline will depend crucially upon our ability to develop explicit psycho-physiological hypotheses that go well beyond mere correlation.

Let us hope that this excellent compendium will inspire future workers to deepen what is correct in current theory, overthrow what is false and reach a new synthesis that will benefit the countless individuals estranged from their native language.

REFERENCES

1. Albert, M. L. & Obler, L. K. (1978) *The Bilingual Brain*. New York: Academic Press.
2. Basso, A., Capitani, E. & Vignolo, L. A. (1979) Influence of rehabilitation on language skills in aphasic patients: a controlled study. *Archives of Neurology*, **36**, 190–196.
3. Benton, A. L. & Joynt, R. J. (1960) Early descriptions of aphasia. *Archives of Neurology*, **3**, 205–221.
4. Breasted, J. H. (1930) *The Edwin Smith Surgical Papyrus*. Chicago: University of Chicago Press.
5. Chadwick, J. & Mann, W. N. (1950) *The Medical Works of Hippocrates*. Oxford: Blackwell Scientific Publications.
6. David, R., Enderby, P. & Bainton, D. (1982) Treatment of acquired aphasia: speech therapists and volunteers compared. *Journal of Neurology, Neurosurgery and Psychiatry*, **45**, 957–961.
7. Elvin, M. B. & Oldfield, R. C. (1951) Disabilities and progress in a dysphasic university student. *Journal of Neurology, Neurosurgery and Psychiatry*, **14**, 118–128.
8. Goldstein, K. (1948) *Language and Language Disturbances*. New York: Grune & Stratton.
9. Hollander, B. (1920) *In Search of the Soul*. London: Kegan Paul.
10. Jackson, J. H. (1874) On the nature and duality of the brain. *Medical Press and Circular*, **1**, 19–41.
11. Marshall, J. C. (1980) The new organology. *Behavioral and Brain Sciences*, **3**, 23–25.
12. Newcombe, F. & Marshall, J. C. (1973) Stages in recovery from dyslexia following a left cerebral abscess. *Cortex*, **9**, 329–332.

John C. Marshall

The Radcliffe Infirmary
Oxford, England

Introduction to the English Edition

During the early 1970s the number of students of various disciplines showing interest in acquired speech and language disorders rapidly increased in Europe and North America (as is now the case, although on a lesser scale, in other parts of the world). It was the opinion of those with whom we interacted on a regular basis—most of them students in speech pathology, psychology, linguistics and a very few residents in neurology—that the difficulties they often experienced when reading articles and books on aphasia and related entities essentially stemmed from having lacked access to a basic teaching work in the field of aphasiology. In 1973 to 1975, when we began making plans, writing outlines, gathering documents and considering the names of eventual collaborators with a view towards the preparation of the French manuscript of this book, standard teaching on aphasia was therefore our own and François Lhermitte's prime concern. More explicitly, it was our intention to write and publish what we then believed would be the first modern 'textbook' of aphasiology. As a matter of fact, the title that we had then in mind for our intended book was *Traité d'aphasiologie*, which we renounced—in favour of *L'Aphasie*[1]—when the late Théophile Alajouanine (1890–1980), undoubtedly one of the major contributors to twentieth-century aphasiology, told one of us, with a somewhat disturbing smile, that his own as well as our knowledge of aphasia was superficial and limited to the point of making our use of both words—'treatise' and 'aphasiology'— sound either very naïve or very pretentious. Now we had long been aware that Alajouanine's statements on 'aphasiology' and 'neurolinguistics' were by then largely subserved by his belief that the mutual relationships of brain and language were and would forever remain a mystery, and that this was in the nature of things and therefore good that it should be so. We also knew that Alajouanine established a clear distinction between knowledge and belief and that he did not care whether or not one agreed with him when it came to the latter. Nevertheless, the rolling /r/ of Bourbonnais could sometimes be quite impressive and none of us was ready to choose between being *très naïf* and being *très prétentieux* in the eyes of the Master. We therefore yielded up our title while keeping our objective unchanged: together with our collaborators, we systematically attempted to give our manuscript the form of a textbook; and, as Alajouanine's friend Macdonald Critchley had done before us, we did not avoid the word 'aphasiology' anywhere but in the book's title.

Curiously enough, it turned out to be somewhat easier to decide about the topics of particular chapters in a textbook of aphasiology (and also, to some extent, about the content of each chapter) than it was to decide about proper sequencing of parts within the whole. We thought, however, that one choice remained almost mandatory in this respect: that is, our textbook had to begin with a chapter dealing with the history of aphasiology or at least certain aspects of it. The main motive for this choice was of course that, by laying emphasis on a given name, doctrine or event rather than another—for instance, by siding with Broca rather than Trousseau, or with Dejerine rather than Pierre Marie—one could already show one's colours without being unduly insistent. On the other hand, the main risk we ran was that we would neglect significant contributors to aphasiology, such as William Ogle and William Broadbent, whom we would have emphasized in a different context but who seemed less crucial in relationship to topics we were to discuss in later chapters.

Devoting our second chapter to neurolinguistic terminology was also quite easy. The increasing interest among linguists in aphasia and the correspondingly increased importance of linguistics in aphasiological research in part dictated this choice. It was also the natural consequence of another—somewhat innovative—editorial decision, which was to include numerous, lengthy excerpts of aphasic productions comprising paraphasias and paragraphias of various types, as well as other forms of deviant linguistic segments. Just as terminological consistency is necessary if a pathologist undertaking the description of abnormal cells and tissues is to refer to normal ones, we felt that a sharable lexicon is also an essential tool for the aphasiologist undertaking the description of deviant linguistic units by reference to normal structures.

After this second chapter on terminology, we devoted chapters to clinical and biological aspects of acquired language disorders resulting from brain lesions, and to topics such as taxonomy, aetiology, cerebral dominance, rehabilitation and so forth. The internal organization and sequencing of these further components of our textbook initially gave rise to animated discussions, but we were under the clear overall impression that we had achieved a reasonably coherent sequence of 15 more chapters when the final manuscript was sent to the French publisher in April 1978. For some reason, this impression had lost a great deal of its persuasiveness when we read the first set of galley proofs a year later. When the second set arrived, we could think of at least three parsing strategies of greater merit. Books will be books, all the more if they happen to be textbooks. Yet this one was the source of considerable pleasure and pride for its authors when it was delivered, only slightly post-mature, in December 1979, and the way *L'Aphasie* was greeted by French-speaking aphasiologists and students was indeed gratifying.

If the notion that we were writing a book of potential utility for those learning or teaching aphasiology provided powerful motivation while we had this piece of work on the drawing board, it is no longer a major issue for us whether or not *L'Aphasie* has indeed been the 'first modern textbook' of aphasiology. As a matter of fact, somewhat paradoxically, what we now find most striking about our book is that it might well turn out to be the last of its kind. Not that we believe—thank God!—that it is already outdated or will be in the near future. But this book of the 1970s has obviously been written along conservative lines, from both the neurological and the linguistic standpoints, and a reasonable prediction would no doubt be that aphasiology texts to come shall, without renouncing acquired knowledge, revise a number of traditional concepts and introduce a few new ones, thus attempting to amalgamate classical and modern views on the mutual relationships of brain and language. Let us therefore speculate for a while on the characteristics of a textbook of aphasiology that might be written, say, ten years from now (and published three years later under the best of conditions). In other words, let us speculate for a while on what might be the impact, on the standard aphasiological teaching of the 1990s, of the outburst of new linguistic and neuroscientific approaches that have marked aphasiological research in recent years.

One way to begin speculation about the future of aphasiology and neurolinguistics is to consider the broad problems of the anatomical definition of the 'language zone' on the one hand, and of aphasiological taxonomy on the other. These problems are deliberately tackled rather late in the present book. Definition of the 'language zone' is the subject matter of the last section of Chapter 8 where, although a certain credit is given to Sigmund Freud's[2] views in this respect and a certain emphasis put on the role of subcortical structures, a very classical two-dimensional conception of the language zone is put forward (albeit cautiously) and (more or less) presented as a necessary and universal attribute of mankind. Aphasiological taxonomy is approached in the tenth chapter, which consists of a summation of previous chapters dealing with clinical and biological aspects of the aphasias, on the one hand, and, on the other, of a comparative presentation of various classificatory schemes, including our own. The latter is quantitatively the most important part of the chapter and, on the whole—that is, not taking into account abstruse classifications such as that of Sigmund Freud[2] nor potentially misleading ones such as that of Henry Head[3]—it leads the reader to the conclusion that there exists gross agreement on facts across various modes of classification in spite of widely divergent, often incongruous, sometimes contradictory, and occasionally whimsical, terminology. As we now see things, it is our impression that the current consensus as to the anatomical components of the speech area as well as the relative homogeneity of aphasiological classificatory schemes might, to some extent at least, depend on a historical accident: starting with Paul Broca's[4] teachings on 'the seat of the faculty of articulate language' and with François Baillarger's[5] pioneering taxonomy of the aphasias, both of which were made public in 1865, the progressive constitution of a body of knowledge (and preconceptions) on aphasia has for an overwhelming part been founded on the observation of disturbances resulting from left hemisphere strokes in individuals belonging to a rather homogeneous population of West European stock. From a biogenetic point of view, this population consists of 'right-handed' 'adults' and, from a sociolinguistic point of view, it consists of literate unilingual speakers of languages with specific structural properties, written following alphabetical codes. Going by UNESCO[6] projections, one can estimate at less than 25 per cent the proportion of the human population which falls in this well-studied group[7]. We shall now consider the consequences of going beyond these restrictions, successively considering new data regarding biogenetic, pathological, clinical and psycholinguistic factors as sources of changes in our concepts regarding the neural basis for language and the taxonomy of the aphasias.

BIOGENETIC ASPECTS

The subject matter of this book, as specified in the 'Introduction to the French Edition', is aphasia in adults as opposed to aphasia in children. As far as we can see, this opposition can to this day be kept as a basic guideline of teaching in aphasiology. How long this will remain the case can, however, be questioned here and now. In fact, two complementary research orientations which have already acquired a certain momentum—one related to Eric Lenneberg's *initial equipotentiality* theory[8] and the other to Jason Brown's *microgenesis* theory[9]—might sooner or later bring permanent modifications to current concepts in this respect. Brian Woods and Hans-Lukas Teuber[10,11] are thus quite convincing when they insist that aphasia resulting from right-hemisphere lesions is far less frequent in children than one would expect given the postulates of the initial equipotentiality theory. Moreover, further research into the natural evolution of aphasia in children, although unlikely to eradicate the belief that a very young brain stands a better chance than an older one when functional recuperation is at stake, might well confirm that rather subtle sequellae rather than *restitutio ad integrum* is the rule with regard to oral language production and comprehension[12-14], and that one with a left-hemisphere lesion during early childhood might be expected to experience certain difficulties when later required to learn to read and write[15,16]. All of this tends to fog the once apparently clear-cut opposition between the aphasias of children and those of adults. This being said, the existence of a clinical difference between the two has not, as far as we know, been seriously challenged to this day: whatever the site of unilateral lesions, massive auditory comprehension disorders and fluency in production do not belong with the semiology of childhood aphasia (this remains true, in our opinion, even if an intern of the Massachusetts General Hospital once reported, in the record of a five-year-old patient with a left Sylvian lesion, the existence in this child of certain difficulties in auditory comprehension and oral production of a repetitive 'ga-ga-oo-oo' behaviour which he or she decided to qualify as jargonaphasia[10]). In a way, this one difference is sufficient to maintain the 'childhood'–'adulthood' opposition in aphasiology.

This opposition needs to be reconsidered as *more* age-dependent differences in the clinical manifestations of the aphasias observed during life are brought to light[9,18,19]. Further systematic research is needed to confirm early reports (a) that a (left) thalamic lesion is likely to cause a deeper disorganization of language during early life[17]; (b) that a left temporal lesion is likely to produce conduction aphasia in the young adult and Wernicke's jargonaphasia later in life[9]; (c) that the linguistic characteristics of discourse in Wernicke's jargonaphasia can vary with age[20]; and (d) that the age difference that has been reported between Broca's and Wernicke's aphasics[18,19] cannot be explained on the basis of a difference in cerebrovascular dynamics. If these hypotheses are proved correct, our approach to the problems of cerebral representation of language and of aphasiological taxonomy will certainly be outdated when the time comes to think about another textbook. Theories of both these subjects will have to take the factor of age into account.

In the present book (showing thereby that a *vis inertiae* inherent to words sometimes slackens the expression of ideas), we present, as basic teaching material, a traditional two-dimensional cortical language 'zone' (or 'area' or 'region'). While we insist that the 'central apparatus' of language comprises subcortical components as well, some of them identified by name and to a certain extent by function, and thereafter we express the wish that an explicit three-dimensional conception of language representation in the brain be shortly developed and popularized, we do not develop this theme in any detail. A textbook of the 1990s will conceivably propose, as a consequence of research results yet to come, a four-dimensional representation of the neurological substrate of language in which age will be taken into account from infancy—perhaps even gestation—to senescence. Concepts such as Dennis' 'thalamization' and 'corticalization' as successive stages of the early ontogenesis of the neurological representation of language will probably play important roles in explaining observations such as those just mentioned above. Complementarily, the taxonomical approaches discussed in Chapter 10 of the present book might conceivably belong with the first chapter of a future textbook (if it were still convenient to take history as the subject matter of an initial chapter), and a new taxonomical scheme might be presented as the result of research bearing on a large number of subjects in which age would have been systematically integrated as a major parameter.

If taxonomical research were thus to take on new perspectives in the few years to come, as we expect to be the case, the study of biogenetic parameters other than age might also provide information convincing enough to be integrated to a future textbook. For instance, the clinical forms and natural evolution of the aphasias of non-right-handers, who constitute about 35 per cent of the human population according to Antonio Subirana[21], might by then be sufficiently known to provide the matter of statements going beyond the usual less-predictable-better-prognosis assertion. The same might be said of the clinical forms and natural evolution of the aphasias of right-handers with a clear family history of ambidextrality or left-handedness.

A third biogenetic parameter, sex, has already proved a matter of interesting if somewhat confusing (aphasiological) discussions: some talk of a more ambicerebral representation of language in women, others of the same in men[22]; and Doreen Kimura[23] went and perhaps still goes as far as suggesting that women—as opposed to men—have a predominantly prerolandic representation of language in their left cerebral hemispheres. Clearly, it will take a lot of careful research in this particular paradigm, from both the taxonomical and the anatomo-clinical points of view, before this problem—an important one if it indeed turns out to bear more than the political dimension underlined by Marcel Kinsbourne[24]—receives an answer convincing enough to be presented as acquired knowledge in a textbook meant to be read indiscriminately by students of at least two sexes. Well the 1990s are still far away, and they should last for at least ten years.

ANATOMO-PATHOLOGICAL ASPECTS

If one now turns to parameters pertaining to pathological anatomy, a number of comments come to mind concerning the future of aphasiological research and teaching. A most immediate one has to do with the aetiology of aphasia-producing lesions. As we have mentioned above and as exemplified in Chapters 3 to 5 of this book, standard teaching of clinical aphasiology is currently founded, for the best part, on descriptions of the linguistic abilities and inabilities of stroke patients, some of them observed more than 100 years ago, that is, at a time when the word 'linguistics' itself probably sounded like a neologism to the ears of a majority of those interested in aphasia. And one might add that over 90 per cent of the significant psycholinguistic research papers published in the course of the last 15 years also report observations on the abilities and disabilities of stroke patients. Of course, one hardly hears any longer neurology professors teaching that the notions of aphasia and dementia are mutually exclusive and, of course, once again, everybody knows that prototypical agrammatism and prototypical logorrhoeic jargon never occur as the result of a glioblastoma (unless the neoplastic formation has been the site of sudden bleeding). One could, as we did in Chapter 9 of this book, list a limited number of useful anecdotes of the above type but, with the single exception of the research and ensuing monograph of Andrew Kertesz[25], we know of no important taxonomical study systematically integrating aetiology as a fully-fledged parameter of classification in aphasiology. Clearly, this is likely to change in the next decade. Indeed, if only in view of demographic considerations, one should hope that an important chapter of any future textbook of aphasiology will be devoted to peculiarities and diachronic characteristics of language disturbances in the dementias.

Another, more hypothetical, change that one might expect to take place in aphasiology teaching in relation to the aetiology parameter is linked to the dichotomy opposing 'acquired' and 'developmental' disorders. The latter have often been taken to have no organic pathological basis. As long as no clear evidence of structural anomalies of the brain existed that could be proposed as a plausible biopathological correlate of (at least) certain developmental disorders, one could ignore the suppositions of impenitent organicists and, as we did in the present book, consider it legitimate and convenient to exclude developmental disorders from the proper domain of aphasiology on organic grounds. It so happens, however, that Alberto Galaburda and Thomas Kemper[26] recently documented the existence of left-hemisphere cytoarchitectonic anomalies involving Wernicke's area in what they consider to be a typical case of (familial) developmental dyslexia, and two more cases with similar heterotopias have also recently been studied by these workers. If it were to be confirmed that the existence of characteristic cytoarchitectonic anomalies is the rule in certain developmental disorders, the authors of a future textbook of aphasiology will have to abandon the correspondence: 'developmental'–'non-organic'. The pathological differences between antenatal, perinatal and postnatal lesions at various stages of the life cycle will be one aspect of the pathological lesion which will have to be taken into account in developing a taxonomy of language disturbances.

The last biopathological parameter which we shall consider in this introduction, lesion localization, is also the one in which many pioneers of aphasiology were most interested from the very beginning. Thus Paul Broca[27] had predicted, in 1861, that a 'phrenology of convolutions', founded on the parallel study of clinical and anatomical abnormalities, was soon to replace Franz Joseph Gall's 'phrenology of bumps'. To a large extent, this is just what happened and has persisted to this day. A quite standard contemporary attitude in this respect might be to assert, as a preliminary position, that the classical notion of 'centre' should be denied any credit whatsoever, and thereafter proceed with a description tion of the exact localization of the lesion in one's last case of Broca's aphasia. Indeed, the problem of lesion site has been the object of a powerful renewal of interest among aphasiologists since the mid 1970s, soon after the publication, in England, of the first papers on computerized tomography (CT)[28,19]. We were then among those who believed that the tenets of the classical anatomo-clinical doctrine of aphasia were, before long and at last, going to be rigorously documented on large groups of patients. We were also among those who soon came down a peg or two. Not that nothing has been learned in aphasiology through the CT technique: it is now demonstrated, for instance, that aphasia resulting from deep-seated lesions is quite frequent and (this time concerning the lesions involving the cortical mantle of the left hemisphere) that gross exceptions to the doctrine are not really that infrequent either (respectively, 18.7 per cent and 13.5 per cent of 267 cases of left-hemisphere strokes in adult literate right-handers reported by Anna Basso and her collaborators[30]. Now any postulate or theory or teaching supported by more than 85 per cent of observations certainly deserves first-rate textbook space, and it can therefore be said, if one considers the problem in general terms such as 'left' vs 'right' hemispheres, 'anterior' vs 'posterior' lesions, 'fluent' vs 'non-fluent' aphasias, and so forth, that CT studies published so far have supported, on the whole, classical teaching on the anatomical-clinical correlations of the aphasias (and further evidenced the necessity of integrating certain subcortical structures to one's conception of the neuronal nets governing speech and language). Nonetheless, if one wishes to go beyond these global assertions, one has to face the fact that a CT-image reading that is perfectly adequate for a neurosurgeon who is about to operate within the skull-brain space of a particular patient can remain a somewhat vague and uncertain document for a neuropsychologist interested in knowing precisely whether or not an infarct is limited to the pars triangularis and pars opercularis of the third frontal convolution of the left cerebral hemisphere of a given patient with a given head size and a given head shape. In other words, but for relatively few cases in which the presence of a sufficient degree of cortical atrophy yields unequivocal information on certain superficial landmarks, we have not yet learned—although a number of recent publications are written as if we had—how to read CT images in precise and reliable neuro-anatomical terms. Attempts are currently being made which, resorting both to the technical improvements that have been brought to recent generations of scanners and to anatomical knowledge acquired through stereotactic research, might correct this situation at least in part[31]. It is hoped that image reading methodologies (devices?) will be available in the near future which should be applicable to CT materials.

If so, it is more than likely that a textbook of aphasiology to be written a decade from now will include a fair amount of new anatomo-clinical knowledge. It might, for instance, comprise, besides an anatomically more precise demonstration as to the validity of classical teachings on the location of cortical lesions causing aphasia, enough information on the site of regularly aphasiogenic deep-seated lesions to permit an explicit three-dimensional definition of the 'language zone'. Indeed, it is even conceivable that enough localization data will by then have been gathered for all age groups to permit confident statements in relation to various anatomical-functional stages in the ontogenesis of the neural substrate of language.

Moreover, other imaging techniques offer new possibilities for investigating the loci and nature of the pathology responsible for aphasia and, hence, the neural elements responsible for language. Some of these techniques also offer exciting possibilities for the observation of brain metabolism in particular areas in normal subjects engaged in language-processing activities. PET, NMR and EP studies are the leading technologies in this area at the moment. All reflect metabolic and/or neurophysiological aspects of normal and abnormal brain, and all are beginning to be applied to the study of neural basis for language processing in aphasia. Besides their potential utility regarding the determination of lesion type and site, these techniques can change our concept of aphasia taxonomy. Anatomically significant documents will probably become available regarding recuperation of language functions in the presence of permanent damage to neural structures essential to language in the normal. Our taxonomic schemes, which already allow for the possibility of several clinical labels being successively attributed to the same patient over the course of recovery, could be extended to integrate views of the language zone which explicitly identify brain structures capable of functional takeover in reaction to pathology. Moreover, the cortical locus of pathology in diseases such as Alzheimer's and other degenerative conditions (which so far have been considered inaccessible to systematic studies, when not actually declared irrelevant) could be integrated into both the classification of the aphasias and theories of the neural basis for language.

LINGUISTIC AND PSYCHOLINGUISTIC ASPECTS

Reassessment of various clinical aspects of aphasia and their description and/or interpretation in linguistic or psycholinguistic terms has recently become a major orientation in aphasiological research. The pioneering work of investigators such as Zurif, Marshall, Kean and others[32-34] has begun to exert a significant influence over functional descriptions of the aphasias, and it is quite predictable that research of this type is bound to be developed further and be extensively represented in any future textbook of the aphasias. We might point out that many of the clinical facts to which these studies have been directed are discussed in the chapters of the present book, but many of the detailed results and theories of this approach are not explicitly taken into account, in large part due to the fact that this work had barely begun at the time that we were drafting our original manuscript. We shall attempt to summarize briefly these new directions.

The study of aphasic symptoms, as presented in the majority of chapters in this text, is largely descriptive in nature. By this term, we mean that the goal of many studies reported here has been to provide a preliminary description of the phenomena of aphasic performance in various language tasks. The study of phonemic paraphasias summarized in Chapter 2 exemplifies this approach. In that chapter, the effort was directed towards separating certain types of error from other error types and characterizing some of the linguistic properties of phonemic paraphasias. For example, at a very simple level, phonemic paraphasias were distinguished from semantic paraphasias, and, at a slightly more subtle level, formal verbal paraphasias—in which a phonemic error gives rise to a real word rather than a neologism—were set apart as a subset of phonemic deviations in general, to be analysed with other phonemic deviations under some conditions but perhaps to be considered separately in other circumstances. The descriptive effort was then directed at characterizing these errors. The model used for description characterized each segment in terms of its distinctive phonological features, established a metric for the phonological distance between any two phonemes in terms of the distinctive features of each phoneme and used this distance as the basis for characterizing the nature of so-called 'paradigmatic' influences on phonemic paraphasias—the influences which are exerted by virtue of the intrinsic nature of phonemes themselves. A second influence on phonemic paraphasias was thought to arise from the sequences of phonemes found in 'superior articulation units'—words, in the cases studied. The descriptive framework adopted allows for the statement of how the presence of one phoneme influences a paraphasia affecting another phoneme in the word. This 'syntagmatic' effect was described in terms of the separation of the two phonemes, measured in terms of the number of intervening phonemes and combined with the effect of the similarity of the two phonemes to affect the distribution of substitutions, omissions, metatheses and additions to the phonological segments of individual words.

This work achieves considerable descriptive detail. Clearly, despite its achievements, it is not an end in itself. We would like to know how these errors arise; that is, what are the processes that are employed for the normal generation of relatively error-free repetition and reading, and how do these processes go wrong? The descriptions and generalizations of Chapter 2 are the facts which such psychopathogenic accounts must deal with. They are not, in and of themselves, psychopathogenic mechanisms.

In recent years, a framework for approaching the psychopathogenesis of phenomena such as phonemic paraphasias has emerged. In its essentials, it is based on the idea that one aspect of the normal psychological processes which terminate in performances such as relatively error-free repetition and reading involve the conversion of one type of linguistic representation to another. For instance, in reading a word aloud, one linguistic representation—the orthography of the word—is converted through a series of steps to another representation—the phonological (and phonetic) form of the word. In reading, for instance, one source of the data of Chapter 2, various workers hold the view that the phonological form of a word can be arrived at directly from the orthography without any intervening semantic features being involved in the conversion, or, on some accounts, without the strings even being recognized as words. In addition to this 'non-lexical' or 'non-semantic' route, these workers postulate a second way to convert orthographies to phonologies by recognizing the lexical identity of a string and accessing in the phonology of the string from its lexical representation. On such accounts, phonemic paraphasias can be assigned a locus in a processing model. Suppose, for instance, that a patient makes phonemic paraphasias only when reading irregularly spelled words. Since the spelling of these words is irregular, and does not code the phonology directly, the phonological values for these words must be assigned post-lexically, and the phonemic paraphasias arise in the post-lexical processing of these words.

Work of this sort obviously takes the question of the exact form of the representation of linguistic items and structures very seriously. Consider, again, the question of transcoding orthographies into phonologies, focusing on the hypothesized non-lexical route. What are the orthographic units and phonological units which are matched in this conversion process? Are they individual graphemes or are larger units involved in the conversion? If larger units are involved, are these units to be described in terms of purely orthographic features of words, or can morphological features of words also be involved (determining, for instance, the pronunciation of ph in *shepherd* as opposed to *grapheme*)? Similarly, what phonological representations are the output of this conversion? The actual pronunciation of most English words differs from what many phonologists consider their underlying phonological analysis. In the word 'contrastive', for instance, the first vowel is always reduced to schwa, but its underlying phonological value is /ɔ/ as can be seen in the related noun 'contrast'. Do the transcoding rules produce the underlying phonological value /ɔ/ and allow the general rules of the phonology (which reduce unstressed vowels in English) to give the final /ə/, or do they yield the final /ə/ directly?

This concern for the nature of linguistic representations affects the descriptions of phonemic paraphasias themselves. What are we to consider the first vowel of 'contrastive'—/ə/ or /ɔ/? Our choice will influence generalizations we find regarding phonological regularities in phonemic paraphasias. In this particular case, the differences could be related to whether we are dealing with an underlying or a surface phonological representation, and these two representations could themselves be related to different stages of word and sentence production. These particular questions do not arise in the French data presented in Chapter 2, since vowel reduction is not a feature of French phonology, but similar questions—for instance, the choice of a distinctive feature framework for the description of phonemes themselves—do.

Thus one effect of recent modelling approaches to psycholinguistics being applied to aphasia is a renewed interest in the nature of the representations described in aphasic performances. The choice of representation for the description of aphasic performance was never divorced from theoretical considerations; it could not be, insofar as any descriptive framework presupposes some theory of the phenomena under description. But current approaches make the specific choice of descriptive frameworks more important, since the psychological processes being modelled consist of conversions of representations, and the choice of descriptions interacts with the models of processing being proposed. As these models become more precise, with respect to both the representations postulated and the processes involved in conversion of representations one to another, more complex issues, such as dependencies between different processes, the ordering of different conversions, the relative speed of different processes and the nature of feedback and other 'checking' and control aspects of these mechanisms, can be studied.

In short, linguistic aphasiology is becoming more theoretical in several senses. The choice of descriptive framework for phenomena, and the range of phenomena being described, are increasingly influenced by linguistics and psycholinguistics. However, in a sense this is the least critical way in which aphasiology is becoming more theoretical. The development of models of language processing, and the attempt to explain aphasic performances in reference to these models and to extend and modify these models on the basis of aphasic data, have led to the enrichment of both aphasiological and psycholinguistic theories. This development has required that aphasiology consider its choice of descriptive terms very seriously, as these terms must be compatible with both theories of language structure and theories of language processing. It is remarkable how productive a restricted number of models have been (such as Morton's logogen model[35], and Garrett's sentence production theories[36]) in both normal psycholinguistics and aphasiology.

In our opinion, these developments need to be extended in a number of directions. Perhaps the most pressing requirement is that the empirical basis for generalizations regarding linguistic aspects of aphasia such as phonemic deviations or disorders of comprehension of syntactic form be documented on much larger populations than has already been done. If this is accomplished, we can predict that a major effect of this research orientation on basic teaching of aphasiology will involve our approach to taxonomy. On the one hand, it is likely that the number of classificatory headings—contrary to what occurs in taxonomic approaches which group virtually all the aphasics[25] under a few rubrics—will be greatly multiplied. It is unclear that such classifications as 'Broca's aphasia' can be maintained as single clinical entities when it is established that 'Broca's aphasia' can exist with or without phonetic disintegration, with or without agrammatism, with or without a disorder of syntactic comprehension, and so forth. Second, we expect the taxonomies will increasingly take into account not only the descriptions of pathological linguistic structures which are produced or comprehended by aphasic patients, but also the particular mechanistic disturbances which give rise to these abnormalities. In short, this movement will require that researchers who have not already done so abandon the inappropriate procedure of classifying patients on the basis of pathological criteria ('anterior' vs 'posterior' lesions) or clinical criteria ('fluent' vs 'non-fluent' aphasias) which are gross to the point of obscuring the most interesting results.

These new directions will also affect our understanding of the functional anatomy of the language zone. The functional role of brain tissue in which damage produces disturbances in linguistic representations and their processing must be related to the long-term storage, accessing and transformation of these representations. As descriptions of aphasic symptoms and syndromes become more specific in linguistic and psycholinguistic terms, understanding of the functional role of these areas of the brain will become more specifically linked to linguistic and psycholinguistic processes.

ENVIRONMENTAL ASPECTS

Another axis of research that is of obvious importance in the present context has to do with the investigation of environmental parameters that are likely to determine, at least in part, the cerebral representation of language. The only explicit approach to a problem of this type that is comprised in the present book, although hardly from a linguistic point of view, has to do with aphasia in bilinguals and polyglots (a problem that has also been reviewed in 1978 in a monograph by Martin Albert and Loraine Obler[37]). On the other hand, virtually nothing is said—mostly because virtually nothing is known—about the eventual relationships between a typology of (spoken) natural languages and the linguistic characteristics of the aphasias. In other words, we do not know to what extent teachings that have been shown to be valid in the case of aphasia in speakers of European languages such as French and English can be considered equally valid in the case of aphasia in speakers of languages belonging to fundamentally different families. Several specific questions—such as the reliance of aphasic patients upon word order in languages which do and do not make use of this parameter as a major indicator of semantic functions such as thematic relations—have begun to be investigated, but such research is in its infancy. Given the nature of aphasiological research at the moment, it does not seem likely that certain interesting subjects, such as the aphasiological characteristics of patients who are speakers of tone languages or agglutinating or polysynthetic languages, are likely to be better understood ten years from now than they are at present, but other questions of a similar sort may have received answers clear enough to permit a typology of languages to enter into linguistic aphasiological teaching. One might quote, as an example, the fact that deletion of morphological endings would hardly be expected to belong with the definition of agrammatism in a language such as Hebrew or Arabic where the structure of words is such that lexical components are systematically borne by consonants and morphological ones by vowels[38]. Likewise, the works of Sumiko Sasanuma in Japan[39] and more recently those of Prathibha Karanth in India[40] point to the necessity of explicitly taking a typology of written codes into account if basic teaching on the linguistic characterization of the various disorders observed in literate aphasics is to become less parochial in the future. The sorts of psycholinguistic mechanisms described above may also differ across languages with different structural characteristics (Kanji cannot be subject to prelexical phonological conversion, for instance), and descriptions at the level of mechanisms are also likely to be influenced by cross-linguistic studies in a future text.

As originally surmised by Ernst Weber[41] when he suggested in 1904 that the acquisition of reading and writing skills might play an enhancing role in the process of functional lateralization to the left for language, the 'literacy'-'illiteracy' opposition can itself be considered to constitute a fundamental environmental issue in aphasiology. Several anecdotes have been reported since then which might be taken as supportive of Weber's postulate[42-45] but systematic aphasiological research bearing on groups of patients—which has never so far considered the natural evolution of aphasia as a parameter of study—has only resulted till now in producing contradictory evidences. In Mississippi, on the one hand, Ralph Cameron and his collaborators[46] reviewed the cases of 65 adults with persistent right hemiplegia due to a stroke; aphasia was found to be present in 29 of the 37 'literates', in nine of the 14 'semi-literates', and in only five of the 14 'illiterates'; these authors conclude that aphasia resulting from a focal left-hemisphere stroke is significantly less frequent in 'illiterates' than in subjects who have learned to read and write and thereafter suggest that the acquisition of written language plays a role of some sort in the ontogenesis of left-brain specialization for language. But in Portugal, on the other hand, Antonio Damasio and his collaborators[47] reviewed the cases of 247 adults with unilateral brain lesions of various aetiologies, 38 of whom were 'illiterates'; these authors found no differences between their two groups of patients regarding the frequency and clinical manifestations of aphasia and thereafter suggested that 'brain specialization for language does not depend on literacy'. As far as one can judge, the strong and the weak points of these two studies are such that there are no reasons to attribute more weight to the American rather than the Portuguese one, nor vice versa, and one is therefore brought to conclude that whether or not Weber's postulate was indeed founded remains an open question. Whatever the angle at which one chooses to consider it, this question—which amounts to asking to what extent an environmental factor can interact with a genetic one in the process of language lateralization—remains of paramount importance. One can only wish that current works on the effects of unilateral brain lesions will provide answers clear enough to find a place in a future textbook of aphasiology.

A last prediction concerning current neurolinguistic work that is likely to exert significant influence on aphasiology teaching in a few years is linked to the research now being led by Ursula Bellugi and her collaborators on the linguistic characterization of acquired communication disorders in signers. It is more than likely that this and other investigations of the same type, beside providing a long-needed description of aphasia in the deaf-mutes, will shed new light on the relationships between the aphasias, on the one hand, and the apraxias and the visuo-spatial disorders, on the other, as well as on aspects of neural 'plasticity' relevant to language.

INTERACTIONS

In a future textbook of aphasiology, we anticipate that the various factors we have identified will not only be studied in isolation but will also be seen as components of a neurally based language processing system which interact among themselves and with other psychological processes. We shall briefly present one line of research which exemplifies these sorts of interactions.

We have already indicated that the clinical forms of aphasia evolve with age. One of the possible reasons for this evolution is that the functional organization of the brain evolves with age both for language and perhaps for all cognitive functions. In this connection, one question which arises is whether this hypothesized age-related evolution is entirely a function of a biological factor—age—which is genetically determined, or whether it is determined by age in conjunction with particular environmental exposure.

Various theoretical approaches allow for the statement of testable hypotheses regarding the interactions between genetic and environmental factors influencing neurolinguistic and neuropsychological organization. Goldberg and Costa[48], for example, hypothesize that there are inter- and intrahemispheric constraints on the neural basis for cognitive functions (lateralization and focalization) which depend upon (a) the degree to which a particular activity lends itself to the process of routinization or automatization by the use of a descriptive system or code; and (b) the degree and the frequency of utilization of this descriptive system or code; that is, the degree to which it actually is automatized. Increasing lateralization and focalization in favour of the left hemisphere is postulated for the use of such descriptive systems, and, conversely, the right hemisphere is thought to be predisposed for the elaboration and characterization of non-automatizable and non-automatized codes. This claim is supported by studies which show that a variety of activities which are either not subject to systematic analysis or are not frequently used (such as musical perception in non-musicians, the early stages of second language learning, acquisition of certain codes such as morse, or face recognition) are right-hemisphere based, and that when these activities, or at least some of them, become systematized and frequently employed (as in music appreciation on the part of a professional musician, the utilization of morse code by experienced professionals, and so on) a relative shift of the neural basis for such activity takes place from the right to the left hemisphere[48]. Furthermore, certain activities whose automatization along algorithmic lines is difficult to imagine, such as face recognition, are rarely if ever exclusive left hemisphere functions, according to current neuropsychological studies.

The use of language is perhaps the best example of a descriptive system which is systematic and heavily used. We would therefore expect it to be highly lateralized to the left hemisphere, and increasingly lateralized throughout the life span. It is, moreover, noticeable that language is an activity that needs not only to be interpreted—that is, decoded—but also reproduced—that is, encoded. In view of the right-to-left shift that seems to exist in any activity when it has to be reproduced (e.g., music for musicians, morse code for its users; see above) one might further hypothesize that reproduction of a certain descriptive system could enhance the left hemisphere's participation.

The degree to which an activity based upon a descriptive code can be and is automatized is related to the importance of such automatization to an individual who is producing the code in question. Efficient linguistic communication depends upon the capacity of an individual to produce the elements of the language system to which he is exposed. As mastery of this code increases on the output side, the theory holds that language-related activities become more lateralized and focalized. This theory leads to a variety of predictions. For instance, second languages which are used primarily for receptive purposes ought to be less left lateralized than those which are used for speech and writing. If the theory is right, it can serve to link the functional organization of the brain with psychological tendencies of each individual, such as an individual's tendency to utilize the language code and a degree to which he masters it. These sorts of interactions between the nature of linguistic code, the biological state of the individual measured in terms of his age and personality, and environmental factors which determine the degree of automatization of the language used, may serve to integrate more restricted views of the functional organization of the language area with broader psychological concerns.

APHASIOLOGY AND NEUROLINGUISTIC THEORY

Throughout this Introduction, we have emphasized the significance of studies of a variety of aspects of aphasias for two subjects: the delineation of the 'language zone' and the taxonomy of the aphasias. These two subjects are related, but differ insofar as the latter is concerned with the description and classification of pathological states, while the former is part of the study of normal neurobiology. It could be argued that a textbook of aphasiology need not, and should not, concern itself with the delineation of the language area of the brain, but be restricted to abnormal function. However, as elsewhere in medicine, and perhaps even more specifically in this area, the development of thinking about normal and abnormal structures and functions is so intertwined that no presentation of aphasiology could possibly be adequate if it did not deal with theories of normal language–brain relationships. The controversies over 'localizationist' vs 'holist' models of language representation in brain, for instance, are difficult to separate from the descriptions and taxonomies of aphasic symptoms and syndromes which adherents of these two positions put forward.

However, the two subject areas can be at least partially separated, and many lines of research do so. The study of non-aphasic patients through a variety of techniques which demonstrate aspects of the neural organization of language functions, as well as the nature of the language functions themselves, has revealed features of the neural basis for language. Chief among these techniques is the visual presentation of linguistic stimuli to one of the two half-fields and dichotic presentation of auditory stimuli. The developing expertise with these techniques has revealed a number of sources of artefact and the locus of a variety of effects in these tests[49], and they promise to continue to be useful in the investigation of the neural basis for language. Study of non-aphasic patients who have undergone callosal section for the relief of epilepsy has also provided important insights into the language capacities of the isolated (if not entirely normal) hemispheres[50].

More direct observations of physiological and metabolic parameters during language use are possible in a variety of ways. In a very few centres, stimulation of exposed cortex during neurosurgical procedures is carried out, and the effects of this local and brief electrical stimulation on language function are being explored[51]. The application of new imaging techniques such as PET and NMR scanning to the study of language functioning in normal subjects is also possible in a few centres. Probably the most widespread approach to the measurement of neurophysiological parameters in relationship to language is the use of event-related potential measurements, which have been applied to a variety of problems in language processing[52].

All of these techniques have their problems and limitations. Cortical stimulation, for instance, is limited to a few, very brief, stimulations of individual loci, because of the risk of creating epileptic foci through prolonged or frequent stimulations, and because of the exigencies of the neurosurgical setting. The temporal resolution of existing isotopes in PET scanning is more than a minute and a half, and 6-deoxyglucose has a half-life of 30 minutes—far too long to expect a subject (let alone a patient) to be engaged in a single psycholinguistic task; the spatial resolution of PET images is also less precise than CT scans, whose utility for answering some of the details of neuro-anatomical analysis we have already questioned. This is not to say, we emphasize, that these techniques are not exciting and full of promise. It is to say, rather, that the use of analyses and aphasic performances, in connection with a variety of imaging and post-mortem examinations of brain, is likely to remain an important source of data and theory for our understanding of language–brain relationships.

In particular, the increasing accommodation of studies in aphasiology to studies and models in normal linguistics and psycholinguistics, discussed above, has already led to the formulation of quite specific hypotheses about the psycholinguistic processes carried out by particular areas of the brain. A major direction of research is likely to carry these correlations further on both the psychological/linguistic and neural sides. The former is likely to be increasingly influenced by linguistic and psycholinguistic concepts, as discussed above, and also by new techniques of study, such as 'on-line', timed investigation of aphasic patients' language processing[53]. The latter can be extended by the metabolic and electrophysiological techniques cited above, and also by the correlation of functional impairments with different cellular pathologies in particular areas of the brain, as more detailed studies of different aetiological causes for aphasia become available in conjunction with radiology, neurophysiological and autopsy studies. We relish the thought that these modern studies, phrased in terms of 'the modularity of mind'[54], 'a mental organ for language'[55] and 'right–left asymmetries in the temporal speech areas'[56], in fact are directed at a thesis which Franz Joseph Gall developed on the basis of observations of criminals of his day and for which he was excommunicated and expelled from Vienna. Well, tenure was tough to come by in 1820, too.

The link from an analysis of abnormal brain and abnormal language to the relationships between normal brain and normal language is complex, and a number of considerations other than identifying the different factors which we have discussed in this Introduction, and which are likely to influence the normal relation, must be considered, such as the possibility that an aphasic performance reflects adaptive or new functional mechanisms, which emerge after or are occasioned by brain damage, rather than being due to a deficit in normal functioning. The logic of these different relationships is becoming better understood, and instances of these various pathological mechanisms are coming to light, as more detail is acquired about the functional characteristics of aphasic performances. Future textbooks are likely to deal with these different mechanisms in more detail than the present volume.

It is our intention and hope that the English version of *L'Aphasie* will serve as an introduction to these subjects, and enable students and workers to pursue these new lines of inquiry on the basis of an acquaintance with existing understanding and investigations in this field.

REFERENCES

1. Lecours, A. R., Lhermitte, F. et al (1979) *L'Aphasie*. Paris: Flammarion.
2. Freud, S. (1891) *Zur Auffasung der Aphasien*. Vienna: Deuticke.
3. Head, H. (1926) *Aphasia and Kindred Disorders of Speech*. London: Cambridge University Press.
4. Broca, P. (1865) Du siège de la faculté du langage articulé. *Bulletin de la Société d'Anthropologie*, **6,** 337.
5. Baillarger, F. (1865) *Recherches sur les maladies mentales*. Paris: Masson.
6. Anonymous (1977) *Annuaire statistique*. New York: UNESCO.
7. Lecours, A. R. (1980) Corrélations anatomo-cliniques de l'aphasie; la zone du langage. *Revue Neurologique*, **136,** 591.
8. Lenneberg, E. (1967) *Biological Foundations of Language*. New York: Wiley.
9. Brown, J. W. (1979) Language representation in the brain. In *Neurobiology of Social Communication in Primates*. p. 133. New York: Academic Press.
10. Woods, B. T. & Teuber, H.-L. (1978) Changing patterns of childhood aphasia. *Annals of Neurology*, **3,** 273.
11. Woods, B. T. (1980) Observations on the neurological basis for initial language. In *Biological Studies of Mental Processes* (Ed.) Caplan, D. p. 149. Cambridge, MA: MIT Press.
12. Dennis, M. & Whitaker, M. (1977) Hemispheric equipotentiality and language acquisition. In Segalowitz, S. J. & Gruber, F. A. *Language Development and Neurological Theory* (Ed.) p. 93. New York: Academic Press.

13. Woods, B. T. (1980) The restricted effects of right-hemisphere lesions after age one: Wechsler Test data. *Neuropsychologia*, **18.**
14. Dennis, M. (1980) Capacity and strategy for syntactic comprehension after left or right hemidecortication. *Brain and Language*, **10,** 287.
15. Lawrence, B. (1979) Waiting patterns of the congenitally neurologically impaired adult. *Brain and Language*, **7,** 232.
16. Dennis, M., Lovett, M. & Wiegel-Crump, C. A. (1981) Written language acquisition after left or right hemidecortication in infancy. *Brain and Language*, **12,** 54.
17. Dennis, M. Personal communication.
18. Obler, L. K., Albert, M. L., Goodglass, H. & Benson, F. D. (1978) Aphasia type and aging. *Brain and Language*, **6,** 318.
19. Harasymiw, S., Halper, A. & Sutherland, B. (1981) Sex, age, and aphasia type. *Brain and Language*, **12,** 190.
20. Lecours, A. R. (1982) Simulation of speech production without a computer. In *Neural Models of Language Processes* (Ed.) Arbib, M. A., Caplan, D. & Marshall, J. C. p. 345. New York: Academic Press.
21. Subirana, A. (1969) Handedness and cerebral dominance. In *Handbook of Clinical Neurology* (Ed.) Winken, P. J. & Bruyn, G. W. Volume 4, p. 248. Amsterdam: North-Holland.
22. McClone, J. (1980) Sex differences in human brain asymmetry: a critical survey. *Behavioral and Brain Sciences*, **3,** 215.
23. Kimura, D. (1981) Sex differences in speech organization within the left hemisphere. *Research Bulletin of the Department of Psychology of the University of Western Ontario*, **548,** 1.
24. Kinsbourne, M. (1981) If sex differences in brain localization exist, they have yet to be discovered. *Behavioral and Brain Sciences*, **3,** 241.
25. Kertesz, A. (1979) *Aphasia and Associated Disorders: Taxonomy, Localization, and Recovery*. New York: Grune & Stratton.
26. Galaburda, A. M. & Kemper, T. L. (1979) Cytoarchitectonic abnormalities in developmental dyslexia: a case study. *Annals of Neurology*, **6,** 94.
27. Broca, P. (1861) Nouvelle observation d'aphémie produite par une lésion de la troisième circonvolution frontale. *Bulletin de la Société d'Anatomie*, **6,** 398.
28. Ambrose, J. & Hounsfield, G. N. (1973) Computerized transverse axial tomography. *British Journal of Radiology*, **46,** 148.
29. Ambrose, J. (1973) Computerized transverse axial scanning (tomography): Part 2. Clinical application. *British Journal of Radiology*, **46,** 1023.
30. Basso, A., Lecours, A. R., Moraschini, S. & Vanier, M. (1983) Anatomo-clinical correlations of the aphasias as defined through computerized tomography: on exceptions. In *The Limits of Cerebral Localization* (Ed.) Alter, I. New York: Raven Press.
31. Vanier, M. (1983) *Lecture anatomique des images tomodensitométriques du cerveau*. PhD dissertation, Faculté de Médecine, Université de Montréal, Montréal.
32. Zurif, E. B., Caramazza, A. & Myersen, R. (1972) Grammatical judgements of agrammatic aphasics. *Neuropsychologia*, **10,** 405.
33. Marshall, J. C. & Newcombe, F. (1973) Patterns of paralexia. A psycholinguistic approach. *Journal of Psycholinguistic Research*, **2,** 175–179.
34. Kean, M. L. (1977) The linguistic interpretation of aphasic syndromes: agrammatism in Broca's aphasia, an example. *Cognition*, **5,** 9–46.
35. Morton, J. (1970) A functional model for memory. In *Models of Human Memory* (Ed.) Norman, D. New York: Academic Press.
36. Garrett, M. F. (1980) Levels of processing in sentence production. In *Language Production* (Ed.) Butterworth, B. Volume I. London: Academic Press.
37. Albert, M. & Obler, L. (1978) *The Bilingual Brain*. New York: Academic Press.
38. Grodzinski, Y. (1983) The syntactic characterization of agrammatism. *Cognition*, in press.
39. Sasanuma, S. (1975) Kana and kanji processing in Japanese aphasics. *Brain and Language*, **2,** 369.
40. Karanth, P. (1981) Pure alexia in a Kannada-English bilingual. *Cortex*, **17,** 187–198.
41. Weber, E. (1904) Das Schreiben als Ursache der einseiligen Lage des Sprachzentrums. *Zentralblatt für Physiologie*, **18,** 341.
42. Critchley, M. (1956) Premorbid latency and the pattern of subsequent aphasia. *Proceedings of the Society of Medicine*, **49,** 335.
43. Gurlitzer von Mundy, V. (1957) Zur Frage der paaring veranlagten Sprachzentren. *Der Nervenarzt*, **28,** 212.
44. Wechsler, A. F. (1976) Crossed aphasia in an illiterate dextral. *Brain and Language*, **3,** 164.
45. Metellus, J., Cathala, M. P., Aubory-Issartier, Z. & Bodak, A. (1981) Une observation d'aphasie chez une illettrée (analphabète): réflexions critiques sur les fonctions cérébrales concourant au langage. *Annales Médico-Psychologiques*, **139,** 992.
46. Cameron, R. F., Currier, R. D. & Maerer, A. F. (1971) Aphasia and literacy. *British Journal of Disorders of Communication*, **6,** 161.
47. Damasio, A. R., Castro-Caldas, A., Grosso, A. & Ferro, J. M. (1976) Brain specialization for language does not depend on literacy. *Archives of Neurology*, **33,** 300.
48. Goldberg, E. & Costa, L. D. (1981) Hemispheric differences in the acquisition and use of descriptive systems. *Brain and Language*, **14,** 144–173.
49. Bryden, M. P. (1982) *Laterality: Functional Asymmetry in the Intact Brain*. New York: Academic Press.
50. Gazzaniga, M. S. (1981) Variability in right hemisphere language function after callosal section: evidence for a continuum of generative capacity. *Journal of Neuroscience*, **1,** 323–331.
51. Ojemann, G. & Mateer, C. (1979) Human language cortex: localization of memory, syntax, and sequentia motor-phoneme identification systems. *Science*, **205,** 1401–1403.
52. Otto, D. A. (1978) *Multidisciplinary Perspectives in*

Event-related Brain Potential Research. US EPA 600/9-77-043, pp. 243–288.
53. Bradley, D. C., Garrett, M. F. & Zurif, E. B. (1980) Syntactic deficits in Broca's aphasia. In *Biological Studies of Mental Processes* (Ed.) Caplan D. Cambridge, MA: MIT Press.
54. Fodor, F. A. (1982) *The Modularity of Mind.* Cambridge, MA: Bradford Books.
55. Caplan, D. (1983) On the concept of a mental organ for language. In *Biological Perspectives on Language* (Ed.) Caplan, D., Lecours, A. R. & Smith, A. Cambridge, MA: MIT Press.
56. Galaburda, A. M., Lemay, M., Kemper, T. L. & Gechmevel, N. (1978) Right–left asymmetries in the temporal speech areas. *Science*, **199,** 852–856.

André Roch Lecours
David Caplan
Yves Joanette
Jean-Luc Nespoulous

Laboratoire Théophile-Alajouanine
Montreal, Canada, February 1983

Introduction to the French Edition

'AH! Outipechere redrecheri bi bi bichere glitonbalari di pilodon teledandre. In the pouve triko—well, a reoudi—when I go the power anrere direbe and gui ragalere jo logolatere dulon toreditron orge de lektole dibakan beledi di tombebisse eleto lunchich kalondichevite igue dutombetre deutombere. Gue te lektere she uh . . . gue kontagore deute bitodolore dubois dolore delon gueulere gue guetrompre deber she elgue de tonkonteguere di tonkontedere any to me arandeze sleeve uh . . . beleri jatanduisse ilabe legalonde plandibre new—uh . . . I had however—however she guede tan meille to say to you lantibedri tintintin re disse pile tilelere telere ceumetre.'*

(*Conversation with Mr Me.; October 1967*)

Although responding to innate biological predispositions, human language does not suddenly spring forth but rather emerges gradually during a course of prolonged learning. Such learning involves up to 14 hours of daily immersion in a flow of familial and social linguistic stimuli which, after the age of five years, normally includes an education based essentially on language. The interactions of numerous individual, sociocultural and professional factors are too complex to permit the limits of language learning to be defined precisely. Although it can be stated that, generally, excellent mastery of spoken and written language is usually attained by adolescents around the age of 15, it is noteworthy that adults continue to enrich their vocabulary until late in life, thereby demonstrating continuing linguistic and cognitive development.

What is the relationship between language and thought? How intricate their reciprocal influences! On the one hand, language acquisition appears as a response to a fundamental need to communicate. Language provides a tool permitting man to express his thoughts in a fashion understood by others and to comprehend the thoughts of others to the extent that they are expressed through language. On the other hand, it is primarily because language assigns words to concepts and abstractions that it constitutes a prerequisite to the full development of man's reasoning, judgement, hypothetical-deductive thinking and even emotional stability.

Language acquisition is possible because nature has endowed the human brain with a group of systems whose functional activity is limited at birth but progressively develops to form the substratum of linguistic activities. These systems and language activities are indissolubly linked. The potential activities of these cerebral systems are progressively structured by information received from the external world and by the responses which these systems elaborate. Before becoming a creator man is first created by his culture.

For spoken language, the input pole is located in the temporal lobe of the brain and ensures the reception and perception of auditory stimuli. The output pole, which is located in the frontal lobes, commands the execution of phonoarticulatory movements. The input pole includes the primary auditory area, Heschl's region and a specific association area composed of neighbouring parts of the first or the first two temporal convolutions. The output pole includes the primary motor area, corresponding to the inferior (opercular) third of the precentral gyrus and a specific association area whose principal

*This language sample, and all others introducing subsequent chapters, were obtained from French-speaking individuals. All conventional segments of French have been translated into English and, whenever possible, a plausible English equivalent has been provided for deviant segments.

component is the foot (pars opercularis) and cape (pars triangularis) of the third frontal convolution. The output pole also includes a feedback system corresponding to the inferior (opercular) third of the postcentral gyrus and to its specific association area which is most in the rostral portion of the supramarginal gyrus.

Although written language resembles oral language in many respects, it includes its own particular functional rules. For written language, the input pole is visual and is situated in the occipital lobes (calcarine cortex and lingual and fusiform lobules). The output pole, which directs dominant-hand activities, is located in the contralateral frontal lobe (middle third of the precentral gyrus). It also includes a feedback system corresponding to the middle third of the postcentral gyrus and to its specific association cortex. Between the input and output poles is a vast, non-specific associative system, a cortical–subcortical network which underlies the integration of the phonetic and phonological codes and morphosyntactical rules of a particular language. This network also permits the establishment and recognition of equivalences between verbal symbols and their referents, which is necessary for the production and comprehension of a communal language. The total apparatus, and particularly the associative cortical structures, is known as *the language zone* (see Chapter 8–5) and is located in the left cerebral hemisphere of almost all right-handed individuals as well as in a significant proportion of left-handers (see Chapter 11).

The term *aphasia* (see Chapters 3 to 7) designates the group of language disturbances resulting from a lesion affecting or destroying any or all of the previously mentioned regions. In adults, a lesion disturbs some or all linguistic behaviours at a time when language acquisition is complete or nearly so. In the case of children, aphasia refers to disturbances resulting from lesions acquired during a previously normal course of language development. In the French literature, 'aphasia' is not used as a term designating failures or delays of language acquisition, although it is sometimes so used in English.

The study of aphasia has progressed to a present position at the crossroad of several scientific disciplines. Many acceptable animal experiments are obviously impossible with man so that the study of aphasia remains the principal route to knowledge of language in relation to its anatomo-functional organization. In destroying one or another of the systems underlying language, cerebral pathology separates the language mechanism and permits identification of certain components.* Moreover, the study of aphasia has benefited from the development of disciplines which focus on the study of the brain, the study of language, or both, and can therefore provide insights concerning the cerebral mechanisms which underlie language acquisition, comprehension and production (see Chapter 8).

Because aphasia is one manifestation of cerebral disease, it naturally attracted the attention of physicians and neurologists who described it and interpreted it (and still do so) in physiopathological terms. They identified the causes of aphasia and its different clinical forms, localized the sites of causal lesions, defined the links between aphasia and cerebral dominance, and described the natural evolution of aphasia and its prognosis. Later, psychologists became interested in aphasia, not with the aim of describing the aphasic personality but in an attempt to analyse and apply the methodology of experimental psychology to the pathological aspects of language and other higher cortical functions. During the last decades, linguists made a brilliant entry into the study of aphasia through their attempts to verify, in aphasic populations, their hypotheses about normal language. As a consequence of their work, neurologists have adopted, to different degrees and with greater or lesser success, the methods of linguistics, thus contributing to the birth of the new discipline of *neurolinguistics*. Its identity has now been established through studies, which are both neurological and linguistic, of aphasics, non-aphasic patients and normal speakers. Such studies attempt to elucidate the mutual relationships between the brain and language and are therefore linked to the more general goal of neuropsychology. Computer scientists have also joined the study of aphasia, not only to contribute their techniques to certain psycho- and neurolinguistic studies but also to carry out investigations derived from the field of artificial intelligence and intended to elaborate different theoretical models which lend themselves to experimental simulation and verification. Finally,

* In addition to techniques particular to pathology, we shall also discuss others which permit the exploration of linguistic behaviours (see Chapters 7 and 11).

speech and language pathologists have long attempted to promote the language recovery of aphasic patients. Utilizing an empirical approach to their patients' language, they have developed strong remedial methods based on pathological realities. The interaction of speech pathology, neurology, psychology, computer science and linguistics has led to more elaborate research on remedial programmes and techniques. This converging of different disciplines has also led to an accumulation of data, approaches, techniques and scientific methods which constitute the field of endeavour known as *aphasiology*.

The idea of writing this book came to one of us (A.R.L.) during a clinical anatomy seminar in which the brain of a patient who had displayed a jargon aphasia was to be examined. The seminar was held in the Neurology Department of the Hôtel-Dieu Hospital in Montreal and was attended not only by the neuropathologist and neurologists from the Department but also by professors and students from varied disciplines. The knowledge required and the vocabulary used were such that only some of the neurologists could take part in the discussion. After listening to a prerecorded sample of the patient's language, one of them remarked that his conversation was characterized by a substantial *dyssyntaxic*. The meaning of this term appeared to be clearly understood by the linguists in attendance. However, a lack of adequate comprehension was further revealed when a neurologist later explained, with splendid assurance, that dyssyntaxia in aphasic language is not associated with a lesion of an anatomofunctional entity specific to syntax. This pronouncement was followed by a gale of laughter. Further misunderstandings arose as the discussion turned to other pathological features of the recorded conversation and their anatomoclinical correlates. One of the participants even maintained that the jargoned language of the deceased was easier to understand than that of the neurologists and speech pathologists from the Hôtel-Dieu. Despite this, everyone who attended the seminar displayed a genuine curiosity about aphasia. It became clear that many of them wished to obtain an expository text which would provide an introduction to the major themes of aphasiology and facilitate the later reading of the ever-expanding number and variety of scientific publications. The preparation of such a text thus became the goal which we have strived to attain.

This work was undertaken and followed by a group of neurologists, speech pathologists, psychologists and linguists from university and hospital settings in Montreal, Marseilles, Paris, Quebec and Halifax. Although it is a collective work, the arrangement of the content of the manuscripts and their composition was left to our discretion and principally to one of us (A.R.L.), as the best means of ensuring the unity and cohesion of the entire work. The English translation–adaptation was later undertaken by another of us (B.B.). Since the text discusses aphasia from multiple viewpoints, each specialist will find chapters concerned with his or her own area of expertise as well as other chapters which will allow expansion of the specialist's field of interest. A carefully conceived, cross-referenced index includes headings familiar to specialists in each discipline and provides guidance to individual readers in their course of reading. For example, a linguist interested in the phonological aspects of aphasia would be guided under the heading *phoneme*, to passages of the text dealing with corresponding neurolinguistic terms, physiopathological interpretations of phonemic disturbances, types of aphasia characterized by such disturbances, and remedial procedures for these types of aphasia. Similarly, a neurologist interested in *conduction aphasia* would be guided by this heading to passages of the book defining the concepts of a phoneme and a phonological system, and to other passages discussing phonemic deviations and their linguistic structure.

Having attempted to produce a multidisciplinary text suited to teaching and research, the authors will not consider that they have attained their goal unless professionals and students in neurology, linguistics, psychology, speech pathology and even computer science find reading of the text to be both straightforward and rewarding.

PHYSIOLOGICAL APPROACH TO LANGUAGE

As previously stated, aphasiology remains by far the most appropriate field for the study of rules governing the breakdown of linguistic functions and one which permits a physiological approach to language. We are aware of the hypothetical nature of some of the material presented in the following pages. Nevertheless we consider it essential that the hypothetical constructs be retained by the reader for they constitute prerequisites to the understanding of aphasic language.

ASSESSMENT PROCEDURES FOR APHASIA

Aphasic language frequently misleads or baffles those who attempt to assess it. In order to appreciate the significance of those aspects of language which are lost, disturbed or conserved, it is necessary that the examiner be aware of the physiological mechanisms which are called into play on each type of task or subtest. He or she must also realize that results on a single subtest are meaningful only when considered in relation to all other tasks included in the test battery (see Chapter 15).

The seemingly most elementary language test is that requiring oral repetition of auditory linguistic stimuli. However, even simple repetition involves much spacial-temporal processing by the brain: perception (or decoding, if one prefers a more modern term) of the auditory stimuli; transposition of the perceptual pattern to activate the appropriate neurological correlates of the phonological code, which themselves will selectively activate the sensory-motor neuronal networks of the phonoarticulatory organs leading the subject to reproduce orally what s/he has just heard. As can be seen, the systems which underlie the semantic aspects of languages are not necessarily involved, so that repetition may represent a form of parrot-like speech. This appears to be the case when meaningless stimuli (nonsense words or syllable strings) are reproduced but, in other instances, semantic systems may play a certain role. Repetition is typically most accurate when the stimuli consist of highly familiar words and the meaning of the words or sentences is understood. As a matter of fact, normal subjects can readily repeat long sentences provided that they contain only a few, related ideas permitting the meaning of the entire sentence to be easily apprehended.

The understanding of spoken words or sentences involves an initial stage of auditory decoding, subsequent reference to the phonological code and the participation of other systems—those concerned with syntax and semantics—which provide support to those units* having the dual aspects of form and meaning. Even then we have not considered verbal memory, which permits the recounting of information in a previously-heard story; nor intelligence which permits the synthesizing or summarizing of lengthy texts or entire conferences (acts which certainly involve more than purely linguistic systems). With respect to auditory comprehension, it should be noted that reference to the phonological code may no longer be necessary—at least for words—after a certain degree of language mastery has been achieved; auditory messages may then be immediately processed at the semantic level (semantic analysis).

The production of spoken language presupposes prelinguistic cognitive activity. This activates unknown neuronal mechanisms and results in the selection of dual aspect units (form and meaning) which, in turn, activate the corresponding phonemic units, leading finally to the activation of the sensory motor patterns of verbal articulation. It should be noted that in the case of sentence production, the selection and ordering of lexical items must be carried out in accordance with syntactical rules. Naming an object or picture involves the same productive processes and is distinguished only by the fact that the stimulus is visual and requires identification and a pre-determined specific response. As indicated by this description, we have adopted a linguistic approach in which language production is viewed as a multi-articulated activity with three essential phases: the first concerned with units having the dual aspects of form and meaning, the second with the phonological code and the third with phonetic-articulatory movements.

The principles discussed in reference to spoken language can be readily extended to written language. In this case, the receptive pole is visual and the expressive pole involves finger and hand movements. Features particular to written language reflect its derivation from the spoken form. Thus the graphemic code is strongly linked, in a subordinate fashion, to the phonological code. However, in many languages the rules of spelling are such that writing does not involve straight-

* *Unités à double face* (*signifiant-signifié*).

forward, unequivocal transposition from phonemes to graphemes (for example, the phoneme /u/ can be written in numerous ways) (see Chapter 17). The extraction of meaning from written words and sentences generally requires reference to the phonological code of spoken language and, of course, the activation of semantic systems (whispering or subvocal speech may occur during reading). However, there is undoubtedly a direct pathway, at least in a certain proportion of (literate) individuals, which short circuits the phonological code and allows visual–verbal patterns direct access to the semantic system. Thus, when viewing a written word, normal subjects may extract certain features which permit understanding without verbalization. On the other hand, it is likely that subvocal speech occurs during writing and that no direct semantic–graphemic pathway is involved.

In summary, a language assessment must include exploration of all input and output poles, realizing that between them lies an entire anatomofunctional language network. It is therefore necessary to include subtests in which the participation of the semantic system may be helpful but is not essential: i.e., audiophonatory transposition (repetition); graphographic transposition (copying of written stimuli); audiographic transposition (writing to dictation); and graphophonatory transposition (oral reading). In addition, subtests should be included which require semantic analysis which is dependent on specific input or output modalities (comprehension of spoken and written language, oral and written expression). By using such subtests and elaborating those of greater complexity to gain insights into the nature of particular deficits, it is possible to define certain parameters of disorganized language (which also indicate a certain reorganization of remaining functions) and thus to discern the laws which govern language acquisition, comprehension and production.

Whether or not articulatory (arthric) difficulties constitute an aphasic impairment has been the topic of lively debates and numerous written commentaries. In fact, the question is one of principle and thus invites deduction of the logical consequences. We consider articulatory difficulties to be aphasic in nature because speech results from the activity of sensory-motor assemblies which are formed in parallel with the acquisition of language. In this case, the agraphias and perceptual disturbances in the decoding of auditory or visual messages would also be considered aphasic.*

All lesions affecting the anatomofunctional language network result in an aphasia and all forms of cerebral pathology may cause such lesions. Furthermore, the deficits resulting from a lesion are related to its extent. Small circumscribed lesions result in more limited deficits and therefore provide greater opportunity to appreciate the anatomophysiological substrates of speech and language behaviours.

Finally, it should be noted that, with the exception of pictured objects included in the visual and written naming subtests, we have previously discussed only linguistic visual and auditory stimuli. However, other non-verbal stimuli may be used to examine all sensory or receptive functions including touch, temperature and pain; recognition of colours, musical selections, musical instruments and familiar noises as well as gustatory and olfactory stimuli which are directly related to language because they are identified by names specific to each stimulus. In this regard, we would not consider as aphasic those impairments which affect either the cortical areas where these sensory stimuli are treated (agnosias) or the pathways which conduct patterns derived from the sensory data to the language zone which is itself spared by the lesion.

LOCALIZATION OF A LESION AND LOCALIZATION OF A FUNCTION: A PSYCHOPHYSIOLOGICAL HIATUS

While we shall discuss here only one particular problem of cerebral localization, it is an important one. In short, if it is true that the brain is composed of a group of organs each of which plays a specific psychophysiological role, it is also true that this group of organs constitutes a whole, and that each part, when isolated by pathology, no longer functions in relation to the whole. An example involving language would be a case in which the language zone was isolated

* Oddly enough, most authors accept this point of view with the exception of agnosic alexia without agraphia. This is probably because the decoding of visual linguistic stimuli is mediated by a region remote from the classical language zone and because the cerebral arterial network is such that alexia without agraphia most frequently occurs in the absence of other aphasic deficits, namely in a form known as pure alexia or pure-word blindness (see Chapter 5).

from the rest of the brain (as may exceptionally occur in certain anoxias and bilateral occlusions of the internal carotid arteries). Speech remains possible, but nearly empty of relevant content. Sentences may be correctly formed and articulated but have little sense and bear no obvious relation to the patient's thoughts or experiences (see Chapter 4). The psycholinguistic function no longer exists. We have already said that the language zone is linked to all sense organs and to mental life but the latter cannot be localized within the brain. At most, we are now aware of the initiating and coordinating roles of the frontal lobes in linguistic production. Nevertheless it must be recognized that certain functions are represented in certain cerebral regions: for example, those concerned with phonetic articulation, and with writing, as well as those concerned with visual and auditory decoding. Viewed in a broad perspective, it appears that the more a function is *instrumental* (we could have said elementary were this term not so ill-suited to activities which are already extremely complex), the easier it is to identify the brain region or regions which underlie it. Conversely, the higher the level of a particular function, up to and including thought, the greater the difficulty in its localization. From another point of view, it is correct to state that the integrity of a particular part of the brain is essential for normal performance of a particular function since a lesion in that part of the brain impairs the function in question. However, this does not imply that the function is located in that part of the brain. Such faulty reasoning could be refuted by numerous biological analogies, particularly those concerning major metabolical functions. However, we have selected an illustration which requires no medical knowledge and can be easily understood. Consider a large city, Paris for example. In it there are numerous physical elements which fulfil specific roles. Although it can immediately be recognized that certain physical elements are clearly related to particular functions, where, precisely, can 'cultural functions', 'religious functions', 'political functions', etc. be located? Surely no one would think of maintaining that the 'traffic function' in Paris is located at the Concorde Bridge on the basis that its destruction would be followed by horrendous traffic jams. It could be said only that an intact Concorde Bridge is necessary for normal 'traffic function' in that city (see Insertion 8.6).

There is, moreover, a missing link between linguistic productions and their biological foundations which can also be illustrated by a comparison. An electronic machine is composed of well-known physical components, including receivers, memory cells and elementary logic circuits, but, depending on the arrangement of the components, the machine is able to perform widely diverse functions. It may perform mathematical computations, make forecasts and projections, translate a language and even play excellent chess. However, the reasoning underlying its moves during a chess game could not be revealed by inserting different electrodes into the machine (and depends, in fact, on its programmer). At most, such electrodes would detect electrical signals and perhaps indicate how they are treated and stored. In the same way, neither microelectrodes nor microprobes will allow direct penetration of human language. Microelectrodes could yield data only on potential changes and microprobes could monitor only the biochemical modifications of mediating processes as indicated by on–off neuronal states. Such data would nevertheless be of value, could they be obtained through medically ethical procedures.

FROM WORD IMAGES TO PATTERNS: ACTIVATION, INHIBITION AND SERIATION

In considering the biological foundations of language further, we must return to the end of the nineteenth and the beginning of the twentieth century. At this time, different writers interpreted aphasic impairments in terms of 'word images' stored in one or several neurones. Later, the word 'engram' became fashionable. Pathological deficits were interpreted either in terms of a 'verbal amnesia' or in terms of interruptions of the pathways between different centres. This orientation was later followed by a globalistic view challenging, when not denying, the notion that separate functions are integrated ('represented') in specific groups of neurones (see Chapter 1).

Which orientation predominates today? One sees a clear rejection of a holistic theory and a return to the idea of functional localization and the association of different functions through longer or shorter axonal pathways. However, the terminology and concepts have changed. Our previous discussion of cerebral localization of function illustrates the differences between contemporary thought and that of the early associationists.

The term 'amnesia' is still employed with reference to amnesic aphasia and other aspects of acquired language disorders but its meaning today is more restricted. We could not, in fact, conceive of knowledge acquired through learning without recourse to the idea of stored physical counterparts in the form of long-term 'traces'. In right-handers, traces of verbal acquisitions are primarily stored in the left temporoparietal region and non-verbal acquisitions are stored in other areas. However, language does not simply involve word memory which is preserved in normals and disturbed in aphasia. Language also implies syntactical knowledge of the permutations and combinations permitted within the limits of acquired conventions. Language involves a highly differentiated activity which is dependent on memory as well as on what is broadly defined as intelligence. In addition, the selection of words —and also ideas—depends upon the speaker's personality. In other words, Shakespeare's works depended somewhat on his verbal memory, even more on his linguistic talents, and most of all on his intelligence and emotional sensitivity.

As for 'word images' and their constituents, they have been banished from contemporary usage and replaced by terms inspired by substantial neurophysiological data. Although the label 'engram' is appropriate in some respects, it is old-fashioned and vague, and does not correspond to physiological reality. Certainly a word must have a physical correlate but it should, in our opinion, be conceived as a specific pattern involving a considerable number (presently unknown) of neurones forming an individual functional configuration. In these neuronal assemblies and subassemblies, each nerve cell may participate in a large number (which also cannot be specified) of patterns, with each of the patterns being specific to a given word. Such a description appears appropriate for the different spatial-temporal aspects of language up to actual articulatory acts as well as for hierarchical levels of spoken language from repetition to the formulation of highly complex thoughts. The same statements may also be applicable to written language.

It must also be added that repetition, comprehension and reading may normally be accomplished in the absence of complete stimulus perception, a fact which may be verified by modifying stimuli by lesser or greater degrees. This implies that neuronal assemblies may actualize patterns from less than the total amount of information conveyed by a stimulus. This is accomplished on a probabilistic basis and may sometimes lead to an erroneous response. This probabilistic mode of operation is not exclusive to language and may well be characteristic of other sensory-motor processes.

This conceptual approach to neurophysiology illuminates the mechanisms underlying aphasic impairments. In *phonemic paraphasias* (see Chapters 2 and 4), certain sounds do not haphazardly replace the target sounds whose grouping forms a word. A qualitative analysis of replacing and replaced phonemes shows many of them to be related in terms of the similarity of phonoarticulatory movements involved in their oral production, or what we call *paradigmatic similarity*. The same concept applies to *formal verbal paraphasias* in which the substituting word shares common phonemes with the substituted word (see Chapter 2). We note in passing that these two types of errors are also made by normal subjects and that some so-called slips of the tongue could also be defined as paraphasias (see Chapter 14). From a physiological viewpoint, it can easily be understood that neighbouring patterns share a large number of common neurones and that, in pathological states, phoneme or word substitutions would most probably occur between adjacent patterns or those which are partly identical. At a higher productive level involving words rather than sounds, the same physiological principle holds with regard to semantic similarity (see Chapter 2). The substituting word shares semantic features (e.g., the same conceptual class, category of use, causal linkages) with the substituted word. Here we are not referring to phrases which patients may produce when they are unable to retrieve a name and resort, for example, to descriptions of use. Rather, we are speaking only of words easily produced in a most natural manner during the course of conversation, picture naming, the description of pictured scenes, etc. They suggest that in the brain, words are anatomofunctionally represented in semantic fields with close proximity between synonyms and words which share common semantic features or conceptual or practical attributes. Consequently, word substitutions will more probably occur between those in the same semantic field than between those whose meanings and semantic features have nothing in common.

The types of errors so far discussed do not

account for all of the paraphasias involving either phonemes or words. An additional factor which must be considered is the serial ordering of linguistic units. For isolated words (as elicited in naming, repetition, oral reading), a major proportion of phonemic paraphasias involve the reiteration of phonemes already pronounced or the anticipatory production of phonemes which would normally be produced at a later moment in the phoneme sequence. These phenomena can be understood in terms of the neurophysiological concepts of activation and inhibition. In the production of a given word, the brain must activate as many specific patterns as there are phonemes in the word and the pattern activated for one phoneme must be immediately inhibited to allow activation of the pattern associated with the subsequent phoneme in the sequence. If inhibitory mechanisms are disturbed by a cerebral lesion, evoked patterns remain active too long and therefore may replace those of a subsequent target phoneme, giving rise to the phenomenon of reiteration (a form of perseveration). On the other hand, when a speaker starts to pronounce a word, the patterns of the last phonemes in the word are already primed but remain partially inhibited until the moment the corresponding phonemes must be produced. Thus it can readily be understood how disturbances in this pairing of activation and inhibition may result in anticipatory phonemic errors, especially when the substituting phoneme strongly resembles the substituted phoneme of the series. The same phenomena of reiteration and anticipation occur at the sentence level and are seen in the production of words similar or identical to a word previously produced and, perhaps to a lesser extent, the production of words which would normally be produced later in the sentence.

This interpretation is clearly not based on neurophysiological research of human language. It is, however, consistent with numerous experimental findings showing that all neuronal activation systems are paired with an inhibitory system which cancels or modulates the initiation of neural activity. This can be illustrated by two very different examples. First, movements of the fingers of one hand are accomplished by activation of neurones in the hand and finger areas of the motor cortex as well as in an inhibitory zone which surrounds the activated region. It appears that this double event facilitates the unequivocal selection of the group of neurones which enter into action. Second, pain signals transmitted by certain peripheral nerve fibres to the posterior horn of the spinal cord encounter a complex neuronal organization made up of peripheral neurones and, especially, neurones descending from the central nervous system. Acting as inhibitors and modulators, they provide a form of gate control regulating, or sometimes blocking, the influx of noxious stimulation or, conversely, permitting excitation and discharge of the spinothalamic systems.

DISCONNECTIONS

The associationists described pathways linking different 'centres' and the syndromes which resulted from the interruption of these associative fasciculi. Their principles were generally sound although they are stated somewhat differently today. We would now say that information is conveyed to the cerebral cortex where it is first processed by the specific association areas and is then transferred, via longer or shorter pathways in the white matter, to a non-specific association area. There, the information is further processed, resulting in a new form of neural activity which commands an appropriate response, which is itself elaborated through successive associative relays. It is tempting to say that, in the final analysis, the outcome of this activity affects muscles and viscera, or else it affects thought processes.

Cerebral pathology does not spare the associative pathways of the white matter. Although their anatomical reality is fairly well established, much less is known about the nature of the information which they convey. For example, the posterior temporal region is one of the cortical areas giving rise to an axonal pathway—the arcuate fasciculus—which terminates in the motor region (frontal). This pathway clearly connects the auditory realm to the motor region (in particular, the buccophonatory zone). Does it, however, transmit phonemic encoding from its point of origin in the temporal region? Or does the phonemic encoding occur in the large region of temporoparietal cortex which surrounds the arcuate fasciculus and continually sends new fibres to it? This question cannot easily be answered because lesions typically involve both the cortex and subcortical regions (see Chapter 8-4). We shall be able to learn more on this subject only after sufficient rigorous anatomoclinical observations have been carried out on cases with extremely limited lesions. Until now such observations have been extremely rare. In any case it is clear that the physiopathological interpretation of those impairments which are known today as disconnection syndromes must consider the role of the cortex as well as that of the associative pathways.

Since axons are, in fact, parts of a neurone, it might first be thought that the disturbances resulting from disconnections are equivalent to those resulting from lesions affecting cortical cell bodies, or from lesions affecting the cortical regions from which the axons originate (or to which they project), the cortex being unable to process information which it no longer receives. However, this interpretation is only partially true because it ignores an important variable, namely the extreme complexity of cortical operations. We can illustrate this in a simplified way, using three black boxes labelled (A), (B) and (C). Box (A) emits information which is transferred via a pathway to (B) which processes this input and emits new information which is transferred to (C). Interruption of the pathways (B→C) impedes activity in (C). But what is normally happening in (B)? First of all, the reception of information from (A), then processing of this information and, finally, the encoding of new information destined for (C). In other words, (B) is not a simple relay station but the site of at least two activities, decoding and encoding (and the operations actually occurring in the cortex are probably infinitely more complex). In any case, damage or destruction of (B) will clearly result in more complex impairments than interruption of the pathways (B→C). In our opinion, this is in fact what is demonstrated by pathology. Consider the case of alexia without agraphia, in which the left occipital lobe no longer receives visual stimulation from the outer world, although such stimuli are still received by the right occipital lobe. The question is whether the observed alexia results from a callosal lesion which interrupts the relay of information from the right occipital lobe to that of the left cerebral hemisphere where it would normally be processed, or whether the reading deficit is caused by impairment of the left occipital cortex (lingual and fusiform lobules). The latter interpretation is suggested by the typical profile of deficits which will later be described (see Chapters 5 and 8-3). The deficits observed in callosal lesions, which effectively separate the two hemispheres so that graphic stimuli are received only by the right occipital lobe, do not correspond precisely with those observed in alexia without agraphia. This disorder cannot therefore be explained solely in terms of an interruption of occipito-occipital pathways.

LANGUAGE RECOVERY AND CEREBRAL PLASTICITY

At present, very little is known about the biological mechanisms underlying recovery of language by aphasic individuals. We can, however, outline the questions of major significance.

In adults with strongly lateralized language representation, one of the principal factors underlying language recovery is the eventual reversibility of lesions affecting neurones of the language zone. Although this process, when it occurs, is no doubt accelerated by language therapy, it is clear that recovery of pre-morbid functioning by all, or nearly all, of the neurones will be accompanied by recovery of all pre-morbid linguistic behaviours. Such cases are indeed rare, if not exceptional, in comparison with those which involve permanent destruction of many neurones and the formation of scar tissue which is devoid of any functional capacity. Nevertheless language therapy may be clearly effective in these cases, even years after the formation of scar tissue. Thus there is no doubt that substantial improvement may result from language therapy even though a ceiling is frequently reached and recovery remains incomplete.

In the not-so-distant past psychologists considered each part of the brain to be equipotential, a view which was supported by findings from research on rats. Today this view is no longer maintained with respect to either rats or animals more primitive on the phylogenetic scale and the concept is clearly inapplicable to man. It is nevertheless true that the human brain shows astonishing plasticity. The irreversible destruction of certain portions of the brain necessary for the performance of certain highly complex functions may be compensated by the activities of the undamaged hemisphere. The brain's capacity to compensate for previously acquired functions is related to age, being greatest in younger subjects but much reduced in older ones. This is demonstrated by observations of hemispherectomized patients as well as by the recovery of language seen in aphasic children, for whom it can be logically supposed that recovery is mediated, in right-handers, by circuits developed in the right hemisphere (see Chapter 11). Note that, in discussing cerebral plasticity, we have considered only the possible compensation for a damaged lobe in one hemisphere through transfer of function to the corresponding lobe of the other hemisphere. We are not referring to the possibility that the frontal lobe might compensate for temporal or parietal functions, a notion which is, strictly speaking, inconceivable. Thus the question of interest concerns the possible importance of the right hemisphere in the recovery of language by right-handers. This is unknown at present (although we can logically speculate that the influence of the right hemisphere varies with the degree of functional lateralization for language, which itself most probably varies as a function of genetic, and possibly cultural, factors). In addition, the role of the right hemisphere could not previously be determined (even the injection of sodium Amytal into the right carotid artery would not permit an answer because, when carried out on a patient with a left-hemisphere lesion, it would result in the well-known symptoms of bilateral lesions). However, it appears possible that this question will soon be answered through progress in techniques which can be applied in conformity with medical ethics (evoked cortical potentials, implanted electrodes, electrical stimulation, non-invasive cerebral blood flow measurements).

Can language therapy activate circuits which are damaged but not permanently destroyed, or even circuits which have recovered a normal or near-normal functional capacity which remains unutilized? The answer appears to be yes. Although further research is needed, we think that this process plays a major role in the recovery of long-established abilities which are severely disturbed by an aphasia-producing lesion.

A final question concerns the possibility that language therapy may create new patterns and circuits in the left hemisphere of right-handers. Nothing rules out this possibility provided that it is recognized that new learning is limited in adults and is probably insignificant in old age. It is often said that man does not utilize all of his brain's functional capacities, which is undoubtedly true. Many contemporary scientists know much more than did Aristotle or the physicists of ancient Egypt, thus implying current involvement of a much larger number of representational patterns and probable use of an increased number of neurones. With regard to contemporary language, vocabulary size varies greatly with socio-economic level and may range from 2000 to at least 10 000 words. These two extremes most certainly reflect differences in the number of neurones and dendrites which enter into play, and it seems to us quite conceivable that new circuits could be created through language therapy. The authors of this introduction cannot forget a patient who received therapy and was followed for some years after the onset of an aphasia caused by a cerebral embolus. He finally possessed two modes of language which alternatively appeared in his conversation. The first was ineffective, consisting of a large proportion of recurring ready-made expressions; some lengthy, and all normally articulated. The second permitted effective communication but was laboured, syllabic and required constant attention to the choice of words and their articulation which nevertheless remained defective. The second mode of expression was, in our opinion, the result of language therapy depending, at least partially, on the establishment of new cerebral circuits.

François Lhermitte
André Roch Lecours

Paris, July 1978

1. Historical Review

'I help myself with some French languages, some French works and also some works in French from English and certain ones are by a German. And then I have some books come from countries north of France, Norwegian and Swedish. They are pretty complicated texts with some words which are not always very very very common and I have to get accustomed to them and get them accustomed. I'm very happy with this work. Right now, I understand just about everything but I am slow to make myself understood. I write slowly and I write especially very slowly.'

(Conversation with Mr Co.; November 1969)

1 FROM FRANZ GALL TO PIERRE MARIE

Despite the progress achieved through increasingly empirical anatomical research, eighteenth-century scientists continued to regard the brain as a homogeneous mass which, under the influence of the *will*, indifferently distributed *vital energy* to all parts of the body. The nerves, descending directly from the brain, were thought to function as channels through which this energy flowed. However, at the end of the eighteenth and the beginning of the nineteenth century, Franz Gall (1758–1828) formulated a new doctrine, one noteworthy for its teaching that man's cerebral hemispheres are composed of several independent organs which subtend his various *moral and intellectual faculties*[1]. Among these faculties is one concerned with verbal memory and located in the 'anterior lobules' of the brain. Gall's original deductions on this matter were based on his observation of several people who, in conjunction with marked protrusion of the eyeballs ('*à fleur de tête*', he wrote), showed an equally remarkable talent for memorizing verbal material. In these subjects, the orbital region of the 'anterior lobules' of the brain, namely the organ of verbal memory, is abnormally enlarged and pushes outside the posterior part of the sockets, thus causing the eyes to protrude (*yeux de boeuf*: ox eyes) as well as—for reasons which are perhaps less clear—the formation of a palpebral pocket (*yeux pochetés*: pocketed eyes). Gall subsequently specified that 'people whose eyes are thus-shaped possess not only an excellent word memory but [that] they feel a particular disposition towards the study of languages, criticism, in general for everything which is related to literature'. It is not generally known that Gall believed his theories to be confirmed by observations of linguistic behaviour in patients whose speech was impaired by a severe reduction following traumatic lesions of the anterior lobes of the brain. Based on these two different types of clinical findings, Gall's work was to give birth to two disciplines. One was *phrenology*, or the study of man's character and faculties in relation to the external configuration of his skull. Although its practitioners are now few in number, if any in fact remain, a trace of its influence on popular language remains in the expression '*la bosse des mathématiques*' (an innate talent for mathematics). The second discipline was *neuropsychology*, or the study of behaviour in relation to the anatomy and physiology of the brain. Interest in this discipline is continually increasing and its name is now listed in recent editions of better dictionaries.

From 1807 onwards, Gall carried out his work in Paris where his doctrine was widely discussed in meetings of the medical profession. Some, who were no doubt repelled by the occult nature of phrenology, considered Gall's work to be that of a charlatan. Others, who did not attach much importance to the bumps of the skull, nevertheless perceived the significance of the concept of cerebral localization and attempted to illustrate it through clinical and anatomical studies. Among this group, the best known was Jean-Baptiste Bouillaud (1796–1881) who taught, beginning in 1825, that the location of a cerebral lesion can be deduced from knowledge of the signs and symptoms which it causes. In the same year Bouillaud published a report entitled *Recherches cliniques propres à démontrer que la perte de la parole correspond à la lésion des lobules antérieurs du cerveau et à confirmer l'opinion de M. Gall sur le siège de l'organe du articulé,** a title which clearly defined the author's positive views of the concept of cerebral localization and Gall's work. The text contains a clear formulation of Bouillaud's conception of speech and its production under the direction of a specific part of the brain. 'I wished only to demonstrate that the organs for the articulation of sounds draw in the anterior lobules of the brain the principle of their complicated movements, and I believe that I have succeeded'[2].

At a medical convention held in Montpellier in July 1836, another of Gall's admirers, Marc Dax (1770–1837), gave a presentation entitled *Lésions de la moitié gauche de l'encéphale coincidant avec l'oublie des signes de la pensée.*† Supported by about 40 clinical and anatomoclinical reports, Dax argued: 'not that all left hemisphere diseases necessarily impair verbal memory, but that, when this memory is impaired by brain disease, the cause of the disorder should be sought in the left hemisphere and still sought there if the two hemispheres are both diseased'. Dax's presentation, which was not published, went unnoticed for almost 30 years. Its significance was finally recognized when his son had the text published in *La Gazette Hebdomadaire de Médecine et de Chirurgie*[3, 4].

In 1861, Paul Broca (1824–1880) used the term *aphemia* to designate an acquired disturbance of the *faculty of articulated language* (which he was careful not to confuse with the *general faculty of language*)[5]. From 1861 to 1865, Broca reported several anatomoclinical case studies in which he stressed the fact that aphemia is caused by lesions of the postero-external parts of the anterior lobes of the brain and not by lesions of their orbital surfaces[6–8]. A competent anatomist as well as clinician, Broca of course noted that the subjects of his autopsies had lesions of the left cerebral hemisphere. However, it was only in 1865, within a few weeks of the publication of Dax's article, that Broca clearly stated his conclusions concerning the lateralization of lesions causing aphemia in *La Bulletin de la Société d'Anthropologie*[9]: 'I have reported to you ... ten case studies of aphemia in which autopsies showed various lesions of the third frontal convolution ... I persist in thinking, until further enquiries have been made, that genuine aphemia, that is the loss of speech without paralysis of the organs of articulation and without the destruction of intelligence, is related to lesions of the third frontal convolution. But it is not about this fact that I have come to speak to you. My address is related to the particular preference of the lesions of aphemia for the left hemisphere of the brain.' Broca tried to explain the lateralization of cerebral structures governing speech production by relating it to the idea of manual dominance: 'There is a certain number of left-handers everywhere; but nearly all men are right-handed ... The most difficult role, the one which demands the most skill, precision, expression or force, in one word the predominant role, is very generally assigned to the right hand.' Although imitation and education no doubt must be considered in the origin of this right-hand dominance, Broca considered the determining factor to be biological: 'in the development of the brain, the left hemisphere convolutions are more advanced than those of the right hemisphere. The first are already delineated at a moment when the others are not yet visible. The left hemisphere, which determines movement of the right limbs, is thus more precocious in its development than the opposite hemisphere' (Fig. 1–1). The embryological studies of Louis-Pierre Gratiolet (1815–1865)[10] provided the basis of Broca's theory that 'the more precocious development of the left hemisphere predisposes us, in our first gropings, to carry out with this half of the brain the most complicated physical and intellectual acts, among which must certainly be included the expression of ideas by means of language and, more particularly, by articulated language.' The parallel with manual dominance enabled Broca to suggest an explanation of the exceptional

---

* *Clinical Research Able to Show that the Loss of Speech Corresponds to a Lesion of the Anterior Lobules of the Brain and to Confirm Mr Gall's Opinion on the Seat of Articulated Language.*

† *Lesions of the Left Half of the Brain Coinciding with the Forgetting of the Signs of Thought.*

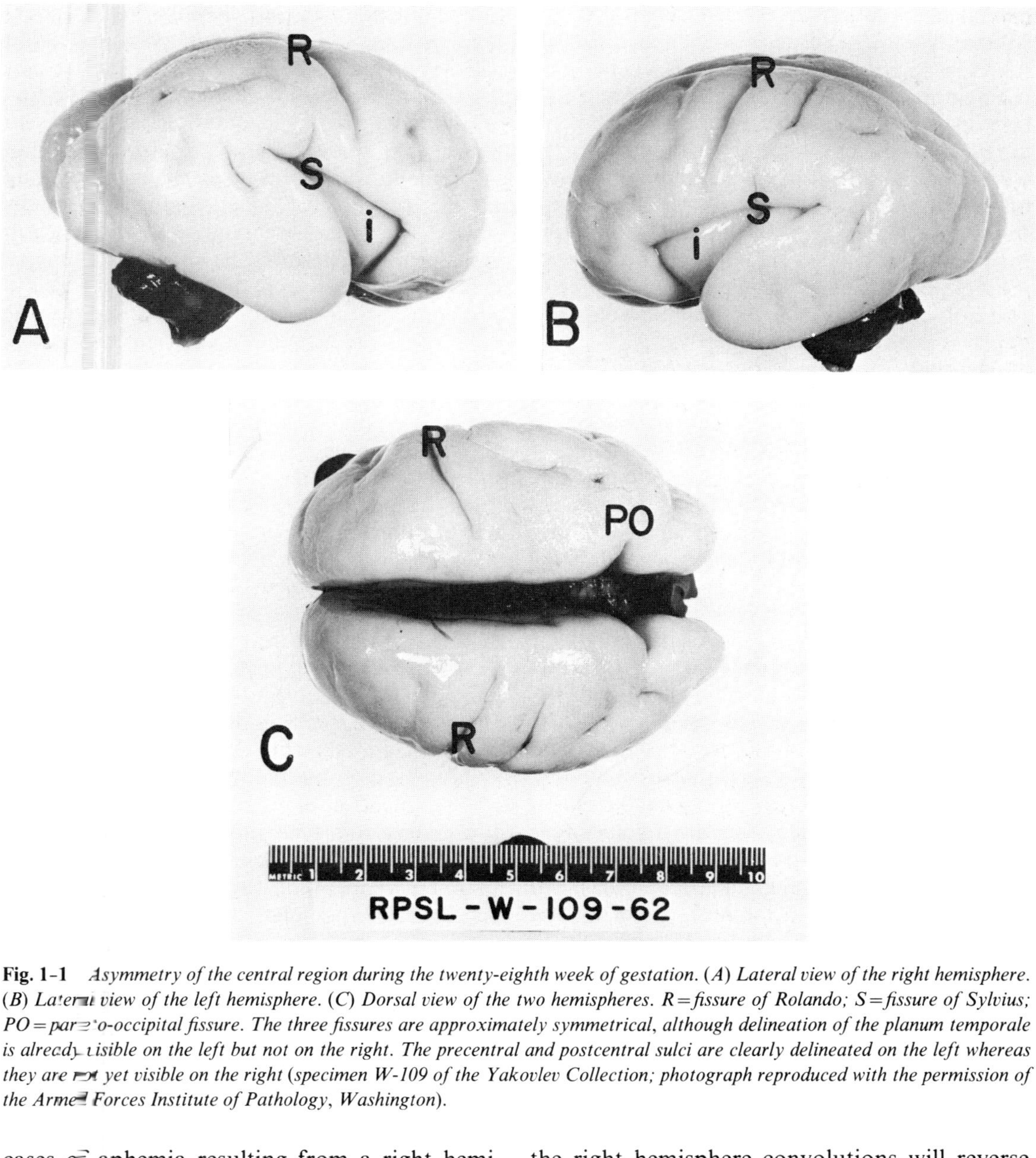

Fig. 1-1 *Asymmetry of the central region during the twenty-eighth week of gestation. (A) Lateral view of the right hemisphere. (B) Lateral view of the left hemisphere. (C) Dorsal view of the two hemispheres. R = fissure of Rolando; S = fissure of Sylvius; PO = parieto-occipital fissure. The three fissures are approximately symmetrical, although delineation of the planum temporale is already visible on the left but not on the right. The precentral and postcentral sulci are clearly delineated on the left whereas they are not yet visible on the right (specimen W-109 of the Yakovlev Collection; photograph reproduced with the permission of the Armed Forces Institute of Pathology, Washington).*

cases of aphemia resulting from a right hemisphere lesion, cases which some considered to refute his theory: 'In the same way that there are left-handed individuals, in whom the natural pre-eminence of the motor forces of the right hemisphere confers a natural and incorrigible pre-eminence on left-hand functions, so is it conceivable that there may be a certain number of individuals in whom the native pre-eminence of the right hemisphere convolutions will reverse the order of the phenomena that I just pointed out, [individuals] in whom the faculty of coordinating the movements of articulated language will then become ... permanently monopolized by the right hemisphere.' It was thus in his 1865 paper that Broca presented his final conception of aphemia and his conclusion that it is caused by a lesion of the 'posterior portion'* of the third

* As far as we know, Broca himself never restricted this area to the foot, or the pars opercularis, of the third frontal convolution.

frontal convolution of the left cerebral hemisphere; the left hemisphere dominance for the function of articulated language is of the same nature as its dominance for manual motor functions in right-handers; in the same way that there are left-handers, exceptional individuals in whom the right hemisphere assumes dominance of manual motor functions, so are there exceptional individuals in whom dominance for the function of articulated language is a property of the right hemisphere;* the phenomenon of cerebral dominance has biological foundations; and aphemia does not affect intelligence[9].

Although not directly concerned with the major anatomoclinical questions of his day, Jacques Lordat's (1773–1870) contribution to the study of aphasia, which he named *alalia* in 1820, is of obvious interest and undeniable originality since it is partially based on Lordat's own experience of a transient aphasia (brief suppression of language followed by a gradually improving disturbance of expression and comprehension).

In a physiology course which he taught at Montpellier during the 1842–1843 academic year, Lordat began by identifying the ten 'distinct successive acts' which take place from 'thought up to the sounds which serve as its vehicle'; in his opinion, 'each one required a special study'[11, 12]. The metaphysical flavour of the vocabulary used in Lordat's statements renders their meaning somewhat obscure. Nevertheless, it is clear that he explicitly distinguished linguistic thought from the idea of words, and that he was concerned, ahead of his time, with the fact that a linguistic message is processed according to a group of phonological, morphological and syntactic rules 'in accordance with the laws of a language which is common to us'. As for alalia, it particularly disturbs the organization of the 'distinct successive acts' which Lordat labelled 'incorporation of ideas into sounds or recollection of previous sounds retained in memory' and no doubt also disturbs the 'act of the syntactic disposition of sounds'. It was from his own experience that the professor informed his students that 'The thought was completely ready, but the sounds which should have imparted it to the medium were no longer at my disposal . . . The difficulty increased rapidly and, within the space of twenty-four hours, I found myself deprived of the worth of nearly all words. If I retained some, they became nearly useless because I no longer remembered the ways in which they had to be coordinated in order that they would express a thought. Thus I found myself suffering from an incomplete alalia. I was no longer able to receive others' ideas, because all the amnesia which prevented me from speaking left me incapable of understanding the sounds which I heard quickly enough to be able to grasp their meaning. It would have required time to make an attempt at remembering each sound and conversation is too flowing for me to have been able to understand a sufficient number of words . . . Do not think that there was the least change in intellectual ability. I always felt the same internally. The mental isolation I speak about, the sadness, the perplexity, and the resulting slow-witted appearance made many think that there was a weakening of my intellectual faculties. This error, which caused sorrow to some, [brought] satisfaction to others.' Today, we are still far from understanding the neurocybernetic significance of a fact pointed out by Lordat, namely that the comprehension difficulties of aphasics are, in numerous cases, clearly related to the time available to the patient for the analysis of the message (see Chapter 4).

No present or future review of the history of aphasia and aphasiology would be complete without mention of Armand Trousseau (1801–1867) whose influence probably owes more to his prestige than to his hellenic culture or the originality of his work. Trousseau attempted to disparage Broca's work and ideas and succeeded in discrediting the word *aphemia*—which was, according to him, an etymological synonym of the word infamy—and replacing it with the word *aphasia*[13]. In addition to giving it a name, Trousseau peremtorily classified aphasia as an intellectual disturbance, clearly rejecting Lordat's introspective considerations on this matter ('Would that the illustrious professor from Montpellier would allow me to say it to him: is he not deceiving himself?'). At the Hôtel-Dieu in Paris, Trousseau taught that 'the aphasic has lost everything at once, to a more or less considerable degree, the memory for words, the memory for acts by the aid of which words are articulated, and intelligence: but he has not lost all these faculties in a parallel manner, and as much as intelligence may be impaired, it is less so than the memory of phonatory acts, and this less than the memory

* Broca clearly pointed out that the same hemisphere is not necessarily dominant for both handedness and language.

for words'. Thus Trousseau initiated a polemic in which the final word has not yet been said (see Chapters 16 and 19).

The writings of Jules-Gabriel-François Baillarger (1806–1891) are remarkable for their clarity. In one of them, published in 1865 under the title *De l'aphasie au point de vue psychologique*,* he distinguishes between simple aphasia, involving a loss of speech and writing or of speech only, and aphasia with perversion of the faculty of language, that is, one in which the patients 'pronounce words unrelated to their thoughts'[14]. Baillarger's ideas on the various clinical forms of aphasia are summarized as follows: '(a) in patients who can neither express their thoughts through speech nor through writing, the aphasia is explained in the most simple way by an amnesia; (b) for patients who are deprived of speech but who can translate their thoughts through writing, it seems to me that the aphasia cannot be explained, as it has been attempted, either by an amnesia for movements, or by a lesion of the coordinating organ of speech; (c) the analysis of the phenomena led to the recognition that, in certain cases of this type, the involuntary verbal incentive continues to exist but the voluntary verbal incentive is abolished; (d) as for the perversion of the faculty of language characterized by the pronunciation of incoherent words, the dysfunction again lies in the substitution of automatic speech for the voluntary verbal incentive'. According to Baillarger, there are thus two major clinical forms of aphasia, one in which language is lost and another in which it is perverted. Having recognized the possibility of an automatic–voluntary dissociation[15] in the first type and its usual existence in the second type, he considered this dissociation to be fundamental, attesting to a certain physiopathological unity of aphasia.

The English neurologist Henry Charlton Bastian (1837–1915) also believed it possible to identify two types of acquired language disorders[16–21], the first resulting from an *amnesia* and the second from an *aphasia*. He considered that amnesia was a manifestation of a lesion which especially affected the grey matter of the cortical mantle, producing a deterioration of thought as well as of language. 'In amnesia, there is an inability to recall words, i.e., they cannot properly be revived in the auditory perceptive centres, and there is an almost proportional impairment of the thinking power'[21]. On the other hand, in aphasia, strictly defined, it is the white matter of the hemispheres which is chiefly affected, particularly the 'efferents', in such a way that even if linguistic expression is abnormal in some aspect or another, comprehension of language as well as thought remain unaffected. Bastian was particularly concerned with the explanation of aphasia, strictly defined. He hypothesized that four cerebral centres are involved in (normal) linguistic functioning: two are receptive in nature, the *verbal auditory* centre and the *verbal visual* centre; and two are expressive, the *glossokinaesthetic* centre and the *cheirokinaesthetic* centre. The two receptive centres are linked to each other by associative fibres, and each receptive centre is similarly linked with each of the two receptive centres. Bastian considered that reference to this model, which was one of the first associationist models, permitted exact localization of the cerebral lesions causing the different clinical forms of aphasia, and it is said that he did not hesitate to make very precise predictions concerning lesion sites. Bastian's talents may have led him to prefer theoretical reflection to the exhaustive description of clinical symptoms and of cerebral lesions. Whatever the case, he was forced to confront the complexity of the problem when a patient whom he had many times presented as having a very circumscribed cerebral lesion was found at autopsy to have sustained nearly total destruction of the territory of the left middle cerebral artery (see Chapter 9). Although Bastian's work later became the object of some disparagement, he is generally recognized for his accurate description of disturbances which he identified, in 1869, by the names of *word deafness* and *word blindness*[16] (see Chapter 5).

The associationist model of the German neurologist Carl Wernicke (1848–1905) was simpler and closer to anatomoclinical reality than that of Bastian and was to have a far more enduring influence. It was an outstanding moment in the history of aphasia when Wernicke reported, in 1874, the discovery of a causal link between a left hemisphere lesion of the first temporal convolution and one of the clinical forms of aphasia[22, 23]. According to Wernicke, such a lesion causes a loss of memory for the auditory image of words, resulting in a primary

---

* *Aphasia From a Psychological Point of View.*

disturbance of language comprehension. Wernicke named this disorder *sensory aphasia* and contrasted it to *motor aphasia*, or *Broca's aphasia*, resulting from a lesion of the left third frontal convolution. Wernicke surpassed his predecessors in extricating the essential symptom configurations of aphasia: motor aphasics speak little but understand language: sensory aphasics speak a great deal but their language is inappropriate and their comprehension of others' language is impaired; in *total aphasia*, which results from a lesion affecting the entire *language area*, the patient's behaviour resembles that of a motor aphasic in terms of his or her expression and that of a sensory aphasic in terms of comprehension. Wernicke incorporated information from Theodore Meynert's (1833–1892) anatomophysiological teachings on the associative fasciculi of the cerebral hemispheres[24] into a theoretical model which led him to hypothesize a further form of aphasia. In a monograph entitled *Der aphasische Symptomencomplex: eine psychologische Studie auf anatomischer Basis*[22], Wernicke postulated the existence of a type of aphasia resulting from a lesion of the associative fibres connecting the first temporal convolution and the third frontal convolution of the left hemisphere. In this form of aphasia, which he named *Leitungsphasie* (*conduction aphasia*), the patient would understand the language of others but his own would be almost similar in form to that of a sensory aphasic.

It is certain that many contemporary aphasiologists consider Wernicke's original ideas on conduction aphasia to be generally accurate. Although Wernicke himself did not substantially change his original views, they were subsequently modified in two ways. The first concerned the precise anatomical localization of fibres connecting the first temporal convolution with the third frontal convolution. Wernicke first thought these fibres to be subinsular so that his hypothesized form of aphasia would be expected to be seen after a lesion of the left insula. However, on the basis of the anatomical studies of Constantin von Monakov (1853–1930), whose views nevertheless extended well beyond an associationist framework[25] (cf. p. 21), these fibres were later considered to belong to the arcuate component of the superior longitudinal fasciculus. Wernicke consequently modified his hypothesis in conceding that conduction aphasia would eventually be observed in right-handers having a left opercular lesion. The second modification was necessary because Wernicke had apparently not realized all the implications of his own model concerning the clinical symptoms of conduction aphasia. It was left to Ludwig Lichteim (1845–1928) to identify a third essential component of conduction aphasia[26, 27] when, in 1884, he described a case of aphasia in which a severe repetition disturbance was associated with the two characteristics predicted by Wernicke. It appears that Wernicke, who usually had the wisdom not to consider his hypotheses confirmed without autopsy evidence, remained sceptical about the reality of conduction aphasia for a long time. It was not until 1904, when one of his students presented a particularly conclusive anatomoclinical case study, that he allowed himself to be convinced.

Ludwig Lichteim found Wernicke's monograph convincing but considered his hypotheses incomplete and, some years later, extended the associationist model to its most complex form. In addition to motor aphasia and sensory aphasia, which appear after lesions of the corresponding *centres*, Lichteim also identified two *central* forms and three *peripheral* forms of *commisural or conduction aphasia*. Furthermore, he added other centres and supplementary connections to his model in an effort to explain aphasic disturbances of written language[27]. A certain excess of enthusiasm may be reflected by assertions that Lichteim was able to observe clinically, in a pure state, the occurrence of all the forms of aphasia which his model had led him to predict.

Compared with the significance of his other contributions to knowledge of nervous system diseases, both from a clinical and neuropathological point of view, Jean-Martin Charcot's (1825–1893) contribution to aphasiology appears relatively modest[28–30]. Nevertheless, he put forward ideas which might one day be reconsidered in spirit rather than in letter: in hypothesizing that the modalities of language learning are of prime importance in determining the clinical manifestations of aphasia, Charcot provided an idea which could conceivably lead to fruitful research in aphasiology. Like Bastian, Charcot assumed the existence of four cerebral *centres* related to linguistic function. According to *the patient's psychic type*, which is determined by his education, his academic knowledge, his linguistic habits, etc., a lesion of one centre may or may not have repercussions on the functioning of the others. In other words, there is no reason to expect that the clinical expression of a lesion in a particular centre will inevitably be the same in all people. Dejerine gives the following résumé of Charcot's position (in which he does not appear to have a great deal of confidence): 'Should the lesion affect the centre which in a given individual takes the greatest part in language, all of language will be disturbed; should it affect a secondary centre, only the language

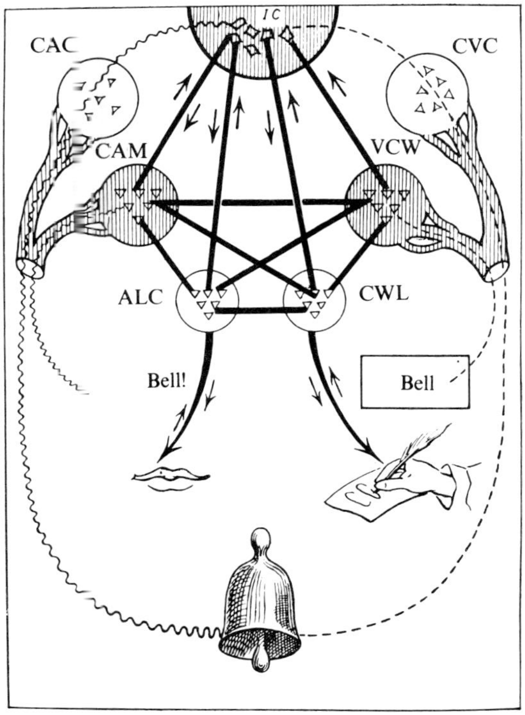

Fig. 1-2 *Charcot's Bell. Schematic illustration of the anatomical foundations of language according to Jean-Martin Charcot. IC = structures underlying ideation (for Charcot this does not involve an anatomically localizable centre nor structures specifically concerned with the governing of linguistic functions); CAC = common auditory centre. CAM = auditory centre for words; ALC = articulatory language centre; CVC = common visual centre; VCW = visual centre for words; CWL = centre for written language.*

made dependent on this centre will be impaired. The same lesion must therefore result in different clinical syndromes, following its occurrence in a motor, a visual, an auditory or a graphic centre' (Fig. 1-2).

The influence of the associationists' hypotheses, particularly those of the German school, is evident in the direction of Joseph-Jules Dejerine's (1849–1917) noteworthy anatomoclinical research. Basing his work on these ideas, Dejerine identified two forms of motor aphasia[31–33]: *cortical motor aphasia*, or *Broca's aphasia*, which is due to a lesion of *Broca's centre* and involves an impairment of *inner language*; and *subcortical motor aphasia*, or *pure motor aphasia*, or else *aphemia*, which is due to a lesion of the projections from *Broca's centre* and is characterized by the complete preservation of *inner language*. Dejerine also distinguished between two types of alexia[34–39], one resulting from lesions of the angular gyrus and accompanying a sensory aphasia and the other appearing as an isolated disturbance following lesions of the fibres associating the visual areas to the region of the angular gyrus (see Chapter 5). In 1914, Dejerine resumed his own contribution to the study of aphasia as follows[40]: 'In a series of clinical and anatomopathological investigations, I studied, for my part, the different forms of aphasia. In 1891, I showed that the hypothesis of a graphic centre was unable to explain the writing disturbances that are seen in aphasics and that these disturbances must be regarded as an impairment of inner language. The same year, I contributed evidence to the study of sensory aphasia and I showed that an isolated lesion of the angular gyrus is manifested by word blindness with total agraphia and paraphasia. In 1892, I showed, again by the anatomoclinical method, that there are two types of word blindness, having different symptoms and localizations—word blindness with agraphia, a type of sensory aphasia, and pure word blindness with preservation of writing—easy to differentiate from each other in the clinic. In 1893, I contributed new material to the study of subcortical motor aphasia, and in 1898 I showed with Sérieux[41] that in certain cases, the localization of pure word deafness was cortical and that the lesion was located in the two temporal lobes.' Although perhaps surprising in tone, which is no doubt more characteristic of the place and the age than of the individual, Dejerine's self-evaluation nevertheless provides evidence of his major contribution to knowledge of aphasia.*

Although a contemporary of the early associationists, John Hughlings Jackson (1835–1911) was nevertheless to develop a view of language and aphasia and, in fact, of the general functioning

* It does not, however, acknowledge the influence of his brilliant American wife, Augusta Klumpke.

of the human nervous system, in which the idea of centres and connections assumed only a very secondary role[42–44]. Jackson conceived of language as a form of mental activity which depends upon the integrity of the brain but is not confined to particular regions. Cerebral lesions which cause aphasia result in two types of phenomena: negative signs and positive signs. The former consist of functional deficiencies, partially linked to the presence of the lesion, which disturb the most developed and most voluntary linguistic processes. The positive signs are attributable to the isolated functioning of released, non-lesioned regions which govern the most primitive and most automatic linguistic processes. Thus aphasia particularly disturbs higher language (the ability to combine words into original propositions) whereas lower language (which is produced in a nearly reflexive manner as, for example, in highly emotional states) remains possible. According to Jackson, there is no reason to believe that the aphasic has lost the memory of one or the other of the forms of word images. What he or she has lost is rather the ability to use words in creating more complex linguistic units which are coherent and adapted to a given situation, that is, propositions: 'It is not enough to say that speech consists of words. It consists of words referring to one another in a particular manner; and, without a proper interrelation of its parts, a verbal utterance would be a mere succession of names embodying no proposition ... Loss of speech is, therefore, the loss of the power to propositionalize. It is not only loss of power to propositionalize aloud (to talk) but to propositionalize either internally or externally.' After having established the distinction between propositional and automatic language, Jackson of course acknowledges that left hemisphere lesions in different locations give rise to different forms of aphasia and that the phenomena of *automatic-voluntary dissociation* may also be manifested in different ways. Alajouanine notes that Jackson 'never neglected to attribute the smallest fact which he used to its author, even when a simple grain of wheat gave birth, because of him, to a rich harvest'[45]. Thus Jackson readily acknowledged that the direction of his work had been influenced by ideas developed some years earlier by Baillarger.

Like the scientific work of his professor Charcot, that of Sigmund Freud (1856–1939) was so extensive that his contribution to the study of aphasia appears comparatively modest. Moreover, the monograph which Freud wrote on aphasia, *Zur Auffasung der Aphasien; eine kritische Studie*[46], had only a very limited distribution and influence at the time of its publication in 1891. However, this work, which was published in English in 1953[47], is remarkable in several respects. In a series of comments which may be seen as a prelude to certain later psychoanalytical writings[48], Freud appears as a forerunner of neurolinguistics in defining different types of paraphasic transformations of language (see Chapter 2) and in discussing their psychophysiological significance. In a period and in a country where it was generally taught that *centres*, or particular zones of the cerebral hemispheres, were the specific and exclusive sites of well defined *functions*, Freud undertook a critical analysis of localizationism, one which was primarily inspired by reflection on the work of Wernicke and Lichteim. He concluded his analysis with the suggestion that the neuroanatomical foundations of speech and language must be conceived as 'a continuous cortical region of the left hemisphere extending from the ends of the acoustical and optical pathways to the beginning of the motor pathways governing the buccophonatory and manual muscles' (see Chapter 8-5 and Fig. 8-32). Thus, according to Freud, the concept of a centre is meaningful only from a pathological point of view but it bears no necessary relation to normal brain functioning. The common distinction between aphasias resulting from lesions of a centre and the conduction aphasias is thus irrelevant: wherever their location, lesions causing aphasia interfere with the interplay of the varied associations which underlie comprehension and the production of articulated language. Consequently it can be maintained that all aphasias are 'conduction aphasias; that is to say, aphasias due to the interruption of associative networks'. Thus Freud found himself in outright disagreement with most of the aphasiologists of his day, with the exception of Hughlings Jackson whose works he knew and admired. The latter fact may be particularly important, given the importance which would be accorded to the idea of *regression* in Freud's later works.

While Hughlings Jackson had formulated his conception of aphasia with relatively little concern for the teachings of the localizationists, and Freud had pointed out their weakness to a limited audience, the most effective denunciation of this orientation[49–56] was to be that of Pierre Marie (1843–1940). Geographical proximity no doubt explains why Marie gave particular attention to the work and opinions of Dejerine (who readily supplied them to him). Marie maintained that aphasia resulted from a lesion in only one region of the left hemisphere, namely *Wernicke's region*, which he considered to be composed of the supramarginal gyrus and the angular gyrus as well as the first two temporal convolutions. Similarly he maintained that there is only one form of aphasia ('aphasia is one'), namely Wernicke's aphasia: 'It is an error to strive, at least by the anatomoclinical method, to divide this area into different centres, of which some would be in charge of hearing words (word deafness), others of reading (alexia), etc., etc. Nothing allows us clinically, to attempt such a division: Wernicke's aphasia is a syndrome which appears with all of its components as soon as there is a lesion, even limited, of Wernicke's zone, in no matter which one of its points'[49]. Clinically the aphasia may vary in severity: 'the severity of the aphasia is proportional to the size of the lesions of Wernicke's zone or the fibres arising from it'[49].

Although Marie considered aphasia a unitary disorder he noted that another clinical entity might be observed, namely *anarthria*, a disorder of speech rather than language. His description of this disorder corresponds closely with that described by Dejerine under the name of subcortical motor aphasia. Marie speaks as follows about the site of lesion: 'For anarthria, there is no problem and everyone agrees to localize its lesion in the region and neighbourhood of the lenticular nucleus, either in the nucleus itself, in the anterior portion and the knee of the internal capsule, or in the external capsule. One fact should be noted, which is that anarthria is not exclusively associated with damage to the left hemisphere and may also be seen when the lesion is located in the right hemisphere involving the zone at the lenticular nucleus. That is an essential difference from aphasia which is exclusively associated with left hemisphere lesions. Another fact to be noted is that when it is due to a lesion of a single hemisphere, anarthria may show a spontaneous tendency towards recovery or, at least, considerable improvement no doubt following the substitution of the healthy hemisphere'[49]. After large left-hemisphere lesions, the clinical association of anarthria and aphasia is, in fact, frequently observed and it is this symptom complex which clinicians have designated since 1865 as *Broca's aphasia*. As for the pathological implications of Marie's last statements, he searched an initial proof—a rather spectacular one!—in the Dupuytren museum. In Broca's original case (Leborgne case) the lesion had destroyed a large part of Wernicke's area: 'Destruction of F3 in its posterior half. Destruction of the rolandic convolutions in their inferior half. Destruction of T1 in most of its extent but especially in the anterior half. The foot of T1 is also affected by softening at the level of the posterior extremity of the fissure of Sylvius which moreover the lesion encircles. The supramarginal gyrus is destroyed to a notable extent'[53].* In Marie's view, the facts were such that he considered it possible to summarize his conclusions by the equation:

'Broca's aphasia = Wernicke's aphasia + anarthria'.

He added that the causal lesions were situated only in Wernicke's area and/or in the lenticular zone. As indicated by the title of an article published in *La Semaine Médicale* of 23 May 1906: *La troisième circonvolution frontale gauche ne joue aucun rôle dans la fonction du langage*[49],† lesions in Broca's zone do not cause, according to Marie, either anarthria or aphasia.

It was not only by his anatomoclinical conception of aphasia but also by his view of the underlying psychopathology that Marie rejected the opinions of most clinicians of his time. He conceived of aphasia not as a primary disturbance of language but rather as an intellectual disorder: 'In aphasics there is something much more important and much more serious than the loss of the sense of words; there is a very marked decrease of the intellectual capacity in general. This idea of aphasics' intellectual impairment must, in my opinion, dominate the doctrine of aphasia; it is because they neglected it that the authors have misinterpreted the essential nature of aphasic disorders, and although that would certainly agree with prevailing ideas, it is impossible for me to accept that, in their definitions of aphasia, most clinicians state that "intelligence is intact". If, for my part, I had to give a definition

* At a Broca's Centennial Conference held in Paris on 19 June 1980, Jean Louis Signoret presented recent photographs of Leborgne's brain. Although they clearly showed a large lesion, it was not as extensive as Pierre Marie had claimed.

† *The Left Third Frontal Convolution Plays No Role in Language Functioning.*

of aphasia, the fact that I would especially aim to highlight would be the decrease in intelligence'[49]. While Marie did not acknowledge the existence of several cerebral areas related to language—at least before the period of his work with Charles Foix (1882–1927) on wartime aphasias (see Chapter 1-2)—he did however specify, in reply to Dejerine's remarks, that intelligence could be considered from different angles and be affected in different ways by neurological pathology: 'Is it therefore necessary to stress this point that the specialized intellectual deficit of the aphasic is in no way comparable to the generalized impairment of certain demented patients or those with advanced general paresis? ... What separates us here, from M. Dejerine, is that my colleague does not seem to want to admit that there can be possible dissociations of intelligence'[49].

To this, Dejerine replied that 'in crossing out with a stroke of a pen all the works accumulated on aphasia since 1825', Marie had turned the problem back to where it had been 'more than eighty years earlier'[37]: to the time when Bouillard was carrying out research able 'to confirm Mr Gall's opinion on the site of the organ of articulated language'[2].

2 FROM PIERRE MARIE TO NORMAN GESCHWIND

After having rejected the associationists' theories of different forms of aphasia as well as the notions of *centres* and *images*, Pierre Marie—the 'iconoclast', according to Henry Head's[57] expression—continued to maintain that there was but one clinical form of aphasia, namely *Wernicke's aphasia*, and that it was an intellectual disorder rather than a specific impairment of language. However, his conception of aphasia as a unitary disorder was to be somewhat modified during the First World War[58], when Marie and his student Charles Foix (1882–1927) had the opportunity to observe young aphasics whose impairments were associated with very circumscribed cerebral lesions caused by gunshot injury. After observation of these cases, Marie conceded that a particular component of the aphasic syndrome may be clearly predominant and that differences in the predominant features of an aphasia constituted the clinical manifestations of different sites of a lesion within *Wernicke's area* (cf. p. 19). However, Marie did not consider the observed variations in symptomatology of sufficient importance to justify the existence of essentially different forms of aphasia. On the other hand, his observations of brain-damaged veterans served to confirm that anarthria, a different entity from aphasia even though the two frequently coexist, may exist in a pure form.

While remaining faithful to his mentor's basic conceptions, Charles Foix nevertheless attempted to demonstrate that three interacting processes were involved in aphasia. Thus he described *verbal amnesia*, which was not a loss of mental word images but rather the forgetting of scholastic knowledge; *agnosia*,* or a disorder involving the recognition—and secondarily the comprehension—of sensory messages, especially those of spoken and written language; and *dysphasia*, consisting of an inability to conceptualize the movements required for speech production.

Aphasia research carried out during the first half of the twentieth century was far more greatly influenced by Marie's original conclusions on aphasia than by his subsequent and, generally speaking, minor modifications of his earlier views. The work of Pierre Marie, like that of Hughlings Jackson and Sigmund Freud, was undoubtedly a primary source of inspiration to researchers who would give full vent to the holistic theory of aphasia.

Arnold Pick (1851–1924), a psychiatrist from the German University of Prague, was among the first clinicians systematically to study language disorders from a purely psychological perspective[59–62]. Like Jackson, Pick based his study of language on its propositional use which he considered to involve two distinct moments: a *psychological moment*, corresponding to the structuring of thought, and a *linguistic moment*, corresponding to the formulation of articulated language. The transition from one to the other occurs through a sequence of stages which is somewhat reminiscent of Lordat's earlier scheme. Pick identified a stage of undifferentiated *intuitive thought*; a *proposition stage* cor-

* A term introduced by Sigmund Freud, who also used it to refer to one of the three clinical types of aphasia which he believed to exist, namely *verbal aphasia*, *asymbolic aphasia* and *agnosic aphasia*.

responding to structured ideas; a stage involving the *formulation of the grammatical scheme of sentences*; and a stage of *explicit verbal formulation*, involving the selection of words. In stressing that language involves psychological processing, Pick concluded that aphasia is not the loss of any particular faculty but rather an interruption, at some point of the process, in the transition from undifferentiated thought to explicit verbal formulation[50]. In addition to emphasizing the psychological dimension of aphasia, Pick also attempted to define *agrammatism*[62] (see Chapter 2), a problem which had attracted the attention of Adolf Kusmaul (1822–1902), beginning in 1873. Pick viewed agrammatism as an inability to formulate sentences in accordance with the syntactic rules governing certain formal aspects of normal language production, and considered it a deficit which specifically impairs the use of words whose function is to indicate the relationships between the lexical elements of a sentence. Even in this early work on agrammatism, Pick outlined a parallel between this type of aphasic disturbance, which interrupts the process described above as the *formulation of the grammatical scheme of sentences*, and certain stages of language acquisition in normal children. Pick considered the anatomoclinical correlation of agrammatism of fundamental interest. Although he did not postulate the existence of a grammatical *centre* in the left temporal lobe of the brain, he contended that agrammatism could result from a lesion in this area.

In his monumental work entitled *Aphasia and Kindred Disorders of Speech*[57], Henry Head (1861–1940) developed an aphasiological theory following the path outlined by Jackson's and Marie's teachings. Head's evaluation of his predecessors and contemporaries sometimes took the form of tirades in which he implied his exclusive affinity with the thinking of Hughlings Jackson, an erroneous conclusion since Freud had previously recognized the soundness and importance of Jackson's ideas. In a critique primarily devoted to the work of Bastian and Wernicke, Head adopted Marie's adamant conclusion concerning the irrelevance of the associationists' theories. Head considered aphasia to be a disorder of *symbolic formulation and expression*. Although it naturally impairs verbal comprehension and formulation, the comprehension and use of non-linguistic symbols are also impaired. In certain respects, Head's position appears similar to that of Pick, as he writes that 'In order to understand the morbid phenomena of speech, they must be considered as a disturbance of progressive acts which cannot reach their proper conclusion'[57]. Head considered all aphasics to be impaired in verbal formulation and that the clinical manifestations could be observed as clearly in receptive as in expressive language, thus supporting the conception of aphasia as a unitary disorder. Using Jackson's distinction between *voluntary and automatic language* as well as a certain number of his own case studies, Head maintained that, depending on the extent of the lesion causing aphasia and the period in its evolution, propositional linguistic utterances would be primarily and most severely affected with only secondary involvement of automatic language. He attempted to specify the nature of the voluntary axis of the dichotomy which Alajouanine was to call the *Baillarger–Jackson principle*. According to Head, the greater the complexity and abstractness of verbal formulation preceding an act, the more the accomplishment of this act is likely to be impaired in aphasia. He identified, from the most automatic to the most voluntary, different constituent aspects of language, namely: articulatory and verbal habits, the relationship between symbols and meanings, the use of grammatical forms and the fitting of symbols to an intention in the expression of thought. Recognition of these various aspects allowed Head, when observing the linguistic behaviours of aphasic patients, to identify four 'types' of aphasia, namely *verbal aphasia*, *nominal aphasia*, *syntactic aphasia* and *semantic aphasia* (see Chapter 10). Although Head maintained that 'aphasia is one', this unity was apparently not characteristic of its clinical manifestations.

The work and teachings of von Monakow[25] were to provide a certain degree of anatomophysiological support to the psychological orientation of the times. Like Jackson, Freud, Marie and Head, von Monakow gave little credence to the localizationists' notion of a *centre*. He considered it particularly inappropriate in regard to language production and comprehension because he believed that, as behaviour becomes increasingly complex, its cerebral substratum is increasingly less circumscribed (see Introduction). Performance of the most complex behaviours, of which language is a prime example, requires the participation of many different neuronal networks, each one entering into play at the appropriate moment. A change in this sequence of events, due, for example, to the presence of a cerebral lesion, results in disturbed performance of the behaviours. Von Monakow considered that anatomoclinical studies were of great interest and that careful observation of a disturbed behaviour could permit more or less accurate prediction of the location of the causal lesion. Nevertheless he thought that the interest of this approach was limited to pathology and that it was logically unjustified to infer the existence of a lesion affecting the specific site, that is, *centre*, of the function which was clinically observed to be disturbed. One of von Monakow's major contributions was his conclusion that a lesion of a given cerebral area results in the temporary reduction or suppression of the activity of neurones which may be more or less remote from the lesioned area but which are directly or indirectly related to it through anatomical or physiological links. Convincing evidence of this phenomenon, which he called *diaschisis*, is provided by comparisons of the clinical manifestations of cerebral lesions during the acute phase with those observed after a certain period of evolution.

Given the primacy of Gestalt theory in the early part of twentieth-century psychology, it was natural that it had a pronounced influence on aphasiological research. Considering language production and comprehension within the general framework of the characteristics of the human organism, the Gestalt psychologists, most notably Ignace Gelb and Kurt Goldstein (1878–1965), derived the implications of this perspective for aphasia theory[63]. Thus aphasia was not conceived as a disorder which specifically affects language, but rather as a manifestation in linguistic behaviour of a global reaction of the organism, a reaction aimed at re-establishing an equilibrium disturbed by the presence of a cerebral lesion. This lesion is, of course, the source of a particular functional disturbance but at the same time, and often to a greater degree than the specific effects of the lesion, the observed clinical picture attests to the reaction of the whole brain to a state of distress. Goldstein's works present the most developed form of the psychological extension of the globalist theory of aphasia. While von Monakow relied on physiological and anatomical arguments to refute the idea that circumscribed cerebral centres were the specific sites of precise symbolic functions, Goldstein contributed psychological arguments formulated on the basis of Gestalt theory[64–66]. According to Goldstein, the essential characteristic of aphasic language is its *concretism*. Abstract propositional activity, or the highest form of language in normal subjects, is no longer possible in aphasia. Thus there is a regression to a more concrete level of behaviour and effective linguistic production is only possible in relation to objects and events in present situations and/or in relation to the patient's emotional state. Aphasia may be clinically expressed in different forms, but no matter how it is manifested there is always a loss of the *categorical attitude* (*abstract attitude*, *conceptual attitude*) (see Insertion 10.2). Goldstein nevertheless considered that the clinical study of aphasia could not be undertaken without making a preliminary distinction between deficits related to the disturbance of sensorimotor processes, that is, the instrumentalities of language, and disorders affecting the psychological function governing the relationship between thought and language. Of these two types of disturbances only the first can be attributed to the presence of a precisely localized cerebral lesion. Having set forth these holistic principles and their limits, Goldstein nevertheless devoted a large part of his aphasiological writings to the description of different clinical forms of aphasia and the psychopathological significance which he attributed to the abnormal behaviours observed in each form of aphasia. Some readers may find it (superficially) paradoxical that the nomenclature of this globalist included more than two dozen nosological headings[65] (see Chapter 10).

Kurt Conrad[67] also referred to Gestalt theory when attempting a nosological analysis of aphasic symptomatology. He began by making a distinction between *Gestalten* (the forms of linguistic segments) and their *Vorgestalten* (preforms: according to Conrad, the *Vorgestalten* are unorganized entities which are imprecise and fluctuating in character; something like a *Gestalten* in gestation) which have attributes and qualities but in an incompletely structured state. The *Gestalten* thus arise from the *Vorgestalten*. From these premises, Conrad maintained that aphasic disturbances of language production are attributable to various abnormalities in the formation of *Gestalten*, whereas aphasic disturbances of language reception and comprehension are related to abnormalities in their auditory perception. An *amnesic aphasia* (see Chapter 4) occurs when the production of words cannot progress, in propositional (voluntary) linguistic usage, beyond the stage of *Vorgestalten*.

The influence of Jackson, Head and Goldstein is evident in the direction of André Ombredane's (1859–1959) aphasiological research and in his attempt to consider, in his method of assessing aphasia, 'the principle of response inconsistency in subjects whose cerebral cortex is lesioned'. Ombredane maintained that 'from a functional point of view, aphasia is a syndrome of the disintegration of the elaboration of verbal propositions whose essence is, according to Jackson's idea, a dissociation between the most voluntary uses of language, which are more or less severely impaired, and its more automatic uses which are not only conserved but even released'[68]. In Ombredane's view, the basic question in aphasia concerns the precise nature, and especially the interaction, of three factors, namely 'the deterioration of symbolic operations, the impairment of sensorimotor components, and the global psychic modification'[68]. He considered this last factor to be an inherent characteristic of aphasia and that the effects of the psychic modification are invariably observed not only in the language behaviours of aphasics, but also in non-linguistic acts. However, the severity of the psychological disturbance may vary widely, depending on the clinical form of aphasia, the moment of evolution and, in certain cases, on whether or not management of the linguistic disturbance had been attempted through a programme of language therapy (see Chapter 17). Ombredane's work and teaching on this matter uphold and detail Marie's earlier conclusions: 'In the aphasic, intellectual activities are normal with regard to those determined by the emotional and practical context and by single and concrete representations. It is when the activities must be initiated from representations removed from the context and particularly from schematic and conventional representations that their cycle of elaboration meets with obstacles which cannot be easily overcome'[68]. Ombredane adds that the abnormal behaviours related to the characteristic modification of adult aphasics' psychological status show certain resemblances to normal childhood behaviours described by the Piagetian school: 'All this can be considered from the angle of a regression of intellectual behaviour to a more primitive, infantile, developmental level'[68].

The work of Marie and then Head inspired a psychological approach to the study of aphasia through the application of test batteries which permitted objective observation of the impairment of higher mental functions in patients with certain cerebral lesions. Further testing methods were developed both by Ombredane and by Weisenberg and McBride[69]. These latter investigators compared the performance of aphasic subjects with that of neurological patients without language disorders, as well as with that of normal subjects on both verbal and non-verbal tasks. They were thus able to demonstrate in a systematic manner that intellectual performance, as indicated by results on non-verbal tests, may be affected in aphasia. This approach to aphasia research, characterized by the application of the methodology of experimental psychology, was later to become more refined and widely adopted through investigations carried out by Joseph Wepman, Ward Halstead, Arthur Benton, Ennio de Renzi and Luigi Vignolo, Klaus Poeck, Ralph Reitan and others (see Chapter 16).

With the exception of the German neurologist Eberhard Bay, Pierre Marie's scientific heirs, particularly those of the Salpêtrière school, were to abandon the *unitary* dimension of his teaching while retaining his empirical outlook, that is, while following his approach which emphasized the primary importance of clinical and anatomoclinical studies as well as the physiopathological hypotheses which could be derived from such studies. Having been Pierre Marie's student for a short period, Théophile Alajouanine (1890–1980) was exceptionally well placed to follow the development of Marie's thinking and his (later) theoretical concessions. Until very recently, Alajouanine was certainly the most representative of the French aphasiologists and among the most productive in the world. The following passage, taken from his book on aphasia[70], clearly illustrates the perspective which guided his research efforts: 'Asked to provide a definition of language, the neurologist can only, in effect, propose a physiological type of definition. I proposed this one: language is the result of complex nervous activity which allows emotional and psychological states to be expressed or perceived through signs (auditory, graphic or gestural), thus materializing psychological or psycho-emotional states externally or internally to the subjects, by the adequate use of sensory or motor functions not initially specialized for this purpose.'

Alajouanine's work on adult aphasia was guided by three basic observations: the onset of aphasia in adults follows the acquisition of language, that is, aphasia is a 'disturbance of completely organized language'; it is through the description and study of aphasic symptoms that we can hope to 'grasp the modalities of psycholinguistic activity'; aphasia results from circumscribed lesions of the brain, lesions whose study should yield 'precise information on the cerebral structures necessary for language functioning'. As indicated by his anatomoclinical studies, Alajouanine's research was first of all that of a neurologist; however, it was also that of a psychopathologist. Even during the time of Pierre Marie, Alajouanine had maintained, despite the inevitable controversy with his professor (was Alajouanine able to convince him?) that aphasia in itself does not affect general intelligence even though it is often disturbed in aphasics. Finally, Alajouanine's research was also, and in advance of his time, that of a neurolinguist. He was undoubtedly the first to recognize the relevance of linguistics to aphasiological research and to request the presence of a linguist in the hospital (cf. below). Working in collaboration with one of us (F.L.), he defined the phonemic and semantic components of jargon aphasia, attributing each one to the impairment of a specific anatomofunctional system.

The list of those who unconditionally supported Pierre Marie's (original) doctrine no doubt ends with the name of Eberhard Bay. The essentials of his teachings can be résumed in the four following statements: (1) 'aphasia is one'; the sensorimotor dichotomy itself must be rejected in a peremptory fashion for 'It contains an even more dangerous implication of the classical theory, namely the tacit assumption that all morbid symptoms in the patients concerned belong to the realm of aphasia'[71]; (2) aphasia is an intellectual disorder: 'All these peculiarities of aphasic behaviour strongly suggest that aphasia is definitely not a disorder of speech but rather a disorder of conceptual thinking and of language in so far as language is our indispensable tool for conceptual thinking'[71]; (c) the variety of clinical symptoms seen in aphasic patients is related to the presence of non-linguistic deficits in conjunction with a *genuine aphasia* (*die genuin Aphasie*); (d) Pierre Marie's anarthria, or *cortical dysarthria* in Bay's terminology, is completely separate from aphasia and is a purely motor disorder affecting the articulatory muscles in the same way that spastic paralysis affects the limbs. From this résumé, the reader will readily understand why René Tissot's excellent monograph on neuropsychopathological problems in aphasia[72] includes mention that, in some respects, Bay's teachings 'are very close to dogmatism'.

The influence of psychology on aphasiological research, which was already evident at the start of the century, was soon to be paired with that of linguistics. The publication in 1939 of research results obtained by the neurologist Théophile Alajouanine, the psychologist André Ombredane and the linguist Marguerite Durand (1904–1962) effectively marked the birth of *neurolinguistics*. Although their monograph entitled *Le syndrome de désintégration phonétique dans l'aphasie*[73]* clearly illustrated the opportunities for the systematic application of the resources of experimental phonetics to the study of acquired disorders of articulation (see Chapter 3), this original work did not immediately receive the widespread attention it deserved. Thus it remained for one of the great masters of contemporary linguistics, namely Roman Jakobson, to launch neurolinguistics effectively towards its present position. As early as 1941, Jakobson had referred to one of Alajouanine's hypotheses in outlining the nature of analogies between certain stages of language development and certain characteristics of aphasic disturbances of language. However, it was only in 1956, in a work entitled *Fundamentals of Language*[74], that Jakobson presented his first linguistic theory of aphasia. This theory views language as a bidimensional activity involving a *paradigmatic axis*, governing the selection of linguistic units, and a *syntagmatic axis*, governing sequential ordering (see Chapters 2 and 10). Aphasia acts to abolish this bidimensional character since only one of the two axes remains functional to the exclusion of the other. Hence there are essentially two forms of aphasia, one consisting of a *similarity disorder* and the other of a *contiguity disorder*. 'When the selective capacity is strongly impaired and the gift for combination at least partly preserved, then contiguity determines the patient's whole verbal behaviour, and we may designate this type of aphasia similarity disorder ... The impairment of the ability to propositionize, or, generally speaking, to combine simpler linguistic entities into more complex units, is actually confined to one type of aphasia, the opposite of [similarity disorder] ... This contexture-deficient aphasia, which we could term

* *The Phonetic Disintegration Syndrome in Aphasia.*

contiguity disorder, diminishes the extent and variety of sentences [but] there is no wordlessness, since the entity preserved in most of such cases is the word'[74].

Following publication of Jakobson's linguistic theory of aphasia, certain investigators, including Olivier Sabouraud in Rennes and Harold Goodglass in Boston, attempted experimental verification of its merits and limits. In concluding his study Sabouraud writes that 'disorders of the two dimensions (paradigmatic and syntagmatic axes) are often associated in the same patient'. On the other hand, 'the separation of the two dimensions is not an artefact of analysis because many patients present a predominant, if not exclusive, disorder of one or the other dimension'[75]. Goodglass' initial investigations involved comparisons of performance on different subtests by aphasics selected according to the presence or absence of agrammatism. In general, his results were also consistent with Jakobson's hypothesis; furthermore, they contributed certain relevant findings, especially concerning the effects of a contiguity disorder on the use of grammatical words belonging to different inventories (see Chapters 2 and 12).

In 1964, the Russian psychologist Alexander Luria (1902–1977) proposed an aphasia classification resulting from consideration of neuroanatomical observations in conjunction with descriptions of the different types of linguistic abnormalities seen in aphasia. In this first genuinely *neurolinguistic* classification[76], Luria recognized a disturbance in the retention of audioverbal traces, a disturbance affecting the acoustic analysis and production of phonemes, a disturbance in the kinaesthetic analysis of articulatory movements, a disturbance in the organization of semantic constituents into a coherent whole, etc. (see Chapter 10). Each of these clinical forms of aphasic behaviour corresponds to a precisely localized circumscribed lesion. Luria's classification illustrates his conception of language as the end result of the activity of complex hierarchically-organized anatomophysiological systems corresponding to different cortical zones, each of which possesses its own functional organization and makes its own specific contributions. When discussing Luria's six types of aphasia in 1964, Jakobson reconsidered his own classification: 'Three types of aphasia—the so-called efferent, dynamic and afferent types—are characterized by *contiguity disorder* with a deterioration of the context; whereas the three other types—in Luria's nomenclature, the sensory, semantic and amnestic—display *similarity disorders* with damage to the code. The same two groups, viewed in terms of verbal behaviour, are opposed to each other as *encoding* and *decoding* disturbances'[77]. Jakobson concluded his analysis by introducing two other linguistic dichotomies (see Insertion 10.5).

More recent neurolinguistic research will be reviewed elsewhere (see Chapter 12), but in the present chapter we shall nevertheless mention research by Davis Howes and Norman Geschwind, who studied the frequency of word usage in normal and aphasic subjects and emphasized the importance of certain quantitative features of the speech flow in the clinical classification of aphasia[78]; studies by René Tissot, Georges Mounin and one of us (F.L.)[79] and by Harold Goodglass, which contributed to the specification of the linguistic characteristics of agrammatism; investigations by Henri Hécaen and Jean Dubois, who contributed a neurolinguistic description of aphasic impairments in spoken and written language using the methods and techniques of modern linguistics (see Chapters 10 and 12); the work of Harry Whitaker and of Yvan Lebrun, for whom the linguistic study of aphasic behaviour constitutes the source of neurolinguistic hypotheses concerning the cerebral mechanisms governing language, etc. We have carried out neurolinguistic research since 1966, research which has been described as follows by Henri Hécaen in his *Introduction à la Neuropsychologie*[80]: 'The research carried out by F. Lhermitte and A. R. Lecours was essentially inspired by structural linguistic models in acknowledging the qualitative differences among the various levels where the elements combine to produce higher level units. Language is defined as a double (or triple) phased system. The description sought of the qualitative and quantitative aspects of aphasic language is based on the hierarchical relationships formed by different linguistic units in normal language. From the descriptions of various levels of analysis, hypotheses are formed concerning actual functioning. From these theoretical bases, these authors call upon computers for the analysis and simulation of aphasic transformations.'

Influenced by psychological theories and methodology, and later by those of linguistics, present-century aphasiology appeared for a time unconcerned with the anatomopathological findings which had constituted the bases of the classical associationist theory. Given the triumph of holistic theory, some no doubt considered the classical views as destined to be permanently neglected. However, they continued to retain the support of some ardent defenders, notably S. Henscher, K. Kleist and J. M. Nielsen, for whom the accumulation of anatomoclinical data and their correlation with particular focal lesions of the brain remained a primary concern in the study of aphasia as well as in that of other acquired neuropsychological disorders. It should also be noted that even though they rejected the notion of *centres* and always spoke of aphasia in the singular, certain of the most fervent and ardent globalists, particularly Head and Goldstein, also contributed to some extent to the maintenance of some important concepts of the localizationists. A significant proportion of their writings was, in fact, devoted to the localization of lesions causing different clinical manifestations of aphasia. More recently, research carried out at the Montreal Neurological Institute re-emphasized the importance to neurolinguistics of anatomophysiological investigations and studies concerning cerebral dominance and cerebral localization (see Chapters 8 and 11). It was through this approach that Wilder Penfield and Lamar Roberts[81] described disturbances of speech, and especially of vocalization, in relation to the functioning of the *supplementary motor area* and that Brenda Milner, after a particularly elegant series of experiments, reopened discussion of the cerebral lateralization of language in left-handed and ambidexterous individuals[82].

Discarded, but not demolished, the localizationists' hypotheses were to return to the limelight with Norman Geschwind's vigorous arrival upon the aphasiological scene. It was no doubt through reflection on the works of Dejerine, Liepmann and Wernicke, and from a wish to provide a clear and simple interpretation of numerous phenomena observed in clinical neuropsychology, that Geschwind was led to rethink the associationist theory, particularly in the form presented by Wernicke, and to conclude that, with few exceptions, it was generally sound. In papers published in *Brain* in 1965, Geschwind presented his conception of a 'disconnection syndrome'[83], a form of neuropsychological disorder of which the aphasias are prime examples. They are, in effect, caused by a lesion of cortical association areas or by a lesion of fibres which connect these areas to each other. Without returning to the original notion of *centres*, Geschwind nevertheless establishes rigorous anatomophysiological parallels between those linguistic components whose impairment is manifested in the various clinical forms of aphasia and the localization of cerebral lesions observed at autopsy (see Chapter 8). As the prototype of a 'disconnection syndrome', Geschwind, with M. Fusillo, presented pure alexia, which they attributed to a left calcarine lesion in association with a lesion of the splenium of the corpus callosum[84] (see Chapter 5). Thus, by 1965, Geschwind thought it time explicitly to challenge the predominant holistic orientation[83]: 'For the past forty years there have been schools of thought which have stressed the importance of thinking of the patient as a whole, of seeing his responses as those of an integrated unitary structure, even in the face of damage ... It should be clear from much of our discussion that this principle, while it may be useful in some cases as a stimulus, may be actively misleading when it is regarded as a philosophical law'. With regard to his case of pure alexia: 'We constantly found that many confusions about the patient in our own minds as well as those of others resulted from failure to do the exact opposite of what the rule to look at the patients as a whole demanded, i.e., from our failure to regard the patient as made of connected parts rather than as an indissoluble whole'. An associationist approach does not necessarily exclude a holistic approach: 'I am not advancing "the atomistic approach" as a basic philosophical postulate to replace "the holistic approach", but am rather suggesting that failure to consider the applicability of either type of analysis will in one situation or another lead to errors. It should be pointed out that the usefulness of sometimes considering animals or humans not as a unit but as a union of loosely joined wholes need not apply only to disease states although probably it will find its greatest use in that situation'. Some of the recent research by Roger Sperry and his collaborators on the language of subjects who have undergone surgical sectioning of the corpus callosum provide support to the hypotheses of Geschwind and his predecessors[85].

Since Geschwind's 1965 publication[83], no one has yet claimed, in a parody of Dejerine's comments on Marie, that 'in crossing out with a stroke of a pen all the works accumulated on aphasia' since the end of the last century, Geschwind had turned the problem back to where it had been 'eighty years earlier'.

REFERENCES

1. Gall, F.J. (1825) *Sur les fonctions du cerveau et sur celles de chacune de ses parties*. Paris: Baillière.
2. Bouillaud, J.B. (1825) Recherches cliniques propres à démontrer que la perte de la parole correspond à la lésion des lobules antérieurs du cerveau et à confirmer l'opinion de M. Gall, sur le siège de l'organe du langage articulé. *Archives générales de Médecine*, **8,** 25.
3. Dax, M. (1865) Lésions de la moitié gauche de l'encéphale coincidant avec l'oubli des signes de la pensée. *Gazette hebdomadaire de Médecine et de Chirurgie*, **33,** 259.
4. Joynt, R.J. & Benton, A.L. (1964) The memoir of Marc Dax on aphasia. *Neurology*, **14,** 851.
5. Broca, P. (1861) Remarques sur le siège de la faculté du langage articulé, suivies d'une observation d'aphémie. *Bulletin de la Société d'Anthropologie*, **6,** 330.
6. Broca, P. (1861) Perte de la parole. Ramollissement chronique et destruction partielle du lobe antérieur gauche du cerveau. *Bulletin de la Société d'Anthropologie*, **2,** 235.
7. Broca, P. (1861) Nouvelle observation d'aphémie produite par une lésion de la troisième circonvolution frontale. *Bulletin de la Société d'Anthropologie*, **6,** 398.
8. Broca, P. (1863) Remarques sur le siège, le diagnostic et la nature de l'aphémie. *Bulletin de la Société d'Anthropologie*, **8,** 379 and 393.
9. Broca, P. (1865) Du siège de la faculté du langage articulé. *Bulletin de la Société d'Anthropologie*, **6,** 337.
10. Gratiolet, L.P. (1854) *Mémoire sur les plis cérébraux de l'homme et des primates*. Paris: Bertrand.
11. Lordat, J. (1843) Analyse de la parole pour servir à la théorie de divers cas d'alalie et de paralalie (de mutisme et d'imperfection de parler) que les neurologistes ont mal connus. *Journal de la Société pratique de Montpellier*, **7,** 333 and 417; **8,** 1.
12. Lordat, J. (1969) Analyse de la parole pour servir à la théorie de divers cas d'alalie et de paralalie (de mutisme et d'imperfection de parler) que les neurologistes ont mal connus. In *La naissance de la neuropsychologie du langage* (Ed.) Hécaen, H. & Dubois, J. p. 130. Paris: Flammarion.
13. Trousseau, A. (1877) De l'aphasie. In *Clinique médicale de l'Hôtel-Dieu de Paris*. Vol. 2, p. 669. Paris: Baillière.
14. Baillarger, J. (1890) De l'aphasie au point de vue psychologique. Aphasie simple. Aphasie avec perversion de la faculté du langage. In *Recherches sur les maladies mentales*. p. 584. Paris: Masson. (First edition in 1865.)
15. Alajouanine, Th. (1960) Baillarger and Jackson: the principle of Baillarger and Jackson in aphasia. *Journal of Neurology, Neurosurgery and Psychiatry*, **23,** 191.
16. Bastian, H.C. (1869) On the various forms of loss of speech in cerebral disease. *British and Foreign Medico-chirurgical Revue*, **43,** 209 and 470.
17. Bastian, H.C. (1887) On different kinds of aphasia, with special reference to their classification and ultimate pathology. *British Medical Journal*, **2,** 931.
18. Bastian, H.C. (1896) *The Brain as an Organ of the Mind*. New York: Appleton.
19. Bastian, H.C. (1897) Some problems in connection with aphasia and other speech defects. *Lancet*, **1,** 933, 1005, 1131 and 1187.
20. Bastian, H.C. (1897) The Lumelian lectures on some problems in connection with aphasia and other speech defects. *Lancet*, **1,** 933.
21. Bastian, H.C. (1898) *Treatise on Aphasia and Other Speech Defects*. London; Lewis.
22. Wernicke, C. (1874) *Der aphasische Symptomenkomplex*. Breslau: Cohn and Weigert.
23. Wernicke, C. (1966) The symptom complex of aphasia. In *Boston Studies in the Philosophy of Science* (Ed.) Cohen, R.S. & Watofsky, M.W. Vol. 4, p. 34. Boston: O. Riedel.
24. Meynert, Th. (1866) *Anatomische Begründung gewisser Arten von Sprachstörungen. Oesterreichische Zeitschrift für Heilkunde*, **10,** and *Zeitschrift des Ges. der Aerzte*. Vienna.
25. Monakow, C. von & Mourgue, R. (1928) *Introduction biologique à l'étude de la neurologie et de la psychopathologie*. Paris: Alcan.
26. Lichtheim, L. (1885) Uber Aphasie. *Deutsche Archiv für klinische Medizin*, **36,** 204.
27. Lichtheim, L. (1885) On aphasia. *Brain*, **7,** 433.
28. Charcot, J.M. (1883) Des différentes formes de l'aphasie. I. De la cécité verbale; II. Aphasie motrice. *Progrès médicale* (Paris), **11,** 441, 469, 487, 521 and 859.
29. Charcot, J.M. (1884) *Differente formi d'afazia; lezioni fatte nella Salpêtrière nel semestre d'estate del l'anno 1883*. Antica casa editrice Dr Francesco Vallardi, Milan.
30. Charcot, J.M. (Ed.) (1887) Un cas de suppression brusque et isolée de la vision mentale des signes et des objets (formes et couleurs). In *Œuvres complètes*. Vol. 3, p. 176. Paris: A. Delahaje and E. Lecrosnier.
31. Dejerine, J. (1901) *Anatomie des centres nerveux*. Paris: Rueff.
32. Dejerine, J. (1906) A propos de la localisation de l'aphasie motrice. *Presse médicale*, **56,** 742.
33. Dejerine, J. (1906) L'aphasie motrice; sa localisation et sa physiologie pathologique. *Presse médicale*, **57,** 453.
34. Dejerine, J. (1891) Sur un cas de cécité verbale avec agraphie, suivi d'autopsie. *Mémoires de la Société de Biologie*, **3,** 197.
35. Dejerine, J. (1892) Des différentes variétés de cécité verbale. *Mémoires de la Société de Biologie*, **4,** 1.
36. Dejerine, J. (1892) Contribution à l'étude anatomo-pathologique et clinique des différentes variétés de cécité verbale. *Mémoires de la Société de Biologie*, **4,** 61.
37. Dejerine, J. (1906) L'aphasie sensorielle; sa localisation et sa physiologie pathologique. *Presse médicale*, **55,** 437.
38. Dejerine, J. & Pelissier, A. (1914) Contribution à l'étude de la cécité verbale pure. *Encéphale*, **7,** 1.
39. Dejerine, J. & Thomas, A. (1904) Un cas de cécité verbale avec agraphie suivi d'autopsie. *Revue neurologique*, **12,** 655.
40. Dejerine, J. (1914) *Séméiologie des affections du système nerveux*. Paris: Masson.

41. Dejerine J. & Sérieux, P. (1898) Un cas de surdité verbale pure terminée par aphasie sensorielle. *Revue de Psychiatrie*, **2,** 7.
42. Jackson, J.H. (1915) Hughlings Jackson on aphasia and kindred affections of speech, together with a complete bibliography of his publications on speech and a reprint of some of the more important papers. *Brain*, **38,** 1.
43. Jackson, J.H. (1874) On the nature of the duality of the brain. *Medical Press and Circular*, **1,** 19, 41 and 63.
44. Jackson, J.H. (1958) *Selected Writings of John Hughlings Jackson*. New York: Basic Books.
45. Alajouanine, Th. (1968) Le principe de Baillarger–Jackson dans l'aphasie. In *L'aphasie et le langage pathologique*. p. 243. Paris: Baillière.
46. Freud, S. (1891) *Zur Auffasung der Aphasien*. Vienna: Deuticke.
47. Freud, S. (1953) *On Aphasia; a Critical Study*. New York: International Universities Press.
48. Freud, S. (1960) Slips of the tongue. In *Psychopathology of Everyday Life*. p. 53. London: The Hogarth Press and the Institute of Psycho-analysis.
49. Marie, P. (1906) Révision de la question de l'aphasie: la troisième circonvolution frontale gauche ne joue aucun rôle spécial dans la fonction du langage. *Semaine médicale* (Paris), **26,** 241.
50. Marie, P. (1926) La troisième circonvolution frontale gauche ne joue aucun rôle spécial dans la fonction du langage. In *Travaux et mémoires*. Vol. 1, p. 3. Paris: Masson.
51. Marie, P. (1906) Révision de la question de l'aphasie: que faut-il penser des aphasies sous-corticales (aphasies pures)? *Semaine médicale* (Paris), **26,** 493.
52. Marie, P. (1926) Quė faut-il penser des aphasies sous-corticales (aphasies pures)? In *Travaux et mémoires*. Vol. 1, p. 31. Paris: Masson.
53. Marie, P. (1906) Révision de la question de l'aphasie: l'aphasie de 1861 à 1866: essai de critique historique sur la genèse de la doctrine de Broca. *Semaine médicale* (Paris), **26,** 565.
54. Marie, P. (1922) Existe-t-il chez l'homme des centres préformés ou es innés du langage? In *Questions neurologiques d'actualité* (Ed.) Wilson, S.A.K. & Chatelin, C. p. 527. Paris: Masson.
55. Marie, P. (1926) Sur la fonction du langage. In *Travaux et mémoires*. Vol. 1, p. 93. Paris: Masson.
56. Marie, P. (1926) Un cas d'anarthrie transitoire par lésion de la zone lenticulaire. In *Travaux et mémoires*. Vol. 1, p. 153. Paris: Masson.
57. Head, H. (1926) *Aphasia and Kindred Disorders of Speech*. London: Cambridge University Press.
58. Marie, P. & Foix, Ch. (1917) Les aphasies de guerre. *Revue neurologique*, **1,** 53.
59. Pick, A. (1892) Beitrage zur Lehre von den Storungen der Sprache. *Archiv für Psychiatrie ünd Nervenkrankheiten*, **23,** 896.
60. Pick, A. (1931) *Aphasia*. Springfield, IL: Thomas.
61. Pick, A. & Thiele, R. (1931) Aphasie. In *Handbuch der normalen und pathologischen Physiologie* (Ed.) Bethe & von Bergmann. p. 1416. Berlin: Springer.
62. Pick, A. (1933) *Die agrammatischen Sprachstörungen*. Berlin: Springer.
63. Goldstein, K. & Gelb, I. (1918) Psychologische Analysen hirnpathologischer Fall auf Grund von Untersuchungen Hirnverletzter. *Zentralblatt für die gesamte Neurologie und Psychiatrie*, **41,** 1.
64. Goldstein, K. (1939) *The Organism*. New York: American Book.
65. Goldstein, K. (1948) *Language and Language Disturbances*. New York: Grune and Stratton.
66. Goldstein, K. (1933) L'analyse de l'aphasie et l'étude de l'essence du langage. *Journal de Psychologie*, **30,** 430.
67. Conrad, K. (1951) Aphasie, Agnosie, Apraxie. *Fortschritte der Neurologie und Psychiatrie*, **19,** 291.
68. Ombredane, A. (1950) *L'aphasie et l'élaboration de la pensée explicite*. Paris: Presses Universitaries de France.
69. Weisenburg, T.H. & McBride., K.E. (1935) *Aphasia*. New York: Commonwealth Fund.
70. Alajouanine, Th. (1968) *L'aphasie et le langage pathologique*. Paris: Baillière.
71. Bay, E. (1964) Principles of classification and their influence on our concepts of aphasia. In *Disorders of Language* (Ed.) de Reuck, A.V.S. & O'Connor, M p. 122. London: Churchill.
72. Tissot, R. (1966) *Neuropsychopathologie de l'aphasie*. Paris: Masson.
73. Alajouanine, Th., Ombredane, A. & Durand, M. (1939) *Le syndrome de désintégration phonétique dans l'aphasie*. Paris: Masson.
74. Jakobson, R. (1956) Two aspects of language and two types of aphasic disturbances. In *Fundamentals of Language* (Ed.) Jakobson, R. & Halle, M. p. 55. The Hague: Mouton.
75. Sabouraud, O., Gagnepain, J. & Sabouraud, A. (1965) Aphasie et linguistique. *Revue pratique* (Paris), **15,** 2335.
76. Luria, A.R. (1964) Factors and forms of aphasia. In *Disorders of Language* (Ed.) de Reuck, A.V.S. & O'Connor, M. p. 143. London: Churchill.
77. Jakobson, R. (1964) Towards a linguistic typology of aphasic impairments. In *Disorders of Language* (Ed.) de Reuck, A.V.S. & O'Connor, M. p. 21. London: Churchill.
78. Howes, D. & Geschwind, N. (1962) Quantitative studies of aphasic language. *Research Publications, Association for Research in Nervous and Mental Diseases*, **42,** 229.
79. Tissot, R., Mounin, G. & Lhermitte, F. (1973) *L'agrammatisme. Etude neuropsycholinguistique*. Brussels: Dessart.
80. Hécaen. H. (1972) *Introduction à la neuropsychologie*. Paris: Larousse.
81. Penfield, W. & Roberts, L. (1959) *Speech and Brain Mechanisms*. Princeton, NJ: Princeton University Press.
82. Milner, B., Branch, C. & Rasmussen, Th. (1966) Evidence for bilateral speech representation in some non-right-handers. *Transactions of the American Neurological Association*, **91,** 306.
83. Geschwind, N. (1965) Disconnexion syndromes in animals and man. *Brain*, **88,** 237 and 585.
84. Geschwind, N. & Fusillo, M. (1966) Color-naming de-

fects in association with alexia. *Archives of Neurology* (Chicago), **15,** 137.
85. Sperry R.W. (1962) Some general aspects of interhemispheric integration. In *Interhemispheric Relations and Cerebral Dominance* (Ed.) Mountcastle, V.B. p. 43. Baltimore, MD: Johns Hopkins.

BIBLIOGRAPHY

Alajouanine, Th. (1952) Pierre Marie et l'aphasie. *Revue neurologique* (Paris), **86,** 753.

Benton, A.L. (1964) Contributions to aphasia before Broca. *Cortex*, **1,** 314.

Benton, A.L. & Joynt, R.J. (1960) Early descriptions of aphasia. *Archives of Neurology and Psychiatry* (Chicago), **3,** 205.

Benton, A.L. & Joynt, R.J. (1963) Three pioneers in the study of aphasia. *Journal of the History of Medicine and Allied Sciences*, **18,** 381.

Benton, A.L. & Joynt, R.J. (1973) Primeras descripciones de la afasia. *Acta Audiologica y Foniatrica Hispanoamericana*, **10,** 1.

Broca, P. (1888) *Mémoires sur le cerveau de l'homme*. Paris: Reinwald.

Broca, P. (1969) Sur les mots aphémie, aphasie et aphrasie. Lettre à M. le professeur Trousseau. In *La naissance de la neuropsychologie du langage* (Ed.) Hécaen, H. & Dubois, J. p. 267. Paris: Flammarion.

Coers, C. (1974) Histoire de l'aphasie et tentatives de classification des troubles du langage. *Le langage et l'homme*, **24,** 7.

Cole, M. (1968) The anatomical basis of aphasia as seen by Pierre Marie. *Cortex*, **4,** 172.

Critchley, M. (1961) Head's contribution to aphasia. *Brain*, **84,** 551.

Critchley, M. (1964) Dax's law. *International Journal of Neurology* **4,** 199.

Critchley, M. (1964) The origins of aphasiology. *Scottish Medical Journal*, **9,** 231.

Ebstein, E. (1923) Gall in defense of his theory. *Medical Life*, **30,** 369.

Eliasberg, W.G. (1950) A contribution to the pre-history of aphasia. *Journal of the History of Medicine and Allied Sciences*, **5,** 96.

Foix, Ch. (1928) Aphasies. In *Nouveau traité de médecine* (Ed.) Roger, G.H., Widal, F. & Teissier, P. J. Fascicule XVIII, p. 135. Paris: Masson.

Geschwind, N. (1964) The paradoxical position of Kurt Goldstein in the history of aphasia. *Cortex*, **1,** 214.

Goldstein, M.N. (1974) Auditory agnosia for speech ('pure word-deafness'). A historical review with current implications. *Brain and Language*, **1,** 195.

Head, H (1920–1921) Aphasia: an historical review. *Proceedings of the Royal Society of Medicine*, **14,** 1.

Head, H (1963) *Aphasia and Kindred Disorders of Speech*. Vol. I, Part I. New York: Hafner.

Hécaen, H. & Dubois, J. (1969) *La naissance de la neuropsychologie du langage*. Paris: Flammarion.

Joynt, R.J. (1961) Centenary of patient 'Tan'; his contributions to the problem of aphasia. *Archives of Internal Medicine*, **108,** 953.

Kann, J. (1950) A translation of Broca's original article on the location of the speech center. *Journal of Speech Disorders*, **15,** 16.

Meunier, L. (1924) *Histoire de la médecine depuis ses origines jusqu'à nos jours*. Paris: Le François.

Meyer, A. (1970) A review of works on aphasia by Pierre Marie and François Moutier. *Psychological Bulletin*, **4,** 180.

Meyer, A. (1974) The frontal lobe syndrome. The aphasias and related conditions—a contribution to the history of cortical localization. *Brain*, **97,** 565.

Mills, C.K. (1907) Discussion on aphasia, especially with reference to the views of Marie. *Journal of Nervous and Mental Diseases*, **34,** 459.

Moffie, D. (1953) History of aphasia theory. *Nederlandse Tijdschrift voor Geneeskunde*, **97,** 2206.

Moutier, F. (1908) *L'aphasie de Broca*. Paris: Steinheil.

Nielsen, J.M. & Friedman, A.P. (1942) The quadrilateral space of Marie. *Bulletin of the Los Angeles Neurological Society*, **7,** 131.

Quercy, P. (1943) Les Fondateurs de la doctrine française de l'aphasie. *Annales médico-psychologiques*, **7,** 161.

Quercy, P. & Bayle, I. (1940) Les fondateurs de la doctrine française de l'aphasie. *Annales médico-psychologiques* **4,** 297.

Quercy, P. & Bayle, I. (1941) Les fondateurs de la doctrine française de l'aphasie. Annales médico-psychologiques, **5,** 209.

Revesz, G. (1950) *Origine et préhistoire du langage*. Paris: Payot.

Riese, W. (1947) The early history of aphasia. *Bulletin of the History of Medicine*, **21,** 322.

Riese, W. (1955) Hughlings Jackson's doctrine of aphasia and its significance today. *Journal of Nervous and Mental Diseases*, **122,** 1.

Riese, W. (1965) The sources of Hughlings Jackson's view on aphasia. *Brain*, **88,** 811.

Riese, W. & Hoff, E.C. (1951) A history of the doctrine of cerebral localization: two methods and main results. *Journal of the History of Medicine and Allied Sciences*, **6,** 457.

Souques, A. (1928) Quelques cas d'anarthrie de Pierre Marie: aperçu historique sur la localisation du langage. *Revue neurologique*, **2,** 319.

Teuber, H.L. (1966) Kurt Goldstein's role in the development of neuropsychology. *Neuropsychologia*, **4,** 299.

Wilkins, R.H. & Brody, I.A. (1970) Wernicke's sensory aphasia. *Archives of Neurology*, **22,** 279.

2. Neurolinguistic Terminology

'When we try it, the holy bronne of bad hole when the news which lets go of an end in the other. It etabords at first a strong in which it was. In each etome respults, behaves and compuls as all of a holy audiforme like nobody. Our goal, know all at first its consistent with includes the sebelsion. First, as everything overflows in the massive debolesse like a symbol marsie to the theoretic treforms. Like in each sibande, Sir, which does not travel nor of a fashion, like the symbol hole prasuve can, itself, be gone somewhere.'

(*Miss Pe.; oral reading of a text; April 1970*)

Although the term *neuropsychology* is listed in the most recent edition of French dictionaries (the study of psychic phenomena in relation to neurophysiology)[1], and in major English dictionaries[2], the word *neurolinguistics* has not yet been included. However, this term is being increasingly employed to refer to that branch of neuropsychology which is specifically concerned with the study of language (Insertion 2.1) in relation to the anatomy and physiology of the human brain. Although ultimately aimed at an understanding of the biological mechanisms underlying normal linguistic functioning, neurolinguistics began with the study of disordered speech and language and much current work still remains within these confines. Neurolinguistics and aphasiology are overlapping domains and, within an introductory text, these terms can be defined to share a common meaning. *Both refer, on the one hand, to the study of all established correlations among the clinical, anatomopathological and physiopathological features of acquired speech and language disorders and, on the other hand, to the study of their purely linguistic characteristics.*

The terminology of neurolinguistics is now quite varied, although a fair number of terms have been precisely defined. Given the roots of the word, it is not surprising that neurolinguistic terminology has been influenced both by the classical vocabulary of neurology and by certain strictly linguistic terms, particularly those of structural linguistics. The organization of the present chapter reflects these two sources of vocabulary. We shall begin by providing summary definitions of certain terms borrowed directly from linguistics. Although generally invented without regard to neurological considerations, these terms are all useful—if not indispensable—when describing pathological language and discussing it with respect to cerebral activity. The definitions which we shall propose for these terms have, in general, been based on those suggested by Martinet in his *Eléments de linguistique générale*[5]. However, several have been reformulated in view of specifically neurolinguistic considerations[6], while others explain the meanings of new terms generated by reflection on the structure of abnormal language. In the second part of the chapter we shall complete this vocabulary listing by reviewing those aphasiological terms drawn from clinical neurology which must be known if subsequent chapters are to be easily understood. In certain cases, definitions which have been generally accepted despite (or because of) their vagueness have been rejected or replaced by others which we considered more adequate, even though they are sometimes more restrictive. Definitions of neuroanatomical terms will be provided in another section (see Chapter 8).

Insertion 2.1

Despite the obvious difficulty, we think it appropriate to attempt a definition of language which specifies its biological aspects. Borrowings from Alajouanine's definition[3] (see Chapter 1-2, pp. 23–24) are evident in the terms included in our proposed definition: that is, '*Language is* (*a*) *the result of complex nervous activity* (*b*) *which permits inter-individual communication* (*c*) *of psychological states* (*d*) *through the actualization* (*e*) *of multimodal signs* (*f*) *which symbolize these states* (*g*) *in accordance with the established conventions of a linguistic community*'[4].

(a) *Complex nervous activity*: refers to the biological foundations of language considered in regard to their anatomical, physiological and biochemical aspects.
(b) *Inter-individual communication*: refers to the dual nature, receptive and expressive, of linguistic communication.
(c) *Psychological states*: the result of a confrontation between present experience (the arrival of information at the brain) and a group of past experiences (i.e., groups of data stored and organized in the brain). Fortunately, the present context does not require us to attempt to identify the respective roles of the emotional and intellectual components of psychological states.
(d) *Actualization*: physical signals, whether auditory or visual, change from external to internal in the case of a message receiver. They change from internal to external in the case of a message sender.
(e) *Multimodal signs*: refers to the availability of two usually receptive modalities, auditory and visual, and of two usually expressive modalities, phonatory and manual. The received auditory signs result from the production of signs through phonatory movements. The received visual signs result from the production of signs through manual movements.
(f) *Symbolize these states*: refers to the fact that linguistic signs or combinations of such signs are ultimately intended to permit both internal and external representation of an individual's psychological states.
(g) *In accordance with established conventions*: these conventions include lexical agreement, represented by the inventory of words learned by a community of individual speakers, and common application of combination rules represented in the phonetic, phonological and morphosyntactical systems of this community.

TERMINOLOGY OF LINGUISTIC ORIGIN

LINGUISTIC UNITS OF SPOKEN LANGUAGE

The number of different types of linguistic units referred to when attempting to describe language segments will vary, to a certain extent, depending on particular viewpoints and interests. The study of language, whether in the context of conversation, narration, or other activities such as naming, repetition, oral reading, etc. (see Chapter 15) produced by individuals with acquired disorders of speech and language, led us to conclude that four principal types of linguistic units are particularly relevant. They are, in order of increasing complexity[7]: features, phonemes, monemes and syntagms.

Features

Although current phonetic terminology is not always explicit on this point, a feature is first of all a matter of functional anatomy, that is, a well-defined state of the buccophonatory apparatus resulting from the action or the non-action of buccophonatory muscles. An expiratory movement may be a feature, as may be the momentary occlusion of the buccal cavity by the action of the tongue on the alveolar ridge (upward and forward projection of the lingual apex); the audible vibration of the vocal folds; or the contraction of the soft palate if sufficient to prevent the passage of air into the nasal cavities. While recognizing that it is theoretically possible to analyse the various muscular activities in

A

/p/	as in /pæt/	(pat)	/f/	as in /fæn/	(fan)	/i/	as in /it/	(eat)
/b/	as in /bæt/	(bat)	/v/	as in /væn/	(van)	/u/	as in /mun/	(moon)
/m/	as in /mæt/	(mat)	/s/	as in /so/	(so)	/e/	as in /ed/	(aid)
/t/	as in /tu/	(two)	/z/	as in /zu/	(zoo)	/o/	as in /o/	(owe)
/d/	as in /du/	(do)	/ʃ/	as in /ʃu/	(shoe)	/ɛ/	as in /ɛb/	(ebb)
/n/	as in /no/	(no)	/ʒ/	as in /vɪʒən/	(vision)	/ɔ/	as in /ɔ/	(awe)
/k/	as in /ki/	(key)	/l/	as in /lɛt/	(let)			
/go/	as in /go/	(go)	/j/	as in /jɛt/	(yet)			
/ŋ/	as in /rɪŋ/	(ring)	/w/	as in /wi/	(we)			

B

/θ/	as in /θɪn/	(thin)	/ʊ/	as in /fʊl/	(full)	/ɪ/	as in /ɪt/	(it)
/ð/	as in /ðɛn/	(then)	/æ/	as in /æd/	(add)	/ɝ/	as in /ɝn/	(earn)
/tʃ/	as in /tʃɪn/	(chin)	/ə/	as in /əbaut/	(about)	/ɚ/	as in /nɛvɚ/	(never)
/dʒ/	as in /dʒæm/	(jam)	/ʌ/	as in /wʌn/	(one)	(aɪ/	as in /aɪl/	(aisle)
/h/	as in /hæt/	(hat)	/ɒ/	as in /wotʃ/	(watch)	/au/	as in /aul/	(owl)
/hw/	as in /hwɛn/	(when)	/ɑ/	as in /fɑr/	(far)	/ɔɪ/	as in /ɔɪl/	(oil)
/r/	as in /rʌn/	(run)						

C

/ʀ/	as in /maʀ/	(*mare*)	/ø/	as in /fø/	(*feu*)	/œ̂/	as in /ʒœ̂/	(*jeun*)
/ɥ/	as in /tɥil/	(*tuile*)	/œ/	as in /pœʀ/	(*peur*)	/ɑ̃/	as in /ʒɑ̃/	(*gens*)
/y/	as in /tyk/	(*touque*)	/a/	as in /pat/	(*patte*)	/ɔ̃/	as in /ʒɔ̃/	(*jonc*)
			/ɛ̂/	as in /ʒɛ̂/	(*geint*)			

Fig. 2-1 *International Phonetic Alphabet (IPA) symbols used in the transcription of: (A) English and French; (B) English but not French; (C) French but not English.*

greater detail, and that such an analysis might eventually prove useful in a more exhaustive study of speech disorders, within the context of the present work we shall consider features to be the most elementary linguistic units.

Phonemes

A phoneme is the audible result of the coordinated realization of a well-defined group of features. It can be produced and recognized by all members of a linguistic community. For instance, in the francophone community all members can effect the quasi-concomitant realization of the five features listed above and, in listening, they will recognize the phoneme /d/ or at least the auditory equivalent of the letter (D). Although incomplete, this definition of a phoneme will be sufficient to permit understanding of subsequent discussions and was, in fact, formulated for this purpose. This definition presupposes the existence of a stock of asemantic units which are relatively stable even in their contextual variations. These units are contrasted with each other and, within a given community at a particular period, their number is almost invariable.

The aspects of language discussed in the pages of this book are illustrated by phonemic transcriptions using characters from the International Phonetic Alphabet (IPA) (Fig. 2-1). Examples* of units or of phonemic sequences will always appear between oblique lines, for instance, /d/ and /dʌzən/, and their written equivalents between parentheses, for instance, (d)

---

* Unnumbered examples within the text are not quotations but were devised by the authors to illustrate particular points. All numbered examples are direct quotations which, in most cases, were originally spoken or written in French. In the present chapter, all such quotations have been translated into English. In subsequent chapters we have not translated examples transcribed in IPA and illustrating only phonetic and/or phonemic transformations (cf. pp. 41–42) or examples illustrating only orthographic deviations (cf. p. 47). All examples illustrating verbal transformations (cf. p. 46) are shown both in the original French and in translation.

and (dozen). In certain examples, hyphens will appear between symbols representing the transcribed units, for instance, /d-ʌ-z-ə-n/ or /dʌzən/.

Monemes*

A moneme is the smallest linguistic sign, that is, the smallest unit which has meaning. Although monemes may occasionally consist of a single phoneme, for example, /æ/ = (a), and /o/ = (owe), in the vast majority of cases monemes are composed of a linear series of several phonemes.

Syntagms

This term designates all groups of monemes which are sequenced according to morphological and/or syntactical rules and which have a unified meaning. Thus it includes linguistic units of varying degrees of complexity, units which will subsequently be classified according to different parameters (cf. p. 38).

LINGUISTIC UNITS OF WRITTEN LANGUAGE

Written language is acquired relatively late both in the development of individuals and of societies. It duplicates spoken language so that the units of written language are symbols of symbols. For these reasons, the linguist may consider it a marginal phenomenon of interest only in terms of its (limited) influence on spoken language. The aphasiologist cannot adopt this point of view because observations of certain patients will lead to the recognition that some disorders may specifically affect written language.

The differences between writing and speech are related on the one hand to the use of different sensorimotor systems to achieve the same communicative ends and, on the other hand, to all the conventions which are more or less specific to each of the two expressive modalities. Despite these differences, written language still shows a hierarchical organization which parallels that just discussed in regard to spoken language.

Features

In spite of innumerable individual variations, a *phoneme* is described in terms of movements of the buccophonatory apparatus or *phonetic features*. In the same way letters, within the context of a homogeneous graphic code (e.g., cursives), can theoretically be analysed in terms of elementary hand movements or *graphic features*. However, an important difference exists because the constituent features of letters, given the nature of writing, are recorded in a linear temporo-spatial array whereas the constituent features of phonemes are co-temporal or very nearly so.

Letters and graphemes

Many languages, including French and English, are written in an alphabetic code whose symbols often do not bear a one-to-one correspondence to the sounds or phonemes which are to be transcribed. Consequently a written word can be analysed in two ways, depending on whether or not it is considered without regard to its spoken equivalent. From one point of view, a written word can be considered as a series of letters assembled according to the rules of conventional spelling so that there are five letter units (W), (R), (I), (T), and (E) in the word (WRITE). In this perspective, a letter results from the articulation of a specific group of graphic features in the same way that a phoneme results from the articulation of a specific group of phonetic features: the complexity of the letter units of written language is equal to the complexity of the phonemic units of spoken language. However, from another point of view, a letter is not the written equivalent of a phoneme. One might wish to analyse the written word with reference to the phonemic pattern of its spoken equivalent. In this case, the word is divided into its constituent *graphemes*, that is, into letters or letter groups, each of which (usually) corresponds to a single phoneme. In the word (WRITE) there are three graphemic units: (WR) = /r/, (I) = /aɪ/, (TE) = /t/. When considered with reference to the phoneme that it represents a grapheme can thus be viewed as a single unit, but when considered with reference to its written production it can nevertheless be viewed as the result of a combination of several literal units. In certain languages the problem of analysing graphemes becomes even more complex because numerous phonemes have several conventional graphemic equivalents (see Insertion 17.4): (WRITE)—(WR) = /r/, (I) = /aɪ/, (TE) = /t/; (RIGHT)—(R) = /r/, (I) = /aɪ/, (GHT) = /t/. In addition, there are also cases in which a single letter corresponds to more than one phoneme,

* The term 'moneme' is synonymous with morpheme in English.

that is, it constitutes more than one grapheme: (X) = /ks/ (as in apex) as well as /gz/ (as in example).

In describing the written language of asphasics, it may be tempting to confine the analysis only to letters on the grounds that letters, like phonemes, result from a combination of specific features and therefore represent the constituent units of written words, that is, the units of the second phase of written language (cf. p. 35). It might also be tempting to restrict the analysis exclusively to graphemes on the grounds that the written code is essentially a secondary representation of the oral code. Nevertheless, in actual practice, it may be necessary to carry out either of these two forms of analysis. In certain cases the majority of spelling errors involve letters when, for example (2.1), *fard* (paint) is written as (*frad*) or (*farad*) or (*fraf*); in other cases the errors clearly involve graphemes, for example (2.2) (*fard*) is written as (*far*) or (*fare*) or (*phard*).*

Monemes and syntagms

The semi-autonomy of writing is primarily related to instrumental factors and is mainly seen during the study of simple units. However, it is much less evident when more complex units are considered, that is, dual-aspect units involving both form and meaning. In these cases, the segmentation of written language samples closely corresponds to the segmentation of spoken language samples. However, in the context of a work on the linguistic productions of aphasics, it should be noted that written language marks, through the absence of a separation, a close connection that exists between certain monemes: for example, in French and other Latin languages, between the verb stem and ending and between the root and affix of a derived word. It should also be noted that, for many people, syntax and vocabulary are markedly richer and more diversified in written than in oral expression.

A FOUR-UNIT-THREE-PHASE MODEL

The idea that language is a multiphased activity was developed by contemporary linguists[5–8] as a result of the following considerations: the number of possible features is restricted by limits on the capacity of the sensorimotor mechanisms which govern their perception and production; the number of phonemes which can result from systematic feature combinations† is finite and relatively restricted; the number of words which can result from systematic phoneme combinations† is theoretically unlimited, but that of words which actually exists is finite, although considerable, and the number of words actually used is even more restricted; the number of sentences which can result from systematic word combinations† is theoretically unlimited, and that of sentences which are actually used is very high. Thus language processing shows a tendency towards maximal *economy*, with each of the less complex linguistic units participating in the structuring of several more complex units. During the use of language by speakers of the different human linguistic communities, this hierarchical organization of verbal gestures, which is no doubt akin to that of many other activities carried out through normal neurophysiological control, does not attain its theoretical limits of saturation (i.e., the possible number of units) at any of the processing phases.

Two points regarding our approach to aphasic language emerge from the definitions which we have provided. First, for reasons primarily related to the priority of oral productions over written productions, we preferred a division into monemes and syntagms[5] rather than into words and sentences. Second, for the descriptive study of aphasic language, we have elected to refer to a model involving four types of linguistic units and three phases‡ (Fig. 2-2). This model is more closely allied to Buyssens'[7] thinking than to Martinet's concept of a double articulation[5].

First phase or *morphosyntactical level*: this phase involves selection of a certain number of monemes and their serial integration, according to conventional, syntactic and morphological (word syntax) systems, into progressively more complex units, that is, syntagms.

*The numbers preceding examples identify them for purposes of all subsequent references. The first figure indicates the chapter and the second indicates the number of the example within the chapter. In cases where examples are subsequently mentioned within the same chapter, the chapter number will be omitted; in all other cases the complete reference number will be given.

† Phonetic, phonological and morphosyntactic systems (cf. this page and p. 35).

‡ Called *articulations* in the original French text.

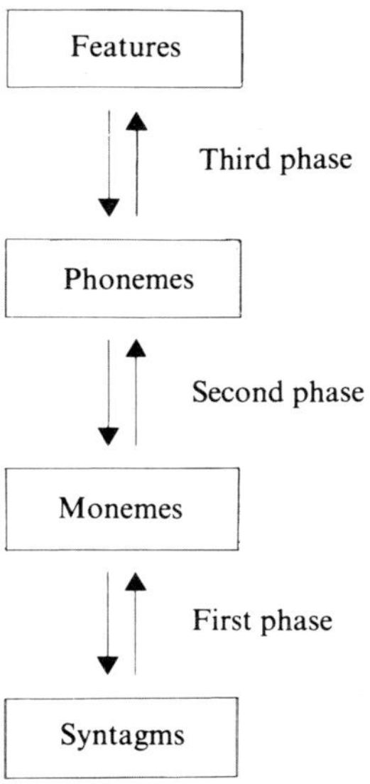

Fig. 2–2 *Postulated linguistic phases: a four-unit, three-phase model. Features combine to form phonemes (third phase), the phonemes form monemes (second phase) and the monemes form syntagms (first phase). Ascending arrows suggest the general direction of decoding and the descending arrows suggest the general direction of encoding.*

Second phase or *phonemic level* or *phonological level*: this phase involves selection of a certain number of phonemes and their serial integration, according to a conventional phonological system, into monemes and other more complex units.

Third phase or *phonetic level*: this phase involves selection of a certain number of features and their integration, following phonetic conventions, in quasi-concomitant constituent groups of more complex units, that is, phonemes.

In our opinion, reference to this model permits an adequate description of spoken-language sequences in terms of simpler units which are *phased* into more and more complex units.

Depending on the point of view adopted, or rather on the nature of the material which is to be described, the second phase of written language is either the selection of a certain number of letters or the selection of a certain number of graphemes, and their integration, following the rules of a conventional orthographic or graphemological system, into monemes and other more complex units. Within the (ideal) context of a homogeneous alphabet, an inventory* of graphic traits could conceivably be described. The third phase of the graphic code would then be defined as the selection of a certain number of features and their spatial integration into a conventional linguistic unit, that is, a letter.

HIGHER- AND LOWER-PHASE UNITS

In liaison with concepts already introduced and with the aim of providing the neurolinguistic lexicon with terms to facilitate functional considerations, the moneme will be designated as the *first phase unit*, the phoneme or the letter† as the *second phase unit* and the feature as the *third phase unit*. A particular unit is itself constituted by other *lower phase units* (LPUs). Similarly, any particular unit may participate in the constitution of *higher phase units* (HPUs). Thus, for phonemes, the LPUs are features and the HPUs are monemes. Similarly for monemes, the LPUs are phonemes and the HPUs are simple syntagms (cf. p. 38, notion of a syntagm-I).

DESCRIPTIVE AND DISTINCTIVE UNITS

All linguistic units can be considered as *descriptive* or as *distinctive*. The term 'descriptive' implies an analysis since a HPU is *described* by listing, in order when appropriate, its constituent LPUs. The term 'distinctive' implies a contrast between two units or groups of units[5]: two HPUs are *distinguished* by those LPUs which they do not share.

Expiratory movement, occlusion, lingual-alveolar articulation, audible vibration of the vocal folds and soft palate contraction are the *descriptive features* of the phoneme /d/. Expiratory movement, occlusion, velar articulation, audible vibration of the vocal folds and soft-palate contraction are the *descriptive features* of the phoneme /g/. When comparing /d/ and /g/, the places of articulation, lingual-alveolar and velar, are *distinctive features* or *pertinent features*, which

* Inventory: a general term designating a homogeneous group of linguistic units. Thus one may speak, for example, of an inventory of phonemes, an inventory of consonants, an inventory of prepositions, etc.

† This does not imply the existence of a correspondence between phonemes and letters but only that the letter is the written unit which results from a specific combination of graphic features.

Third Phase

voiced—oral—stop— [bilabial
voiced—oral—stop— lingual alveolar } *Paradigm:* distinctive features
voiced—oral—stop— velar]

Field: groups of descriptive features constituting phonemes (here /b/, /d/ and /g/).

Second Phase

b—æ [—d
b—æ —g
b—æ —k } *Paradigm:* distinctive phonemes
b—æ —n
b—æ —t]

Field: groups of descriptive phonemes constituting monemes [here (bad), (bag), (back), (ban) and (bat)].

First Phase

ðə—bɪg— [bɔɪ
ðə—bɪg— kʌp } *Paradigm:* distinctive monemes
ðə—bɪg— naɪf]

Field: groups of descriptive monemes constituting syntagms [here (the big boy), (the big cup) and (the big knife)].

Fig. 2–3 *Illustrations of paradigms and fields. No matter how complex the units considered, a paradigm is composed of distinctive LPUs which are defined by reference to an invariable context. A field is composed of HPUs which resemble each other in sharing an invariable context and are contrasted to each other by their LPUs belonging to the paradigm.*

permit the two phonemes to be contrasted. The same distinctive features also permit the contrast, for example, of the phonemes /t/ and /k/.

The phonemes /k/, /æ/ and /t/, in this order, are the *descriptive phonemes* of the English moneme /kæt/ (cat). The units /p/, /æ/, and /t/, in this order, are the *descriptive phonemes* of the moneme /pæt/ (pat). In reversed order, the phonemes are descriptive of the monemes /tæk/ (tack) and /tæp/ (tap). The units /k/ and /p/, in the initial position, are *distinctive phonemes* which permit the contrasting of /kæt/ and /pæt/; and, still in the initial position, of /kæn/ (can) and /pæn/ (pan). In the final position, /k/ and /p/ are the *distinctive phonemes* of /tæk/ and /tæp/.

The units /ðə/, /bɪg/, and /bɔɪ/ are the *descriptive monemes* of the English syntagm /ðəbɪgbɔɪ/ (the big boy). Similarly, /ðə/, /bɪg/ and /kʌp/ are the *descriptive monemes* of the syntagm /ðəbɪgkʌp/ (the big cup). In a comparison between /ðəbɪgbɔɪ/ and /ðəbɪgkʌp/ the units /bɔɪ/ and /kʌp/ are the *distinctive monemes* which permit the two syntagms to be contrasted.

PARADIGMS AND FIELDS

Within this book, the word 'paradigm' will be used only in its strictest linguistic sense, that is, to designate all distinctive units which may appear at a particular position* within a fixed context* provided by other units of the same phase (Fig. 2–3). Each of the distinctive LPUs of the paradigm can appear in a specific position

* Theoretically, the words *position* and *context* are applicable only to the first and second phases where units are integrated in linear series. We have extended their use to the third phase with the aim of emphasizing points common to all phases.

within a fixed context of descriptive LPUs and thereby constitute a HPU. When understood in this sense, the word 'paradigm' leads to a definition of the word 'field'. This term is used to designate all of the HPUs constituted by the association of distinctive LPUs belonging to the paradigm with the fixed context of descriptive LPUs (Fig. 2–3).

Paradigms are defined solely through an appropriate relationship to a particular fixed context: outside this context the units of a paradigm may or may not be similar in form and/or meaning. In contrast, a field is defined within an inventory and without any reference to context. The units of a field, as here defined, are necessarily similar since they share a certain number of common LPUs. As a preliminary to definitions to be introduced in the second part of this chapter and to considerations relevant to aphasia therapy (see Chapter 17), we shall label a group of HPUs which share a number of their LPUs a *field of forms* (*champs de signifiants*). It may be contrasted to a *field of meanings* or *semantic field* (*champs de signifiés*), which refers to a group of units sharing a certain number of common semantic constituents (semes). Thus /ti/, /ki/ and /bi/ would be said to belong to the same field of forms whereas 'bee', 'fly' and 'mosquito' would be said to belong to the same semantic field.

PARADIGMATIC AND SYNTAGMATIC FUNCTIONS

The formation of a HPU requires the *selection*, for each position or moment of the HPU, of a single LPU and the exclusion of all other items within the same inventory as the selected LPU. This process of selection is known as the *paradigmatic function*. The study of aphasic language shows that, in the neurophysiological mechanisms underlying this selection process, the units which should be excluded are not all equivalent. As an illustration of this problem, consider three aphasic errors, all of which, at first glance, can be described as interphonemic substitutions: (2.3) /s-e-k-a-t-œ-ʀ→s-e-n-a-t-œ-ʀ/ (*sécateur→sénateur*: pruning shears→senator), (2.4) /s-e-k-a-t-œ-ʀ→s-e-g-a-t-œ-ʀ/ and (2.5) /s-e-k-a-t-œ-ʀ→s-e-s-a-t-œ-ʀ/. In the transformation* in (3), the substituting phoneme bears little resemblance to the substituted phoneme (they share few of their consecutive LPUs) but they belong to the same paradigm. Thus one word is transformed to another word belonging to the same field of forms (cf. p. 42, notion of a formal verbal paraphasia). In (4), the substituting phoneme does not belong to the same paradigm as the substituted phoneme but the two phonemes are highly similar. (They share all but one of their LPUs.) Thus one phoneme is transformed into another phoneme within the same field. In (5) the substituting and substituted phonemes do not belong to the same paradigm nor to the same field and the substitution involves the duplication of a unit in the immediate phonemic context. In terms of cerebral physiology, it must therefore be recognized that, during normal production, the paradigmatic function controls not only the selection of a particular unit of a paradigm but also the exclusion of certain units which may or may not belong to this paradigm.

The formation of a HPU also presupposes the *integration* in a linear series (first and second phases) or in a nearly contemporal *cluster* (third phase) of all the LPUs which constitute the HPU. This process of integration is known as the *syntagmatic function*. The integration is carried out in accordance with (acquired) rules involving the morphosyntactical system during the first phase, the phonological system during the second phase and the phonetic system during the third phase.†

CONSOLIDATED UNITS

Use of the word *syntheme* will here be restricted to the designation of a particular type of syntagm, namely one whose constituent monemes form a derived word (affront, frontier, frontage) or a compound word (sunshine, football). Martinet[5] considers the units composing synthemes to be consolidated monemes and postulates that a syntheme acts as a single unit in the speech chain. In other words, synthemes, like monemes, correspond to a single choice by the speaker.

When extended beyond the first phase and

* Transformation or aphasic transformation: a general term utilized to designate segments of different complexity in aphasic language. In the transcription of aphasic language, an arrow (→) appears between the conventional item and the transformed item.

† Additional material on this topic is included in the section dealing with Jakobson's theories of aphasia (Chapter 10).

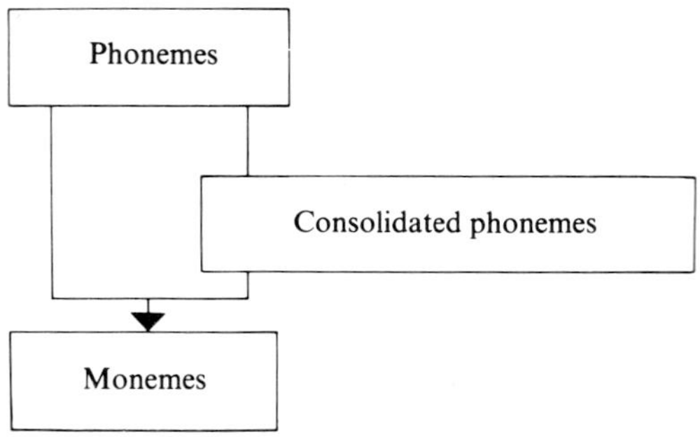

Fig. 2–4 *Consolidated phonemes. A group of two or more phonemes may temporarily act as a single phonemic unit, thereby forming a contingent intermediate phase between phonemes and monemes* [*see examples* (*2.6*) *to* (*2.8*)].

enlarged and modified for the second phase, the concept of consolidated units appears useful in the analysis of all types of aphasic transformations. In certain second-phase aphasic transformations, two or more phonemes, which we shall call *consolidated phonemes*, seem to act temporarily as a single phonemic unit and thereby form a contingent intermediate phase between phonemes and their HPUs (Fig. 2–4). In the transformations

(2.6) (sad) *triste* /t.ʀ-i-s-t →t.ʀ-i-s-t.ʀ/

(2.7) (shrewish) *acariâtre* /a-k-a.ʀ-j-ɑ-t-ʀ→ɑ.ʀ-k-a.ʀ-j-ɑ-t-ʀ/

(2.8) (weakness) *faiblesse* /f-ɛ-b-l.ɛ-s →f-l.ɛ-b-l.ɛ-s/

the phonemic groups /t.ʀ/, /a.ʀ/ and /l.ɛ/* are considered to be consolidated phonemes within the specific context of these transformations. Consolidated phonemes often correspond to a syllable, but this is not necessarily so, and it is doubtlessly more accurate simply to state that they are usually of the form CV, VC, CS, SC, SV, VS, or CSV (C = consonant, V = vowel, S = semi-vowel).

The concept of consolidated letters is also useful when describing orthographic errors commonly seen in written productions of aphasics. Thus in the following examples

(2.9) (traffic) (C-I-R.C-U-L-A-T-I-O-N → C-I-R.C-U-L-R.C-A-T-I-O-N)

(2.10) (rubber) (C-A-O-U-T-C.H-O-U-C → C-A-O-U-T-C-O-U-C.H)

(2.11) (abundance) (A-B-O.N-D-A.N-C-E → A-B-O.N-D-O.N-C-A.N)

the letter-groups (R.C.), (C.H.), (O.N), and (A.N)* are considered to be consolidated letters within the specific context of these transformations. The groups of letters which may correspond to a grapheme frequently appear to be consolidated [see (10) and (11)], and when describing errors of the type illustrated in (2), it is usually assumed as a matter of course that all graphemes composed of more than a single letter are, in fact, composed of consolidated letters.

MAJOR TYPES OF SYNTAGMS

Certain authors, particularly Companys[9], use the terms *phonic word*, *group* and *sentence* to distinguish three types of syntagms of increasing complexity. Thus the sentence 'The new mayor of Montreal did not react to statements in the local papers' is first divided into groups: 'The new mayor of Montreal—did not react—to statements in the local papers.' Although this division appears to correspond to a psycholinguistic reality, we prefer to replace the terms *phonic word*, *group* and *sentence*, respectively, by *syntagm-I*, *syntagm-II* and *syntagm-III* (Fig. 2–5). These terms are more neutral, more obviously related to each other and seem to us more suited to discussion of aphasia in terms of cerebral functioning. As seen in the above example, a syntagm-III is centred on a single predicate, and a syntagm-II is composed of one to *N* syntagms-I. This last type will be further discussed later.

As we have previously mentioned, a syntheme corresponds to a single choice by the speaker. Synthemes occupy a position between monemes and syntagms-I which is analogous to the place of what we have called consolidated phonemes between phonemes and monemes (see Fig. 2–4). Other monemic associations, which are neither derived words nor compound words, no doubt also represent single choices in the majority of speakers. Thus we shall use the term 'consolidated moneme' to designate synthemes and other simple monemic associations ('and then', 'once in a while', 'just a minute') of a similar type (Fig.

* In the transcription of these transformations, periods, rather than hyphens, will appear between the units considered to be consolidated.

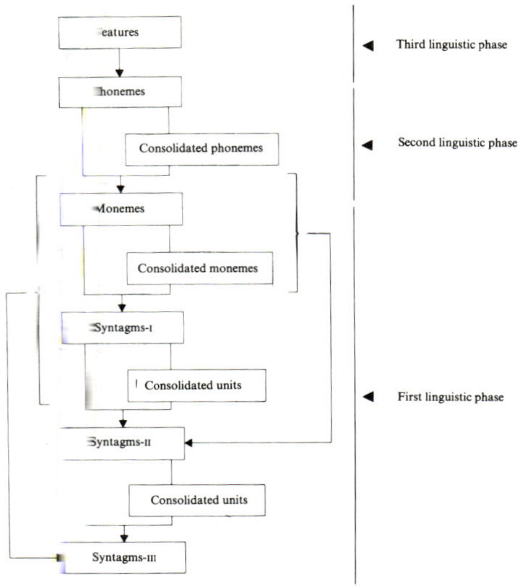

Fig. 2-5 *Complete schema of postulated linguistic phases. Linguistic production is considered as a hierarchical and economic activity involving repeated combinations in accordance with phonetic, phonological, morphological and syntactical conventions. Less complex units from relatively restricted inventories permit the formation of progressively larger inventories of more complex units. Consolidated units may enter into play at any level of the second and first phases. The latter involves several levels as simple syntagms are combined according to morphosyntactical rules into progressively more complex syntagms. Brackets and lateral arrows indicate that all different levels of complexity may not necessarily be involved in each phase.*

2-5). Similarly, other consolidated units can be introduced into this general, multiphased schema of language between syntagms-I and syntagms-II and between syntagms-II and syntagms-III (Fig. 2-5). The concept of consolidated units is even more useful in the study of aphasics than in the case of normal speakers because it permits separate consideration* of ready-made expressions or fixed syntagms ('if you please', 'how shall I put it', 'let's go', 'take it easy') which may constitute most of the language produced by certain patients. Unfortunately, it is difficult to conceive of a systematic procedure to identify which productions are, in fact, ready-made expressions (or fixed syntagms). In our opinion, the only criterion possible (although very subjective) is the high frequency of a particular segment in an adequate sample of the language produced by a particular aphasic individual.

MONEME INVENTORIES

The term 'inventory' refers to a group of homogeneous linguistic units so that we may speak of an inventory of phonemes, or of monemes, or of prepositions, etc. In the case of monemes, an inventory is said to be *open* or *unlimited* when, as a consequence of new realities, newly discovered realities or new perspectives on reality, new units may be added to the inventory without changing the morphosyntactic system of the language. Such is the case for verb stems, attributive adjectives, etc. In contrast, an inventory is said to be *closed* or *limited* when new units cannot be added because this would result in a change in the morphosyntactic system of the language, as would be the case, for example, for personal pronouns, verb endings, etc. Although their number tends to remain stable, affixes are generally considered to belong to an inventory which is *potentially open*. This view appears consistent with observation since, in certain language disorders, the behaviour of affixes resembles that of monemes belonging to an open inventory rather than that of monemes belonging to a closed inventory.

CLASSIFICATION OF MONEMES ACCORDING TO INVENTORIES

The classification presented below is similar to that suggested by Martinet[5]. It provides details on several linguistic terms which will be used frequently throughout this book.

(a) An item belonging to an open inventory is called a *lexical moneme* or a *lexeme*. The equivalent terms, *lexical morpheme* and *semanteme*, will not be used here.

(b) An item belonging to a potentially open inventory is called an *affix*. In French, for example, this term is used to designate all affixes and suffixes except those marking gender or number; verb endings are also excluded.

* Failure to consider consolidated units separately when studying aphasic language will automatically result in inaccurate estimates of the actual frequency of determinative adjectives, adverbs of time, use of the conditional, imperative, interrogative and other structures and, especially, of the easy propositional use of these various types of linguistic segments.

(c) An item belonging to a closed inventory is called a *grammatical moneme*. Other precise terms are used to refer to certain subinventories of grammatical monemes. For example, in French (and this classification can be largely applied to English as well):
- —the term *functional* or *functional moneme* refers to subordinates (subordinate conjunctions, prepositions, relative pronouns and adjectives);
- —the term *morphological marker* refers to verb inflections and suffixes which mark gender and number;
- —the term *determiner* is applied to articles and other determiners (possessive adjectives, demonstratives, etc.);
- —closed subinventories other than those included in the above classes are referred to using the terminology of conventional grammar: for example, coordinating conjunctions, personal pronouns, auxiliaries, etc.

Certain consolidated monemes can be included in the above moneme inventories. Thus conjunctive, subordinate and prepositional locutions are included in the inventory of functional morphemes. Similarly, ordinal numerical adjectives can be classified with the determiners.

SUBTYPES OF SYNTAGMS-I

When studying the conversational language of aphasics or describing the linguistic materials included in remedial exercises for specific aspects of language, it is often useful to carry out an initial analysis in terms of syntagms-I. To describe these units we shall use the following four labels as needed: *nominal syntagm* (NS), *prepositional syntagm* (PS), *verbal syntagm* (VS) and *accessory syntagm* (AS). When a NS is centred on a substantive noun it is called a *nominal nominal syntagm* (nNS); the substantive may or may not be accompanied by one or several determiners (cf. above). A NS may also be formed with a pronoun (pNS), an infinitive (iNS), etc. A PS is composed of a preposition or prepositional phrase followed by a NS (PS = P + NS). In the analysis of syntagms-I, the VS designates the predicate without possible accompanying completions (either essential or non-essential). Finally, the AS is composed of an adverb, an adverbial phrase or an interjection which may be either a word or phrase. The division of a syntagm-III into its constituent syntagms-I is illustrated by the following example of aphasic language: (2.12) '*Il est exactement dans l'* /ɔʀsjal/ *pour certains étudiants jeunes de la* /fɔʀsjal/ *jeune de Paris*.' ('He (pNS) is (VS) exactly (AS) in the /ɔʀsjal/ (PS) for certain young students (PS) of the young /fɔʀsjal/ (PS) in Paris (PS)').*

It follows, from this manner of division based on syntactical aims, that single monemes may function as syntagms, as in the case of the pNS included in the previous example (Fig. 2-5, lateral arrows).

FUNCTIONAL CLASSIFICATION OF MONEMES AND SYNTAGMS

When studying aphasic language and preparing remedial exercises, it is also useful to distinguish among units involved in the organization of the first phase of language according to the varied syntactic function of these units. Depending on its situation in an utterance, a moneme or syntagm may be qualified by a label which specifies its role.

(a) It is said to be *autonomous* when its function does not depend on its position in the utterance. When understood in this sense, the description *autonomous* applies to all ASs and many PSs (cf. above).
(b) It is said to be *functional* when it indicates the function of another moneme or syntagm (or group of monemes or of syntagms).
(c) It is said to be *dependent* in all other cases. According to its syntactical function, the dependent unit may be *governed*, when it has a primary function such as that of a substantive subject or object, or *modifying*, when it accompanies a governed unit. In the latter case, it may be a *lexical modifier*, such as a qualifying adjective, or a *grammatical modifier*, such as a possessive or demonstrative adjective.

---

* It should be noted how neologistic segments (cf. p. 2-44) invented by aphasics can be likened to units of a specific inventory—in this case the inventory of substantives—on the basis of their location in the utterance.

TERMINOLOGY OF NEUROLOGICAL ORIGIN

Under this heading we shall review a certain number of terms belonging to the classical vocabulary of aphasiology. We shall particularly emphasize certain ones which, like *paraphasia* and *paragraphia*, refer to segments of abnormal language in the same way as names of linguistic units (cf. pp. 31–33) designate segments of normal language. We shall also review some terms such as *jargonaphasia*, *dyssyntaxia* and *agrammatism*, which refer to a general quality of pathological language behaviour.

The term *transformation*,* or *aphasic transformation*,* will serve to refer, in a general manner, to any erroneous linguistic unit or series of units produced by an aphasic individual. This term may be qualified to indicate the type of error: *phonetic transformation*, *phonemic transformation*, *verbal transformation*, etc. By our selection of these terms, the reader will quickly recognize our attempts to refer to the multiphased model of language presented in the preceding part of this chapter. It schematically suggests the notion that the articulatory difficulties seen in many aphasics attest to a disorganization of the third linguistic phase, that is, of the phonetic level; that the various errors observed in the selection and serial integration of phonemes constituting words attest to a disorganization of the second linguistic phase, that is, of the phonemic level; and that the various errors observed in the selection and serial integration of monemes and words constituting sentences attest to a disorganization affecting the first linguistic level (morphology and syntax), that is, of the semantic level. Although simple, and even simplistic in certain regards, this conception is partially validated by the occurrence of exceptional cases: either at onset or at a given moment during evolution, certain aphasic syndromes are observed to affect one or another of these phases[10, 11] in a quasi-exclusive and specific manner (see Chapters 3 to 5).

PHONETIC TRANSFORMATIONS—PHASE III TRANSFORMATIONS

The articulatory disturbance seen in right-handers following certain left-hemisphere lesions of the brain belongs, according to some, to the symptomatology† of aphasia. Others maintain that it should be distinguished from aphasia, as strictly defined, while emphasizing that it frequently accompanies aphasia. The interest of this argument is limited since the majority of those holding either of these views recognize that this particular type of articulatory disturbance can exist, even though it is a rare occurrence, in an isolated or nearly-isolated state (see Chapters 3, 5 and 10).

Calling the disturbance the *phonetic disintegration syndrome*, Alajouanine, Ombredane and Durand[12] described the phonetic abnormalities which characterize the speech of approximately one-half of aphasic individuals (see Chapter 1-2, p. 24). These investigators concluded that the phonetic disintegration syndrome represents the effects of a triple dysfunction, that is, paretic, dystonic and dyspraxic, and also stressed that any of these three components may dominate the clinical picture. The contemporary neurological glossary does not contain terms designating the group of abnormal linguistic segments resulting from the articulatory disturbances of aphasics. Thus we shall group them here under the name 'phonetic transformations'. They include more or less partial or complete (and inappropriate) devoicing, nasalization, occlusion, etc., abnormalities involving pseudo-diphthongization or pseudo-polythongization, the more or less complete omission of consonant phonemes in consonant clusters, etc. The common characteristic of phonetic transformations is that they can be adequately described by reference to the unit of the third linguistic phase, namely in terms of abnormalities in the realization of certain constituent features of the phonemes produced (see Chapter 3).

PHONEMIC PARAPHASIAS—PHASE II TRANSFORMATIONS

A phonemic series which constitutes a word, or a sentence fragment more complex than a word, may be abnormally spoken despite the absence of any articulatory difficulty. In this case the

* The synonyms *deviation* or aphasic *deviation* are sometimes used instead.

† The term sémiologie was used in the original French. In English semiology is listed as a synonym for symptomatology (*Dorland's Illustrated Medical Dictionary*, 25th edn, W. B. Saunders, Philadelphia, 1974).

210	**(2.13)** (complex)	*complex*	/k-ɔ̃-p-l-ɛ-k-s	→k-ɔ̃-p-l-ɛ-s/
212	**(2.14)** (sauntering)	*déambulant*	/d-e-ɑ̃-b-y-l-ɑ̃	→d-e-b-ɑ̃-b-y-l-ɑ̃/
214	**(2.15)** (inactive)	*inactif*	/i-n-a-k-t-i-f	→i-n-a-k-t-i-k/
216	**(2.16)** (psychology)	*psychologie*	/p-s-i-k-ɔ-l-ɔ-ʒ-i	→p-s-i-k-l-ɔ-s-ɔ-ʒ-i/
218	**(2.17)** (poultry farmer)	*aviculture*	/a-v-i-k-y-l-t-œ-ʀ	→v-a-t-i-k-y-l-t-œ-ʀ/
220	**(2.18)** (grocery store)	*épicerie*	/e-p-i-s-ʀ-i	→e-s-i-p-ʀ-i/
	(2.19) (notaries public)	*notariat*	/n-ɔ-t-a-ʀ-j-a	→n-a-ʀ-j-a-t-a/
223	**(2.20)** (unskilful)	*malhabile*	/m-a-l-a-b-i-l	→a-m-a-l-a-b-i-m/.

abnormalities are seen in the omission and/or addition, displacement or substitution of phonemic units. This type of aphasic transformation is known by the name of *phonemic paraphasia*[13, 14]. In certain types of aphasia, it can be observed during repetition or reading tasks, during conversation, etc. (see Chapters 4 and 15). The above phonemic paraphasias were produced by one of our subjects during a single-word repetition subtest.

When phonemic paraphasias occur in the absence of an associated articulatory disturbance, each phoneme spoken, whether or not it was correctly selected or occupies its conventional position in the series, is completely normal in terms of its phonetic realization (third linguistic phase).

The examples (13) to (20) illustrate two facts of sufficient importance to be explicitly mentioned in the definition of paraphasias. They show how the phonological rules of the aphasic speaker's linguistic community are respected in phonemic paraphasias and also show how the meaning of the transformed words is not directly affected by phonemic paraphasias. They occur during the (asemantic) second linguistic phase and meaning conveyed to the listener is not lost unless the complexity and the number of transformations centred on a particular segment exceed a certain threshold. For example, the listener can easily recognize the sense of a patient's statement that he was (2.21) 'helped by a/aplazɑ̃-dœ-plɔtis/ [instead of /aʒɑ̃-dœ-pɔlis/(policeman)]. Beyond this threshold, phonemic paraphasias can be recognized as such only when they are produced during repetition or oral reading. In other contexts they cannot be identified definitely as phonemic paraphasias and are therefore designated by the less precise name of neologism (cf: p. 44). When, in an aphasic's conversation, the word (2.22) *inhabituel* (unusual) /inabityɛl/ is transformed to /ibatiyɛl/, there is not a loss of meaning for the listener and the transformation can confidently be identified as a phonemic paraphasia. However, if the segment produced is (2.23) /ɛanitabjebitil/, there is, unless the contextual cues are particularly rich, a complete loss of meaning and the observed transformation cannot confidently be stated to be a phonemic paraphasia.

FORMAL VERBAL PARAPHASIAS—PHASE II TRANSFORMATIONS

Verbal paraphasias are usually defined as the erroneous use of a word belonging to an inventory of the language in place of another word which also belongs to one of the language inventories. This definition will be reformulated below because it appears inadequate or at least incomplete. Nevertheless, it is sufficient in terms of the information which we shall provide concerning formal verbal paraphasias, aphasic transformations in which the substituting word and the substituted word are similar in terms of their form (and not in terms of their meaning): that is, they belong to the same field of forms (cf. p. 37). When present in the clinical picture of an aphasia, the production of formal verbal paraphasias is typically associated with the production of phonemic paraphasias. This association, which is particularly obvious during conversation,* is illustrated in the following excerpt from a conversation with a patient. The formal verbal

* In the quotations excerpted from conversation, all phonemic transformations are transcribed in IPA. Phonemic paraphasias appear between oblique lines and formal verbal paraphasias appear between vertical lines. The vertical arrows (↓) indicate the end of a faulty segment which is usually incomplete and is often followed by an attempt at correction.

paraphasias are seen in the substitution of /gã/ (glove) and /blã/ (white) for /bã/ (benches).

(2.24) '*On recevait ca dans des* /sk/↓ *quelquefois des* /saʃk/↓ ... *sacs en jute qui* /saRt/↓ *qui sentaient le* /tRava/↓ *le* /kavjaR/↓ *le* /kadRav/↓ *le cadavre ... On entrait dans cette* /gRas | *dans cette grande salle* /pɛRpãdidylɛRmã/. *Puis il y avait des* | gã | *des* | blã | ↓—*Non! Attendez! Je le sais.—des bancs. Et puis, devant, il y avait une* /ɛspa/↓ *une* /ɛstaR/↓ *une* /ɛstaR/↓ /tRak/↓ *une estrade.*'

'We received that in some /sk/↓ sometimes some /saʃk/ ↓ ... jute sacks which /saRt/↓ which smelled of the /tRava/↓ the /kavjaR/↓ the /kadRav/↓ the cadaver ... We went in this /gRas/↓ in this large room /pɛRpãdidylɛRmã/. Then there were some | gã | some | blã—No! Wait! I know it.—some benches. And then, in front, there was an /ɛspa/↓ an /ɛstaR/↓ an /ɛstaR/↓ /tRak/↓ a platform.'

In our opinion, verbal paraphasias of a formal type constitute a particular category of phonemic paraphasias (see Insertion 8.4). Thus they can be considered, like phonemic paraphasias, as evidence of a disturbance of the second linguistic phase: that is, the physiopathology of formal verbal paraphasias is not essentially different from that of phonemic paraphasias (see Insertion 8.4).

PHONEMIC TRANSFORMATIONS—PHASE II TRANSFORMATIONS

From the above considerations, it follows that phonemic paraphasias and formal verbal paraphasias can be grouped under the name of phonemic transformations. There is a particular clinical form of aphasia in which the observed disturbance of oral expression is essentially confined to the production of phonemic transformations (see Chapter 4, conduction aphasia, and Chapter 15).

MONEMIC PARAPHASIAS—PHASE I TRANSFORMATIONS

The term 'monemic paraphasias' designates a particular type of neologism (cf. below) in which the monemic paraphasia is used in the place of a word and is composed of an association, which does not appear in dictionaries of the language, between monemes belonging to any of the language inventories. Although this type of aphasic transformation is relatively rare, there are some cases in which the clinical picture is dominated by the production of monemic paraphasias, especially during conversation language[15]. This is clearly seen in the following excerpts from a conversation with one of our aphasic patients. All of the monemic paraphasias in this particular series are composed of a lexical moneme and a suffix:*

(2.25) '*entre les artilleurs* /ital-ar/.'
'Between the /ital-ar/ artillerymen.' (Lexical component as in *ITALIEN* /italjɛ̃/.)

(2.26) '*on me donne des* /fɔrm-œtyR/, *d'accord.*'
'They give me some /fɔrm-œtyR/, agreed.' (Lexical component as in *FORMATION* /fɔRmasjɔ̃/.)

(2.27) '*Je n'ai pas moi-même de ca, personnellement, en grand* /dɔRs-aʒ/.'
'I don't myself have any of that, personally, in large /dɔRs-aʒ/.' (Lexical component as in *DORSAL* /dɔRsal/.)

(2.28) '*Nous voulons avoir deux fois moins de* /fɔRs-aj/.'
'We want to have twice as little /fɔRs-aj/.' (Lexical component as in *FORCE* /fɔRs/.)

(2.29) '*On me donne que les* /pRɔm-yR/ *que ca peut.*'
'They give me only the /pRɔm-yr/ that that may.' (Lexical component as in *PROMOTION* /pRɔmɔsjɔ̃/.)

(2.30) '*En* /alʒeR-ik/, *non, je n'ai pas vu.*'
'In /alʒeR-ik/, no, I didn't see.' (Lexical component as in *ALGERIEN* /alʒerjɛ̃/.)

(2.31) '*Mon* /sɔld-aʒ/—*si vous voulez—s'emploie différemment.*'
'My/sɔld-aʒ/—if you like—is used differently.' (Lexical component as in *SOLDAT* /sɔlda/.)

(2.32) '*Mon âge actuel, c'est* /fRãs-i/, *si vous voulez.*'
'My age now, it's /fRãs-i/ if you like.' (Lexical component as in *FRANCAIS* /fRãse/.)

Given the choice of the lexical monemic components of these transformations, it is interesting to know that our patient was a professional soldier. On the basis of their structure, the abnormal segments appearing in examples 25 to 32 can be referred to as derived monemic paraphasias. They can thus be contrasted with compound monemic paraphasias[16] which are abnormal segments consisting only of lexical monemes, as in the case in (2.33) 'day-night', (2.34) 'summer–

* The monemic paraphasias are transcribed in IPA and appear between oblique lines. A hyphen may be inserted between the constituent monemes.

winter', (2.35) 'winter–summer', (2.36) 'cold–hot', and (2.37) 'hot-cold' in the following excerpt from a conversation with a schizophasic patient.

(2.38) '*Le vrai calendrier est différent du faux ... Ils l'ont fait du nuit et jour, et de JOUR–NUIT. Et le quinze avril est au quinze octobre, pour l'ÉTÉ–HIVER, et le quinze octobre est au quinze AVRIL-RE-AVRIL pour l'HIVER–ÉTÉ. De telle sorte qu'on passe un ÉTÉ–HIVER et un HIVER–ÉTÉ ... de FROID–CHAUD ou de CHAUD–FROID.*'

The real calendar is different from the false ... They made it from night and day, and from DAY–NIGHT. And the fifteenth of April is on the fifteenth of October, for the SUMMER–WINTER, and the fifteenth of October is on the fifteenth of APRIL–RE–APRIL for the WINTER–SUMMER. In such a way that you spend a SUMMER–WINTER and WINTER–SUMMER ... of COLD–HOT or of HOT–COLD.'

NEOLOGISMS—PHASE I AND PHASE II TRANSFORMATIONS

In the aphasiological lexicon, the connotations of the word 'neologism' refer to the form of the segments so designated (i.e., to their formal aspect) and not to their meaning (their semantic aspect). In essence, neologisms are linguistic segments which are used as words even though they do not appear in the dictionary of a given language community. Thus phonemic and monemic paraphasias are, strictly speaking, neologisms. Nevertheless, we prefer to reserve this label for those neologistic segments which cannot be identified as phonemic paraphasias (because the word 'transformed' cannot be specified), monemic paraphasias (because monemes of the language cannot be recognized), or still other types of less well-defined transformations[17]. In certain forms of aphasia (see Chapter 4, Wernicke's aphasia proper) neologisms may be particularly abundant in productions obtained during naming tasks and, as in (39), during conversation. The patient is answering the question 'How long have you been in the hospital?'*

(2.39) '*Je crois, Mademoiselle, je crois que je suis ici depuis cinquante* /dɔno/↓ *cinquante* /dɔno/ *le* /swɛn/ *dernière ... Ca doit etre cinquante-sept* /i/ *que je suis restée ici, où j'ai été* /pɛji/ *pour le petit* /sɑ̃plɔ̃/, *ici, et que dont je suis restée quinze jours complètement dans le* /oki/. *Pourquoi? J'en sais rien. Pour le* /oka/? *J'en sais rien. Je ne sais pas pourquoi. Cela faisait quatre ans que j'étais ... quatre ans passé que j'étais chez un* /feli/, *là-bas, oùj'* /ɑ̃bit/*↓ *ou je m'* /ɑ̃tid/ *tous les jours de*↓ *de* /sɔtim/.'

'I believe, Miss, I believe that I am here since fifty /dɔno/↓ fifty /dɔno/ the last /swɛn/ ... that must be fifty-seven /i/ that I've stayed here, where I've been /pɛji/ for the little /sɑ̃plɔ̃/, here, and that of which I've stayed fifteen days completely in the /oki/. Why? I know nothing about it. For the /oka/? I know nothing about it. I don't know why. That made four years that I was ... four years ago that I was in the home of a /feli/, over there, where I /ɑ̃bit/†↓ where I /ɑ̃tid/ myself everyday of ↓ of /sɔtim/.'

SEMANTIC VERBAL PARAPHASIAS—PHASE I TRANSFORMATIONS

The term 'formal verbal paraphasia' is used to designate aphasic transformations in which the substituting and substituted words are similar in regard to their form: that is, they belong to the same field of forms (cf. p. 42). In contrast, the term 'semantic verbal paraphasia' is used to designate aphasic transformations in which the substituting and substituted words are similar in meaning: that is, they belong to the same semantic field (cf. p. 37). The same term is used regardless of the nature of the semantic association existing between the two words in question. For example, the words may be associated through membership in the same class as in (2.40) '*pomme*'→'*poire*' ('apple'→'pear'); through opposition, as in (2.41) '*bon*'→'*mauvais*' ('good'→'bad'); through usual proximity in the environment, as in (2.42) '*pipe*'→'*allumette*' ('pipe'→'match'), etc.

Because oral reading and naming tasks allow an obtained response to be evaluated with reference to a specified stimulus, they facilitate the study of semantic paraphasias. However, if one wishes to study material obtained under less restricted conditions, it is best to rely on the narration of certain well-known stories since the traditional version provides a standard of reference (see Chapter 15). For example, semantic paraphasias are obvious in the narration of a patient who successively spoke of a (2.43) '*sac*', '*bourse*', '*saquet*' and '*sachet*' ('bag', 'purse',

* Neologisms are transcribed in IPA and appear between oblique lines.

† Probably a phonemic paraphasia: J' /abit/ (I live)→J' /ɑ̃bit/.

'sackette', then a 'sachet') when referring to the 'basket' carried by Little Red Riding Hood. The identification of semantic paraphasias in conversational language is often difficult because the observer lacks sufficient confidence about what the aphasic subject wished to say. One of our patients made the following statements* when commenting on a recent presidential election in the United States:

(2.44) '*On s'est surtout occupé de la partie intérieure et on s'est aperçu que, partout ailleurs, ils ont mis de PETITS COLPORTEURS et ils ont pu, avec un VESTON ... —Non! C'est pas un "Veston"—avec de la POUDRE ... —"des POUDRES" et du "VESTON", j'allais dire—avec un MANTEAU COLPORTÉ de la MEILLEUR POUDRE pour former de SUPRÊMES JUGEMENTS.*'

'Above all we took care of the internal part and we realized that, everywhere else they put LITTLE PEDLARS and they were able, with a JACKET ... No! It's not a "JACKET"—with POWDER ... —"POWDERS" and a JACKET, I was going to say—with a PEDDLED JACKET of the BEST POWDER in order to form SUPREME JUDGEMENTS.'

The impression of incoherence which emerges from this type of discourse may be at least partially related to the abundant production of semantic paraphasias. However, they are difficult to identify with absolute certainty and it is impossible to specify which words have appeared in the corresponding normal series.

It is important to realize that semantic paraphasias may involve grammatical monemes[11], a point illustrated by the substitutions of prepositions appearing in the following sentences: (2.45) '*Elle portait une gallette SUR sa grand-mère*' ('She was carrying a cake ON her grandmother'), (2.46) '*Ma soeur, elle travaille DANS un docteur*' ('My sister works IN a doctor'), (2.47) '*Ils s'habillent AVEC cette boutique*' (They get their clothes WITH this shop'). We shall return to this type of semantic paraphasia when later defining the concept of dyssyntaxia (cf. p. 49).

PREFERRED WORDS—PHASE I INVOLVEMENT

Use of a preferred word constitutes a particular form of verbal paraphasia, one which is especially noticeable in conversational productions and sometimes in oral reading of passages, where the preferred word may unexpectedly replace any other word belonging to the same inventory. As indicated by the following excerpts from a tape-recorded conversation with one of our patients, the recurring word is almost always a substantive.

(2.48) '*Il était—Comment on appelle ca?—un CURÉ qui cherche tous les crochets qu'il trouve.*'

(2.49) '*Elle s'est enfermée dans une maladie terrible par un CURÉ qui l'a soignée justement aussi terriblement.*'

(2.50) '*C'était un marchand de CURÉ qui ecrivait des lettres.*'

(2.51) '*Alors voyez, les CURÉS, je suis obligée de le laver, cela, de temps en temps pour pas le déchirer.*'

(2.48) 'He was—what's it called?—a VICAR who looks for all the hooks that he finds.'

(2.49) 'She was enclosed in a terrible disease by a VICAR who treated her exactly as terribly.'

(2.50) 'He was a VICAR dealer who wrote some letters.'

(2.51) 'So you see, the VICARS, I have to wash it, that, from time to time, in order not to tear it.'

It often happens that the productions of a particular aphasic attest to a preference for several words rather than for only one. In this case, the preferred words almost always belong to the same semantic field so that it is appropriate to speak of a preferred field or a preferred theme. In addition to the word '*curé*' (vicar), the patient who produced the above sentences also used, although somewhat less frequently, the words '*prêtre*' (priest), '*abbé*' (abbot), '*père*' (father) and 'église' (church) in the same fashion. We note in passing that at the present time, in the age group most affected by aphasia and within the geographical regions of our patients, women's preferred words are often related to religion or the family whereas men's are often related to work.

VERBAL PARAPHASIAS—PHASE I AND II TRANSFORMATIONS

An observer may sometimes recognize that a word has been substituted without being able to specify which word has been replaced. Since it then cannot be determined whether the substitution involved a formal paraphasia, a semantic paraphasia or another less-well-defined form of aphasic transformation, the observed

---

* In quotations taken from conversations, the verbal paraphasias (probably or positively identified) are transcribed in capital letters.

transformation should be designated by the more general term 'verbal paraphasia'.

VERBAL TRANSFORMATIONS—PHASE I TRANSFORMATIONS

From the above considerations it follows that all forms of verbal paraphasias, with the exception of formal paraphasias, can be grouped under the name of verbal transformations.

A PARALLEL BETWEEN THE DEFINITIONS OF PHONEMIC AND VERBAL PARAPHASIAS

The definition of a phonemic paraphasia (cf. p. 43) explicitly mentioned that the omission, tion and displacement of phonemes are possible although simple interphonemic substitutions are by far the most frequent abnormality. This implies that phonemic paraphasias cannot be adequately described without consideration of the relations existing between the phoneme or phonemes directly involved and the other constituent phonemes of the word giving rise to the transformation. Similarly a complete definition of a verbal paraphasia must also specifically mention that the omission, addition and displacement of words are possible, although simple word substitution is by far the commonest type of abnormality. This implies that verbal paraphasias cannot be adequately described without consideration of relations existing between the word, or the words, directly involved and the other constituent words of the sentence giving rise to the transformation. This need for systematic reference to contextual units in the description of all types of aphasic transformations will become clearer during subsequent discussions of the notions of *selection errors* and *sequencing errors* (cf. pp. 48–49).

SYNTAGMIC PARAPHASIAS—PHASE I TRANSFORMATION

Another type of transformation, which is generally apparent only in oral reading and repetition tasks, involves substitutions between linguistic units which are more complex than words: (2.52) *'ùn éclairage intime'*→*'la lumière tamisée'* ('cosy lighting'→ 'filtered light'); (2.53) *'l'opium du peuple'*→*'l'argent des contribuables'* ('the opium of the people'→'the taxpayers' money'). Such transformations can logically be designated as syntagmic transformations[11]. However, it must be noted that the meaning given here to the root syntagm is not the same as in the term syntagmatic function which was defined in the first section of this chapter.

PARALEXIAS

All the types of paraphasias discussed so far may appear during oral reading; they can then be referred to as paralexias[18].

GRAPHIC DISTURBANCES—PHASE III TRANSFORMATIONS

The written language productions of aphasics may include all the types of transformations just discussed in regard to their oral productions. One speaks of a graphic* disturbance—and sometimes, inappropriately, of agraphia—to designate in a global fashion the various deformations of written linguistic symbols observed in certain clinical forms of aphasia (see Chapter 3). A graphic disturbance attests to a disorganization of the third phase of written language (cf. p. 35); in other words, it does not affect the selection of letters but rather their execution. Thus there is a clear parallel between an articulatory disturbance in oral language and a graphic disturbance in written language[19].

LITERAL AND GRAPHEMIC PARAGRAPHIAS—PHASE II TRANSFORMATIONS

Aphasic disorganizations of the second phase of written language are manifested through the production of *literal paragraphias* and *graphemic paragraphias*. Although these two types of paragraphic transformations are frequently seen in the productions of the same patient, a (quasi) exclusive production of one of these two forms may sometimes be observed.

The unit involved in literal paragraphia is the

* Throughout this text, graphism is used in a limited sense to refer to the graphic aspects of handwriting.

(2.54)	(to look for)	(C-H-E-R-C-H-E-R	→C-H-E-C-H-E-R)
(2.55)	(talkative)	(B-A-V-A-R-D	→B-A-V-A-B)
(2.56)	(to furnish)	(F-O-U-R-N-I-R	→F-O-U-R-F-I-R)
(2.57)	(cold)	(F-R-O-I-D	→F-O-R-I-D)
(2.58)	(tornado)	(T-O-R-N-A-D-E	→T-O-R-N-A-R-D-E)
(2.59)	(agricultural)	(C-U-L-T-I-V-A-T-E-U-R	→C-U-R-V-I-L-A-T-E-U-R)
(2.60)	(library)	(B-I-B-L-I-O-T.H-E-Q.U.E	→B-I-B-L-I-O-T-E-C)
(2.61)	(domain)	(D-O-M-A.I-N.E	→D-O-M.M-E-N)
(2.62)	(French)	(F-R-A.N-C-A.I.S	→F-R-A.N-C-A.I.T)
(2.63)	(beginning)	(C-O-M.M-E.N-C.E-M-E.N.T	→C-O-M-A.N-S.E-M-E.N.T)
(2.64)	(red)	(R-O.U-G.E	→R-O.U-C.H.E)
(2.65)	(Sunday)	(D-I-M-A.N-C.H.E	→T-I-M-A.N-C.H.E)

letter. The linear structures observed in these transformations duplicate, in written language, all the characteristic aspects of phonemic paraphasias [compare the structures of examples (13) to (20) to those of (1) and (54) to (59)]. Thus literal paragraphias are appropriately described in terms of omissions, additions, displacements and/or substitutions of letters[20]. This can be clearly seen in examples (54) to (59), which were written by one of our patients during a subtest involving dictation of isolated words.

The unit involved in graphemic paragraphias is the grapheme (cf. p. 33). Graphemic paragraphias always involve—and thus are defined as—substitutions between homographs, that is, between graphemes which may represent the same phoneme in different orthographic contexts [see examples (60) to (63)], or substitutions between graphemes corresponding to phonemes having similar constituent features [see examples (64) and (65)]. The samples provided above [(60) to (65)], which are intended to illustrate these concepts, were obtained from one of our patients during a subtest of writing isolated words to dictation.

ORTHOGRAPHIC DEVIATIONS—PHASE II TRANSFORMATIONS

Literal paragraphias and graphemic paragraphias can be grouped under the title 'orthographic deviations'.

VERBAL PARAGRAPHIAS—PHASE I TRANSFORMATIONS

The varied forms of verbal paraphasias, which attest to an aphasic disorganization of the first phase of spoken language, are paralleled by the varied forms of verbal paragraphias which attest to an aphasic disorganization of the first phase of written language[11, 21]. In cases where both spoken and written production remain possible, both paraphasias and paragraphias are usually seen in the same patient. Like verbal paraphasias, verbal paragraphias usually consist of simple word substitutions. However, the abnormalities may involve word omissions, additions or displacements so that verbal paragraphias must therefore be systematically studied in the context of the sentence in which they occur. The two sentences shown below [see (66)], written by one of our patients, contain numerous verbal paragraphias. The repetition of 'from the north' in the first sentence illustrates the phenomenon of verbal transformation by addition.

(2.66) *'Ceux-ci entrent en ville par le sud de sa richesse et tout aussitôt se développe un asseau brutal sur la ville du nord, où justement arrivaient les pétroles du nord de la guerre. Ce brutal est violent; les Norvégiens font leur guerre, se difficilent autant qu'ils peuvent, mais malgré l'envoi de militaires anglais et même des militaires français, ce n'est pas un long et difficile combat.'*

'These ones enter the city by the south of its riches and all as soon as spread out a brutal assault on the city from the north where, as it happened, the oils were arriving from the north of the war. This brutal is violent. The Norwegians make their war difficulting themselves as much as they can but, despite the dispatching of English soldiers and even French soldiers, it's not a long and difficult combat.'

SELECTION ERRORS AND SEQUENCING ERRORS

The concept of selection errors and sequencing errors can be applied to all types of paraphasias and paragraphias[21]. Consider, for example, the utterances (15), (30) and (67) to (72):

(2.67) v-ɛ-ʀ-t-i-ʒ/→/f-ɛ-ʀ-t-iʒ/ ('vertigo'→'fertigo')

(2.30) '*En* /amer-ik/'→ '*En*/alʒer-ik/' (in America'→in Algeria')

(2.68) '*le petit SENTIER dans la foret*'→ '*le petit TROTTOIR dans la foret*'* ('the little PATH in the forest'→'the little SIDEWALK in the forest')

(2.69) '*au milieu de*'→'*le centre d'une chose*'† ('in the middle of'→'the centre of a thing')

(2.15) /i-n-a-k-t-i-f/→/i-n-a-k-t-i-k/ ('inactive→inactick')

(2.70) '*On remBALlait à l'arriere; c'était un* /bal-aʒ/ *assez dur*.'‡ ('They rePACKed at the back; it was a pretty tough (?) job.')

(2.71) '*sont differents de ce qu'on a appris à des GOSSES. On leur a appris des tas de GOSSES*.'z‡ (' are different than what was taught to KIDS. They were taught lots of KIDS.')

(2.72) '*J'ai un hélicoptère comme TOUT LE MONDE qui etait avec TOUT LE MONDE*.'‡ ('I have a helicopter like EVERYONE who was with EVERYONE.')

Each of these paraphasias, whether it be phonemic, monemic, verbal or syntagmic, occurs through a simple substitution. In examples (30) and (67) to (69), the substituted and substituting units belong to the same fields of forms or of meanings and the errors are thus called selection errors. In examples (15) and (70) to (72) the substituted and substituting units are not similar (do not belong to the same field) but the substituting unit is identical to another LPU of the same HPU (anterograde assimilation) so that a pair of identical units is thus created. These errors are therefore called sequencing errors.

The examples (15) and (70) to (72) do not illustrate all the possible linear structures of sequencing errors. The term 'sequencing errors' is, in fact, used to designate all aphasic transformations, regardless of the linguistic phase, which indicate at least a single displacement of a linguistic unit or the creation or destruction of at least one pair of identical or similar linguistic units. Sequencing errors may thus involve: (a) transformations resulting from an elementary operation [simple omission (73), simple displacement (74), simple addition (14)]; (b) transformations resulting from complex processes entailing a combination of two elementary operations [omission and displacement (75), omission and addition (76), displacement and addition (17)]; (c) transformations resulting from complex processes entailing a combination of three elementary operations [omission, displacement and addition 77)].

As seen in example (77), any aphasic transformation may simultaneously show the characteristics of both a selection and a sequencing error. Moreover, the same aphasic individual produces

(2.73)	(descending)	*descendant*	/d-ɛ-s-ɑ̃-d-ɑ̃	→d-ɛ-s-d-ɑ̃/
(2.74)	(hen house)	*poulailler*	/p-u-l-a-j-e	→a-p-u-l-j-e/
(2.14)	(sauntering)	*déambulant*	/d-e-ɑ̃-b-y-l-ɑ̃	→d-e-b-ɑ̃-b-y-l-ɑ̃/
(2.75)	(security)	*securité*	/s-e-k-y-ʀ-i-t-e	→s-y-k-ʀ-i-t-e/
(2.76)	(solidarity)	*solidarité*	/s-ɔ-l-i-d-a-ʀ-i-t-e	→s-ɔ-l-e-d-a-ʀ-i-t-e/
(2.17)	(poultry farmer)	*aviculteur*	/a-v-i-k-y-l-t-œ-ʀ	→v-a-t-i-k-y-l-t-œ-ʀ/
(2.77)	(abominable)	*abominable*	/a-b-ɔ-m-i-n-a-b-l	→a-m-ɔ-n-i-n-a-b-l/§

* Narration (*Little Red Riding Hood*).
† Oral reading (stimuli isolated from context).
‡ Conversational language.
§ All the transformations quoted to illustrate the concept of literal paragraphia are also sequencing errors [(54) to (59)]; several also appear in the passage illustrating the concept of verbal paragraphia [(66)].

both types of errors and there is no reason to suppose that the physiopathology of selection errors is essentially different from that of sequencing errors. In both cases, there appears to be involvement of the paradigmatic function (cf. p. 37); see also Insertion 8.4; and Chapter 10, section dealing with Jakobson's theories of aphasia).

DYSSYNTAXIA (OR PARAGRAMMATISM)

The term *dyssyntaxia*[22] refers to the overall quality of pathological linguistic productions characterized by a larger or smaller proportion of sentences which violate the normative rules of the common morphosyntactical convention. Verbal and syntagmic paraphasias and paragraphias, especially when they involve grammatical monemes and/or result from processes other than simple substitutions, often constitute dyssyntactic transformations. Some examples are:

(2.45) '*Elle portait une galette CHEZ sa grand-mère.*'→'Elle portait une galette *SUR* sa grand-*mère*.'* 'She was carrying a cake TO her grandmother's.'→'She was carrying a cake ON her grandmother.'

(2.78) '*J'étais dans la couturE; j'ai toujours fait des robes.*'→'*J'étais dans la couturIÈRE; j'ai toujours fait des robes.*'† 'I was in dressmakING; I've always made dresses.'→'I was in dressmaKER; I've always made dresses.'

(2.79) '*Avec quoi fabrique-t-ON de la brique?*'→'*Avec quoi ON fabrique-t-ON de la brique?*'†
'With what does ONE make bricks?'→'With what ONE does ONE make bricks?'

(2.80) '*Le plus QUE JE PEUX*'. + '*Le plus POSSIBLE*'.→'*Le plus QUE JE POSSIBLE.*'†
'As much AS I CAN' + 'As much as POSSIBLE'.→'As much AS I POSSIBLE.'

(2.66) '*Cet assaut est brutal et violent.*'→'*Ce brutal est violent.*'‡
'This attack is brutal and violent.'→'This brutal is violent.'

It is important to note that the structure of these paraphasias and paragraphias is not essentially different from that of paraphasias and paragraphias which do not involve dyssyntactic transformations. In other words, it is important to realize that the term 'dyssyntaxia' does not designate a specific disorder of syntax. Rather it serves to describe certain segments of aphasic language further and, in particular, certain verbal paraphasias and paragraphias.

Other characteristic features of certain clinical forms of aphasia (see Chapter 4)—repetition of determiners, of prepositions, etc.; difficulty or failure in producing certain essential words of the sentence, etc.—may be the source of dyssyntactic behaviour. In general, the proportion of dyssyntactic sentences is relatively small in conversational productions (as far as we know, a maximum of 20 per cent of the utterances) but may be much larger in written productions. The latter point is well illustrated by an exceptional passage written by a patient of B. de Ribaucourt-Ducarne (description, during a therapy session, of a picture of a street fair).

(2.82) '*Les bizarres excès sont droit toutes tentes des forains. Sur après-midi les enfants ravient le fête et pour l'amusent dans un manège des chevaux-bois, les balançoires et fauteuils des chaînes tournent d'un axe.*

Peut voir les roulottes qui vient des romanichels, forains et acrobates? Ils au public travaillent du cirque et endroit a vouloir le inouï vêtement d'un pitres clown aussi merveilleusement d'un écuyer et autre envers, ici la caravate, est à pauvre habit, a un gilet et vertes blouson qui tendent de acrobatic aux chevaux, chiens et ses enfants.'

'The bizarre excesses are right all tents of the itinerants. On afternoon the children are delighting the festival and to entertain it in a roundabout of horses-

---

* Narration (*Little Red Riding Hood*).

† Conversational language. See also examples (46) and (47). Example (80) illustrates a particular type of error in which elements belonging to two different syntagms are combined, producing a dyssyntaxic transformation. [This same structure may be seen, at the second linguistic phase, in certain neologisms, for example in (2.81) /afymet/ which, presumably, is a telescopage of '*fumée*' (smoke), '*allumette*' (match) and '*cigarette*'.]

‡ Written response; the conventional utterance was provided by the patient's corrections.

wood the swings and armchairs of the chains turn on an axis.

Can see the trailers which come from the gypsies, itinerant and acrobat? They to the public work of the circus and place has to want the unheard of clothes of a buffoon clown also marvellously of an equestrian and other here the caravate is at poor dress, at a vest and green wind-breaker which makes of acrobatic at the horses, dogs and his children.'

JARGONAPHASIA

The term 'jargonaphasia'[11, 13] designates related types of pathological linguistic productions which are characterized by normal articulation and prosody, normal or exaggerated fluency (logorrhoea), and an abundance of paraphasias. Some dyssyntactic transformations are always observed in the conversation of jargonaphasics and when they are particularly numerous, which is quite rare, the output is sometimes labelled dyssyntactic jargon. In most cases, all types of paraphasias are produced and many abnormal linguistic segments must be grouped under the name 'neologisms' because they cannot be more precisely identified. Repetition of determiners, prepositions, etc., and incompleted (aborted) sentences, are more or less common and no doubt reflect the reduced availability of words (word-finding difficulty) (see Chapter 4), especially lexical words. These features are illustrated by the following excerpt from a conversation with one of our patients.

(2.83) '*Madame*↓—*la dame qui est venue après, une dame que j'aime beaucoup, qui est très* /ɛlɛmabl/, *une* /ɛmɛbl/ *dame* /menizɛʀ/, *qui est venue chez ce monsieur, là; elle est venue après puis je l'aime beaucoup parce qu'elle est*↓ *elle est très*↓ *très* /sumɛl/; *elle est*↓ *elle a une* /tɛ̃til/ *euh bleue, une* /ɛ̃tid/ *ordinaire, quoi! elle est*↓ *elle est vraiment très bien, elle m'a ACHETÉ plusieurs* /plɛʀ/, *elle dit: "Mais*↓ *mais je*↓ *je ne sais pas quoi lui ÉPLUCHER." Il dit: "Je ne sais pas, moi. Comment vous appelez ça?" Ben, je dis: "Comme ça." "Comment vous appelez ça?" Ben, je dis: "Une très jolie* /kaʀezɛʀ/, *je dis, vous avez quelque chose de très bien* /ɔkɔnɔzi/, *de très* /ʒɔdi/ *sur votre* /kis/." *Il dit: "oui, mais qu'est-ce que vous voulez que je fasse?" Effectivement, monsieur, je suis absolument sans* /ʀɛʀ/ *... Toujours! Mais alors, ou j'ai été vraiment* /kɔʀɛkte/, *c'est quand je suis arrivée ici, que j'ai eu tombé, que je m'étais esquinté, ici, un bout*↓ *un bout de*↓ *de* /sɔty/—*enfin* /sɔty/, *je ne sais pas si c'etait* /sɔty/ *enfin, je ne crois pas—euh, que j'ai trouvé ici et euh, que je suis* /ʀɛte/ *pendant dix-huit jours mais absolument dans*↓ *dans* /l/↓ *complètement dans la*↓ *dans la* /sɔ/↓ *dans la* /sɔ/↓ /sɔlɛtvegi/. *Il y a*↓ *il y a*↓ *J'ai personne. J'avais de la* /vegi/.'*

'Madam↓—the lady who came after, a lady that I like very much, who is very /ɛlɛmabl/, a /ɛmɛbl/ lady who came to this man's home, there; she came after then I like her very much because she is↓ she is very↓ very /sumɛl/; she is↓E she has a /tɛtil/ uh, blue, an ordinary /ɛ̃tid/ what! she is↓ she is really very good, she BOUGHT me several /plɛr/, she says: "But↓ but I↓ don't know what TO PEEL to her." He says: "I don't know. What do you call that?" Then I say: "Like that." "What do you call that?" Then I say: "A very pretty /kaʀezɛʀ/, I say: you have something very good /ɔkɔnɔzi/, very /ʒɔdi/ on your /kis/." He says: "Yes but what do you want me to do?" Effectively, Sir, I'm absolutely without /ʀɛʀ/ ... Always! But then, where I was really /kɔʀɛkte/ it's when I came here, that I had had fallen, that I had tired myself out, here, a bit↓ a bit of↓ of /sɔty/—finally /sɔty/, I don't know if it was /sɔty/ finally, I don't believe so—uh, that I found here, and uh, that I am /ʀɛte/ during the sixteen days but absolutely in↓ in /l/↓ completely in the↓ in the /sɔ/↓ in the /sɔ/↓ /sɔlɛtvegi/. There is↓ there is↓ I have nobody. I had the /vegi/.'

In certain patients, the paraphasic output consists (almost) entirely of phonemic and formal verbal paraphasias and is therefore called phonemic jargon [see example (24); see also Chapter 4, section dealing with conduction aphasia]. In other patients, the paraphasic output consists (almost) entirely of semantic paraphasias, preferred words, other types of verbal transformations (with almost a total absence of formal verbal paraphasias) and syntagmic paraphasias; a type of production which is referred to as semantic jargon [see examples (44) and (90); see also Chapter 4, section dealing with Type II Wernicke's aphasia]. This form of Wernicke's aphasia is usually characterized by an abundant production of fixed syntagms.

GLOSSOLALIA

Curiosity alone is sufficient to prompt mention of the conversational output of certain jargonaphasics which, while abundant and without prosodic abnormalities, is entirely or almost entirely neologistic. This type of output is known as *glossolalia*[17]. Example (84) was taken from a recorded conversation with a patient whose pro-

* See also examples (4.20) and (4.21).

sody clearly created the impression that he was speaking in words and sentences. Longer pauses are indicated by oblique lines and shorter ones by spaces.

(2.84) Q: 'How old are you, sir?'
R: '/celɛdʀœdebit pʀɔbablœʀe mepɔ̃dʀe digetʀumɛt/ /celœlœdœʀe di ki-tʒ-ke dis gɔdɛtœʀe/'

Q: 'Do you have any children?'
R: '/delɛ̃dʀœdebit pʀɔbablœʀe mepɔ̃dʀe digetʀu-mɛt/ /lœdepʀɛt delœlœdœʀe œ e œ ɛlzekute ɛlnœpuʀi-makɔ̃te tɑ̃ tut e dœgʀedœgʀe dis gy lateʀe digelotere/.'*

JARGONAGRAPHIA

The term 'jargonagraphia'[11], or written jargon, refers to the written productions of aphasics which contain numerous paragraphic transformations. These transformations, which include many verbal paragraphias and usually a fair number of dyssyntactic transformations [see examples (66) to (82)], may be produced despite complete intactness of graphic activity and preservation of written automisms. The passage shown below, example (85), was written, without the least hesitation, by one of our patients and illustrates that written jargon may also include neologisms.

(2.85) '*Il y a parfois des conrénent, tandis que je n'ai ras leurie très vitement. Peut-être étager intifrend, ou bien ne fabribiant sans avoir une gâte suferieure. J'aime faucout à me montrer ce qu'auprès peut-être une condamte pour aller rapis dans une sache d'avie. Il aventut recarge les conseils.*

Je ne fais pas toujours de condemner mais poúr auger je serais falus senti que je devrais mes afficant et tremper nos peu audent. Saura-t-il me sendre si je dois avoir plus de décousite?'†

'There is sometimes some concrenent while I have not short leurie very quickly. Perhaps to carry out in stages intifrend, or else not fabribant without having a suferior scribbler. I like faucot to show myself what near perhaps a condamte to go rapis in a know of avie. He aventut reçarge some advice. I don't always do of condemner but to auger I would be falus smelled what I should my afficant and to soak our little audent. Would he know to sendre to me if I must have more décousity?'

GLOSSOMANIA

With the exception of phonetic transformations, all types of abnormal segments may be found in glossomania[16]: phonemic transformations, monemic transformations, verbal transformations and neologisms. In its usual form, which is referred to as formal glossomania, linguistic output is characterized by the production of utterances whose units are selected according to their similarities in form rather than by their relevance to the subject of conversation. Alliteration‡ and assonance§ are frequently seen in this type of production. Example (86)—which was not written by an abstruse poet or lover of puns but spoken by a schizophasic subject—illustrates the formal relations between the different segments of the utterance: [ɔʀlɔʒʀi], [ɔʀaʒ], [œʀ-aʒ], [ɔʀ-aʒ], [tɔn-aʒ], [dɛzepɔkdɛʀ], [dezɛʀdepɔk].

(2.86) '*Il y a donc des plans ... d'horlogerie et d'orage. Vous appelez ça des heures-âge, des ors-âge, d'où des tonnes-âge ... le calendrier possède des↓ des époques d'ères, déserts d'époque.*'

'There are thus some plans of clock-making and of storm. You call that the hours-age the nows-age, from which the tons-age. The calender possesses [*des*] epochs, [*d*] eras, deserts of epochs.'

Glossomania may also be evident in utterances in which the segments are selected, as in certain word games, according to semantic associations diverging from the conversational topic, a type of linguistic behaviour called semantic glossomania. In the prototypical case, the utterance showing semantic glossomania includes a segment with a potential for homonymy: this then generates associations related to several of the possible meanings. This is seen in example (87), where [fɛrm] generates associations to both its meanings FARM (city, village, country) and CLOSE (to open–to close).||

* See also Insertion 13.3, example (13.44).

† See also examples (4.19) and (4.27) and Fig. 4–2.

‡ Alliteration: repetition of initial consonants (and, by extension, of medial consonants) in a series of consecutive words.

§ Assonance: repetition of the same sound (in poetry, the last accentuated vowel in each line). These definitions are borrowed from *Le Petit Robert*[1].

|| See also example (44). An element of glossomania can be considered to be present in this example where the words *colporteur* (literally, a carrier of a collar), *veston* (jacket) and *manteau colporté* (peddled jacket) appear successively.

(2.87) '*Ce sont des campagnes. On appele ça des campagnes. C'est appelé ainsi: des villes, des villas-campagnes. Des villas-campagnes sont les fermes d'ouvre-ferme. Le vrai nom de ferme: ce sont des j'ouvre-ferme.*'

'They are countries. One calls that countries. It is named thus: some cities, some country houses. Some country houses are farms of open-close. The real name of farm: they are some I open-close.'

AGRAMMATISM

The word agrammatism refers to a particular type of pathological linguistic behaviour which is characterized by a slowed rate of speech, a general reduction of available vocabulary, a reduction in the number and complexity of available syntactical structures; shortened utterances showing a tendency to juxtaposition; and omissions and substitutions specifically centred on grammatical monemes[23]. One of our patients, who was an amateur archaeologist and architect, made the following comments on his hobbies:

(2.88) '*Ah! mon vieux, l'archéologie! Oh! attention parce que moi euh, euh, trois mois ou quatre mois, la petite bêche et la euh, la région euh, Provins. Trouver les↓ les↓ les pots, etc. ... Alors, deux architectes deux architectes, comme ça. Alors portion là, moi et l'autre architecte, l'autre. Après, zut! parce que moi, je peux pas, là ... Là, rien du tout moi, rien du tout. Là, a côté, euh, la, comme ça, architecte, bon architecte. Ah zut alors! ... Rien du tout, moi, rien du tout, dans mon champ. Tout↓ tout petit peu à côté, bien, bien, bien, bien! Ah zut alors!*'

'Ah! Old chap, archaeology! Oh! Be careful because I ah, ah, three or four months, the little spade and the↓ uh, uh, Provins region. To find the↓ the↓ jugs, etc. ... So, two architects↓ two architects, like that. So, that part, me and the other architect, the other one. Afterwards, darn it! Because I, I can't, there ... There, nothing at all me, nothing at all. There, beside, uh, there, like that, architect, good architect. Ah darn it anyway! ... Nothing at all, me, nothing at all, in my field. All↓ a little bit beside, well, well, well, well! Ah, darn it anyway!'

On the semantic level agrammatic discourse differs from jargonaphasia by its much greater efficiency in terms of information conveyed. Compare, for example, the following two commentaries on political events in Paris in May 1968. The first illustrates agrammatism and the second jargonaphasia:

(2.89) '*Ah oui! Grèves euh, grèves, euh, drapeaux rouges. Euh, euh, matraques, enfin matraques, Facultés. Euh, ah oui! Dix pour cent euh, salaire. Euh, bah! c'est tout.*'

'Ah yes! Strikes uh, strikes, uh, red flags. Uh, uh, bludgeons, finally bludgeons, universities. Uh, ah yes! Ten per cent, uh, wages. Uh, oof! That's all.'

(2.90) '*Mais un jour, euh, vous aurez, dans la France entière, reparti dans la France↓ Vous aurez, dans la France↓ Vous aurez la France. Vous aurez Paris qui sera, vraisemblablement, euh, une partie qui sera difficile à tenir, puis tout le reste sera↓—Je ne veux pas dire tout dans l'ensemble—sera l'ensemble de la France, mais l'ensemble de la France sera a peu pres convenable.*'

'But some day, uh, you will have, in the whole of France spread through France↓ You will have, in France↓ you will have France. You will have Paris which will be, probably, uh, a part which will be difficult to hold, then all the rest will be↓—I don't mean all—on the whole, will be the whole of France, but the whole of France will be about normal.'

LINGUISTIC REDUCTION

Quantitatively, the flow of aphasic speech may be greatly reduced as a consequence, for example, of significant articulatory impairment or severe word finding difficulty (*quantitative reduction*): it may also be normal or even logorrhoeic. When judged in terms of the number of words produced per unit time, these quantitative characteristics are extremely important to the definition of the different clinical forms of aphasia[24] (see Chapter 4). Qualitatively, aphasics may produce a wide variety of words, whether or not they are correctly used. However, the variety of productions may also be severely limited (sometimes to the extent that the aphasic repeatedly uses the one or few words remaining at his or her disposal). This latter case illustrates the concept of a *qualitative reduction*. It is almost always seen in cases with slowed laboured speech: that is, in cases showing a *quantitative reduction*. Patients with normally fluent speech or logorrhoea may or may not present a qualitative reduction.

REFERENCES

1. Robert, P. (1969) *Le Petit Robert*. Paris: Société du Nouveau Littré.
2. Burchfield, R.W. (Ed.) (1976) *A Supplement to the Oxford English Dictionary*. Vol. II, A–N. Oxford: Clarendon Press.
3. Alajouanine, T. (1968) *L'aphasie et le langage pathologique*. Paris: Baillière.
4. Lecours, A.R. (1974) Le cerveau et le langage. *Union médicale du Canada*, **103,** 232.
5. Martinet, A. (1967) *Eléments de linguistique-générale*. Paris: A. Colin.
6. Lecours, A.R., Dordain, G. & Lhermitte, F. (1970) Recherches sur le langage des aphasiques. 1. Terminologie neurolinguistique. *Encéphale*, **59,** 520.
7. Buyssens, E. (1967) *La communication et l'articulation linguistique*. Paris: Presses Universitaires de France.
8. Saussure, F. (de) (1967) *Cours de linguistique générale*. Paris: Payot.
9. Compernys, E. (1968) Les jonctions. *Le français dans le monde* **57,** 20.
10. Lecours, A.R. & Lhermitte, F. (1976) The 'pure form' of the phonetic disintegration syndrome ('pure anarthria'); anatomo-clinical report of a historical case. *Brain and Language*, **3,** 88.
11. Lecours, A.R. & Rouillon, F. (1976) Neurolinguistic analysis of jargonaphasia and jargonagraphia. In *Studies in Neurolinguistics* (Ed.) Avakian-Whitaker, H. & Whitaker, H. Vol. 2, p. 95. New York: Academic Press.
12. Alajouanine, T., Ombredane, A. & Durand, M. (1939) *Le syndrome de désintégration phonétique dans l'aphasie*. Paris: Masson.
13. Alajouanine, T. & Lhermitte, F. (1964) The phonemic and semantic components of jargon aphasia. *Journal of Neurology*, **4,** 277.
14. Lecours, A.R. & Lhermitte, F. (1969) Phonemic paraphasias; linguistic structures and tentative hypotheses. *Cortex*, **5,** 193.
15. Lecours, A.R. & Lhermitte, F. (1972) Recherches sur le langage des aphasiques: 4. Analyse d'un corpus de neologismes; notion de paraphasie monemique. *Encéphale*, **61,** 295.
16. Lecours, A.R. & Vanier-Clément, M. (1976) Schizophasia and jargonaphasia. A comparative description with comments on Chaika's and Fromkin's respective looks at schizophrenic language. *Brain and Language*, **3,** 516.
17. Lecours, A.R. & De Kock, J. (1977) Sprachlich neugebildete Segmente und Glossolalie. *Review of Applied Linguistics*, **37,** 3.
18. Lhermitte, F., Lecours, A.R. & Ouvry, B. (1967) Essai d'analyse structurale des paralexies et des paragraphies. *Acta Neurologica Belgica*, **11,** 1021.
19. Lecours, A.R., Bérubé, L., Courtois, G. & Lhermitte, F. (1972) Recherches sur le langage des aphasiques: 3. Désorganisation de l'expression orale et désorganisation de l'expression ecrite. *Encéphale*, **61,** 208.
20. Lecours, A.R. (1966) Serial order in writing—a study of misspelled words in developmental dysgraphia. *Neuropsychologia*, **4,** 221.
21. Lecours, A.R. (1974) Linguistic analysis of paraphasias. *Neurosciences Research Program Bulletin*, **12,** 555.
22. Ducarne, B. & Preneron, C. (1976) La dyssyntaxie. *La Linguistique*, **12,** 33.
23. Dordain, G. (1968) *Contribution à l'étude neurolinguistique de l'aphasie. Analyse comparative des performances grammaticales de 28 aphasiques dont 14 agrammatiques.* Medical thesis, Paris.
24. Alajouanine, T. & Lhermitte, F. (1963) Les désorganisations des activités expressives du langage dans l'aphasie. *Encéphale*, **52,** 5.

BIBLIOGRAPHY

Bach, E. (1964) *An Introduction to Transformational Grammar*. New York: Holt, Rinehart and Winston.

Berelson, B. (1952) *Content Analysis in Communication Research*. New York: Free Press.

Bloomfield, L. (1962) *Language*. London: Allen and Unwin.

Chomsky, N. (1957) *Syntactic Structures*. The Hague: Mouton

Chomsky, N. (1969) *Structures syntaxiques*. Paris: Seuil.

Chomsky, N. & Halle, M. (1968) *The Sound Pattern of English*. New York: Harper and Row.

Critchley, M. (1967) Aphasiological nomenclature and definitions. *Cortex*, **3,** 3.

Critchley, M. (1970) *Aphasiology and Other Aspects of Language*. London: Edward Arnold.

Darrault, I. (Ed.) (1976) *Langages 43: Modalités*. Paris: Didier-Larousse.

Delage, J. (1977) *Glossaire anglais-français de l'aphasiologie*. Thesis, Faculté des Arts et des Sciences, Université de Montréal, Montréal. (*Dorland's Illustrated Medical Dictionary*; Saunders, Philadelphia and London, 1957.)

Etienne, L. (1957) *L'art du contrepet*. Paris: Pauvert.

Etienne, L. (1965) *L'art de la charade à tiroirs*. Paris: Pauvert.

Fillmore, C. & Langerdoen (Ed.) (1971) *Studies in Linguistic Semantics*. New York: Holt, Rinehart and Winston.

François, D. (1966) Le contrepet. *La Linguistique*, **2,** 31.

François, D. & François, F. (1967) L'ambiguité linguistique. *Word*, **23,** 150.

Garnier, M. & Delamare, V. (1970) *Dictionnaire des termes techniques de médecine* (*18ᵉ* édition, *revue et augmentée par J. Delamare et J. Delamare*). Paris: Maloine.

Geets, W. (1974) Définir l'aphasie et ses épithètes. *Le Langage et l'Homme*, **24,** 3.

Gleason, H.A. (1969) *Introduction à la linguistique*. Paris: Larousse.

Greimas, A.J. (1966) *Sémantique structurale*. Paris: Larousse.

Greimas, A.J. (1970) *Du sens: essais sémiotiques*. Paris: Seuil.

Grévisse, M. (1964) *Le bon usage*. Gembloux: Duculot.

Guiraud, P. (1956) Les champs morpho-sémantiques. *Bulletin de la Société de Linguistique*, **1,** 265.

Halle, M. (1964) On the bases of phonology. In *The Structure of Language* (Ed). Fodor, J.A. & Katz, J.J. p. 324. Englewood Cliffs, NJ: Prentice-Hall.

Harris, Z. (1968) *Mathematical Structures of Language*. New York: Interscience Publishers.

Hécaen, H. & Angelergues, R. (1965) *Pathologie du langage*. Paris: Larousse.

Hjelmslev, M. (1954) La stratification du langage. *Word*, **10,** 163.

Hockett, C.F. (1958) *A Course in Modern Linguistics*. New York: Macmillan.

Jakobson, R. (1963) *Essais de linguistique générale*. Paris: Minuit.

Jakobson, R. (1966) Linguistic types of aphasia. In *Brain Function, Speech, Language and Communication* (Ed.) Carterette, E.C. Vol. III, p. 67. Los Angeles, CA: University of California Press.

Jakobson, R. (1969) Saussure's unpublished reflections on phonemes. *Cahiers Ferdinand de Saussure*, **26,** 5.

Jakobson, R. & Halle, M. (1956) *Fundamentals of Language*. The Hague: Mouton.

Jakobson, R., Fant, G. & Halle, M. (1969) *Preliminaries to Speech Analysis*. Cambridge, MA: MIT Press.

Juilland, A. (1965) *Dictionnaire inverse de la langue française*. The Hague: Mouton.

Katz, J.J. & Fodor, J.A. (1964) The structure of a semantic theory. In *The Structure of Language* (Ed.) Fodor, J.A. & Katz, J.J. p. 479. Englewood Cliffs, NJ: Prentice-Hall.

Kock, J. de & Bossaert, W. (1974) Una segmentación morfológica formal y automática del español. *Boletin de la Real Academia Española*, **54,** 17.

Kussmaul, A. (1884) *Les troubles de la parole*. Paris: Baillière.

Ladefoged, P. (1971) *Preliminaries to Linguistic Phonetics*. Chicago, IL: University of Chicago Press.

Longerich, M.C. & Longerich, E.B. (1945) German–English speech terminology. *Journal of Speech Disorders*, **10,** 39.

Comtesse M. de la F. (1967) *L'album de la Comtesse. Le général est arrivé à pied par la Chine*. Paris: Pauvert.

Marouzeau, J. (1961) *Lexique de la terminologie linguistique (français, allemand, anglais et italien)*. Paris: Geuthner.

Martinet, A. (1966) Les choix du locuteur. *Revue philosophique*, **156,** 271.

Martinet, A. (1967) *A Functional View of Language*. London: Oxford University Press.

Martinet, A. (Ed.) (1968) *Encyclopédie de la Pléiade: le langage*. Paris: Gallimard.

Martinet, A. (1969) *Langue et fonction*. Paris: Gonthier.

Miller, G. (1951) *Language and Communication*. New York: McGraw-Hill.

Miller, G. (1956) *Langage et communication*. Paris: Presses Universitaires de France.

Moor, L. (1969) *Lexique français-anglais-allemand des termes usuels en psychiatrie, neuropsychiatrie infantile et psychologie pathologique*. Paris: L'Expansion scientifique française.

Mounin, G. (1965) Essai sur la structuration du lexique de l'habitation. *Cahiers de Lexicologie*, **1,** 9.

Mounin, G. (1965) Un champ sémantique: la dénomination des animaux domestiques. *La Linguistique*, **1,** 31.

Mounin, G. (1970) Quelques observations sur la notion d'articulation en sémiologie. In *Introduction à la sémiologie* (Ed.) Mounin, G. p. 135. Paris: Editions de Minuit.

Mounin, G. (1972) *Clefs pour la sémantique*. Paris: Seghers.

Mounin, G. (1974) *Dictionnaire de la linguistique*. Paris: Presses Universitaires de France.

Nielsen, J.M. (1942) Epitome of agnosia, apraxia and aphasia with proposed physiologic-anatomic nomenclature. *Journal of Speech Disorders*, **7,** 105.

Perceau, L. (1963) *La redoute des contrepèteries*. Paris: Briffaut.

Porot, A. (1969) *Manuel alphabétique de psychiatrie clinique et thérapeutique*. Paris: Presses Universitaires de France.

Ruwet, N. (1967) *Introduction à la grammaire générative*. Paris: Plon.

Santerre, L. (1975) Le français parlé à Montréal. *Chercheurs (Université de Montréal)*, **1,** 7.

Saussure, F. (de) (1949) *Cours de linguistique générale*. Paris: Payot.

Tesnière, L. (1959) *Eléments de syntaxe structurale*. Paris: Klincksieck.

Clinical Study of Aphasia

3. Articulatory and Graphic Disturbances of Aphasics

'Doctor,
I shall try to explain to you the reason why I have to speak syllabically. In the normal state, thought is expressed through speech automatically. One pays little or no attention to articulation; through the force of habit articulation becomes "mechanical" ...

Four weeks ago, all that came out of my mouth when I wanted to say a word was a raucous sound. One day I managed to pronounce A, I, and later A, E, I, O, U. In the following days I managed certain syllables and words beginning with a vowel. It was only about ten days ago that I was able to say "yes". Since I've been here I have pretty well mastered J, G, L. Three days ago I was unable to say my son's name, "Jean"; I could not say "le", "la", "les".*

I have to speak syllabically because my articulation is lazy, it is no longer automatic but has to be commanded, directed. I have to think of the word I am going to say and how to say it, to articulate it. If I want to say "Bonjour", habit no longer takes over, it is no longer automatic, if I don't pay strict attention, I'll say Beuseau. If I want to say "Le", "La" without paying attention, I'll say "De", "Da".

Because of that, I must articulate each vowel, each consonant, in short, each syllable.'

(*Letter from Mr Fri.; January 1948*)†

Each *articulatory* and *graphic disturbance* of aphasics affects one of the two usual modes of linguistic expression. In certain cases, which are of major theoretical interest, one or the other of these two disturbances may predominate, or even occur in a (quasi) isolated form. Despite this, as well as the need to consider these disturbances separately when carrying out a symptomatological description, it should be borne in mind that, in the great majority of cases, these two disturbances are not only associated with each other but occur in the context of an aphasia characterized by many other symptoms (see Chapter 4). These two disturbances of linguistic *expression*, as well as the corresponding disturbances of linguistic *reception*, namely *word deafness* and *word blindness* (see Chapter 5), raise three questions of obvious theoretical interest: should they, or should they not, be considered *aphasic*? Can they exist in a strictly isolated state in the absence of any other neuropsychological disturbance, and particularly in the absence of any (other) aphasic impairment? Can they be attributed to an impairment of a specific neuronal network which is functionally quite independent from the rest of the cerebral systems underlying speech and language (see Chapter 8)? Although these questions are reminiscent of those which sparked major aphasiological disputes between Dejerine, Marie and others at the start of the century[1–3], they remain of interest today. Without claiming to provide definitive answers, we note that in the case of articulatory disturbances the clinical and anatomoclinical evidence[4] suggests that the answer to each of these questions tends to be affirmative rather than negative.

* Forms of the article 'the'.

† See Chapter 8–4.

ARTICULATORY DISTURBANCES OF APHASICS

The aphasiological glossary contains many terms which designate an articulatory disturbance, terms referring to clinical phenomena which may overlap but are not necessarily superimposed (see Chapter 10). In certain cases the designated clinical phenomena include not only the articulatory disturbance but also other aphasic symptoms of *Broca's aphasia* (as this term has been understood by the French school since the time of Pierre Marie), *motor aphasia*, *cortical motor aphasia*[5], *verbal aphasia*[6], *apraxia of speech*[7], or *aphasia of phonematic realization*[8]. Other terms are used to designate only the articulatory disturbance itself: *pure motor aphasia*[5], *subcortical motor aphasia*[5], *aphemia* (as used by Dejerine[5]), *cortical dysarthria*[9], *pure anarthria*, *anarthria*, *phonetic disintegration syndrome*[10].* All terms in this latter group, with the exception of anarthria or phonetic disintegration syndrome, not only refer exclusively to an articulatory disturbance but also imply that it exists in an isolated state. In usual French terminology, *anarthria* and *phonetic disintegration* are used to refer to an articulatory disturbance which may or may not be associated with other symptoms of aphasia. The clinical phenomena designated by these two terms are, in fact, quite similar. However, common usage has led to a tendency to employ the term *anarthria* when referring to the purest and/or most severe cases (at the extreme, oral expression may be reduced to automatic expressions or stereotypes with a total absence of propositional language) whereas the term *phonetic distintegration* is used, in general, when referring to patients whose oral expression is quantitatively sufficient to permit recognition of a majority of characteristic *phonetic transformations*, usually in association with other manifestations of aphasia.

The phonetic disintegration syndrome in aphasia was first described by Alajouanine, Ombredane and Durand in a monograph whose publication, in 1939, marked the birth of neurolinguistics[10] (see Chapter 7). These authors characterized the articulatory disturbances of aphasics as a selective deficit of the elocutionary phase of verbal expression and drew a parallel between these disturbances and certain features of phonetic development in children. They also provided, through use of the methodology of experimental phonetics, a detailed description of symptoms which served as a major reference for many of the following paragraphs.

As we have already mentioned, articulatory disturbances are commonly seen in the context of a Broca's aphasia (see Chapter 4). In this case, they are associated with other impairments of oral expression (stereotype(s), reduction, agrammatism, word-finding difficulty) which may impede demonstration of an articulatory disturbance, at least in the period soon after onset. In fact, the most characteristic elements of the phonetic disintegration syndrome, in Broca's aphasia, are usually observed only after a certain period of evolution. They may then still be associated with other aphasic impairments of varying severity, but they may also appear as an isolated disturbance. An *anarthria*, said to be *pure*, is sometimes a residual of a Broca's aphasia. It is also possible, although exceptional, for an isolated articulatory disturbance to be immediately evident at onset, which may be either sudden or progressive, depending on the nature of the causal hemispheric lesion (see Chapter 9).

Despite their rarity, the isolated disturbances are of great theoretical interest. In these cases, as well as in those where the associated aphasic deficits are relatively mild, the most adequate auditory samples can be obtained for the systematic study of phonetic deviations, that is, for the study of the aphasic disturbance of the third phase of oral language[11] (see Chapter 2).

SYMPTOMATOLOGY OF ARTICULATORY DISTURBANCES—NEUROLOGICAL ASPECTS

The presence of an articulatory disturbance can usually be identified with relative ease. However, in some cases it may be absent or hardly notice-

---

* *Student's Lament*: Some aphasics coin words by the score.
It seems experts invent even more.
Linguistic profusion
Leads to such confusion,
I understand less than before. [B.B.]

able in *automatic language* (curses, prayers, naming the days of the week, productions linked to immediate emotional states or other elements of concrete situations). In contrast, the articulatory difficulty becomes clear in repetition, oral reading, conversation, etc. and becomes more severe as the psycholinguistic situation requires increasingly *voluntary* and *propositional* production. The presence or absence of this form of automatic-voluntary dissociation is probably related to differences in the physiopathology of the observed disturbances and in the localization of the causal lesions (see Chapters 8 and 15).

Alajouanine and his collaborators identified three types of motor impairment—*paretic*, *dystonic* and *dyspraxic*[10]—which can selectively affect the muscles of the larynx, pharynx, velum, tongue, lips or face. These three types of motor impairment of the buccophonatory organs, which correspond to three levels of motor system disorganization, may coexist in different combinations with or without a clear predominance of any single type. In certain exceptional cases, usually after a period of evolution rather than at onset, one or another of these types of impairment may be observed in a nearly isolated form which is then referred to as *paralytic anarthria*, *dystonic anarthria* or *apraxic anarthria*.

Paresis

The phonetic disintegration syndrome is related to the abnormal functioning of axial muscles, that is, those of the buccophonatory apparatus. Thus there is no need to introduce here the concept of left or right lateralization of the involved musculature, an assertion which applies to the paretic aspects of phonetic disintegration as well as to the dystonic and dyspraxic aspects. However, it is necessary to distinguish between articulatory deficits possibly related to right facial paralysis of the central type, which is usual during the first stages of evolution of the neurological disease, and the paretic impairment of phonetic disintegration. In our opinion, facial paralysis (right-sided, in the present case) results in noticeable articulatory impairment only in very severe cases. As for the paretic impairment of phonetic disintegration, it is especially evident, in speech behaviours, in the weakness of articulatory movements and in an inadequate tracheal airflow. In addition, certain patients may show the effects of weakness in movements of the velum and/or laryngeal muscles. When the disturbance is not related to the presence of a progressive disease, the paretic impairment may decrease in severity after a relatively short period. Progressive improvement is usually seen, leading to full recovery, a mild persisting disturbance or, most frequently, to the gradual appearance of a dystonic impairment.

Dystonia

Dystonic impairments may be evident at onset but this is unusual. In most cases, their appearance follows initial paretic phenomena, thus suggesting the occurrence of post-paralytic functional reorganization[12]. With the appearance of the dystonic impairment, the most characteristic speech productions of phonetic disintegration can be clearly observed, that is, the constituent movements of features are exaggerated in force and duration; the contraction and relaxation of muscles underlying speech production is, on the whole, delayed, brutal, global, synkinetic* and does not permit the fine gradations (simultaneous or rapidly successive) required for normal speech. Certain types of language therapy probably promote the transition from the paretic phase to the dystonic phase or at least accelerate the emergence of the latter and accentuate its characteristics (see Chapter 17). If well managed, this effect of therapy may be desirable as the productions are often more audible to the listener in the dystonic phase than in the paretic phase.

Articulatory disturbances of a paretic or dystonic type may appear as a result of brainstem lesions (*dysarthrias*) and, in this case, are often more severe than in most cases of phonetic disintegration. The problem of differential diagnosis will be discussed in a later section of this chapter.

Dyspraxia

The existence of a dyspraxia is presumed to explain the varying degrees of difficulty shown by some patients in the *voluntary* execution of fine articulatory movements, sometimes despite the absence of any evident paretic or dystonic

* Synkinetic movement: involuntary muscle contraction accompanying voluntary movement in another muscular area, for example, elevation of the lateral labial commissure during a wink.

involvement.* Since paresis and dystonia are not unique to the articulatory disturbances of aphasics, dyspraxic impairment is the most specific feature of phonetic disintegration. In other words, the phenomenon of automatic–voluntary dissociation which may be seen in phonetic disintegration, and sometimes in a striking fashion, is far more characteristic of its dyspraxic component than of its paretic or dystonic component (indeed, all impairments related to the presence of a dyspraxia are characterized by obvious variability).

Buccofacial apraxia

It is interesting, and no doubt significant from a physiopathological point of view, to compare the dyspraxic component of the phonetic disintegration syndrome, which is limited to movements of speech production, with the dyspraxic nature of buccolingual–facial movements during non-speech acts, phenomena which are grouped under the term buccofacial apraxia[13]. This type of apraxia, which by definition occurs in the absence of elementary sensory or motor disturbances, is apparent during the voluntary execution, in response to a verbal command or on imitation, of certain movements involving the muscles of the mouth and the face. Thus certain acts such as: protruding the tongue; blowing softly; whistling; pointing the tongue towards the nose, the chin, the edge of the lips; puffing the cheeks; sending a kiss; clacking the tip or the blade of the tongue against the alveolar ridge; making a noise to call a cat; imitating different emotional states, etc., may be very poorly performed whereas the same elementary movements are normally carried out in different *automatic* or *reflexive* acts (kissing a loved one, blowing out a match, licking the lips while eating, chewing, swallowing, etc.). A buccofacial apraxia is commonly associated with the phonetic disintegration syndrome whether it exists in a pure, or nearly pure state, as in anarthria, or whether it occurs in the context of a Broca's aphasia. In either case, a clear *clinical* distinction must be made between buccofacial apraxia and phonetic disintegration. This distinction is based on several different facts: there are cases, even though rare, in which buccofacial apraxia is not observed during the evolution of phonetic disintegration; in the usual (regressive) evolution, buccofacial apraxia decreases and disappears far more quickly than the articulatory disturbance; although very infrequent, the opposite dissociation may also be seen, namely the persistence of a buccofacial apraxia despite rapid regression or even the disappearance of phonetic disintegration; a buccofacial apraxia, different in certain respects from that seen in Broca's aphasia, one in which the phenomenon of automatic–voluntary dissociation (cf. p. 77) is particularly clear, may be associated with certain forms of Wernicke's aphasia and thus is not, strictly speaking, accompanied by any form of articulatory disturbance (see Chapter 4); in certain exceptional cases, subjects who are not, nor have ever been, aphasic may present a buccofacial apraxia. Thus a clinical distinction can be made between the dyspraxic component of phonetic disintegration and buccofacial apraxia. Nevertheless, a *physiopathological* distinction is not possible in all cases and, in the most characteristic patients, the dyspraxic component of phonetic disintegration appears to be the manifestation of a buccofacial apraxia within a group of particularly precise and complex acts, namely those of speech. In these patients, a buccofacial apraxia which is considered to have 'disappeared' can usually be seen to reappear as soon as the tasks are complicated by requiring the execution, not of elementary, isolated non-linguistic acts, but rather of arbitrary sequences involving the alternation of two or three of these elementary acts.

A clinical distinction should also be made between buccofacial apraxia and limb apraxia since they may, and frequently do, exist independently.

SYMPTOMATOLOGY OF ARTICULATORY DISTURBANCES—LINGUISTIC ASPECTS

General speech characteristics

At the onset of the phonetic disintegration syndrome, voluntary utterances may be totally impossible; in attempting speech, the patient shows desperate facial movements whose only result is the production of a hoarse and undifferentiated sound. If this is to be distinguished from language suppression and from a severe lin-

* This difficulty may be the source of transformations which are sometimes difficult or even impossible to distinguish from phonemic paraphasias on the basis of purely linguistic criteria (see Chapters 2 and 4).

guistic reduction (cf. pp. 52 and 78), then this severe form of anarthria—the only form that actually corresponds to the etymological meaning of the term—is extremely rare and its persistence is even rarer. In less severe forms, which are more distinctive because oral expression is possible and can be studied, speech is also usually accompanied by exaggerated and apparently irrelevant facial movements. The initiation of articulatory movements is clearly laborious and is often preceded by aborted movements (*phonetic approximations*). Most frequently, the movements are abandoned because they were inadequate but in some instances the beginning of a normal movement may also be aborted. When the dysfunction is dystonic, the output is irregular and explosive and the speech is syllabic and stressed. The flow of speech is considerably slowed and normal speech inflection is obliterated by the more or less uniform brusqueness of intersegmentary pauses. Besides this lack of inflection, and to a certain extent because of it, those prosodic features signalling emotional state or suprasegmental conventions (e.g., rising intonation at the end of a question) may be reduced or absent. These features are grouped under the name *aprosody* or *dysprosody* (cf. p. 79). However, it characteristically varies to a certain extent within the same individual and some patients present no, or very little, prosodic impairment either at onset or during the course of evolution. This is illustrated by a patient who, with the help of a wide repertoire of intonation patterns, was able to effect a significant increase in the amount of (suprasegmental) information conveyed by his impaired and laborious utterances. When a dysprosody is evident, it does not usually affect the individual characteristics of speech, nor those of regional accents. However, there are cases in which the latter may be more or less profoundly altered, sometimes giving rise to a *pseudo-accent*. For example, a French-speaking aphasic may gradually acquire an English pseudo-accent (if the articulatory disturbance is predominantly paretic) or else a German pseudo-accent (if the articulatory disturbance is predominantly dystonic). These rather spectacular prosodic transformations do not usually occur in the initial stages of anarthria. Rather, they are seen after more or less prolonged evolution and particularly, it seems to us, in patients who have participated in an intensive programme of articulation therapy (see Chapter 17). In certain patients, the pseudo-accent may constitute the final residual of the phonetic disintegration syndrome.

Phonetic transformations

The three following statements are generally true in regard to the phonetic transformations (see Chapter 2) seen in the most typical cases:

(a) Their frequency of occurrence is extremely variable in a particular patient at any given moment in the evolution of his disease. Phonetic transformations are greatly influenced by psycholinguistic conditions and their frequency increases as the language productions become increasingly propositional. However, the occurrence of any particular transformation is not obligatory even in the most propositional linguistic productions[7, 14]. Each is more or less probable—and this probability may be extremely high—depending on the phoneme considered, its contextual environment, and the respective severity of the dyspraxic, dystonic and paretic impairment. This variability emphasizes the difference in the meaning of these last two terms depending on whether they are applied to phonetic disintegration or to other types of articulatory disturbances (cf. pp. 65–69).

(b) They represent a simplification of articulatory motor production [(3.1)*/ɛksplwa→ ≃ɛspwa/, (3.2) /spɛktakl→≃pɛstak/or /≃paktak/†]. While undoubtedly corresponding to clinical reality, this classical statement must, in our opinion, be moderated. In fact, patients with phonetic disintegration may produce or attempt to produce phonemic sequences of considerable motoric difficulty (contextual phonetic complexity) [(3.3) /lavabo→≃alvalbo/, (3.4) /espjɛgl→≃ɛksplɛgl/, (3.5) /kapitalism →≃katila - lapitalikstœ/]. This is especially true of cases showing predominant dystonic and dyspraxic factors and in relation to aborted phonemic approximations followed by attempts at correction.

* All transcribed phonemic sequences preceding an arrow represent conventional words or phrases in French.

† In the written representation of phonetic transformations, the symbol ≃ appearing after an arrow indicates the approximate nature of the transcription of the abnormal segment.

(c) The patients are generally aware of the defective nature of their productions.

The articulatory simplifications of phonetic disintegration typically affect phonemes which can be described as *fragile*[10]. This characteristic may involve *natural fragility*, which is related to the complexity of the articulatory movements constituting a particular phoneme, or *positional fragility* subtended by remoteness from the syllable carrying the primary stress, by inclusion in a consonant cluster, particularly when the places of articulation of the juxtaposed phonemes are relatively distant from each other, etc. It follows that the conjunction of natural and positional fragility would increase the probability of a phonemic transformation of a given phoneme.

No matter how complex the context in which they occur, those phonemic transformations which are more or less clearly perceived as interphonemic substitutions are essentially described by reference to the constituent features of the phonemes considered individually (see Chapter 2, concept of the third linguistic phase[11]). The feature, or features, involved in the transformations are first identified and the nature of their abnormality is specified. The other phonemes in the immediate context are then considered and the factor, or factors, which could have promoted the transformation of the phoneme under consideration are identified. Consider, for example (3.6), the /b/ of /tɔ̃bato/ (*ton bateau*) in the case where the production would be, approximately /tɔ̃pato/ [/b→ ≃p/]. First, we would point out that the abnormality hinders the functioning of largyngeal muscles responsible for the adduction and vibration of the vocal folds (feature: *voiced*; natural fragility). Then we would define the characteristics of this abnormality—total absence of vibration, delayed onset of vibration, intermittent vibration, etc.—and subsequently ask whether this could be attributed to weakness of muscular contraction (paretic factor) or, conversely, to the occurrence of contractions which are poorly differentiated, too intense and/or too sustained (dystonic factor). We would next consider the possibility of an additional (assimilation) effect which the two *unvoiced* phonemes in the immediate context, /t - - t/, may exercise on this transformation through *devoicing* /t - - b - - t→≃t - - p - - t/ (contextual fragility: dyspraxic factor?).

Among the phonetic transformations which the listener perceives as interphonemic substitutions, those involving vowels are primarily seen in cases with predominant paretic and/or dystonic impairment. In the most typical patients, the transformations attributable to paresis, that is, to muscular activity which is too weak and/or regressive, are most frequently observed soon after the onset of the disturbance. Thus paresis provides an explanation of the tendency to produce *low* vowels in place of *high* vowels* or to *nasalize* vowels[15]. Because of the regressive nature of palatal buccolingual muscular activity, these vowel transformations may sometimes result in the production of *pseudodiphthongs* and *pseudopolyphthongs*[4, 10]. In contrast, the transformations observed in the prototypic phase† of phonetic disintegration are usually subtended by dystonia. They are therefore related to movements which have increased in intensity, often to the point where their force is excessive, and are characterized by buccophonatory muscular action which is too brusque, poorly differentiated, poorly synchronized and synkinetic. Thus dystonia provides an explanation of the phenomena of vowel *glottalization* or a tendency to produce *higher* vowels rather than normally *low* vowels as well as transformations of (French) *nasal* vowels into the corresponding *oral* vowels. In this last case [(3.8) /bɛ̃→ ≃bɛ/], it is probably the effects of the synkinesis which prevent differentiation of laryngeal and velar muscular activity. The dystonic vowel transformations may also result, although through a mechanism opposite to that characteristic of the paretic phase, in the production of *pseudodiphthongs* and *pseudopolyphthongs* [(3.9) /kɔ̃stitysjɔ̃→ kaɔɔ̃stitysjɔ̃/]. These often appear related to the behaviour of patients who attempt, as far as possible, to correct their phonetically abnormal productions as they occur.

Whether they are approximate or very clear, the interphonemic permutations or substitutions of patients with articulatory disturbances affect

* The articulation of many vowels may thus result in the production of a more 'neutral' sound [≃/œ/; 3.7) /ʀepyblik→ʀœpyblik/].

† Prototypic phase, in the sense used here, refers to that period of evolution in which the clinical picture includes symptoms recognized as characteristic.

consonants more frequently than vowels. The occurrence of approximate consonant transformations may be seen soon after onset when the articulation is dominated by a significant paretic component which has not yet been compensated by a dystonic post-paralytic reorganization, as well as in rare cases which show a persisting, nearly-isolated paretic impairment (paralytic anarthria). In these cases, the productions typically involve the approximate transformation of *stops* into *fricatives*, *orals* into *nasals* or even *unvoiced* into *voiced*.* The approximate nature of those paretic productions is easily seen in many transformations of the type *stop*→ ≃ *fricative*. Rather than an unequivocal fricative, the sound produced is often more of an *affricate* (initial occlusion followed by constriction). In contrast, difficulty in sustaining an intermediate position when the dystonic component later becomes predominant results in the replacement of *fricatives* by *stops* having the same place of articulation [(3.10) /siRo→≃tiRo/] or neighbouring places of articulation [(3.11) /ʃimi→≃kimi/]. Similarly, the dystonic factor explains the tendency *to oralize nasal consonants* which is seen in many patients with phonetic disintegration. The difficulty in maintaining the velum in an intermediate position or in terminating velar activity adds to the effects of the synkinesis between the velum and the larynx [(3.12) /m-a-ŋ-a-n-i-m-i-t-e →≃m-a-g-a-d-i-b-i-t-e/]. The replacement of *voiced* consonants by their *unvoiced* cognates, already illustrated in example (6) is also a usual feature of the dystonic phase of phonetic integration. This *devoicing* which is often partial or intermittent, is especially related to difficulty in the distribution of muscular effort between the larynx and the place of articulation. The tendency to transform consonants into *affricates*, which is analogous to the transformation of vowels into *pseudodiphthongs* continues during the dystonic phase. However this typically no longer occurs during the attempted production of *stops* but rather during the production of *fricatives*. Indeed, the approximate nature of dystonic productions is therefore particularly clear in transformations of the type *fricative*→*stop*. An initial occlusion, which creates the impression of an approximate substitution, is, in fact, frequently followed by more or less adequate constriction which is relatively too brief [(3.13) /s-a-k-R-i-f-i-s→≃s-a-k-R-i-f-i-ts-œ/, (3.14) /y-z-a-ʒ→≃y-dʒ-a-ʒ/]. In this type of dystonic transformation, the occlusion may occur after the constriction [(3.15) /p-ɔ-l-i-t-ɛ-s→≃p-ɔ-l-i-t-ɛ-st-œ/].

In general, phonetic transformations leading to approximate substitutions are often fostered by one or more occurrences of the substituting phoneme in the immediate context of the transformation [see example (6)]. This phenomenon is known as assimilation. The term *anterograde assimilation* or *reiteration* is used when the assimilating phoneme precedes the assimilated phoneme in the normal phonemic sequence [(3.16) /klaRte→≃klaRke/]. The terms *retrograde assimilation* or *anticipation* are used when the assimilating phoneme follows the assimilated phoneme in the normal phonemic sequence [(3.17) /dekuvɛRt→≃tekuvɛRt/]. In French-speaking aphasics, retrograde assimilation is usually more frequent than anterograde, perhaps because the tonic syllable in French is generally at the end of the word. The probability that assimilation—or all other phenomena determining the positional fragility of a given phoneme—will play a role in an interphonemic substitution is increased if the phoneme which may be assimilated is itself naturally fragile. The converse is equally true and also merits statement: there is an increased probability that a naturally fragile or *difficult* phoneme will be replaced by a non-fragile or *easy* phoneme having the same or a neighbouring place of articulation when the immediate context contains one or more easy phonemes which could act as assimilators.

The preceding discussion of pseudodiphthongs and affricates illustrated how certain transformations must be described in terms of *additions* as well as *substitutions*. There are other types of phonetic transformations, usually suggestive of a tendency towards the (physical) simplification of articulatory movements, which are described in terms of phoneme *additions*, *displacements* (*metatheses*) or *omissions*. The need for solid articulatory support at the start of a segment may, for example, explain the more or less systematic transformation of *vocalic initiation* into *consonantal initiation*[10]. This type of transformation may result from the omission of an initial vowel [(3.18) /ipɔtɛk→≃pɔtɛk/], the addition of a consonant before the initial vowel [(3.19) /yzaʒ→≃ʒyʒaʒœ/] or, again, the

* With regard to this last point, it is conceivable that certain phenomena involving the more or less complete devoicing of consonants, sometimes observed during the paralytic phase, may be related to insufficient vocal fold adduction.

displacement of a consonant to the initial position [(3.20) /admisjɔ̃→ ≃damisjɔ̃/]. Because the abrupt termination of sound production is particularly difficult for patients with phonetic disintegration, final consonants are frequently transformed into final vowels[10]. The transformation most often results in the addition of a vowel, usually /œ/ or a neighbouring one in French [see examples (5), (13) and (15)] but may also result in consonant omission or, less frequently, displacement. The particular difficulty associated with the production of clusters of consonants or vowels also results in omissions, displacements or additions which often produce a simpler phonemic sequence [for example, of the type consonant–vowel–consonant–vowel, etc.; see examples (20), (22), (23), (24), (26) and (27)]. With the exception of clusters in the syllable receiving the tonic accent (which are relatively preserved) the omission of consonants from clusters is a common phenomenon [(3.21) /admisjɔ̃→≃amisjɔ̃/, (3.22) /ɔgmɑ̃tasjɔ̃→ ≃ omɑ̃tasɔ̃/] but displacements are relatively infrequent [example (20), cited with regard to vocalic initiation, is equally applicable here]. Finally, the addition of a vowel, which in this precise case is called *epenthesis*, is very common [the added vowel is often /œ/ or a neighbouring one; (3.23) /ɔbʒe→ ≃ɔbœʒe/, (3.24) /klaʀte→ ≃klaʀœte/].

Although there is some variation among individual cases, a fair proportion of the deviations leading to phonemic additions entail the duplication of a phoneme in the immediate context. This phoneme, which is more often a consonant than a vowel, may precede or follow the position of the addition [(3.25) /afʀø→ ≃fafʀø/, (3.26) /kʀeatœʀ→ ≃kʀekatœʀ/]. These two examples illustrate, this time without substitution–assimilation, the phenomena previously described under the names of anticipation and reiteration. Inversely, in deviations involving phoneme omissions, the omitted unit is often one of two identical units appearing in close proximity [(3.27) /ɛ̃tɛstɛ̃→ ≃ɛ̃tesɛ̃]. The structural relationships between the phonemic constituents of the same word or simple syntagm clearly affect these different types of additions and omissions. The influence of structural relationships is also evident in displacements, in anterograde and retrograde assimilations and, a fortiori, in the more curious transformations which may result from a combination of several of these elementary operations [(3.28) /tʀaktœʀ→ ≃kʀatœʀ/: both displacement and assimilation]. Such transformations appear attributable to what Alajouanine and his collaborators called the dyspraxic component of phonetic disintegration[4, 10] and cannot, in any case, be considered the result of elementary paretic or dystonic impairment. As we have pointed out and illustrated by numerous examples [see examples (1), (2), (20) to (24), (27) and (28)], these transformations frequently result in articulatory simplification in the same way as most of the transformations which can be attributed to the paretic and dystonic components of phonetic disintegration. However, we have also mentioned and illustrated at the start of this section [see examples (3) to (5)] that such transformations do not always simplify articulatory acts and may even increase their apparent complexity. In some patients with phonetic disintegration, a certain number of these displacements, additions by anticipation or reiteration, assimilations and other forms of *sequencing errors* (cf. pp. 48–49) quite often occur in segments whose phonemic units, when considered individually, are perfectly pronounced. In our opinion there are then no available linguistic criteria to permit a distinction between these particular transformations and the phonemic paraphasias of certain Wernicke's aphasics (see Chapters 2 and 4). Stated more explicitly, the production of phonemic paraphasias attesting to a disturbance of the second linguistic phase is as characteristic of certain Broca's aphasias as it is of certain Wernicke's aphasias. A quasi-dogmatic position may be taken with regard to this subject, that is, it may be considered a particular application of Pierre Marie's law: *Broca's aphasia = Wernicke's aphasia + anarthria*[15].

ARTICULATORY DISTURBANCES IN APHASIA AND THE PROBLEM OF SO-CALLED PURE ANARTHRIA

There is no doubt that, in the vast majority of cases, phonetic disintegration constitutes only one of the elements of a Broca's aphasia. It is then associated with an aphasic disturbance of oral expression, a disturbance of writing and/or a buccofacial apraxia[13] as well as with other deficits. A Broca's aphasia entailing various disturbances besides impaired articulation may nevertheless evolve in such a way that, after a certain period, the phonetic disintegration exists in isolation. In very exceptional cases, pure anarthria (Insertion 3.1) may have a sudden onset, with preservation of written language (cf. pp. 204–209) and sometimes even without buccofacial apraxia. A progressive transition from pure anarthria to a more complete, but usually atypical, form of Broca's aphasia is also seen in the rare case of progressive lesions (see Chapter 9). These observations suggest that the articulatory realization of oral language is subtended by neurophysiological mechanisms, and therefore by neuronal nets, which are relatively distinct from those subtending symbolic formulation. The lesions causing anarthria have not yet been precisely determined[4], no doubt because of the scarcity of well-documented anatomoclinical studies (see Chapter 8–4).

DIFFERENTIAL DIAGNOSIS OF PHONETIC DISINTEGRATION AND THE DYSARTHRIAS

Only in very exceptional cases would a neurologist's diagnosis of aetiology and lesion site be based primarily on the analysis of an articulatory disturbance. The nature of speech disturbances is certainly considered but almost always in conjunction with other deficits (especially motor) observed during the neurological examination and with information reported in the anamnesis.* Thus the above heading is somewhat spurious in regard to medical diagnostics but does provide an opportunity to mention and briefly describe articulatory disturbances other than phonetic disintegration. This extension beyond the domain of aphasiology is explained by the general interest of most aphasiologists in non-aphasic speech disorders and by the possibility that students in speech pathology and phonetics may find it a useful elementary guide. Before turning to the *dysarthrias strictly defined*[17–20] we shall briefly discuss two concepts which we consider to merit separate treatment, namely *dysphonia* and *cortical dysarthria.*

Dysphonia

The dysphonias are disturbances of sound production affecting non-articulated sounds as well as speech sounds. They affect the quality of the voice and not that of articulatory production itself. They are mentioned here only as a reminder that dysphonia may accompany an articulatory disturbance in many cases of dysarthria.

Cortical dysarthria†

As used by certain authors, particularly Bay[9] (see Chapter 10), the term 'cortical dysarthria' refers to cases of pure or nearly pure anarthria in which the articulatory disturbance resulting from a left hemisphere lesion is characterized almost exclusively by paretic and/or dystonic impairment [i.e., cases showing very few abnormalities resembling phonemic paraphasias (cf. pp. 41–42)]. Other authors reserve the same label, and thus raise the issue of the differential diagnosis of cortical dysarthria,‡ for articulatory disturbances, usually of the paretic type, which sometimes occur in right-handers following certain right-hemisphere lesions.§ In both cases, the articulatory deficits grouped under the name of cortical dysarthria (slowed speech, imprecise articulation of consonants and consonant clusters, mild nasalization of certain consonants and vowels, etc.) do not vary between automatic and voluntary production, or at least are said not to vary in a striking manner. This being stated, it should nevertheless be noted that these abnormalities do not show the extreme regularity characteristic of the articulatory disturbances seen in dysarthrias resulting from brain stem lesions. This is probably related to the bilateral hemispheric representation of the phonoarticulatory organs. Bilateral representation may also

---

* Anamnesis: case history, that is, information provided by the patient or informant regarding his or her medical past and the history of the ailment.

† This term implies the existence of a dysarthria whose clinical characteristics are sufficiently definite that it can be unequivocally attributed to a cortical lesion. In our opinion, use of this term is rarely justified without radiological or necropsic verification.

‡ The term 'cortical dysarthria' merits reflection. From an etymological point of view, use of the word 'dysarthria', in place of 'anarthria', is fully justified. The reasons we have opted to use the latter are related to the traditions of the francophone community which, since Pierre Marie's time, contrasts anarthria, an articulatory disturbance frequently associated with aphasia and resulting from a left hemisphere lesion, with the dysarthrias, that is, other types of articulatory disturbances, especially those resulting from (various) brain stem lesions. Although use of the adjective 'cortical' corresponds to demonstrated clinical facts in certain cases, it is not always used appropriately (see Chapter 8).

§ Marie[21] long ago pointed out the occurrence of articulatory disturbances in right-handers following right- or left-hemisphere lesions (cf. p. 8). In both cases, he attributed them to subcortical lesions.

underlie the trend towards at least partial recovery which is seen in the majority of articulatory disturbances resulting from a unilateral hemispheric lesion.

The *dysarthrias, strictly defined*, show the following three characteristics:

(a) The disturbances are related to defective functioning of muscular groups involved in speech production. Thus a diagnosis of dysarthria implies the existence of a disturbance, usually organic but sometimes functional, of nerve structures which, with the exception of the cerebral cortex and its immediate afferents and efferents, participate in the control of the phonoarticulatory organs. The lesion of the nerve structures is usually bilateral.
(b) The disturbance is permanent and consistent and does not show a dissociation between automatic and voluntary productions.
(c) The patient is totally aware of the phonetic abnormalities in his speech.

Several different areas are normally assessed in the clinical examination of the dysarthric patient[18]: (a) respiration (intensity, amplitude, regularity, blockages, voluntary control, expiratory emission preceding the initiation of articulation, etc.); (b) voice (pitch, intensity, timbre, etc.); (c) resonance (hypernasality, nasal emission, hyponasality, etc.); (d) articulation (inaccurate place, insufficient occlusion or constriction, etc.); (e) fluency and (f) prosody. Clearly the examination of the buccophonatory organs is of prime importance. The discovery of a palatal cleft, trismus* or luxation† of the temporomaxillary joint occasionally provides a simple explanation of an articulatory disturbance which appeared disconcerting on casual observation.

The symptoms of dysarthria may have three different aspects: *paralytic*, *extrapyramidal* and *cerebellar*. Depending on the aetiology, a single aspect may be observed in isolation or, in the more usual case, the different aspects may be grouped in various combinations.

Paralytic dysarthria

Paralytic dysarthria results from lesions (generally bilateral) of the pyramidal tracts‡ and/or of certain bulbar motor nuclei or from a lesion of certain cranial nerves. The phonetic abnormalities observed are related to the weakness of buccophonatory muscles and to inadequate tracheal airflow. The principal speech characteristics shown by a patient having a paralytic dysarthria are: (a) a generally slow rate of speech resulting from the prolongation of individual phonemes, particularly vowels; (b) possible acceleration of the speaking rate during brief periods; this no doubt reflects the patient's deliberate attempts to 'say it all' in the course of a short expiration; (c) the beginning and end of phonemic segments are poorly defined and progressive, which explains the undifferentiated character of speech; the melodic line is always disturbed and the intonation is monotone (lack of variation in vocal intensity and timbre); (d) nasal resonance is excessive during production of nasal phonemes and weak contraction of the velar musculature may result in generalized hypernasality; (e) the vowels, which are excessively prolonged, are often modified or diphthongized; (f) consonants in running speech are also altered, voiceless phonemes may be replaced by voiced approximations and stops may be distorted by leakage of air at the place of articulation and/or by nasal emission.

In the most severe cases, the lack of phonetic differentiation, the weakness of articulatory movements and the monotonous intonation result in almost, if not totally, unintelligible mumbling. All the consonants tend towards the same nasalized sound resembling a /n/ without complete occlusion, and all the vowels, which are also nasalized, resemble the central nasalized (≃/œ̃/].

Partial paralytic dysarthrias may result from lesions of the cranial nerves involved in the motor control of the buccophonatory apparatus[22].

Among other functions, the facial nerve controls lip muscles and the buccinator muscle of the cheek which, on contraction, retract the labial commissure. Thus *facial nerve* lesions especially impair production of bilabial consonants (/p/, /b/, and /m/) and vowels requiring lip rounding (/u/, /ʊ/, and /o/). In severe bilateral paralysis, bilabial stops are produced as fricatives and

* Trismus: tonic contraction of the muscles of mastication.
† Luxation: displacement of organs or articular surfaces.
‡ An articulatory disturbance resulting from bilateral lesions of the rolandic cortex or of pyramidal fibres leaving the rolandic cortex is often called *pseudobulbar dysarthria* (cf. p. 68).

the labiodental fricatives (/f/ and /v/) are often omitted. These phenomena are related to insufficient intra-oral pressure, resulting from the weakness of the peribuccal musculature. Generally speaking, labial sounds are least impaired in the final position of a segment. The plosive element is then less important and a simple approximation of the lips may be sufficient to produce the vowel modification required to give rise to perception of a consonant (*coarticulation*).

Among others, the *glossopharyngeal nerve* innervates the superior constrictor muscle of the soft palate. Although isolated lesions of this nerve may result in disturbed deglutition, with regurgitation of foods into the nasal cavities, speech is usually unaffected even in the case of bilateral lesions. However, hypernasality may be observed if the lesion also affects the vagus nerve.

The *vagus nerve* provides part of the motor innervation to the pharynx (pharyngeal nerves) and larynx (superior laryngeal nerve, inferior or recurrent laryngeal nerve). Lesions of the vagus may result in voice disorders as well as in other impairments.

The *hypoglossal nerve* provides motor innervation to the tongue. A unilateral lesion gradually produces a slight, and transitory, distortion of consonants requiring particularly fine movements of the tongue tip, especially /s/ and /z/ (and, in certain francophone patients, of /ʀ/). Bilateral lesions result in a dysarthria of much greater severity and cause distortion of all tongue-tip consonants as well as a slowed rate of speech.

Extrapyramidal dysarthrias

The extrapyramidal dysarthrias are as varied as the numerous neurological syndromes which can be grouped for convenience under the label of *extrapyramidal syndromes*. The dysarthria appears as a parallel to disorders of motor automaticity affecting the rest of the body. Two major types of extrapyramidal dysarthrias can be distinguished, namely, hypokinetic and hyperkinetic dysarthrias.

Hypokinetic dysarthria, or *parkinsonion dysarthria*, is the commoner type. At onset, the disturbance is very mild and the speech appears monotonous, showing only occasional aphonia and acceleration of rate as well as some degree of articulatory imprecision. These cases are said to show *monotone tachyphemia* or *loss of the melody of language*. As the disease advances, speech becomes more severely affected, generally in parallel with (other) akinetic phenomena. The disturbance of speech, as of movement, involves difficulty of initiation, of accomplishment and of termination. The initiation is always laboured and characterized either by a type of blocking which results in silence despite the patients' evident attempts to express themselves, by a discontinuous, rapid vocalic utterance (most often: ≃/u-u-u . . ./) or by repetitive production of the first syllable of the word. Once speech is initiated, evident abnormalities include *tachyphemia*, a faint and somewhat high-pitched voice, and a near-total lack of prosody (utterances are produced in a single spurt with the phonemes nevertheless remaining fairly distinct). These rushes of speech, which are very characteristic of parkinsonian dysarthria, do not result in an overall increase of the rate of speech. The average number of words per minute is in fact reduced because of abnormally long pauses which are unrelated to the content of the utterances. The end of words or sentences may give rise to involuntary repetition of the last word or words. This phenomenon, known as *palilalia*, may be characterized by decreasing vocal intensity (*aphonic palilalia*).

In *hyperkinetic dysarthria*, as may be seen in bilateral athetosis, the predominant symptoms consist of synkinetic phenomena. When the patient speaks, synkinetic movements may affect not only the phonoarticulatory muscles but also spread to the face, neck or even limbs. Articulation is inadequate, weak and indistinct. The flow of speech is irregular, hesitant, slowed and subject to unpredictable involuntary variations. The voice is weak and abnormal in quality.

Cerebellar dysarthria

Resulting from certain lesions of the cerebellum and/or cerebellar pathways, cerebellar dysarthria is characterized by a slowed rate of speech and abnormalities of laryngeal functioning and of movements occurring at the place of articulation. Patients with cerebellar dysarthria display considerable difficulty in controlling laryngeal valving. Thus, during production of a single word or simple syntagm, the voice may be initially feeble and suddenly increase in intensity and remain at this level, or the voice may be abnormally loud at the start of the utterance and remain so through the entire segment. These excessive variations are distributed throughout the flow of speech and bear no relation to the normal prosody of the sentences. In some cases, the rate of speech is considerably decreased by the prolongation of almost all phonemes and by the abnormal lengthening of pauses. Other observed phonetic abnormalities are as follows: (a) voiced consonants, particularly stops, are totally or partially devoiced; (b) as a result of prolongation, the plosive burst of voiceless stops is exaggerated; (c) vowels are frequently diphthongized; and (d) the last phoneme of a segment is often prolonged by a faint sound. In certain patients the inability to achieve the required placement of the tongue results in successive and more or less accurate attempts at articulation, producing a type of *pseudo-stuttering*. In severe cases, the articulatory imprecision may result in almost totally unintelligible speech.

Several different neurological disorders may accompany a dysarthria or be manifested by dysarthria. A pragmatic dichotomy can be established between those which are observed frequently, almost daily, in neurology clinics, and those whose occurrence is much rarer or even exceptional.

Frequently occurring disorders

Five diseases or groups of diseases should be noted:

(a) *Pseudobulbar palsy* results from bihemispheric lesions, usually ischaemic vascular lesions (see Chapter 9), affecting pathways originating from the rolandic region and/or affecting this cortical region itself; more or less marked involvement of the grey matter nuclei is also fairly common. It is sometimes called the 'biopercular syndrome' when the lesion especially affects the two rolandic opercula. The dysarthria, which is one of the constituent features of the pseudobulbar syndrome (pseudobulbar dysarthria), is usually mixed, that is, is both paralytic and extrapyramidal.

(b) *Parkinson's disease* has a high incidence and the dysarthria which constitutes one of its manifestations is the prototype of the hypokinetic dysarthrias (cf. p. 67).

(c) Explosive scanning speech is one of the classically recognized symptoms of *multiple sclerosis*, especially in cases where the disease has evolved over a long period. The dysarthria of multiple sclerosis frequently shows associated paretic and cerebellar elements and its high frequency is related to the high incidence of pyramidal and cerebellar involvement in this disease.

(d) *Vascular or tumoral lesions* of the brain stem and/or cerebellum may be accompanied by a paralytic, cerebellar or mixed dysarthria.

(e) *Amytrophic lateral sclerosis* (Charcot's disease) generally affects nuclear and supranuclear bulbar structures, most commonly near the end of the disease progression but sometimes at an earlier stage. In either case, involvement of these structures is associated with a characteristic dysarthria which is at first paretic and spastic, resulting primarily in distortion of tongue-tip consonants, but which rapidly becomes paretic. Lingual atrophy may be substantial so that speech assumes a characteristic resonance. In the final stage of this progressive disease, the patient is often unable to produce any articulated sounds.

Less frequent or rare disorders

A dysarthria whose characteristics will vary according to the aetiology of the disease and site of lesion may be a feature of the clinical picture observed in a large number of relatively infrequent neurological diseases. Thus the following list is not exhaustive:

(a) *Complete bulbar pathology* (bulbar poliomyelitis, bulbar syringomyelitis, progressive bulbar palsy, etc.) generally results in a severe paralytic dysarthria.

(b) In *Parkinson's syndromes* of varied aetiology (vascular, toxic, tumoral, traumatic, infectious), both the dysarthria and the akinesis are less striking than in Parkinson's disease.

(c) *Cerebellar atrophies* of varied aetiology as well as *spinocerebellar heredo-degeneration* may cause the purest forms of cerebellar dysarthria.

(d) *Choreic syndromes, athetoid syndromes and hepatolenticular degeneration* (Wilson's disease) may include a hyperkinetic dysarthria whose characteristics reflect the motor disturbance affecting the body.

(e) In the absence of any lesions affecting the neural structures themselves, a dysarthria may be caused by a dysfunction at the level of the neuromuscular junction (*myasthenia gravis*). Myasthenic dysarthria is in many ways similar to paralytic dysarthria. However, a pathognomonic feature of myasthenic dysarthria is its usual disappearance after a period of rest (particularly on awakening in the morning) and its progressive accentuation as speech continues. It is only necessary to ask the patient to read a passage or recite a series of numbers in order to observe the appearance of the dysarthria and its progressive increase in severity, sometimes to the extent that the voice becomes totally inaudible.

(f) Finally, speech impairments observed during the course of *general paresis* (diffuse syphilitic meningoencephalitis) should also be noted and, in fact, merit separate consideration. Speech abnormalities, which may be absent during the repetition of syllables and short words and scarcely observable during the usual picture-naming tasks, are especially noticeable during the production of longer words and sentences. The abnormalities are often most marked at the middle of a word or sentence and typically appear as a hesitation, stumbling, or indistinct mumbling or, sometimes, a stop in speech production. In very severe cases speech may be totally unintelligible. Although elementary motor disturbances (particularly a nearly-constant labiolingual tremor) can certainly be observed in these cases, we do not consider use of the word 'dysarthria' to be particularly appropriate. It is, in effect, being applied to patients who also present deficits, which are often severe, of memory, attention, 'intelligence', and who often demonstrate writing disturbances which bear a curious resemblance to those of oral expression. In addition, articulatory disturbances showing characteristics quite similar to those of syphilitic 'dysarthria' may be observed during the course of other processes leading to diffuse brain pathology.

GRAPHIC DISTURBANCES OF APHASICS

In the preceding pages, the articulatory disturbances of aphasics were considered as a behavioural manifestation of an aphasic disorganization of oral expression (or more precisely, as a disorganization of the third phase of spoken language). Graphic disturbances will now be considered in an analogous fashion, that is, as a behavioural manifestation of an aphasic disorganization of written language (or more precisely, as a disorganization of the third phase of written language). We are aware that our linguistic subdivisions are somewhat artificial in regard to written language. However, we believe that they are supported by certain case studies and that this analysis is particularly useful in leading to clearer definitions of the behaviours studied. Thus the term 'graphic disturbance' will be used to designate a disturbance of the ultimate stage of writing, that is, of the gestural process through which a linguistic programme is executed with the help of a pen and a sheet of paper. Thus graphic disturbances are distinguished from literal, verbal or other types of paragraphic transformations which may also attest to a disorganization of written expression (see Chapters 2 and 4).

Certain precautions must be taken in the clinical examination of graphic disturbances. For example, it is essential to consider the patient's educational level and habitual use of writing as a means of linguistic expression, as well as the nature of premorbid writing (as judged from a sample of writing produced before onset of the disease). In addition, if there is an associated right hemiplegia, it is necessary to consider that left-handed writing in right-handers is generally inferior to that of the dominant hand (i.e., it is slower, more hesitant, laboriously executed, shows awkward graphic features, a tendency towards letter reversals,* etc.).

No matter which phase of written language is of interest, written productions are examined as closely in spontaneous writing as in transposition activities (copying, writing to dictation). It must also be determined whether patients can copy in transcribing the graphic code (for example reproduce a printed sentence in cursives), whether they can spell orally, whether they can 'write' with the aid of mobile letters, whether they show a parallel disturbance in the writing of words and letters as opposed to that observed with figures and numbers, etc. Finally, it is frequently

* Letter reversals, for example, S→Ƨ, B→ᗺ, E→Ǝ, etc., also called *mirror writing*. Mirror writing may sometimes be very systematic, involving reversals of all letters within a long passage.

interesting to study and compare productions obtained from the left and from the right hands[23]. These different aspects of the assessment of written language will be discussed in a later section of this book (see Chapter 15).

SYMPTOMATOLOGY OF GRAPHIC DISTURBANCES

In the context of a didactic presentation, we would have preferred to discuss the symptomatology of graphic disturbances according to the same plan as that followed in discussing articulatory disturbances. Two interrelated facts, both open to future neurolinguistic research, make such an approach almost impossible, given our presently limited state of knowledge. Whereas linguists have very precisely identified the inventories of units of the third linguistic phase of spoken language, the contents of the analogous inventories of written language remain unspecified. In addition, the articulatory impairments respectively related to paretic, dystonic and dyspraxic factors which disturb the functioning of the buccophonatory apparatus have been at least partially identified, whereas the graphic impairments respectively related to analogous factors which disturb the functioning of the dominant hand in writing movements remain poorly identified. It is nevertheless recognized that these factors may be associated, appear successively, predominate, or even act in a nearly independent fashion in causing a graphic disturbance. This lack of elementary taxonomic data will necessarily be reflected in our approach to the graphic disturbances of aphasics.

The behaviours observed vary according to the severity of the disturbance. In most severe cases, graphic activity regresses to simple rudimentary forms seen in pictorial attempts as frequently as in apparent attempts at writing. These scribbles, irregular and awkward traces and interwoven loops bear certain resemblances to very early graphic productions in childhood. Even in the most severe cases, it is not unusual that the patients remain able, somehow or other, to sign their names and perhaps even write their address, if it has not recently changed. In other cases, the output is slightly more abundant but production is very slow and laboured, significantly disturbed by a graphic clumsiness, by additions, omissions, displacements and distortions of graphic features

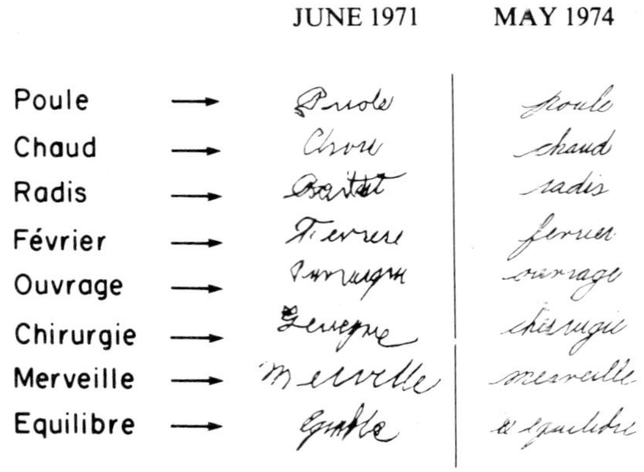

Fig. 3-1 *Graphic disturbance with impaired spelling (Case Ph.B). Cortical–subcortical softening of the left prefrontal convexity in a 49-year-old right-hander. The involved area includes the caudalmost part of the second frontal convolution. Words written to dictation: the first sample was obtained 14 days after the occurrence of a cerebral vascular accident and the second was obtained almost three years later: both samples were written with the right hand (see also Fig. 4-1 and 6-2, and Insertion 6.2).*

(cross-strokes, vertical lines, loops, etc.) which often result in unrecognizable letters (if it is still possible to speak of letters), and by perseverative phenomena which may involve features, letters, word-parts, words or sometimes groups of words. Between this extreme of a major graphic disturbance and normal writing, all intermediate degrees of severity may occur. In certain, infrequent, cases they may all be observed in a single patient, either during the development of a progressive disease (see Chapter 9) or, on the contrary, during an exceptionally favourable course of recovery. The latter was the case of a patient who received therapy and whose written productions are presented as an illustration (Fig. 3-1).

Besides these properly 'linguistic' characteristics, other aspects of graphic disturbances are equally significant from the point of view of clinical neurology and should therefore be noted.

The graphic disturbances of aphasics are almost always observed in the context of a severe quantitative and qualitative reduction of written language. Even in the case of extremely favourable evolution, the premorbid fluency of written language is very rarely recovered. In fact, the patient typically shows a certain, permanent aversion towards writing comparable with that which is often seen in adults presenting a developmental dyslexia–dysgraphia.

In addition to the impaired combination of features into letters, the disturbance frequently affects the spatial arrangements among letters, among words and among lines. In other words, there is often a loss of the *automatisms* of writing (regular linear arrangement, similarity of intervals between letters, words, lines, indentations and alignments, etc.). These phenomena are sometimes referred to as *spatial agraphia.*

An aphasic's written productions may sometimes show occasional letter reversals. Although this is extremely rare, it has been pointed out that during the waning of left-hemisphere disease, a right-hander may spontaneously begin to produce rather long segments of *mirror writing.*

The problem of pure agraphia seldom arises in clinical aphasiology. Observation of different patients generally leads to a conception of graphic disturbances either in relation to a more or less complex configuration of aphasic symptoms (see Chapter 4) or in relation to the presence of an apraxia (see Chapters 4 and 16).

GRAPHIC DISTURBANCES AND APHASIA

Like the articulatory disturbance, the graphic disturbance in Broca's aphasia is usually severe.* In certain patients, at a given period in the evolution of their aphasia, the articulatory and graphic disturbances are of equal severity and constitute the predominant expressive symptoms. In others, the former is very severe and the latter is scarcely observable, this dissociation being most frequently seen during the course of evolution (cf. p. 89, nearly pure anarthria). More frequently, in a patient whose articulatory disturbance is lessening, the graphic disturbance continues to reduce writing to a meagre scribbled production or to perseverative behaviours, regardless of the hand used in writing. In cases where writing shows a more favourable evolution, the output may gradually become more abundant and sufficiently well formed to allow the emergence of other aphasic features to be observed: verbal and orthographic deviations, agrammatism and sometimes even neologisms and jargonagraphia [see examples (4.2) and (4.3), p. 88]. These last cases are of obvious theoretical interest.

In the same way that the production of phonemic paraphasias may be completely dissociated from that of phonetic transformations (cf. p. 41), aphasic misspelling may be completely dissociated from a graphic disturbance[24]. Either or both of these dissociations may be present immediately after the onset of certain forms of Wernicke's aphasia (see Chapter 4): one then sees phonemic transformations in the absence of articulatory difficulty and/or orthographic deviations in the absence of a graphic disturbance. It is not unusual for an analogous tendency to develop during a favourable course of recovery in certain forms of Broca's aphasia. In this case, improvement of articulation is more advanced than recovery from the phonemic disturbance and/or the recovery of graphism is more advanced than that of orthography. In this type of evolution, transformations affecting the second linguistic phase become progressively easier to identify and therefore to study.

The opposite dissociation of written language, namely the occurrence of a graphic disturbance in the absence of aphasic misspelling, is very seldom seen in right-handers with left-hemisphere lesions. Should it be present it is, in fact, difficult to recognize. Frequently occurring graphic transformations involving omissions, additions, displacements and substitutions of features often result in productions similar in form to transformations involving literal paragraphia [(3.29) (G)→(C), (3.30) (V)→(N) or (W), (3.31) (F)→(E), (3.32) (P) or (R)→ (B), etc.]. Their physiopathological significance does not appear essentially different from that of the omissions, additions, displacements and substitutions of features which result, in the same patients, in the production of literal neosegments such as a four-legged 'M', an 'E' with an extra horizontal line, a 'Q' with two cross strokes, etc. Although many written 'spelling' errors may thus result from a graphic disturbance, it is generally not the case that all the spelling errors of patients with such a disturbance can be attributed to their graphic difficulty. Misspellings are also apparent, although less numerous than in conventional writing, in oral spelling and in writing with the help of mobile letters.

Even though a qualitative and quantitative reduction of written expression is the rule in the different clinical forms of Wernicke's aphasia, and may sometimes be as severe as in Broca's aphasia, graphic activity itself is less frequently

* Broca's aphasics often have a right hemiplegia and sometimes a left-limb apraxia. Thus the study of graphic disturbances may be very difficult.

disturbed. When a graphic disturbance is present, it can generally be attributed to an associated apraxia. There is, however, an exception to this rule involving the possible production of literal neosegments as well as various other types of paragraphic and neologistic transformations. This will be discussed in a later section of this book (see Chapter 4, Type III, Wernicke's aphasia) as will the effects—which are generally very mild—of *word blindness* on graphic activity (cf. p. 116).

GRAPHIC DISTURBANCES AND APRAXIA

Various disturbances of movement may be seen in the neurology clinic. They are identified as an apraxia when they are unrelated to deficits of muscular strength, muscle tone or coordination, to the presence of involuntary movements (tremors, etc.) during performance of the intended movement or to disturbances of sensitivity or auditory language comprehension. This apraxic type of abnormal behaviour affects only the execution of voluntary movements. Ideally, it is necessary to observe that a movement may be carried out in certain circumstances but not in others in order to conclude with absolute certainty that the movement is apraxic. Thus it may be impossible for a patient to demonstrate a grasping movement in response to a verbal command (which was understood), although his hand movements are normal when spontaneously grasping an object, thereby attesting to the integrity of the elementary sensorimotor systems subtending this gestural production.

In many respects, the abnormal buccophonatory or manual linguistic movements constituting the various aphasic expressive disturbances appear to parallel the abnormal non-linguistic movements constituting the various clinical forms of apraxia[13]. Moreover, there are certain cases in which the distinction established between these groups of disturbances appears more related to the clinically convenient vocabulary used to label them than to a demonstration of their essentially different nature. While we think it relevant to present the problem in these terms, the role of apraxia in the origin of the expressive disturbances observed in aphasia is even more difficult to specify because the usual distribution of cerebral lesions is such that the different clinical forms of aphasia are often associated with those of apraxia. In the first section of this chapter, buccofacial apraxia was discussed in relation to the articulatory disturbance of Broca's aphasics. The apraxia which frequently affects movements of their upper limbs can be similarly discussed in relation to their graphic disturbance[25]. When the apraxia is considered in conjunction with right-handed writing by a right-hander with a left cerebral lesion (see Chapter 8), it must be asked whether or not the praxic component adds to the effects, which vary during the course of evolution, of a more elementary disturbance determined by the usual presence of an associated right hemiparesis.

The relationship between apraxia and the other forms of aphasia are equally intricate. In regard to graphic disturbances, the different aspects of the problem would ideally be delineated by case studies in which such disturbances affect all modalities of writing and drawing in the absence of an associated impairment of oral spelling. If such cases exist, they are extremely rare. In fact, the left parietal lesions which are often the source of apraxias in right-handers typically cause an aphasic disorder as well, so that the interpretation of writing deficits in terms of aphasia and apraxia then becomes very tenuous. We shall return to this problem when discussing those forms of Wernicke's aphasia which may be accompanied by a major graphic disturbance (see Chapter 4). In the meantime we should point out that the distinction between aphasic and apraxic disturbances remains valid from a clinical point of view since clear dissociations are sometimes observed. Thus a limb apraxia may be seen in the absence of a significant graphic disturbance or graphic activity may be impaired in the absence of a significant disturbance in non-linguistic movements of the limbs.

THE PROBLEM OF SO-CALLED PURE AGRAPHIA

It is undeniably true that the vast majority of graphic disturbances observed in clinical aphasiology constitute only one symptomatological element of aphasia which includes many others. However, since the 1881 publications by the Austrian physiologist, Siegmund Exner[26], there has been discussion concerning the possible occurrence of an isolated disturbance of written expression in a right-hander following a left hemisphere lesion of the caudalmost part of the

Insertion 3.1

When considered from a theoretical point of view, pure anarthria and pure agraphia are each defined by a triple dissociation in linguistic behaviour.

In *pure anarthria*

Language comprehension is normal but linguistic expression is disturbed.

Within the domain of linguistic expression: written expression is normal but oral expression is disturbed.

Within the domain of oral expression: the first and second phases of spoken language are normal but the third phase is disturbed.

In *pure agraphia*

Language comprehension is normal but linguistic expression is disturbed.

Within the domain of linguistic expression: oral expression is normal but written expression is disturbed.

Within the domain of written expression: the first and second phases of written language are normal but the third phase is disturbed.

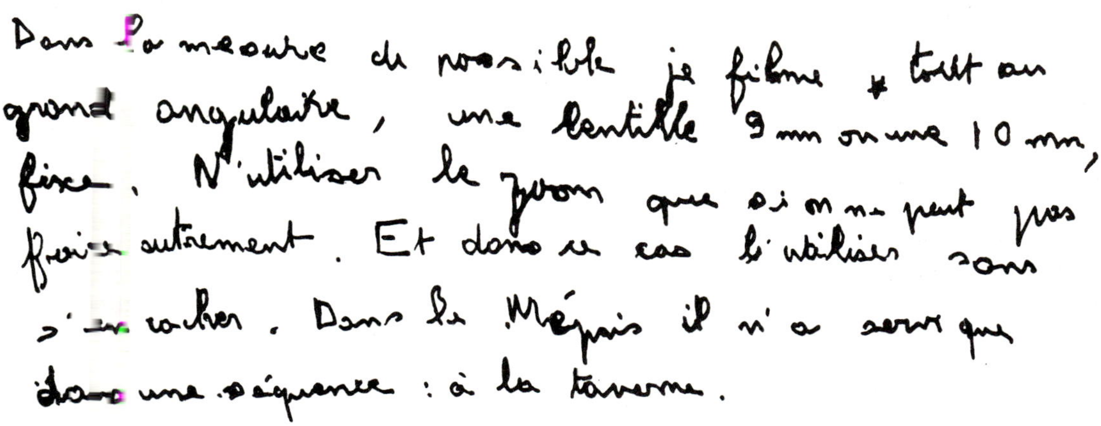

Fig. 3-2 *An isolated writing disturbance: pure agraphia (Case R.M.). A small haemorrhage of the left internal capsule in a 45-year-old right-hander. Attempted writing with the right hand three days after the occurrence of a cerebral vascular accident.*

second frontal convolution (see Chapters 6 and 8), a disturbance which would be seen in writing produced by either hand and would not be accompanied by any other aphasic or apraxic disturbance. Such would be, according to certain authors, the clinical picture of *pure agraphia*. In this conception, the ideas of aphasia and agraphia are compared and the latter is viewed as the equivalent to a Broca's aphasia which only affects written language. In our opinion, this conception of pure agraphia does not correspond to clinical reality.* At most, it can be argued that, after a period of favourable evolution, the graphic disturbance of certain Broca's aphasics is clearly predominant in the general clinical picture† (see Chapter 6). On the other hand, the ideas of anarthria and agraphia have also been compared and the latter viewed as the equivalent, in written language, of pure phonetic disintegration, that is, as a disorder affecting only graphic

* If one insists that this conception of pure agraphia is theoretically valid, then it must be conceded that the probabilities of cerebral lesions are such that it almost never occurs.

† More often, as has already been mentioned, the predominance of the writing disturbance is shared with that of the articulatory disturbance.

activity (Insertion 3.1). We have observed such a clinical picture on some occasions[24] (Fig. 3-2). Certain left parietal lesions (partial involvement of the angular region) may also give rise to a clinical picture which is clearly dominated by a graphic disturbance; one which will be discussed elsewhere in this book (cf. p. 94).

REFERENCES

1. Klippel, M. M. (Ed.) (1908) Compte rendu de la réunion de la société neurologique de Paris du 11 juin 1908: discussion sur l'aphasie. *Revue neurologique*, **16,** 611.
2. Klippel, M. M. (Ed.) (1908) Compte rendu de la réunion de la société neurologique de Paris du 9 juillet 1908: discussion sur l'aphasie (suite). *Revue neuroligique*, **16,** 974.
3. Klippel, M. M. (Ed.) (1908) Compte rendu de la réunion de la société neurologique de Paris du 23 juillet 1908: discussion sur l'aphasie (fin). *Revue neurologique*, **16,** 1025.
4. Lecours, A. R. & Lhermitte, F. (1976) The 'pure form' of the phonetic disintegration syndrome (pure anarthria); anatomo-clinical report of a historical case. *Brain and Language*, **3,** 88.
5. Dejerine, J. (1914) *Sémiologie des affections du système nerveux*. Paris: Masson.
6. Head, H. (1926) *Aphasia and Kindred Disorders of Speech*. London: Cambridge University Press.
7. Donnel, F. J. & Darley, F. L. (1970) Phonemic variability in apraxia of speech. *Journal of Speech Research*, **13,** 556.
8. Hécaen, H. (1972) *Introduction à la neuropsychologie*. Paris: Larousse.
9. Bay, E. (1957) Theorie und Empirie bei der Klassifikation und den Untersuchungsmethoden der aphasischen Störungen. *Psychiatrie und Neurologie*, **134,** 298.
10. Alajouanine, Th., Ombredane, A. & Durand, M. (1939) *Le syndrome de désintégration phonétique dans l'aphasie*. Paris: Masson.
11. Buyssens, E. (1967) *La communication et l'articulation linguistique*. Paris: Presses Universitaires de France.
12. Twitchell, T. E. (1951) The restoration of motor function following hemiplegia in man. *Brain*, **74,** 443.
13. Alajouanine, Th. & Lhermitte, F. (1960) Les troubles des activités expressives du langage dans l'aphasie; leurs relations avec les apraxies. *Revue neurologique*, **102,** 66.
14. Marcie, P., Hécaen, H., Constans, J. P. & Chodkiewicz, J. P. (1969) Etude spectographique de la parole chez deux malades après ablation de méningiome de la région du pied de la troisième circonvolution frontale gauche. *Revue neurologique*, **120,** 350.
15. Malmberg, B. (1966) *La phonétique*. Paris: Presses Universitaires de France.
16. Poncet, M., Degos, C., Deloche, G. & Lecours, A. R. (1972) Phonetic and phonemic transformations in aphasia. *International Journal of Mental Health*, **1,** 46.
17. Darley, F. L., Aronson, A. E. & Brown, J. R. (1969) Differential diagnostic patterns of dysarthria. *Journal of Speech Research*, **12,** 246.
18. Darley, F. L., Aronson, A. E. & Brown, J. R. (1969) Clusters of deviant speech dimensions in the dysarthrias. *Journal of Speech Research*, **12,** 462.
19. Grewel, F. (1957) Classification of dysarthrias. *Acta Psychiatrica Scandinavica*, **32,** 325.
20. Peacher, W. G. (1950) The etiology and differential diagnosis of dysarthria. *Journal of Speech Disorders*, **15,** 252.
21. Marie, P. (1926) *Travaux et mémoires*. Vol. I. Paris: Masson.
22. Bastron, J. A. and the Neurologists of the Mayo Clinic (1956) *Clinical Examination in Neurology*. Philadelphia and London: W. B. Saunders.
23. Geschwind, N. & Kaplan, E. (1962) A human cerebral deconnection syndrome. *Neurology*, **12,** 675.
24. Lecours, A. R., Bérubé, L., Courtois, G. A. & Lhermitte, F. (1972) Recherches sur le langage des aphasiques: 3. Désorganisation de l'expression orale et désorganisation de l'expression écrite; une étude comparative de deux cas d'aphasie. *Encéphale*, **61,** 208.
25. Liepmann, H. & Maas, O. (1907) Fall von linksseitiger Agraphie und Apraxie bei rechtsseitiger Lähmung. *Journal für Psychologie und Neurologie* (Leipzig), **10,** 214.
26. Exner, S. (1881) *Untersuchungen über die Lokalisation der Funktionen in der Grosshirnrinde des Menschen*. Vienna: Wilhelm Braumuller.

BIBLIOGRAPHY

Arseni, C. & Botez, M. I. (1960) Considérations physiopathologiques sur l'apraxie faciale. *Revue neurologique*, **102,** 664.

Assal, G., Chapuis, G. & Zander, E. (1970) Isolated writing disorders in a patient with stenosis of the left internal carotid artery. *Cortex*, **6,** 241.

Bouman, I. & Grunbaum, A. A. (1930) Uber motorische Momente der Agraphie. *Monatschrift für Psychiatrie und Neurologie*, **77,** 223.

Clément, M. & Twitchell, T. E. (1959) Dysarthria in cerebral palsy. *Journal of Speech Disorders*, **24,** 118.

Critchley, M. (1952) Articulatory defects in aphasia. *Journal of Laryngology*, **66,** 1.

Dordain, M., Degos, J. D. & Dordain, G. (1971) Troubles de la voix dans les hémiplégies gauches. *Revue de Laryngologie* (Bordeaux), **3–4,** 178.

Dubois, J., Hécaen, H. & Marcie, P. (1969) L'agraphie 'pure'. *Neuropsychologia*, **7,** 271.

Geschwind, N. (1964) Non-aphasie disorders of speech. *International Journal of Neurology* (Montevideo), **4,** 207.

Herrmann, G. & Pötzl, O. (1926) *Uber die Agraphie und ihre lokaldiagnostischen Beziehungen*. Berlin: Karger.

Leanderson, R., Persson, A. & Ohman, S. (1970) Electromyographic studies of the function of the facial muscles in dysarthria. *Acta Oto-laryngologica* (Stockholm), **263**, 89.

Lebrun, Y. (1967) An articulation problem. *Handelingen van het 26ste Vlaams Filologenkongres*, **279.**

Lebrun, Y. (1957) Remarks on dysarthria. *Acta Neurologia Belgica*, **67,** 835.

Leischner, A. (1950) Uber Störungen des Stenographieren. Ein Beitrag zur Agraphie. *Archiv für Psychiatrie und Nervenkrankheiten*, **185,** 271.

Leischner, A. (1957) *Die Störungen der Schriftsprache* (*Agraphie und Alexie*). Stuttgart: Thieme Verlag.

Lenneberg, E. H. (1964) Speech as a motor skill with special reference to nonaphasic disorders. *Monographs of the Society for Research in Child Development*, **29,** 115.

Mahoudeau, D. (1950) Considérations sur l'agraphie, à propos d'un cas observé chez un traumatisé du crâne porteur d'une lésion des deuxième et troisième circonvolutions frontales gauches. *Semaine des Hôpitaux de Paris*, **26,** 1598.

Mahoudeau, D., Davis, M. & Lecœur, J. (1951) Un nouveau cas d'agraphie sans aphasie révélatrice d'une tumeur métastatique du pied de la deuxième circonvolution frontale gauche. *Revue neurologique*, **84,** 159.

Marce, L. V. (1856) Sur quelques observations de physiologie pathologique tendant à démontrer l'existence d'un principe coordinateur de l'écriture. *Mémoires de la Société de Biologie*, **3,** 93.

Mounin, G. (1970) *Introduction à la Sémiologie*. pp. 135–148. Paris: Editions de Minuit.

Nathan, P. W. (1947) Facial apraxia and apraxic dysarthria. *Brain*, **70,** 449.

Ottonello, P. (1949) Contributo alla conoscenza dell'aprassia costruttiva. *Rivista di Patologia Nervosa e Mentale*, **70,** 475.

Sabouraud, O., Gagnepain, J. & Chatel, M. (1971) Qu'est-ce que l'anarthrie? *Presse médicale*, **79,** 675.

Shankweiler, D. P., Harris, K. S. & Taylor, M. L. (1967) Electromyographic studies of articulation in aphasia. *The Haskins Laboratories Status Report on Speech Research*, *SR-9*, 1 and 16.

Vendrell Brucet, J. & Vendrell Gomez, P. (1974) Una aproximación metodológica al estudio de la praxis bucofonatoria en la afasia. *Revista de Neurologia*, **5,** 123.

Whitty, C. W. M. (1964) Cortical dysarthria and dysprosody of speech. *Journal of Neurology, Neurosurgery and Psychiatry*, **27,** 507.

4. Clinical Forms of Aphasia

'Uh! I still can't talk! Four languages: impossible! Italian: still a half. German: ... English: me, the first language, but impossible! Why? I can't. While me ... my, son, him, he's ... English: perfectly. And Russian. Russian: but like me! And now, me, impossible! Why? Yes, of course, I know words but sentences have had it. While German, it's still good. I was even an interpreter. While English, me to have ... now impossible. I'm blocked or I don't know, me. French, yes. French especially. Some words. I can't unhook. I can't.

(*Conversation with Mr Vi.; September 1969*)

This chapter is intended to familiarize the reader with the symptom complexes characteristic of those forms of aphasia which are most frequently seen in clinical neurology. Preparation of such a chapter naturally presupposes the prior selection of an aphasia classification scheme. Since classifications are almost as numerous as are famous aphasiologists (see Chapter 10), such a selection might at first appear difficult. However, within the context of this book it seemed natural to adopt the empirical classification which is both the oldest and still the most widely used by neurologists. Following the tradition of the French school[1], we shall thus speak, primarily, of Broca's aphasia and of Wernicke's aphasia. In addition to perpetuating the memory of two great pioneers in aphasiology (see Chapter 1), the use of these labels has the advantage of avoiding particular prejudices concerning the anatomopathology, the physiopathology or the psychopathology of these two basic forms of aphasic behaviour.*

This chapter will be almost exclusively devoted to clinical aphasiology, that is, to the description of aphasic behaviours. The first of three principal sections will consist of a general review of aphasic symptomatology[2]. In the second section, we shall identify certain clinical subgroups whose identity is more or less obvious. In distinguishing among Broca's aphasics and, even more clearly, among Wernicke's aphasics, we shall borrow heavily from our own publications[3,4] and from those of Hécaen[5] and Geschwind[6]. Finally, we shall provide certain information concerning the neurological and neuropsychological signs which are often associated with aphasia, emphasizing those which influence linguistic behaviour and may occasionally raise problems of differential diagnosis. Having intentionally omitted reference within this chapter to other aphasia classifications, we shall return to them later (see Chapter 10) both to discuss certain theoretical aspects and, because the phenomena classified remain the same, to point out major similarities and differences.

Because of the customary distribution of cerebral lesions which cause the aphasias (see Chapters 8 and 9), their symptomatology is usually composite. However, certain disturbances may be clinically present in a nearly isolated state. It will be readily understood why we shall attach great importance, both here and elsewhere in this text (see Chapters 3 and 5), to the discussion of those forms of aphasia which involve a partial

* We should no doubt explain why we avoid use of the terms 'motor aphasia' and 'expressive aphasia' as synonyms for Broca's aphasia and the terms 'sensory aphasia' and 'receptive aphasia' as synonyms for Wernicke's aphasia. Although it is true that Broca's aphasics usually present a severe disturbance of linguistic expression, it can also be demonstrated, through the use of appropriate tests, that many of them are also impaired in language comprehension. Similarly, while it is true that a marked comprehension disturbance is observed in the most frequent forms of Wernicke's aphasia, several different expressive aspects are also clearly abnormal.

and nearly specific disorganization of linguistic behaviour. It is precisely from such cases that one may hope to identify certain aspects of linguistic functioning subtended by (relatively) independent physiological systems. It is also in such cases that conclusive anatomoclinical correlations can usually be established (see Chapter 8).

SYMPTOMATOLOGY OF THE APHASIAS

The symptomatology of the aphasias will be discussed under four headings which have been adopted for expository convenience and not to suggest the absolutely independent existence of the anatomophysiological mechanisms in question, a suggestion which would be clearly erroneous. Thus we shall discuss disturbances of oral expression and then those of spoken language comprehension, disturbances of written expression and then those of written language comprehension. Before following this classic scheme in providing an inventory of recognized signs of aphasia, it is useful to point out certain general features which characterize the whole of aphasic linguistic behaviour and attest to the enormous complexity of underlying physiopathological events.

In the same subject, and at the same moment in the evolution of his or her disease, the aphasic symptomatology may be, wholly or partially, more or less apparent according to certain characteristics of the language produced and the situation in which production occurs. For example, it is well known that certain linguistic segments having a high frequency of usage and a limited propositional value (curses, prayers, social expressions, etc.) may be normally uttered by a patient whose language nevertheless becomes clearly aphasic as soon as its propositional focus becomes more definite (picture description, comments on the news, answers to precise questions, etc.). Clinical aphasiology will also permit observation of the typical case in which a given word cannot be evoked by an aphasic during a somewhat abstract task but is pronounced with no hesitation a few seconds later in the context of a particularly concrete extralinguistic situation. For example, a patient unable to produce the word 'door' during a naming test may tell someone to 'close the darn door' when later bothered by a draft of air. These and related phenomena have long been recognized and grouped by Alajouanine under the name of the *Baillarger and Jackson automatic–voluntary dissociation*[1, 7]. While observation of aphasics will provide some spectacular examples of this automatic–voluntary dissociation, it will also demonstrate that all intermediate points are possible between the *automatic* and *voluntary* poles of linguistic activity. Speaking generally, it can be stated that language related to objects, actions or concrete situations is, on the whole, 'less aphasic' than language expressing more abstract ideas. Similarly, it is also generally true that linguistic productions are increasingly transformed as their semantic and syntactic complexity increases, and are increasingly 'normal' as the words and expressions produced are characterized by a higher frequency of usage in the aphasic speaker's linguistic community.

Other factors also enter into play. For example, the variability of aphasic behaviour in different states of 'fatigue' and the adverse effects of temporal stress are well known. Similarly, the patient's cultural background, particularly his premorbid linguistic habits (e.g., preferred use of a particular branch of the lexicon or of particular grammatical constructions) give his aphasia an individual colour. Thus work-related vocabulary may, for example, be well preserved in a particular patient as a consequence of its high frequency of usage, and perhaps also of a significant emotional investment in work, whereas subordinate and relative clauses are more adequately produced by another patient who enjoyed lectures and discussions. Most of the phenomena mentioned above can be readily recognized as a pathological exaggeration of features commonly observed in the linguistic behaviour of normal subjects (see Chapter 14).

ORAL EXPRESSION

The clinical signs of aphasia are particularly numerous and varied in oral expression. It is important that they be precisely recognized and evaluated, both qualitatively and quantitatively, since a diagnosis concerning the clinical variety of aphasia, and thus the localization of causal lesions (see Chapter 8), is largely based on such an evaluation. Several aspects of spoken language behaviour must be systematically studied.

Suppression and other disturbances of fluency (reduction and logorrhoea)

The term 'suppression' refers to a total absence of linguistic expression. It is observed only in those forms of aphasia associated with an abrupt onset and vascular or traumatic aetiology[8] (see Chapter 9). In the great majority of cases the suppression is transient and typically evolves towards a form of reduction which is both qualitative and quantitative. Thus suppression appears to represent the extreme form of such a reduction[8].

As soon as a certain amount of oral language is produced, objective measurements are desirable and should be taken with regard to the number of words per unit time, phrase length, the number of words produced between pauses, etc.[9]. However, in most cases such measurements are not required in order to judge whether an aphasic's speech is meagre, slow and laboured (*quantitative reduction*), or conversely, is easily produced and quantitatively normal or even—seemingly—more abundant than normal (*logorrhoea*). This simple step indicates one of the essential characteristics of the aphasic disturbance which an observer is attempting to identify.

Qualitative reduction and stereotypes

The term 'qualitative reduction' refers to an immediately apparent decrease in the number of different words remaining available. In certain forms of aphasia, a qualitative reduction is always paired with a quantitative reduction and an associated articulatory disturbance is then the rule, although there are exceptions. In other cases, a qualitative reduction, almost exclusively involving lexical words, coexists with a quantitatively abundant production.

The phenomenon of reduction may be so marked that possible productions are limited to a few phonemes or to one or a few words or automatic expressions which are emitted as soon as the patient attempts to communicate through spoken language. These residual productions are known as verbal stereotypes. Broca's famous patient who could repeat only /tã-tã/[10] illustrates a particularly frequent form of verbal stereotype consisting of a repeated syllable. It is, for example, quite common to see a reduction to a 'yes-yes-yes' as representing a condensation of all the patient's capacities for linguistic expression. With the onset of his aphasia, Baudelaire was reduced to '*Cré nom*' (a French abbreviation for Sacred Name of God); another literary figure treated more recently by Alajouanine[2] could repeat only '*Bonsoir les choses d'ici-bas*' (Good evening, things of this earthly world) during several months; and the key phrase for one of our patients was '*C'est encore mieux ce soir*' (It's even better tonight). Jackson[11] pointed out that the linguistic content of stereotypes may be related to the patient's thoughts or language at the moment he or she suddenly—this characteristic is constant—sustained the cerebral lesion. This fact can sometimes be documented through the case history as, for example, with one of our patients whose stereotype was '*ai bien dit*' (told you so) which repeated the essential idea of the last phrase she said to her husband before the occurrence of a car accident which left her aphasic. Finally, we should note the case of certain aphasics who manage, through a surprising range of prosody, to invest their stereotype with a certain, although very limited, communicative efficacy[1].

Word-finding difficulty

As used in aphasiology, the term 'word-finding difficulty' refers to the patient's trouble, or often failure, in producing the appropriate word in the course of a given linguistic activity. There are several reasons why this phenomenon is particularly evident in relation to nouns and predicative* adjectives[4]: (a) their absence in a sentence is immediately obvious; (b) the use of multipurpose verbs masks word-finding difficulties involving predicates; (c) the absence of attributive† adjectives is usually imperceptible; (d) naming specifically requires the production of substantives, etc. Although partially related, the concept of word-finding difficulty differs in many respects from that of a qualitative reduction. In the clinical varieties of aphasia which include this type of reduction, it is a general characteristic of all forms of linguistic activity. In contrast, word-finding difficulty may predominate in a particular activity, for example, in naming. Word-finding difficulty is always evident when

* Predicative adjective: the house is BIG (*adjectif attribut* in French).

† Attributive adjective: the NEW house ... (*adjectif épithète* or *adjectif qualificatif* in French).

there is a reduction but the converse does not hold (elaborated, but inadequate, linguistic productions, i.e., circumlocutions and periphrases, may constitute a spontaneous attempt to palliate word-finding difficulty which, by definition, is not the case in regard to qualitative reduction).

The clinical situations in which word-finding difficulty becomes obvious can be roughly classified under two headings: either the stimuli leading to the observed linguistic expression are generally imprecise and numerous responses are possible and relatively unpredictable or, conversely, the stimuli are very specific and the possible responses are either unique or very limited in number. Free conversation is the typical example of the first type of situation and naming of stimuli from the external environment is a good illustration of the second. Narration of a well-known story and word evocation guided by a conceptual or formal requirement (e.g., animal names, words beginning with a given letter) constitute intermediate situations.

In conversational language [see example (28)] and in narration, word-finding difficulty is manifested by repetition of determiners, prepositions and other functional units (see Chapter 2), by numerous aborted sentences (the word-finding difficulty is then perceived as a blank in the sentence), by the frequency and length of pauses, as well as by a large number of vocal mannerisms ('uh', for example). It may also be indicated by more or less adequate periphrases and by various verbal and neologistic transformations[12]. On naming tasks involving visual, auditory or tactile stimuli, word-finding difficulty is manifested by delays in responding, circumlocutory responses and by various types of paraphasic and neologistic responses.

The severity of the word-finding difficulty may vary, depending on the abstractness and picturability of the words to be produced, their frequency of usage in the linguistic community or in professional language, their membership in a particular lexical or grammatical category, etc.

When word-finding difficulty is manifested, the examiner can try to facilitate production through different procedures[13]. The common feature of all these techniques is that they are aimed at the elicitation of a productive automatism or at the limitation, to different degrees depending on the word, of the number of possible responses (see Chapters 15 and 17).

Word-finding difficulty forms part of the clinical picture of nearly all clinical forms of aphasia (cf. pp. 86–101). Depending on the case, it predominates in one particular type of linguistic activity rather than in another; it is manifested by silences and delays rather than by paraphasic productions, or vice versa; it is more or less susceptible to facilitation through different procedures; etc. In other words, word-finding difficulty is clearly not related, in all the clinical forms of aphasia, to the same physiopathological mechanisms[2].

Dysprosodies

The word 'prosody' refers to a complex phenomenon which includes several different elements: emotional tone, regional variations, tonic accent in certain languages, other suprasegmental conventions such as the rising intonation at the end of a sentence indicating a question without rearrangement of word order, etc. Although most regional variations are usually resistant to aphasia—only a few words, even distorted, are necessary to distinguish among francophone aphasics from Marseilles, Brussels and Montreal—aphasia may severely alter the melody of the language, a disturbance referred to as dysprosody or even aprosody. It is typically observed in cases of a significant articulatory disturbance. Speech is then slow, syllabic and monotone; emotional tone and suprasegmental melodic conventions are considerably attenuated. During the course of evolution, the predominance of certain types of phonetic transformations may result in the superimposition of a pseudoaccent (cf. pp. 60–61). Even in the absence of an articulatory disturbance, a dysprosody may appear secondarily as the patient realizes that voluntary slowing of speech and a tendency to syllabification increase his control of his linguistic production. This type of phenomenon may often be related to aphasia therapy (see Chapter 17). Finally, it should be noted that patients who produce a great deal of jargon show very rich prosody which sometimes appears inappropriate. For example, a rising interrogative intonation may be observed at the end of a sentence whose content is clearly affirmative. While such instances can rarely be identified with absolute certainty, they are no doubt frequent in certain patients and, in line with the aphasiological vocabulary already discussed (see Chapter 2), can be named 'dysprosodic transformations'.

Aphasic transformations of spoken language

Because of their significance and their great interest for neurolinguistic research, the symptomatology of aphasic transformations of spoken language were treated separately in other chapters of this text. The concept of a phonetic transformation was previously defined and the articulatory disturbance distorting the language of the great majority of Broca's aphasics has been discussed in detail (see Chapters 2 and 3) [see also examples (3.1) to (3.28)]. Phonemic transformations were also discussed and amply illustrated [phonemic paraphasias—see (2.13) to (2.22)—and formal verbal paraphasias—see (2.24)], as were monemic paraphasias [see (2.25) to (2.38)], neologisms [see (2.39) and (2.81)], verbal transformations [verbal paraphasias of a semantic type—see (2.40) to (2.47)—and preferred words—see (2.48) to (2.51), etc.] and syntagmic paraphasias [see (2.52) and (2.53)]. Paralexias [see (2.69) and (5.6) to (5.41)] have either been or will be discussed in detail.

When analysing the patient's behaviour, it is always important to specify which types of transformations are observed and in which types of linguistic behaviours they occur (conversation, repetition, reading, etc.) (see Chapter 15). The predominance of one type of transformation in a particular type of behaviour may provide valuable information concerning the physiopathology of the observed disturbance (see Chapter 8).

Jargonaphasia, dyssyntaxia and agrammatism

For the same reasons mentioned in regard to aphasic transformations of language, the expressive symptomatic features designated as jargonaphasia, dyssyntaxia and agrammatism were defined and illustrated by characteristic examples in another section of this work [see (2.83), 2.88) to (2.90)].

COMPREHENSION OF SPOKEN LANGUAGE

The aphasic behaviours observed in oral expression are remarkable because of their richness, or, more precisely, because of the precision with which they can be described despite their variety. In contrast, the behaviours related to a disturbance of spoken language comprehension are characterized by their scarcity, or rather by the imprecision with which they are usually described by the examiner. To a large extent, this difference depends more on the nature of tasks used in testing language comprehension, and thus on the ingenuity involved in preparing such tasks and the relevance of the analyses carried out, than it does on the patients' generally limited behavioural diversity. Thus the examiner must attempt to differentiate the behaviours in terms of qualitative and quantitative parameters, an undertaking which is particularly difficult because of the numerous and varied factors which must be considered.

As on identification-by-pointing tasks (see Chapter 15), the observed behaviour—although it must be considered with respect to latency, need for stimulus repetition, corrections, etc.—may lend itself to quantitative evaluation in terms of the number of correct or erroneous responses. In other cases, only a global and uncertain judgement may be possible, one which is sometimes as dependent on the experience and insight of the observer as on the patient's actual abilities to understand spoken language. Such is the case, for example, in attempts to evaluate the extent to which the patient considers an interlocutor's interventions during conversation, as indicated by more or less appropriate responses.

A disturbance of spoken language comprehension may or may not be clinically manifest depending on the tests presented[14]. For example, in the case of an identification-by-pointing task, the disturbance may be revealed only if the correct picture must be selected from a group of conceptually related pictures (apple, banana, orange), or pictures whose names are similar in form (pie, fly, tie), whereas the disturbance is not evident, or is much less apparent, when the selection must be made among very different pictures (apple, fly, bolt).

Depending on the type of aphasia, the recognition of the auditory constituents of spoken language may or may not be impaired, that is, there may or may not be an element of word deafness, a form of auditory agnosia (see Chapter 5). When present, this disturbance naturally interferes with comprehension of spoken language. Comprehension may also be disturbed in the absence of any word deafness and repetition is then normal. To facilitate discussion, we shall contrast an *agnosic disturbance* of spoken language comprehension with a *psycholinguistic disturbance*. When the impairment is almost exclusively of the latter type, sentences are generally better understood than are isolated words: this is probably related to the fact that, in sentences, word meanings are specified through their relationship with each other so that the message is somewhat redundant. In contrast, when impaired comprehension is related to an agnosic disturbance (regardless of whether or not it is considered to be aphasic in nature), comprehension of single words, which are simpler sensory messages than are sentences, is generally better than that of sentences.

Sentence comprehension may itself be dependent on numerous factors. There is little risk of error in stating, for example, that there is an optimal rate of speech beyond and above which the aphasic may experience serious difficulties in understanding. Similarly, sentences are generally better understood in the absence of significant background noise, particularly that of general conversation. The grammatical nature of key words which must be identified relative to the task at hand may also be important: for example, the patient must understand substantives when asked to select particular objects whereas understanding of prepositions—a potentially more difficult linguistic unit for all aphasics—is required in the context of a multiple-choice procedure in which the patient must identify the relationship between two objects (the pencil 'on', 'under', 'in' the box). Finally, success or failure may be related to the syntactic and semantic complexity of the stimuli: the use of more or less frequent and automatized expressions, the concrete or abstract nature of the signified concepts, their unity or multiplicity and whether or not the patient must deduce an implicit conclusion from several juxtaposed notions. Thus, when studying the patient's comprehension of a text read to him, it is quite common to observe relatively good understanding of the meaning of the individual sentences but an inability to grasp the general meaning of the entire passage, a phenomenon which is called a *disturbance in the comprehension of wholes* (*trouble de la compréhension des ensembles*).

The patient's ability or inability to repeat to himself, with or without perceptible participation of the buccophonatory apparatus, may certainly influence his response to a relatively complex command. Similarly, success or failure in responding may sometimes depend on the patient's ability or inability to interpret prosodic or gestural cues (if the observer has not taken care to eliminate such cues, as far as possible, from the stimuli), to read the examiner's lip movements (*speech reading* or *lip reading*) to consider any non-linguistic contextual information inherent in the testing situation, etc.

The patient's state of fatigue—that is, the degree of functional exhaustion of the neuronal networks governing residual linguistic functioning—plays a spectacular role in many cases. The patient's performance may be within normal limits during the first part of a test and then deteriorate; he/she then shows an apparent decrease of *attention* and perseverative phenomena appear (repetition of the same behaviour despite the nature of the stimulus). A few seconds of relaxation often permit a temporary return to the initial level of performance.

The time provided for the understanding of directions[15] and their repetition or non-repetition are also crucial factors.

Certain anomalies observed in clinical neurology may be erroneously interpreted as signs of disturbed comprehension. For example, if the patient's behaviour is studied in terms of relatively complex gestural responses to verbal commands, it must be recognized that inadequate responses can result from a praxic disorder[6] (cf. p. 102) as well as from a disturbance of spoken language comprehension.

WRITTEN EXPRESSION

Aphasia is usually present as a disorder which affects linguistic expression in general and is then evident in both written and spoken language for the same reason. Although there are exceptions, whose number and theoretical significance cannot be ignored, written language is often more severely disturbed than spoken language and, in cases of favourable evolution, the recovery of written language is generally slower and less complete. Many of the possible reasons underlying this difference can be readily evoked: (a) written language is acquired later than spoken language and may therefore be more fragile; (b) in quantitative terms, most people produce less written than spoken language so that written language acquisition may be less firmly anchored; (c) written language is generally more propositional than spoken language and often includes a greater variety of words and syntactical devices, with relatively complex syntactical constructions being more frequent and *fixed syntagms* (ready-made expressions) being less frequent.

Even in certain cases of aphasia where it could logically be expected that written language would be relatively spared, the occurrence of a marked disturbance may be partially explained by the fact that a disorganization of spoken language may have greater or lesser secondary effects on the organization of written language. During language development, written language is, in fact, acquired through systematic associative learning which is based, at least for a long period, on reference to the oral code; during adult life, the relative independence of written language from spoken language probably varies among different individuals. If reading and writing are habitual activities in daily life and involve syntactical structures and semantic concepts which are seldom or never included in oral linguistic exchanges, then the anatomophysiological substratum of written language could conceivably acquire, with time, a relative independence from that of spoken language. However, if, as is probably true in the majority of cases even among the generally most literate populations, reading and writing are only rarely practised after a relatively short period of formal education and are used only in repeating the themes and forms of usual conversational language, the anatomophysiological substratum of written language may retain those features which were characteristic during development, that is, it remains highly dependent upon that of spoken language[16] (see Insertion 8.2). Be that as it may, the aphasic symptomatology of written expression includes nearly the same elements as that of oral expression[17].

Disturbances of fluency

The written productions of aphasics who do not present a graphic disturbance may sometimes be quantitatively normal or nearly normal. Although each patient's linguistic background must be considered, it is, however, generally true that the written productions of aphasics are much decreased (quantitative reduction) relative to those of normal subjects. The suppression of written linguistic expression is more frequent and is more often permanent than is that of oral language.

Qualitative reduction

The qualitative reduction of written language is usually similar to that of spoken language in aphasics who show such a reduction. However, it is not exceptional for the former to be immediately more obvious than the latter. A qualitative reduction in the absence of a severe quantitative reduction is less frequently seen in the case of written production than in the case of oral production.

Although relatively rare, two possible dissociations should be mentioned. In the first, which is seen in certain Broca's aphasics, the flow of oral expression is greatly reduced relative to normal, and a severe qualitative reduction is apparent. However, in written expression, the patient's behaviour resembles jargonagraphia, and while a qualitative reduction is certainly present it is masked to some extent by the production of neologisms and all types of paragraphic transformations. The opposite phenomena are seen in the second, and more frequent, dissociation shown by certain Wernicke's aphasics. In these cases, oral production consists of copious aphasic jargon, which may partially mask the presence of a qualitative reduction, whereas written production is meagre and qualitatively very reduced.

Word-finding difficulty

The concept of word-finding difficulty was discussed earlier in this chapter in relation to aphasic disturbances of oral expression. Generally speaking, the same statements are also valid in regard to the symptomatology of written expression. However, we should point out the possibility of a relative dissociation between oral and written production in patients whose difficulty or inability to produce words is primarily related to an instrumental (motor) deficit and is manifested by delays or failures to respond. In such cases, one of the two expressive modalities, usually the oral modality, may then be more effective. Such a dissociation is sometimes particularly evident in naming and word-fluency tasks (see Chapter 15).

Aphasic transformations of written language

For the same reasons cited in regard to oral language, aphasic transformations of written language were also discussed in other sections of this text. Graphic disturbances were the topic of a discussion which paralleled that of articulatory disturbances (see Chapter 3). It was mentioned that they could vary widely in severity and that mild graphic disturbances are characterized by the production of transformed units, although features of normal written language can be recognized and may be sufficiently numerous to permit the identification of most of the transformed letters (Fig. 4–1).

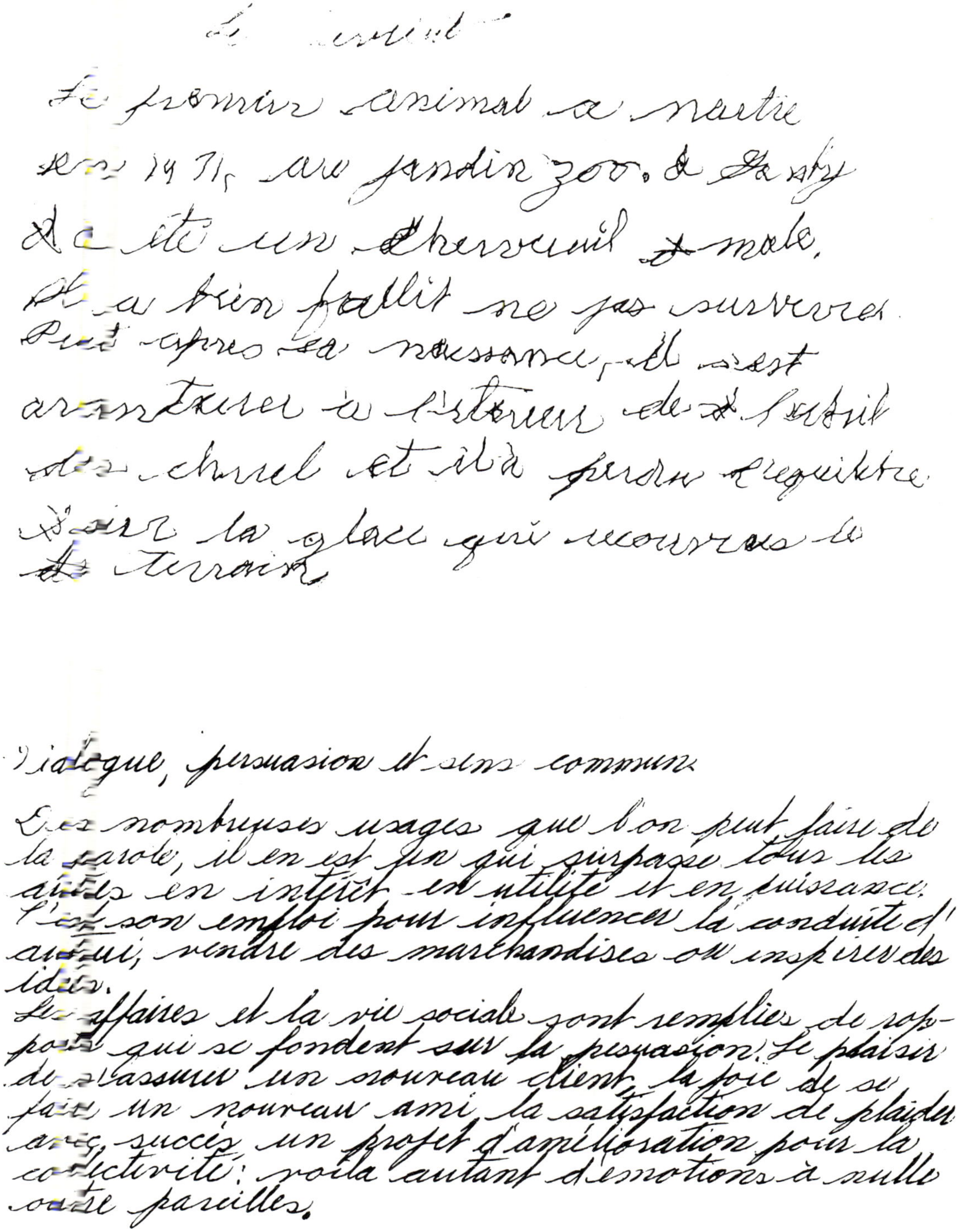

Fig. 4-1 *Graphic and orthographic impairment (Case Ph.B.). Cortical-subcortical softening of the left prefrontal convexity in a 49-year-old right-hander. Texts written to dictation. The first sample was obtained 16 days after the onset of the cerebral vascular accident and the second was obtained almost three years later. Both samples were written with the right hand.* (*See also Fig. 3-1 and 6-2 and Insertion 6.2.*)

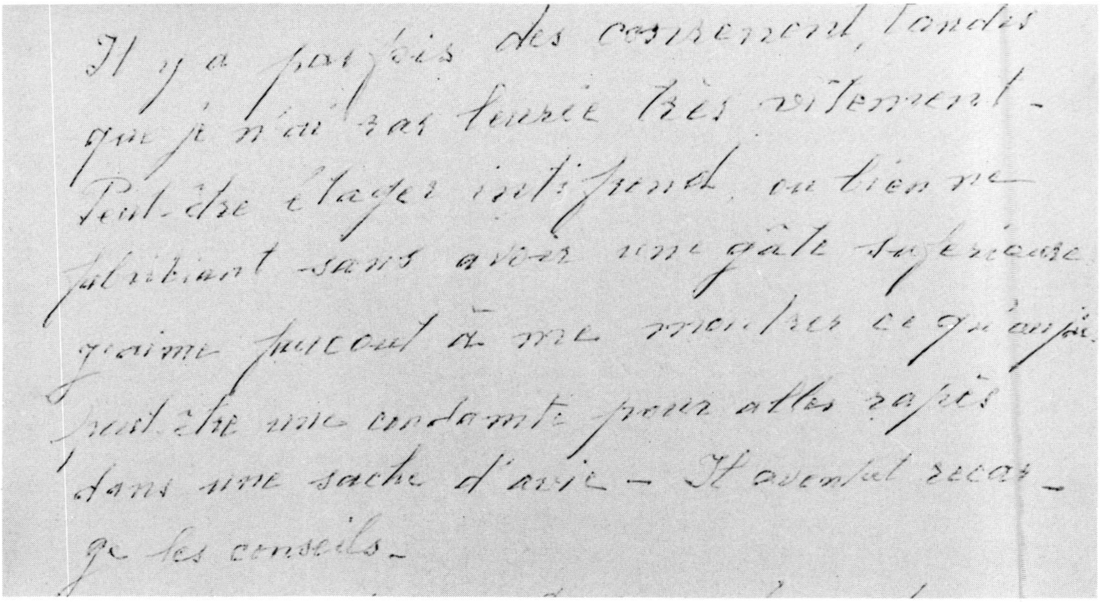

Fig. 4–2 *Jargonaphasia with preservation of graphic skills and automatisms of written language (Case F.F.). Softening in the left, posterior sylvian region in a 76-year-old right-hander. Attempted writing with the right hand. This sample was previously quoted in (2.85).*

In contrast, severe cases are characterized by such gross distortions, and usually by perseverative phenomena, that the production is almost unrecognizable as an attempt at writing. We should also note that graphic activity and automatisms of written language (in several languages, including French and English: horizontal arrangement proceeding from left to right, indentation of the first line of a paragraph, approximately equal spaces between words and between lines, etc.) may be astonishingly well preserved in the productions of patients who nevertheless present a severe jargonagraphia (Fig. 4–2) [see also example (2.85)].

The concepts of orthographic deviations [literal paragraphias—see examples (2.54) to (2.59)—and graphemic paragraphias—see examples (2.60) to (2.65)], verbal paragraphias [see (2.66)], written neologisms [see (2.85)], etc. were also defined elsewhere. When analysing the patient's written productions it is always important to specify which types of transformations are observed and in which types of productions they occur. The predominance of a given type of written transformation in a particular type of production (spontaneous writing, writing to dictation, copying) may constitute, although only in rare cases, the most interesting symptomatological element in the clinical picture of an aphasia. In cases where samples of conversational speech and spontaneous writing are sufficient to permit comparisons, a certain correspondence between the paraphasic and paragraphic transformations can often be seen: the disorganization of the first and/or second phase of written language then parallels the corresponding disorganization of oral language.* Some dissociations are nevertheless possible (cf. p. 99). They are most often seen in transposition activities, particularly when the disorder mainly affects the second linguistic phase. For example, phonemic paraphasias may be rare during repetition whereas literal or graphemic paragraphias are frequent when writing to dictation [see examples (43) to (52)]; or again, the opposite dissociation may be observed when the second phase of oral language is particularly disturbed. As indicated in the preceding chapter, graphic activity is frequently normal despite numerous spelling transformations but the occurrence of the opposite dissociation is exceptional (Fig. 3–1 and 4–1).

* This does not imply that, for a given segment, there is usually a one-to-one correspondence between the units of the spoken and written productions. Such a correspondence is, in fact, extremely rare.

Jargonagraphia, dyssyntaxia and agrammatism

The three terms 'jargonagraphia' (Fig. 4-2), 'dyssyntaxia' and 'agrammatism' were defined elsewhere [see (2.82), (2.85), (2.88) and (2.89)]. When patients with jargonaphasia can write, they usually jargon in writing as well. Here again, surprising dissociations are occasionally observed, as in the case of patients whose conversation includes few paraphasias or neologisms but whose written expression is clearly jargoned [see (31)]; or in the even more exceptional case of patients whose written language contains few segments suggesting jargon but whose spoken language contains so many that it becomes almost totally incomprehensible [see example (30)]. These dissociative phenomena are seldom part of the clinical picture at the onset of an aphasia. Rather, they generally become apparent in the course of evolution and it is likely that, in certain cases, various procedures of aphasia therapy may play a role in their development. Furthermore, the second of the above dissociations has important theoretical implications: it indicates that, in such a case, the phonological code, which determines the graphemic code, is in fact preserved; the oral jargonaphasia is no doubt related to a disturbance of those patterns which originate from the phonological code and serve to activate the sensorimotor networks of verbal articulation, which are themselves spared by the lesion.

In forms of aphasia showing a tendency towards dyssyntaxia (*paragrammatism*), it is not uncommon for this to be immediately more apparent in written than in spoken language [see (2.82) and (4.27)]. In our opinion, this reflects, among other factors, the fact that the syntax of written language is generally more complex than that of everyday speech. On the other hand, when agrammatism forms part of the clinical picture of an aphasia, it is almost always observed to be equally manifest in oral and written expression (provided that sufficient samples may be obtained in each modality, which is not always possible).

COMPREHENSION OF WRITTEN LANGUAGE

The general considerations previously discussed in regard to spoken language comprehension are, on the whole, applicable to written language comprehension. Nevertheless, certain specific features should be pointed out. They are primarily related to the fact that the linguistic stimuli used in studying aphasics' comprehension abilities do not involve the same sensory channel (auditory in one case and visual in the other) for the two usual receptive language modalities.

If the functional mapping of the brain and the usual distribution of brain lesions are such that an isolated agnosic disturbance of spoken language comprehension (*pure word deafness*) occurs only in very exceptional cases, they are also such that the corresponding agnosic disturbance of written language comprehension occurs in a pure state (*pure word blindness*) (see Chapters 5, 8 and 9) somewhat more frequently. Furthermore, it is not uncommon to observe either of these disturbances within a more complex symptomatological context. An agnosic disturbance of written language comprehension is recognized by the fact that the identification of visually presented linguistic units becomes more accurate with increasing simplicity of the sensory message[18]. For example, isolated letters are more accurately identified than words which, in turn, are more accurately identified than sentences. In contrast, in a psycholinguistic disturbance of written language comprehension, simple sensory messages, which convey relatively little information, generally give rise to more abnormal behaviours than do more complex sensory messages which convey more information but are also more redundant. This is well illustrated by the behaviour of certain patients who are able to understand, or partially understand, written sentences but are unable to identify written letters. When patients show near normal comprehension of written language in conjunction with a severe disturbance of spoken language comprehension, or present the opposite dissociation, it can be concluded that the comprehension disturbance is primarily related to an agnosic impairment. In contrast, psycholinguistic disturbances almost always affect the comprehension of spoken and written language in a parallel manner.

When comparing the patient's comprehension of spoken language with that of written language, it is necessary to consider not only his or her cultural background but also certain inherent differences between the tests used to assess comprehension of spoken and written stimuli (see Chapter 15). For example, in tasks involving the matching of pictures and words, or responses to questions through a multiple-choice procedure, the visual stimuli remain exposed while the auditory stimuli do not. The relative permanency of the linguistic stimuli facilitates correct responses—as well as reviews and corrections—in the case of written language but this facilitation is absent in the case of spoken language (even when the examiner repeats the stimuli).

It is obvious that oral reading (i.e., reading aloud) is generally not a prerequisite to the comprehension of written messages. When oral reading clearly facilitates comprehension by an aphasic subject, it may be suspected that he or she circumvents a comprehension difficulty by supplementing the visual information with its auditory counterpart. However, there is often little relationship between the oral reading of a message and its comprehension: aphasics commonly transform written messages at either the phonetic, phonemic or even verbal level and yet clearly demonstrate that the message was understood, or at least sufficiently understood to permit responses which are not clinically abnormal. The opposite dissociation, namely failure to understand despite accurate oral reading, is less common.

BROCA'S APHASIAS

The Broca's aphasic is laconic. The qualitative reduction of his language is obvious. He presents an articulatory disturbance. His speech is slow, laboured, often syllabic and the prosody of his propositional productions may be greatly reduced. He may evolve towards agrammatism. His comprehension of usual, everyday language is normal or nearly so.

THE COMMON FORM OF BROCA'S APHASIA

The clinical picture emerges rapidly, almost always following a cerebral vascular accident or cerebral trauma (see Chapter 9). A complete linguistic suppression is quite common at onset; its duration may be long or short but total and irreversible mutism is exceptional. On the other hand, the permanent reduction of linguistic behaviour to a verbal stereotype is less rare. In some cases showing a verbal stereotype, the patient may achieve control of its production after a period of evolution and progressively reacquire some words and common expressions. These re-acquired units may sometimes, and most often temporarily, behave as stereotypes, that is, they are produced more or less indifferently without regard to the propositional content of the linguistic situation. They may also be related to the situational context through prosodic features. The recovery process may stop at this point and the patient shows no further improvement. In more favourable cases, the inventory of available words is gradually enriched, the reduction becomes less severe and language becomes increasingly propositional. At this time, a certain number of cases begin to evolve towards agrammatism.

Agrammatism is never present at the onset of a Broca's aphasia but is rather a behaviour which emerges during evolution. It is no doubt a manifestation in linguistic behaviour of the brain's adaptation to the presence of the type of circumscribed cerebral lesion which causes Broca-type aphasias (see Chapter 8). Experience has convinced us that intensive language therapy may foster the emergence of agrammatism in patients who, in the absence of therapy, would not have progressed beyond a stage of reduction limited to the production of a few more or less fixed expressions (see Chapter 17). It is often younger patients, those whose articulatory difficulties have disappeared or greatly decreased, who develop the linguistic behaviours characteristic of agrammatism [see examples (2.88) and (2.89)]. These patients may then continue to improve over the years, not so much in terms of increased syntactical proficiency, although this may sometimes happen, but rather in terms of an enrichment of available lexicon through a process which might best be described as cramming. Although agrammatics seldom recover great conversational fluency, their language may nevertheless be quite effective in terms of communication. This is well illustrated by the following description[1] given by an agrammatic patient about the evolution of his disease.

(4.1) *'Euh, hémiplégie, euh, fulgurant, euh, Hôpital Pasteur, Nice, Nice. Euh, Docteur Dupont. Euh, euh, examens↓ enfin, examen, euh, enfin, un coma euh, un petit peu.*

Euh, un mois↓ un mois, euh, pavillon F-3 /dy/↓ euh, Docteur Durand. Les reins. Euh, kinésithérapeute. Marche euh, euh, très bien, enfin, un peu, un peu. Euh, premier novembre, médica↓ Le↓ Giscard↓ Docteur Giscard euh rééducation. Euh, euh, oui, euh, kiné↓ non, huit heures, kiné, euh, un quart d'heure. Euh, mécano, enfin. Euh, euh, euh, huit↓ euh, deux heures, euh, euh, déjeuner. Euh, rééducation, euh, euh, ah oui! euh, parole↓ parole, euh, une demi-heure.'

'Uh, hemiplegia, uh, fulgurant, uh, Pasteur Hospital, Nice, Nice. Uh, Doctor Dupont, uh, uh, examination↓ finally, examinations, uh, finally, a coma uh, a little bit. Uh, a month↓ a month, uh, pavillion F-3 /dy/↓ uh, Doctor Durand. My kidneys. Uh, physiotherapist. Walk uh, uh, very well, finally, a little, a little. Uh, November first, medica↓ The↓ Giscard↓ Doctor Giscard uh, therapy. Uh, uh, yes, uh physio↓ no, eight o'clock, physio, uh, a quarter of an hour. Uh mechano, finally. Uh, uh, uh, eight↓ uh, two o'clock, uh, uh, lunch. Uh, therapy, uh, uh, ah yes! Uh, speech↓ speech uh, a half an hour.'

Ever since Pierre Marie's time (see Chapter 1), many aphasiologists refuse to identify a disorder as a *Broca's aphasia* unless the symptom complex includes an articulatory disturbance. If certain cases showing a severe quantitative and qualitative reduction in the absence of an articulatory disturbance are ignored (Insertion 4.1) there are, in fact, few exceptions to this general rule and phonetic transformations are almost always very obvious in the common form of Broca's aphasia. The adjective *articulatory* emphasizes that the disturbance is one of speech rather than language and one related to relatively peripheral involvement of the sensorimotor networks underlying verbal expression. Such involvement is manifested clinically by anomalies in the force, tonus and/or coordination of the muscles of the buccophonatory apparatus (see Chapter 3), and the most specific manifestation of an articulatory disturbance is the production of individual phonemes which are poorly pronounced (disorganization of the third phase of oral language) [see examples (3.1) to (3.15)]. The articulatory disturbance may be less apparent during transposition activities, repetition and, when possible, oral reading than during more spontaneous and propositional linguistic productions (where the disturbance is not equally apparent at every moment). In certain patients, articulation may appear completely normal during highly automatized utterances [listing days of the week, prayers, sometimes songs (see Insertion 17.3), etc.] or in short sentences produced in highly concrete situations, often under emotional pressure (*automatic-voluntary dissociation*).

A severe articulatory disturbance obviously contributes to the reduced output of speech production in Broca's aphasia. However, as indicated by the definitions previously provided (see Chapter 2), a reduction must not be confused with an articulatory disturbance.* It is, in fact, not uncommon to observe a very clear dissociation between these two phenomena [for example, when a Broca's aphasia evolves towards a clinical picture of nearly pure anarthria (see Chapter 3), the reduction may scarcely still be noticeable while the phonetic disintegration remains severe; in contrast, when the clinical picture evolves towards agrammatism (cf. p. 52), the reduction may still be obvious while the articulatory disturbance has completely or almost disappeared].

Word-finding difficulty belongs to the clinical picture of Broca's aphasia, as it does to that of almost all other aphasias. Quantitatively, it may range from a relatively moderate to an extremely severe impairment. The severity generally decreases during evolution, especially when the patient receives therapy (see Chapter 17). Difficulty in word finding is often more obvious during conversation, narration and word-fluency tasks than on naming tests. The word-finding difficulties of Broca's aphasics are unrelated to their articulatory disturbance although the latter may explain certain delays in word production. On the other hand, word-finding difficulty cannot be distinguished from the phenomenon of reduction in conversation, where it is primarily manifested by delays and absences of production. The presence of word-finding difficulty in Broca's aphasics showing predominantly expressive (not to say *motor*) symptomatology is obvious in the most characteristic cases; *facilitation by phonemic cueing* is then maximally effective (the word which was not produced is uttered as soon as the first phoneme or syllable is supplied).

In the common form of Broca's aphasia, the phonetic transformations are such that they most often (superficially) mask the production of other types of aphasic transformations of oral

* In this regard, it may be useful to reformulate Pierre Marie's Law (see Chapter 1) in the following terms: 'Broca's aphasia = Wernicke's aphasia + anarthria + reduction'.

language, particularly the production of phonemic paraphasias. Nevertheless, a careful study of these patients' productions, especially those obtained during audiophonatory transposition (repetition) and visuophonatory transposition (oral reading) tasks will reveal the presence of errors in the selection and serial ordering of phonemes, errors which cannot be explained on the basis of a purely articulatory disturbance (see Chapters 2 and 3), nor be distinguished from the phonemic paraphasias observed, in the absence of any articulatory disturbance, in other forms of aphasia (cf. p. 64). Although not an invariable feature, the production of phonemic paraphasias may thus be part of the clinical picture of Broca's aphasia. In some cases this phenomenon becomes more obvious (particularly in oral reading) after a certain period of recovery, when the articulatory disturbance has decreased in severity and the obtained speech samples are somewhat more abundant. At this time is it also easier to recognize the presence of some verbal paraphasias and less frequent neologisms in the conversation of certain patients.

If written expression is not completely suppressed in Broca's aphasia, a graphic disturbance is as commonly observed as an articulatory disturbance (see Chapter 3). An assessment of graphic activity, as well as of automatisms of written language, is more difficult in patients who must write with their left hand because their aphasia is accompanied by a right hemiplegia. In cases where a sufficient sample of written language can be obtained, it always shows the effects of a reduction and often those of a stronger or weaker tendency towards agrammatism. Paragraphic transformations are always present, particularly literal and graphemic paragraphias. This last point is well illustrated in the example (2) shown below without the graphic deficits. It involves a written description of a picture showing an accident at a level crossing:

(4.2)

(Tamponnement→) '*Tamponement d'un train et d'une voiture. La cloche* (sonne→) *sone, la voiture semble en* (panne→) *penne sur la voie* (ferrée→) *ferré les* (occupants→) *occupant* (prennent→) *prenent la* (clef→) *voie des champs. Et la locomotive qui fonce sur la voiture.*'

'Collision *of a train and a car. The bell* rings. *The car seems* stuck *on the* railway *track, the* occupants take *to the fields. And the locomotive which rushes towards the car.*'*

Although copying of a written stimulus is usually defective, it is not usually servile.† In certain patients, generally after a period of evolution, the production of written language is not particularly abundant and does not appear particularly easy but nevertheless shows a greater resemblance to jargonagraphia than to the severe reduction which remains obvious in oral expression[19]. Example (3) was taken from the file of a patient who showed this type of evolution.

(4.3) (J'avais→) '*J'aivais 5 (cin) enfant un succend pnenais du'en Mon (a) (a) (a) marie vend des amaus Mon areparition est vide et je ne parle plus* (Mes→) *Mon 4 petits (le) Enfants 2 garçons et 2 filles.*'

'*I* had *5 child a succend pnenais of the in* M*y (a) (a) (a) husband sells some amaus. My areparition is empty and I no longer speak.* M*y 4 little ones (the) Children 2 boys and 2 girls.*'

In typical cases of Broca's aphasia, comprehension of oral language is only mildly disturbed; in some cases, it may even be completely normal. On the other hand, comprehension of written language is often more affected. Those close to the patient in daily life generally claim that he 'understands everything', a statement which will be confirmed on examination if it is limited to an assessment of the comprehension of relatively simple oral and written commands. However, a linguistic examination in depth generally reveals the following comprehension deficits: poor comprehension of grammatical words, inability to follow complex directions, and fragmentary comprehension of *linguistic wholes*, resulting in incomplete understanding of overall meanings of passages read or heard by the patient (see Chapter 15).

BROCA'S APHASIA ALMOST LIMITED TO AN ARTICULATORY DISTURBANCE

The clinical picture may appear suddenly, no doubt as the manifestation of the presence of a

---

* Correct target words appear before an arrow in the French samples. In the English translations of written productions, neologisms appear as they were originally written and orthographically deviant segments appear in print rather than script.
† Servile copying: slavish attempts at a visually exact reproduction as if copying unfamiliar forms.

Insertion 4.1

A clinical picture is sometimes observed which resembles the common form of Broca's aphasia. The similarity is most apparent in the flow of speech which, in both cases, shows a severe quantitative and qualitative reduction. However, the absence of any articulatory impairment in the present case constitutes an essential difference. The observed symptomatology thus appears hybrid: the occasional paraphasic and neologistic productions, not being masked by articulatory difficulties, are suggestive of jargon seen in Wernicke's aphasia whereas the relative mildness of the comprehension disturbance and the quantitative features of the speech flow call to mind the behaviour of Broca's aphasics.

Some aphasiologists show no hesitation in considering this symptom complex as a Broca's aphasia while others prefer to speak of a Wernicke's aphasia with a quantitative reduction (*reduced Wernicke's aphasia*). The former no doubt emphasize the nature of the speech flow and the fact that this clinical picture may sometimes be seen at onset or appear during the evolution of a global aphasia. The latter give greater importance to the absence of an articulatory disturbance and the fact that, in certain cases, the picture represents an evolutionary form of Wernicke's aphasia (cf. p. 94). In certain respects, this clinical picture is reminiscent of that described by Goldstein under the name *central motor aphasia*[21] (*see Chapter 10*).

circumscribed cerebral lesion, or it may emerge gradually in the course of recovery from an initially more severe Broca's aphasia. An articulatory disturbance, which is very marked in certain patients and very mild in others, is present in a nearly isolated state. Occasional hesitations may suggest mild word-finding difficulty but the more or less evident slowing of speech can be primarily attributed to the articulatory disturbance. It may also underlie a decrease in prosodic variation. Performance is normal on naming tests. Paraphasic transformations are infrequent and are mainly or always of the phonemic type. There is usually a mild disturbance of written expression which is seen in graphic deficits and the production of spelling errors. Comprehension of spoken and written language is normal. It is obvious that this form of Broca's aphasia may evolve towards *Pierre Marie's pure anarthria* (see Chapters 1 and 3) and there is, in fact, nearly no qualitative difference between them. In both cases (if the severity of the articulatory disturbance does not preclude conversation) a striking contrast can be observed between the clarity, as well as the semantic and syntactic coherence of the discourse, and its defective articulation. Example (4) is taken from a conversation with one of Alajouanine's[22] patients. Because written expression was completely normal we considered that the patient presented pure anarthria. However, because his discourse included some phonemic paraphasias, others would no doubt prefer to speak of a Broca's aphasia almost limited to an articulatory disturbance. In either case the reader may gain an idea of the patient's conversation by trying to read this passage aloud, slowly and syllabically, exaggerating the force and amplitude of buccophonatory movements, particularly in regard to stop consonants. The patient is answering a question about his occupation.

(4.4) '/mɔ/↓ /mɔm/↓ *Momentanément, je* /sʃ/↓ /sʃ/↓ *je suis* /ʀœ/↓ /ʀœ/↓ *représentant en vins. C'est*↓ *ce*↓ *ce n'est pas mon métier en temps normal. Mais*↓ *Mais*↓ *J'*/eti/↓ *j'étais représentant, mais de*↓ *de* /li/↓ /le/↓ *lincléums.* /ɑ̃/↓ /ɑ̃/↓ *Avant* /li/↓ *la guerre, j'étais agent d'une* /y/↓ /y/↓ *usine de ... d'une* /pa/↓ /pafi/↓ /fabikœ/ *de linoléums et* /twa/ *cirées.*'

'/mɔ/↓ /mɔm/↓ Momentarily, I /sʃ/↓ /sʃ/↓ I'm a /ʀœ/↓ /ʀœ/↓ representative for wines. It's↓ it↓ It's not my work in usual times. But↓ But↓ I /eti/↓ I was a representative, but of↓ of↓ /li/↓ /le/↓ linoleums. /ɑ̃/↓ /ɑ̃/↓ Before /li/ the war, I was an agent for a /y/↓ /y/↓ factory of ... of a ... a /pa|↓ /pafi/↓ /fabikœ/ of linoleums and waxed /twa/.'

WERNICKE'S APHASIAS

During the most characteristic phase of Wernicke's aphasia, the flow of speech is normal and even logorrhoeic and the patient shows no articulatory difficulty. In the 'common form' of this disorder, this phase is also characterized by a severe disturbance of language comprehension and the patient may present an anosognosia regarding his aphasia, that is, he appears quite unaware of his linguistic behaviour.

Under the general heading of Wernicke's aphasia, we shall describe conduction aphasia and the common forms of Wernicke's aphasia. These common forms are Wernicke's aphasia proper, Wernicke's aphasia with preserved repetition, and Wernicke's aphasia with a predominant disturbance of written language. Depending on the nature of the causal cerebral lesion (see Chapters 8 and 9), each of these forms may occur at onset or gradually emerge after a period of favourable or unfavourable evolution. Consequently, numerous intermediate symptom complexes are possible (*mixed aphasias*) and are, in fact, frequently observed.

CONDUCTION APHASIA

Three principal symptoms are associated with the most characteristic phase of conduction aphasia: when evaluated globally, the flow of speech appears normal or near normal but conversational speech includes evidence of word-finding difficulty and numerous phonemic approximations and transformations; repetition is markedly disturbed; language comprehension is normal or nearly so.

The patient's conversational behaviour is very typical [see (2.24)]: although the output is abundant and generally appropriate, it is interrupted by hesitations, pauses and corrections related to the presence of word-finding difficulty and paraphasic productions. These last two behaviours are probably not independent, and it should be noted that the paraphasic transformations often occur on words which are not immediately retrieved. In typical cases, these transformations attest to an almost selective disturbance of the second linguistic phase, that is, they consist almost exclusively of phonemic paraphasias and verbal paraphasias of the formal type (phonemic transformations)[19] (see Chapter 2). They may be so numerous and bewildering at onset of the aphasia that clinicians sometimes refer to the output as *phonemic jargon*[23, 24], a label which appears appropriate in many cases. The patient is generally aware of his expressive disturbance and usually attempts to correct his productions through *phonemic approximations* (*conduites d'approche phonemiques*: the production, often repetitive, of phonemes which may or may not belong to the target word); these attempted corrections are often successful. In other cases, the patient may suddenly abandon the word which is causing trouble and, without any hesitation, utter a semantically related word, an acceptable synonym or a less adequate circumlocution[19]. These various characteristics are illustrated in example (5):

(4.5) Q: '*On me dit que vous allez mieux. Est-ce vrai?*'
R: '*Oui, c'est* |ʀvy|, /sɑ̃du/, *je vous dis,* /dɔktɔʀ/, *si je parle* /pɔʀɛʀ/↓/pozɛʀmɑ̃/↓ *posément, si—euh—je parle lentement. Et si je ne suis pas trop—euh—nerveux ... Vous savez (je suis souvent nerveux), surtout* /da/↓ *depuis quatorze de*↓ *la guerre de* /sa/↓ *la guerre de* |kalis|↓ *de* |galis|↓ *de*↓ *oui, c'est la* /kɛ/ ↓ *c'est la* /gɛ/↓ *depuis la guerre de* /kɔz/↓ *de mille neuf cent* /kasɔz/↓ /kœ/↓ /katʀɔs/↓ ... *quatorze.*'

Q: '*Où étiez-vous au début de la guerre?*'
R: '*J'étaus* à↕ *j'avais* /fiji/↓—*euh—je venais de* /f/↓—*euh*—/fi/↓ *terminer mon droit et j'ai*↓—*euh—j'aidais mon*↓ *mon père à l'*/ɑ̃batal/↓ *a l'* /ɑ̃ba/↓ *a l'* /ɑ̃basald/ *de* |fɔ̃t| *à Berne* ... *J'ai été* /vo/↓/vobi/↓/vo/ /↓—*euh attendez!—oui, j'ai été mobilisé.*'

Q: 'I've heard that you're feeling better. Is it true?'
R: 'Yes it's |ʀvy|, /sɑ̃du/, I tell you /dɔktɔʀ/, if I speak /pɔʀɛʀ/↓ /pozɛʀmɑ̃/↓ carefully, if—uh—I speak slowly. And if I'm not too—uh—jittery ... you know (I'm often jittery), especially /da/↓ since fourteen of↓ the war of /sa/↓ the war of |kalis|↓ of |galis|↓ of↓, yes it's the /kɛ/↓ it's the /gɛ/↓ since the war of /kɔz/↓ of nineteen /kasɔz/↓ /kœ/↓ /ka/↓ /katʀɔs/ ... fourteen.'

Q: 'Where were you at the start of the war?'
R: 'I was in↓ I had /fiji/↓—uh—I had just /f/↓—uh—/fi/↓ finished law and I↓—uh—I was helping my↓ my father at the /ɑ̃batal/ at the /ɑ̃ba/ at the /ɑ̃basald/ of |fɔ̃t| in Berne ... I was /vo/↓ /vobi/↓ /vo/↓—uh wait!—yes, I was mobilized.'

As mentioned by this patient, a voluntary slowing of speech may reduce the number of phonemic transformations. At the onset of his disease the patient usually experiences some difficulty in controlling his speaking rate and generally succeeds only intermittently. However, if the lesion is of vascular origin, as is almost always the case (see Chapter 9), control is frequently achieved after a few weeks of evolution. In certain patients, particularly those who have received aplasia therapy (see Chapter 17), this control is only evident in 'difficult' passages, suggesting that the patient has learned to predict probable transformations. Syllabic speech gradually comes to replace phonemic approximations and transformations except in the case of lengthy and less frequently used words.

As in the case of Broca's aphasia, the word-finding difficulty of conduction aphasics is often more obvious during conversation than during naming tests. Such tests often give rise to phonemic transformations of the correctly selected word. When the patient is unable to retrieve the word required in response to a particular stimulus, production may be facilitated by phonetic placement cues but they may also lead to the production of verbal paraphasias of the formal type. Verbal paraphasias of the semantic type are rare and, if they are produced, it is usually clear that the patient considers them approximate and inadequate responses.

Linguistic behaviour is severely disturbed during repetition. In some cases, the patient is almost totally unable to repeat but, in most cases, the disturbance is manifested through phonemic approximations and numerous phonemic paraphasias [see (2.13) to (2.20)]. Even shortly after onset, the repetition of short words (monosyllables and bisyllables) is often normal. However, the phonemic transformations increase in number as soon as the patient is asked to repeat longer words having a more complex phonemic structure. Such words may sometimes present greater difficulty than the repetition of syntactically simple sentences of medium length. On the other hand, the repetition of longer sentences which include a high proportion of grammatical monemes, particularly functional monemes, represents a particular source of difficulty[6]. Repetition of such sentences generally remains very poor even at the stage of evolution where the other symptoms have considerably regressed (Insertion 4.2).

In qualitative terms, oral reading is usually affected in the same way as repetition. In quantitative terms, the disturbance is frequently* less apparent in visuophonatory than in audiophonatory transposition and, as a general rule, decreases or disappears earlier in oral reading. The examples shown below [(6) to (10)], which were taken from the file of a conduction aphasic, illustrate this relative dissociation which is often immediately evident at onset of the aphasia:

	Stimuli		Repetition	Oral reading
(4.6)	*navet*	/navɛ/	→/natavɛt/	/navɛ/
(4.7)	*esprit*	/ɛspʀi/	→/sɛspʀi/	/ɛspʀi/
(4.8)	*textile*	/tɛkstil/	→/sɛktɛktil/	/stɛkstil/
(4.9)	*spécialité*	/spesjalite/	→/ɛspasjɛl/	/spjesjalite/
(4.10)	*galvanomètre*	/galvanɔmɛtʀ/	→/kalœvalœ/	/galvanɔmɛtʀ/.

Graphic skills and automatisms of writing are usually spared in conduction aphasia but written productions generally show numerous paragraphic transformations. Nevertheless, in certain cases, either at onset or after a period of evolution, written expression is essentially normal or, at any rate, clearly much less disturbed than oral expression. When written language is disturbed, the deficits are particularly evident in spontaneous productions or in writing to dictation whereas copying of writing† is generally less affected. Conduction aphasics characteristically produce orthographic deviations, particularly literal paragraphias [see (2.54) to (2.59)], and may also produce verbal paragraphias, especially those of the formal type. The text shown below [example (19)] was written by a patient who showed a much milder disturbance of spelling than of repetition:

(4.19) '*Etre commissaire dans une grande ouvrière comme Lille est un sujet bien difficile à exposer un peu de mots à un profane ... avoir trent-six patrons: préfet* (procureur→), *procureor, maire, députés, notabilités ... de* (faire→) *faife* (des→) *der rapports qui ne personne ne lira jamais surtout s'ils sont* (originaux→) *origsinaux* (*excusez l'immodestie*) ... *pour vaincre* (délicatement→) *diliactement de préférence, le malfaiteur.*'

'*To be a commisioner in a large industrial city like Lille is a very difficult subject to explain to a layman in a few words ... to have thirty-six supervisors: police chief, public prosecutor, mayor, deputies, prominent people ... to* prepare some *reports which not nobody will ever read especially if they are* original (*excuse the immodesty*) ... *to outdo, preferably* in a delicate manner, *the scoundrel.*'

* Although not always, and there are some cases in which oral reading is more impaired than repetition.

† All subsequent statements about copying will refer to the copying of written stimuli.

Insertion 4.2

A phenomenon resembling the use of synonyms in conversation [see example (5)] occurs quite frequently during repetition tasks. Thus, when repeating an isolated word, the patient attempts to facilitate his production by uttering a word conceptually related to the one he cannot repeat. This is well illustrated by examples (11) to (16) which were taken from the file of a conduction aphasic:

(4.11) sot /so/→ /sœ/↓ /sa/. *Il est* /sa/. *Il n'est pas fin. Un* /sa/. *Non, un* /so/.
fool /so/→ /sœ/↓ /sa/. He's not sharp. A /sa/. No a /so/.

(4.12) *colis* /kɔli/→/kɔ/↓ /kɔdi/. *Un* /kɔdi/. *Un paquet. C'est ça.* /kɔdi/. *Un* /kɔdi/. *Un* /kɔ/↓ *un* /kɔdi/. *Un paquet.*
parcel /kɔli/→/kɔ/↓ /kɔdi/. A /kɔdi/. A bundle. That's it. /kɔdi/. A /kɔdi/. A /kɔ/↓ a /kɔdi/. A bundle.

(4.13) *dégoût* /degu/→/dedu/↓ /debu/↓ /desu/. *Non. C'est pas bon. La, ca veut dire que ce n'est pas bon. Je*↓ *du*↓ *le* /dedju/↓ /djedi/. *J'ai du goût. Il n'a pas de goût. J'ai pas de goût. Du* /degu/.
disgust /degu/→/dedu/↓ /debu/↓ /desu/. No. It's not good. There, it means that it's not good. I↓ of the↓ the /dedju/↓ /djedi/ . . .

(4.14) *maximum* /maksimɔm/ *Au* /maktivœ/. *Au*↓ *au*↓ *Plus gros, ça. Au*↓ *au*↓ *au* /maktimɔm/
maximum /maksimɔn/→to the /maktivœ/. To the↓ to the↓ That's bigger. to the↓ to the↓ to the /maktimɔm/.

(4.15) *décolorant* /dekɔlɔʀɑ̃/→*Un* /dekɔlɔlɑ̃/. *Un* /dekɔʀɔlɑ̃/. *Un*↓ *Non. Pour les cheveux. Un* /dekɔ/↓ /dekɔle/↓ /dekɔlɔʀɑ̃/. *Un* /dekɔlɔʀɑ̃/.
bleaching agent /dekɔlɔʀɑ̃/→A /dekɔlɔlɑ̃/. A /dekɔʀɔlɑ̃/. A↓ No. For the hair. A /dekɔ/↓ /dekɔle/↓ /dekɔlɔʀɑ̃/. A /dekɔlɔʀɑ̃/.

(4.16) *antiquité* /ɑ̃tikite/→/ativite/↓ /ak/↓ /a/↓ *Un* /akti/↓ *Quelque chose de vieux. Un ancien. Un ancien.* /ɑ̃ti/ /ɑ̃tikite/.
antiquity /ɑ̃tikite/→/ativite/↓ /ak/↓ /a/↕. A /akti/↓ Something old. An antique. An antique. /ɑ̃ti/ /ɑ̃tikite/.

Later on in the course of evolution, sentence repetition may give rise to an analogous behaviour, one which is always recognized by the patient. As in the following examples, the repetition responses then include semantic paraphasias:

(4.17) '*Je vous télephonerai quand je serai libre*'→'*Je vous télephonerai quand je pourrai.*'
'I'll telephone you when I'll be free.'→'I'll telephone you when I can.'

(4.18) '*Veut-tu coudre mon pantalon?*'→'*Veut-tu pas tricoter mon pantalon?*'
'Would you sew my trousers?'→'Won't you knit my trousers?'

No matter which type of errors are made, the patient usually becomes aware of his mistakes and then often attempts to correct them. Although phonemic paraphasias and literal paragraphias share basic linguistic structures, there is no obvious parallel between the phonemic paraphasias and the literal paragraphias made by a particular individual on the same words, that is, a word may be written incorrectly just after it has been pronounced without error or vice versa.

Certain conduction aphasics produce a fair number of transformations which suggest a disturbance of morphology and syntax, namely a disorganization of certain aspects of the first linguistic phase is added to the disturbance of the second phase which was just discussed. Performance on transposition tasks shows a number of substitutions which particularly involve affixes and morphological markers and thus result in the production of verbal and monemic paraphasias and paragraphias. Similarly, repetition, oral reading, writing to dictation, as well as conversation and, especially, spontaneous written productions [see (19)] show syntactical errors involving omissions, additions, displacements and replacements of words or short syntagms within the context of sentences. In these patients, grammatical words are no doubt more susceptible to these types of transformations than are lexical words.

Previous statements concerning the comprehension of language in Broca's aphasia are equally valid in the case of conduction aphasia. Whether spoken or written language is considered, comprehension is only mildly or moderately involved. In some cases it may be completely normal, especially when evaluated after a period of favourable evolution and therapy.

COMMON FORMS OF WERNICKE'S APHASIA

We shall now discuss three clinical pictures which, when present in their most typical form, include the common features of easy, fluent speech, a more or less abundant production of paraphasias and/or paragraphic transformations, and a disturbance of language comprehension. The three symptom complexes are discussed separately as much for purposes of convenience as to emphasize their (relative) clinical uniqueness. In fact, the identity of each clinical picture often becomes apparent only during the course of evolution. Here, even more than elsewhere, it is important to emphasize the possible occurrence of various intermediate symptom combinations.

Type I—The first form of Wernicke's aphasia is identified, in its most characteristic phase, by three principal features, namely: a normal or logorrhoeic flow of speech which includes all types of aphasic transformations (jargonaphasia) with the exception of phonetic transformations; extremely poor repetition; and a disturbance of spoken language comprehension. This clinical picture is often designated as Wernicke's aphasia proper (i.e., Wernicke's aphasia strictly defined).

At onset, and sometimes following a (very) brief period of suppression, spoken output is usually copious and rapidly emitted. If the patient is logorrhoeic, that is, speaks incessantly and generally without external stimulation, his general behaviour often conveys an impression of great excitation. The prosody is rich but its sometimes inappropriate nature may sporadically be evident in those sentences whose meaning is approximately clear to the listener. Anosognosia is generally obvious[25] but is rarely absolute. In fact, if attention is given to the content of the patient's discourse, it is almost always possible to note a few more or less direct allusions to the expressive difficulty. Nevertheless, the patient continues to talk a great deal and, apparently, to expect that he will be understood. This expectation can only be partially satisfied despite the impeccable articulation. The patient's productions are, in fact, difficult, and sometimes impossible, to understand because they include all types of aphasic transformations[26] [see (2.83)], particularly verbal paraphasias as well as phonemic paraphasias and other types of neologisms (the output is jargon). The patient may speak without attending to the interlocutor's interventions: he may continue to speak even when his interlocutor is talking or else pause, sometimes with all the external signs of polite attentiveness, and then resume his monologue whose content shows no conceptual relationship to the questions or comments which were just addressed to him. In certain cases, the repeated production of the same preferred words creates an impression of conversation permanently oriented towards the same theme[19]. A certain number of dyssyntactic utterances are always observed but, in the severest cases, they probably do not involve more than 15 to 20 per cent of the sentences produced[27]. The fluency of the speech flow during conversation may superficially mask signs of word-finding difficulty. However, such difficulty is always present, as indicated by the production of verbal paraphasias and neologisms as well as by the large number of aborted sentences and the repetitions of determiners, prepositions and functional monemes. Despite all these abnormalities of linguistic expression, the examiner can usually estimate the extent to which the patient understands questions directed to him. It is not uncommon that his or her productions, particularly when they immediately follow the interlocutor's comments, attest to a fragmentary understanding of the linguistic interventions of others.

This clinical picture undergoes considerable modification with evolution[19, 28, 29] when the course is favourable [compare examples (20) and (21)], as it quite often is in patients who sustained a cerebral vascular accident (see Chapter 9).

After some weeks or months, speech is slower, although remaining fluent, preferred themes are no longer evident, neologisms decrease and then disappear and verbal paraphasias are more often identified as being of the semantic type (the conceptual link between what the patient tries to say and what he actually produces is more obvious). Conscious attempts to retrieve an unavailable word are more frequent (the word-finding difficulty is thus more obvious although less severe), the patient often speaks syllabically when producing a word which was difficult to retrieve, the anosognosia decreases and the understanding of an interlocutor's comments is clearer and less transient. Recorded at an interval of some months, the following excerpts [(20) and (21)] illustrate certain aspects of this type of evolution. In both samples the patient is responding to a question about his family:

(4.20) First interview

'*Oui, j'ai une autre FEMME qui est restée depuis la* /bœtʀe/ *de l'enfant de MA FILS. IL a↓ elle avait dix ans quand mon* |fɛs| *est mort. Et alors, elle est là maintenant. Elle va sur* /syz/ *ans. Elle va toujours à l'école, puisqu'elle se présente les↓ Je l'avais envoyée à l'école puisque, moi, je travaillais bien dans les* /syz/↓*—euh—à la* /faʀmid/ *de↓ de↓ de* /syz/, *n'est-ce pas, de deux* /ɛtmiʀ/. *Et alors, je↓ Cette* /mwazɛ/*—la—euh, GINETTE, elle s'appelle—elle↓ elle* |abil|. *Tous les jours, elle venait à Paris pour* /pale/ *dans les* /kɔsig/ *parce qu'elle prenait pour aussi↓ pour entrer le↓ le PALAIS—le PALAIS normal, bien entendu—le* /namytyʀ/, *la* /tɔktœʀ/ *et l'* /ɑ̃bœtjɛʀ/, *pour qu'elle sache tous ces↓ ces CHOSES, pour qu'elle sache à bien s'* /ɛ̃skʀyme/*ȧbien↓biens'*/ɛ̃/↓*s'*/ɛ̃kyme/. *Et c'est là que je↓ que je suis MORTE, là, cette année. Elle était↓ elle allait toujours à l'école, cette pauvre petite, mais enfin elle↓ elle était pas là. J'étais pas à la PAUSE puisque je la CONNAISSAIS pas. Alors, elle a été chez mon PARENT.*'

'Yes I have another WOMAN who has remained since the /bœtʀe/ of the child of MY SON. HE is↓ she was ten years old when my |fɛs| died. And then, she is there now. She will soon be /syz/ years old. She is still going to school since she presents herself the↓ I had sent her to school since I myself was indeed working in the /syz/↓—uh—at the /faʀmid/ of↓ of /syz/ isn't it, of two /ɛtmiʀ/. And then, I↓ This /mwazɛ/—there uh, GINETTE is her name—she↓ she |abil|. Each day, she came to Paris to /pale/ in the /kɔsig/ because she was taking in order to also↓ in order to enter the↓ the PALACE—the normal PALACE of course—the /namytyʀ/, the /tɔktœʀ/ and the /ɑ̃bœtjɛʀ/, in order that she would know all these↓ these THINGS, in order that she would know to /ɛskʀyme/ herself well, to↓ to↓ /ɛ̃/↓ /ɛ̃kyme/ herself well. And this is when I↓ when I DIED, then, this year. She was↓ she still went to school, poor little thing, but finally she↓ she wasn't there. I wasn't at the pause since I didn't KNOW it. So, she has been at my RELATIVE'S.'

(4.21) Second interview

'*Ah! moi, j'ai deux enfants. J'ai un garçon qui A trente-cinq ans le↓ qui a eu trente-cinq ans le mois↓ oh! ce mois-ci, le↓—euh—le sept ... Ah! alors donc, j'ai un garçon qui a trente-cinq ans, marié, père de deux garçons, et j'ai MON AUTRE FILLE qui va avoir seize ans le trente septembre prochain ... Mon mari aurait eu LE cinquante-trois* [*ans*] *le quatorze. Mon mari est mort il y a six ans, Monsieur. Il est mort de la↓—euh—du du ... du* /k/↓ ... *—C'est comment?—le* |gɛ̃| *le ah! ... le cancer. Voila. Le cancer. Mon mari pesait quatre-vingt-cinq kilos. Quand il est mort, il en pesait trente-huit.*'

'Ah! me, I've two children. I've a boy who IS thirty-five years old the↓ who was thirty-five years old a month↓ Oh! this month, the—uh—the seventh. Ah! So then, therefore I've a boy who is thirty-five, married, the father of two boys, and I've MY OTHER GIRL who will be sixteen years old the thirtieth of next September ... My husband would have been THE fifty-three [years] the fourteenth. My husband died six years ago, Sir. He died of a↓—uh—of a↓ of a↓ ... of a /k/↓—what's it?—a |gɛ̃|↓ a↓ ah! ... a cancer. There it is, a cancer. My husband weighed eighty-five kilos. When he died he only weighed thirty-eight.'

Certain patients are less verbose at the onset of their disorder and, with evolution and the disappearance of the anosognosia, their conversational production may be reduced to a few aborted sentences and fixed syntagms interspersed with automatic expressions indicating failure ('I can't', 'I'm not able', 'I seem stupid', etc.). This behaviour merges with that which has already been described with regard to a *reduced Wernicke's aphasia* (see Insertion 4.1).

Word-finding difficulty is obvious during naming tests (in those cases where the patient willingly attempts such tests). It is less often manifested by failures to respond than by immediate responses which take the form of verbal paraphasias, neologisms, and circumlocutions whose relationship to the stimuli is not always apparent. When such a relationship can be observed as, for example, in the case of a circumlocution including a word having the same root as the appropriate response to the stimulus, production of the former often has no facilitating effect on production of the latter. Moreover, with the exception of written language cues, the various means of facilitation which the examiner might attempt (see Chapter 15) are usually not very effective and, in certain patients, often elicit the production of neologisms. In the case of patients in the logorrhoeic-anosognosic phase, the presentation of stimulus items from a naming test does not typically elicit naming behaviour. Rather, each stimulus elicits a long commentary whose meaning most often escapes the listener.

It may be impossible to test repetition ability immediately after the onset of the aphasia because a demand for any type of linguistic activity elicits logorrhoea: the patient's behaviour cannot be *channelled*. Nevertheless, impaired repetition, which can generally be demonstrated a little later, is an essential characteristic of Wernicke's aphasia proper. In many respects, the repetition disturbance resembles that observed in conduction aphasia and both are probably of the same basic type (see Chapter 8). However, the repetition responses are often less similar to the stimuli than is the case in conduction aphasia. They are, in fact, often so dissimilar that it might be asked whether they would not be more appropriately considered neologisms than phonemic paraphasias, even though these two terms are not mutually exclusive (see Chapter 2). As indicated by examples (22) to (26), performance is generally more accurate on tests of oral reading than of repetition, a feature which is also reminiscent of behaviour observed in conduction aphasia [see examples (6) to (10)] (moreover, a progressive transition from the clinical picture of Type I Wernicke's aphasia to that of a conduction aphasia is not unusual). It can be seen that the transformations occurring during oral reading, in the patient whose productions are quoted as examples, are unequivocably phonemic paraphasias. Consequently, it can be suggested that the transformations occurring in repetition are also phonemic paraphasias (even though the responses are very remote from the stimuli) and that there is not, in these patients during the act of repetition, a qualitative difference between neologism and phonemic paraphasias.

Graphic skills and automatisms of writing are generally spared. However, in typical cases, writing to dictation is severely disturbed. If a sufficient sample of spontaneous writing is obtained, the presence of neologisms and all types of paragraphic transformations can usually be observed [see (2.85)]. They may decrease during evolution and written language may become effective—sometimes clearly more effective than spoken language—in terms of information conveyed[30].

	Stimuli	Repetition	Oral reading
(2.22)	*égalité* /egalite/	→/dekelete/	/egalite/
(2.23)	*combinaison* /kɔbinɛzɔ̃/	→/kubʀɛze/	/kɔlɔ̃binɛzɔ̃/
(2.24)	*projectile* /pʀɔʒɛktil/	→/kɑ̃pʀiɛiʀ/	/pʀɔʒɛktili/
(2.25)	*cinérama* /sineʀama/	→/ʃimeʀagaʀt/	/sineʀama/
(2.26)	*dévouement* /devumɑ̃/	→/fʀɑ̃fʀi	/demɔ/↓ /devumɑ̃/.

At this stage of evolution, the written productions are sometimes very dyssyntactic [see (2.82)]. Some of the features mentioned above are illustrated in the sentences shown below [see (27)], which were spontaneously written by the same aphasic on two occasions several months apart.

	First sample	Second sample
(4.27)	'*Ma dumorale ferdant donc une pouette de péa près.*'	'*J'ai* (langage→) *languege. J'ai a perdu des mots.* (Analphabète→) *Anaphèle.*'
	'*Mes pelits beaubpoud persent des blassisseuses.*'	'*Alors, j'espère la sante d'un cerveau.*'
	'*My dumorale thus ferding a pouette of péa near.*'	'*I have* language. *I've to lost some words.* Illiterate.'
	'*My pelits beaubpoud persent of the blassisseuses.*'	'*So, I hope the health of a brain.*'

Finally, there are some patients—and their number is quite considerable—whose written productions are excessively reduced at onset, both qualitatively and quantitatively. This reduction may be permanent.

Comprehension of spoken language is always impaired at onset of this form of aphasia. The disturbance may vary in severity but many patients fail on even the simplest tests. In certain cases, the comprehension deficits are related, at least in a large measure, to an agnosic type of disturbance (cf. pp. 80–81) (see Chapter 5, *word deafness*) and there may be a dissociation between written comprehension, which is less impaired, and oral comprehension. In such cases, sentences are generally more poorly understood than are isolated words. The patient's behaviour may then resemble that of the hearing impaired, even though auditory sensitivity is normal or nearly so.* For example, on a naming

* An audiogram of pure tone hearing threshold levels may indicate a mild loss at the higher frequencies.

test, the patient may cup his ear, request a repetition of the stimulus or use gestures to indicate that he has difficulty hearing. It is this type of behaviour which is referred to when speaking of the *auditory aspect** of certain Wernicke's aphasics [see (5.5)]. In the case of a regressive evolution, the disappearance of logorrhoea and anosognosia is generally accompanied by a considerable improvement in comprehension. While the disturbance of oral comprehension may remain relatively severe in certain cases, it is not uncommon that only the comprehension of wholes remains as a persisting area of particular difficulty.

The comprehension of written language is frequently impaired with the severity of the disturbance varying among different cases. It may be approximately equal in severity to the disturbance of spoken language comprehension but is sometimes clearly less severe. Such a dissociation becomes increasingly obvious as the disturbance of spoken language comprehension is more closely related to a component of word deafness. When this component is very significant, the comprehension of written language, especially after a certain period of evolution, may be almost normal whereas spoken language comprehension remains severely disturbed. In these cases, written expression is usually relatively intact as well[31]. This dissociation, which favours written language, could conceivably be partially related to the patient's educational and cultural background.

Type II—The second form of Wernicke's aphasia is identified, in its most characteristic phase, by three principal features, namely: the flow of speech is usually normal and the output, which is normal in phonetic and phonemic aspects, includes verbal paraphasias and shows a significant qualitative reduction; repetition is normal or nearly so and echolalic phenomena may sometimes be observed; language comprehension is impaired (both for spoken and for written language). This clinical picture has also been designated by the names of *transcortical sensory aphasia*[21] or *isolation of the speech areas*[32] (see Chapter 10).

Here again, the spoken output may be abundant; the speech rate is normal and articulation is impeccable [see (2.90)]. The prosodic aspects are the same as in Wernicke's aphasia proper. Anosognosia is generally present and may be tenacious. Conversational speech is characterized by a type of jargon but, in the most typical cases, the predominant types of transformations are verbal and syntagmic paraphasias. In many cases, even at onset of the aphasia, patients do not produce phonemic paraphasias or other types of neologisms so that their conversation[19] reflects a nearly exclusive disorganization of the first phase of spoken language (see Chapter 2). With the exception of these differences in the types of abnormal segments, the manifestations of word-finding difficulty during conversation are qualitatively comparable to those observed in Wernicke's aphasia proper. Quantitatively, they are often even more numerous (the number of aborted sentences and circumlocutions may be particularly large). In prototypical cases, the number of dyssyntactic transformations is negligible[19]. Nevertheless, the patients' productions often appear very incoherent. Either at onset or during evolution, a qualitative reduction may be obvious in the vocabulary composing this type of jargon. The output then includes a large number of ready-made expressions (*fixed syntagms*) but a small number of lexical units which are used repeatedly. Several of these features are illustrated in (28):

(4.28) '*J'ai un metier qui à peu pres↓ qui est à peu pres identique a celui des autres, à des↓ Seulement, IL est* /pRɔ/↓ *IL est PROFESSEUR. Enfin, c'est↓ c'est↓ c'est dur. C'est dur pour moi. IL est difficile parce que—euh—je suis↓ je suis chargé de↓—Attendez!—Je suis PROFESSEUR. Comment je pourrais dire? Je fais rien du tout. Je suis chargé de faire mettre de la↓ de la terre cuite en état—euh—pout le↓la↓ la plupart des gens ... Bon! Mais, malgré tout, j'arrive à faire↓—euh—à faire—euh—que le↓ que le total arrive à faire un certain bien↓—ah la la la la!—un certain bien et qu'on arrive à avoir des↓ des marchandises qui sont propres, qui sont nettes et qui sont convenables pout la↓—euh—pour le besoin↓ pour le besoin de↓ des↓pour les besoins de↓ Notez bien que c'est pas mal, hein. Non? Dans les↓ Il est certain que j'arrive à faire quelque chose de bien parce que j'arrive à obtenir que le raisonnement—euh—soit convenable. On arrive déjà à avoir ça, hein. C'est pas toujours↓ Enfin, c'est pas toujours facile mais c'est toujours.*'

'I have a trade that is nearly↓ that is nearly identical to that of others, to that↓ Only, HE'S a /prɔ/↓ HE'S a PROFESSOR. Well it's↓ it's↓ it's hard. It's hard for me. IT's difficult because—uh—I'm↓ I'm in charge of—Wait! I'm a PROFESSOR. How can I put it? I do nothing at all. I'm in charge of seeing to it that↓ that↓ baked clay is prepared—uh—for the↓ the most of the people ... Good! But despite everything, I

* Auditory aspect (*versant auditif*): auditory comprehension is clearly more impaired than visual comprehension.

manage to do↓—uh—to do—uh—that the↓ that the total manages to do something good↓—ah Oh Dear—something good and that we manage to manage to have some↓ some merchandise which is clean, which is neat and which is appropriate for the↓—uh—for the need↓ for the need of↓ of the↓ for the needs of↓ Now that it's not bad eh? No? In the↓ It's sure that I manage to do something good because I manage to get that the thinking—uh—is appropriate. We have already managed to have that eh? It's not always. Well it's not always easy but it's always↓.'

In a certain number of cases, the qualitative reduction may be paired with a quantitative reduction. When this occurs, it is usually after a certain period of evolution and may then be a permanent phenomenon.

After a certain period of evolution if the aphasia results from a cerebral vascular accident, or at onset if it is related to a degenerative disease (see Chapter 9) it is usually easy to engage the patient in repetition behaviour. It will then be seen that audiophonatory abilities are normal or nearly so. Certain patients, particularly those suffering from degenerative diseases, may show a spontaneous tendency to repeat words spoken by others (especially those at the end of a sentence), a phenomenon known as *echolalia*. It is demonstrated in a spectacular fashion by having the patient echo sentences in a foreign language. Some imitate unfamiliar accents and other aspects of prosody in a very natural manner and may even reproduce their interlocutor's gestures (*echopraxia*). Oral reading may also be almost completely intact but in some cases gives rise to the more or less abundant production of all types of paraphasias and neologisms.

Graphic activity and automatisms of writing may be intact. Spontaneous production is typically rather meagre and disorganized in terms of word arrangement. It may include all types of paragraphias and neologisms and perseverative phenomena occur frequently. As in example (29), a qualitative reduction is often apparent:

(4.29) '*une une journée avec les patients une chambre qui est assez* (malade→) *malade une bien malade Chambre avait dans maiche ... J'ai J'ai* (faibli→) *faiblel (J'ai fo) J'ai faible Bien faible.*'

'*a a day with the patients a room which is quite* sick *a very sick Room had in maiche ... I've I've* weakened *(I've fo) I've feeble Very feeble.*'

Writing to dictation may sometimes be less severely disturbed but orthographic deviations are nevertheless numerous. When copying is possible it is usually carried out in a servile fashion.

When the aphasia is caused by pathology having a sudden onset, language comprehension is immediately and severely disturbed. In the case of slowly progressive disease, the comprehension disorder becomes increasingly severe. Simple sentences are generally understood better than isolated words (cf. p. 81, psycholinguistic comprehension disturbance). Comprehension is usually equally impaired for spoken and for written language and this remains true, even when oral reading is possible. Thus some patients may be able to read words aloud, and are sometimes even able to name their corresponding pictures, but are neverthess unable to match the written words with the corresponding pictures.

Type III—Two dissociations in linguistic behaviour are evident during the most characteristic phase of the third form of Wernicke's aphasia. The disturbance of oral expression is primarily confined to word-finding difficulty, whereas the disturbance of written expression is manifested by a suppression or by jargonagraphia. Second, spoken language comprehension is severely disturbed. This clinical picture is sometimes referred to as *Wernicke's aphasia with predominant impairment of written language*. In the very rare cases where oral expression and spoken language comprehension are both completely normal and non-linguistic findings from a neurological examination are negative (see Chapter 16), the clinical picture is referred to as (*Dejerine's*) *alexia with agraphia*[33].

Conversational output is normal or nearly so in regard to quantitative features as well as articulation and prosody. The volubility often seen at the onset of other forms of Wernicke's aphasia is not typical in this case and the patient's discourse clearly indicates his or her attention to the interlocutor's comments and questions. Paraphasias and neologisms are rare (perhaps as rare as in certain normal speakers) or even absent. However, word-finding difficulty is obvious. The patient's discourse is interspersed with hesitations, aborted sentences, repetition of determiners, prepositions, etc., and circumlocutions, and includes many words (thing, matter, gadget, etc.) whose meaning is extremely vague and which generally convey little information. In other words, the qualitative reduction of immediately available vocabulary may be obvious. In some respects, the conversational behaviour in Type III Wernicke's aphasia is comparable with that which is present in amnesic aphasia (cf. p. 100). The patient is invariably aware of his oral expressive difficulty and often complains spontaneously about it. The following comments [see (30)], produced in an ordinary conversational tone, are normal in structure, given the patient's cultural background:

(4.30) *'Bien! des fois, j'essaye à dire quelque chose, je suis pas capable. Des fois, bien! je vais essayer de dire quelque chose, je vais plutôt envoyer une platitude SALE—euh—folle. Ou bien↓ Ou bien donc, je sais pas quoi c'est dire. Ou bien donc, je voudrais dire de quoi à mon mari, tu sais, des fois, là—euh hein hein—je suis pas capable. Je suis pas capable de dire rien.'*

'Well! sometimes, I try to say something, I'm not able. Sometimes, well! I'm going to try to say something. I'm going rather to deliver a DIRTY remark—uh—mad. Or else↓ Or else then I don't know what that's to say. Or else then I would like to say something to my husband, you know, sometimes there—uh eh eh—I'm not able. I'm not able to say anything.'

The clinical picture of spontaneous written expression is strikingly different. In extreme cases, patients are unable to write or their production is limited to a few words, such as their names (*suppression*). As previously mentioned (see Chapter 3, *graphic disturbance*), the strictly graphic aspect of writing, namely the third phase of written language, is sometimes completely disorganized in this particular form of Wernicke's aphasia. The output is generally meagre and made up of combinations of graphic features oriented in various ways so that few letters can be immediately recognized. In the least complex instances, it is sometimes possible to recognize a combination of features borrowed from several different letters, thus forming what might be considered *literal neosegments* (see Chapter 3). More frequently, the production is further complicated by perseverative phenomena and the graphic transformations show very little or no resemblance to the structure of conventional letters. In other cases, graphism and automatisms of written language are relatively intact. Although written productions are then quantitatively limited and the time required for their composition is abnormally long, it is possible to obtain fairly lengthy samples composed almost entirely of recognizable letters. Such samples show the features of a severe jargonagraphia, that is, orthographic deviations, verbal transformations, neologisms, syntactic oddities. In this jargonagraphia, as in all others which may be observed in Wernicke's aphasia, the graphemological system of the patient's language is often fairly intact (see Fig. 4.2). Thus the jargoned productions can easily be read aloud and most are composed of highly probably associations.

The dissociation which is thus observed between oral and written expression seems particularly well illustrated by a comparison, in example (31), between the written jargon and the transcription of the patient's oral comments which were uttered concurrently.

(4.31)

French	English translation
'la charg nos chos moil	*'the charg our chos moil*
"Je prends les voitures neuves.	"I take the new cars.
falleg ma fallon, chagne l'halis	*falleg my fallon, chagne the halis*
Vérifier les poulies. Changement d'huile.	Check the pulley. Oil change.
chee spoko, pliats, s"	*chee spoko, pliats, s"*
Vérifier les pointes, les spark plugs et le distributeur.'	Check the wiring, the spark plugs and the distributor.'

Despite the patient's awareness of his oral expressive difficulty, it is not uncommon that he is anosognosic in regard to his written jargon.

When the disturbance of written expression evolves favourably, the neologistic jargon is gradually replaced by productions which are dyssyntactic and dysorthographic but become increasingly efficient in terms of the information conveyed[19]. Thus, after several months of evolution (and aphasia therapy) the patient quoted in (31) was able to give the following written description of a recent hunting expedition [see (32)].

(4.32) *'La chasse a* (été→) *ete mauvaise, il a pleut toute* (la→) *le journée.* (*no*) *on pas des chevreuils. Un peu des* (perdrix→) *pridix et un*(*e*) (*liv*) *lièvre. On se leve à cinq* (*heures*→) (*heuh*) *heure du matin et* (*sa*) *a chasser pour heures. Je suis* (revenu→) *revenir merdredi soir, à 6 hrs.* (*Je*) *J'ai* (commencé→) *commence a travailler jeudi matin.'*

'Hunting was bad. It has raining all day. We no deer. A few some partridge. *We get up at five* o'clock *in the morning and to hunt for 10 hours. I'm come back Wednesday night at 6 o'clock. I've begin to work Thursday morning.*

Different cases show varying degrees of word-finding difficulty on naming tests. In oral naming, the difficulty is manifested primarily in failures to respond or delayed responses. It may also be manifested by numerous circumlocutions which often indicate that the patient has at least partially apprehended the word which s/he is unable to retrieve. On the other hand, in those cases where writing is possible, written naming often leads to the production of numerous paragraphias and neologisms. Although many no doubt reflect the presence of word-finding difficulty, others may represent possible orthographic transformations of correctly selected words. Certain predominant error patterns are sometimes observed but written naming, as well as writing to dictation (cf. below) usually shows a mixture of literal paragraphias and graphemic paragraphias [see (2.54) to (2.65)]. In short, it is likely that certain segments identified as neologisms during tests of written naming are in fact particularly complex types of orthographic transformations. These different points are illustrated by examples (33) to (42), which were taken from the file of the patient already cited in (30). The words in parentheses identify the photographs presented and those responses consisting of conventional words.

(4.33)	(guitar)	*guitare*	→ *vlolol—violin* (violin)
(4.34)	(snake)	*serpent*	→ *cerfamt*
(4.35)	(chick)	*canard*	→ *un cananr*
(4.36)	(coat)	*manteau*	→ *un mameteau*
(4.37)	(bus)	*autobus*	→ *hauteaubul—hotobuce*
(4.38)	(church)	église	→ *gegirit—herniche*
(4.39)	(dog)	*chien*	→ *un cheval—chain* (horse - chain)
(4.40)	(bread)	*pain*	→ *trapage homte*
(4.41)	(parrot)	*perroquet*	→ *hibout* (owl)
(4.42)	(drum)	*tambour*	→ *tambouir—tamblue.*

Oral facilitation is often effective in instances of word-finding difficulty in these patients. In contrast, written facilitation is almost never effective.

Although abnormal (servile), copying is generally less affected than is writing to dictation. In cases where writing is possible, the orthographic deviations, which we are often tempted to call neologisms, may in fact be sufficiently numerous and complex to justify use of the term 'jargon' in summarizing the patient's behaviour in writing. Nevertheless, the jargoned segments are, in a large measure, composed of letters from the dictated words. In contrast, repetition is much more accurate, if not completely normal. This characteristic dissociation between repetition and writing to dictation is well illustrated by examples (43) to (52) [the same file as in (30) and (33) to (42)]. The patient's task was to write the words immediately after having repeated them.

	Stimuli	Repetition	Writing to dictation
(4.43)	*toxicomane* /tɔksikɔman/	→/tɔksikɔman/	*toucsimea*
(4.44)	*égalite* /egalite/	→/egalite/	*hecalier*
(4.45)	*psychologie* /psikɔlɔʒi/	→/siskɔlɔʒi/	*shicolagie*
(4.46)	*maximum* /maksimɔm/	→/maksimɔm/	*mesiment*
(4.47)	*décolorant* /dekɔlɔʀɑ̃/	→/dekɔlɔʀɑ̃/	*diencoramt—derolara*
(4.48)	*ignominie* /inɔmini/	→/inɔmini/	*himoniemie*
(4.49)	*électricien* /elɛktʀisjɛ̃/	→/elɛktʀisjɛ̂/	*exquiceur*
(4.50)	*thermomètre* /tɛʀmɔmɛʀ/	→/tɛʀmɔmɛtʀ/	*hermoneur*
(4.51)	*neurologie* /nøʀɔlɔʒi/	→/nøʀɔlɔʒi/	*ninirolajeur*
(4.52)	*protestataire* /pʀɔtɛstatɛʀ/	→/pʀɔtɛstatɛʀ/	*prapatateur*

Oral reading is disturbed. In some cases it may be impossible or, in other cases, give rise to paraphasias of all types and to neologisms. A behaviour is sometimes observed which is analogous to that already pointed out in regard to naming. The patient is unable to utter the word presented to him in writing but shows, through his comments, that he has at least partially understood its meaning.

If comprehension of spoken language is nearly normal in typical cases of Type III Wernicke's aphasia, comprehension of written language is always impaired. It may be more or less profoundly affected but a disturbance which was very severe at onset may show considerable improvement with evolution. In general, simple sensory messages are more accurately recognized than more complex ones. The disturbance appears to be primarily of the agnosic type (cf. p. 85) and, according to Dejerine, is related to an element of *word blindness*[33] (see Chapters 5 and 10). Patients readily attribute their failures on tasks assessing comprehension of written language to a purely visual problem, stating that they need glasses or that those which they are wearing are too weak. When presented with visual stimuli, patients move them closer to their eyes or farther away, or else view them from a different angle as if trying to see them in a better light. It is this type of behaviour, plus the fact that spoken language comprehension is relatively better, if not normal, which is referred to when speaking of the *visual aspect** of certain Wernicke's aphasics.

AMNESIC APHASIA

Amnesic aphasia is primarily characterized by more or less severe word-finding difficulty which often defies attempts at facilitation. In the most typical cases, the meaning of words which cannot be retrieved may be only partially apprehended when the patient hears them or reads them.

Fluency is approximately normal and prosody and articulation are completely normal. However, word-finding difficulty, which varies in severity among different cases, is manifested in conversation by the use of circumlocutions, which are often vague, by the selection of inadequate words, which are often acknowledged as such by the patient, and by a large number of sentences which are not completed because of the inability to retrieve the desired word, which is usually a substantive or attribute. Analogous phenomena are apparent in spontaneous written language which is, however, normal with respect to fluency, graphic features and automatisms of writing.

The word-finding difficulty is generally severe as soon as the patient is asked to name objects or pictures of objects. As in all the aphasias, it becomes increasingly obvious as the required lexicon becomes more specific and/or has a lower frequency of usage. For example, a bicycle may be named successfully but not its chain or pedals, a leaf may be named but not its stem or veins, etc. During naming, the word-finding difficulties of amnesic aphasics are manifested by delays and failures to respond as well as by frequent circumlocutory responses.† Paraphasic responses are rare. In certain cases of amnesic aphasia, but not in all, attempts to facilitate production by phonemic cues are almost always ineffective.

Repetition is normal, oral reading is normal or slightly slowed, and copying is normal. Writing to dictation may, and usually does, indicate the presence of a spelling disturbance.

Few difficulties are observed on the simple tests commonly presented to aphasics in an attempt to assess spoken and written language comprehension. However, as Goldstein and Bay have emphasized (see Chapter 10), comprehension of word meanings is not uncommonly seen to be incomplete when more complex tasks are presented. For example, an amnesic aphasic may experience very obvious difficulty in grouping words according to their mutual semantic relationships[34, 35, 36] and, if the trouble is severe, may even fail to recognize certain words as actually existing in the language[37].

Even in severe cases, tests of general intelligence and visual memory are not affected by amnesic aphasia. However, deficiencies are observed in verbal learning tasks[37] (see Chapter 16).

Nearly isolated word-finding difficulty, such as that occurring in amnesic aphasia, may constitute the initial element of a symptom constellation which will become much more complex as the disease progresses. This often occurs, for example, in the case of cerebral tumours or degenerative diseases (see Chapter 9). Conversely, isolated word-finding difficulty may constitute the sole residual, after some months or years of evolution, of an initially more complex clinical picture, particularly that of Types I and III Wernicke's aphasia. In these cases, the aphasia is generally caused by vascular disease (see Chapter 9).

MIXED APHASIA

Although we have mentioned this several times, we think it important to emphasize further that the aphasias may appear—and in fact often do appear at some moment in their evolution—in forms which are somewhere between the classical pictures which we have just described. In general, these intermediate forms bear a fairly clear resemblance to one or another of the classical pic-

* Visual aspect (*versant visuel*): comprehension of written language is clearly more impaired than comprehension of spoken language.

† Often of the type involving description of use: sink—'It's for washing hands'; pencil—'it's for writing', etc.

tures. In any case, there is rarely any hesitation in saying whether the aphasia is clearly of a Broca's or a Wernicke's type. Nevertheless, there are certain cases in which this initial clinical judgement itself is not immediately obvious, even in the case of a relatively mild aphasia. Whatever the case, the problems of terminology are usually solved, after describing the features of all these symptom complexes, by saying that the aphasia is *mixed.* The problem of mixed aphasias is more frequently encountered in ambidexterous and left-handed individuals than in right-handers (see Chapter 11).

GLOBAL APHASIA (OR TOTAL APHASIA)

The expressive disturbance is that of Broca's aphasia in its most severe form, that is, a severe quantitative and qualitative reduction or even suppression, involving all aspects of both spoken and written language. The comprehension disturbance which also affects both spoken and written language, is that of the most severe form of Wernicke's aphasia. In general, expressive language shows little improvement with evolution. In contrast, language comprehension, particularly spoken language comprehension, quite often improves, sometimes to a considerable degree. In the spirit of Pierre Marie's classification[38] (see Chapter 10), this clinical picture is also known by the name of a *full Broca's aphasia* (*grande aphasie de Broca*).

NEUROLOGICAL AND NEUROPSYCHOLOGICAL SYMPTOMATOLOGY ASSOCIATED WITH THE APHASIAS

Because of the mapping of the brain and the functional polyvalence of certain regions (see Chapter 8), and also because of the usual distribution of cerebral lesions, particularly when they result from vascular disease (see Chapter 9), aphasia often coexists with other neurological or neuropsychological disorders. Thus the assessment of an aphasic includes not only the study of his linguistic behaviours (see Chapter 15) but also a neurological examination and, in most cases, a psychometric evaluation (see Chapter 16).

Right-handers, who are of primary concern in the following comments, may show a right *hemiparesis* that is, a right-sided weakness of the face and limbs which varies in severity among different cases. Right hemiparesis usually coexists with a Broca's aphasia and almost always accompanies a global aphasia. As a general rule, the upper limb, and particularly the hand, is more affected than the lower limb. A right *hemihypoaesthesia* that is, a decrease of sensation on the right side, may also be present in these patients. Less commonly, right hemiparesis and hemihypo-aesthesia may occur in association with Wernicke's aphasia, especially when the clinical picture is of the *conduction* type. In these cases, they are usually mild and transitory, and recovery often occurs in a few days or weeks. A deficit of elementary sensation affecting the right half of the body may also coexist with certain forms of Wernicke's aphasia.

Right *facial paresis* is usual in Broca's aphasics (cf. p. 59) but, unless it is extremely severe and its effects thus easily identified, it does not explain their articulatory disturbance. Equally common at the onset of Broca's aphasia, the *buccofacial apraxia*—a non-lateralized disturbance of voluntary buccofacial motricity—is much more closely linked to the articulatory disturbance[8]. The term 'buccofacial apraxia' designates the disturbance of those buccofacial activities which are independent of speech production. This disturbance, which may vary in severity and often does not involve the upper facial musculature, affects voluntary activities carried out on order or in imitation. However, it spares highly automatized movements, such as those of mastication. The dyspraxic movements are characteristically variable and the same movement may be properly executed on one occasion and poorly executed on another. The disturbance is not one of comprehension, is not related to abnormalities of muscle tone or of elementary muscular coordination, and it does not reflect a sensory loss. Buccofacial apraxia is almost always present to some degree, at least in the initial stage, in subjects presenting an articulatory disturbance regardless of whether or not it is associated with other manifestations of Broca's aphasia. The relationships between articulatory disturbances and buccofacial apraxia were discussed elsewhere (see Chapter 3). It was suggested that the dyspraxic component of phonetic disintegration cannot be qualitatively distinguished from buccofacial apraxia and that it constitutes the manifestation of a buccofacial apraxia in the most finely differentiated movements of the lips, tongue, velum, etc. (i.e., in the movements underlying speech production). Milder and less clearly defined forms of buccofacial apraxia may be associated with conduction aphasia and with Wernicke's aphasia proper, that is, it may occur in patients who do not present either a hemiplegia or an articulatory disturbance[8]. Instances of automatic–voluntary dissociation are usually very clear in these cases.

Some degree of *limb apraxia*, especially affecting the upper limbs and often transient in nature, may coexist with most of the clinical forms of aphasia. Whether the movements considered are *transitive* (manipulation of actual objects) or *intransitive* (pretended manipulation of objects, execution of symbolic or arbitrary movements) and are, or are not, *reflexive* (reflected on the body), various types of dyspraxic behaviours may occur: the beginning of a non-specific movement, the use of a body part as if it were the object whose use is being pantomimed (the index finger becomes the toothbrush, the forearm and fist become the hammer), *parapraxic transformations* (replacement of one movement by another), *perseverative phenomena* (they may be partial as when the memory of thumbing the nose is reflected in a military salute by the open-fan position of the fingers[39]). As different as they may be from each other, all these abnormal gestural behaviours have in common that they do not result from failure to understand the task nor from any elementary motor or sensory disturbance. Moreover, the movements are characteristically variable, so that the same one may sometimes be properly executed and sometimes poorly executed; an automatic–voluntary dissociation can usually be demonstrated. In patients presenting a right hemiplegia, as is common in Broca's aphasia, the presence of an eventual apraxia will be manifested mainly or only in the left upper limb[32]. It can be readily understood that it would then provide at least a partial explanation of the difficulties which these patients present in attempts at left-hand writing. Limb apraxia is bilateral when present in Wernicke's aphasia. In certain cases, it takes a very particular form in which the sequential performance of elementary movements is disturbed even though each individual movement of the series can be properly executed (*ideational apraxia*). Thus, when a box of matches and a candle are placed on the table in front of the patient, he will open the box, remove a match and place it on the table and then strike the end of the candle against the frictional surface of the match box. Aware of the ineffectiveness of his action, and sometimes clearly astonished by it, he may attempt correction by re-opening the match box and attempting to insert the candle or by touching the match remaining on the table with the wick of the candle. This behaviour in the execution of non-linguistic acts is reminiscent of that which disorganizes verbal gestures in jargonaphasia and it is therefore tempting to speak of a *jargonapraxia*. Moreover, of all the Wernicke's aphasics, it is especially those with severe jargon who present this type of apraxia in its most spectacular form.

A right *hemianopsia* (or *quadranopsia*) may be *absolute* (the patient does not see stimuli presented in the right half of the visual field) or *relative* (the patient does not report the presence of stimuli presented in the right half of the visual field when concurrent stimuli are simultaneously presented in the left half). A right hemianopsia often coexists with a total aphasia or a mixed aphasia and is also commonly associated with several of the clinical forms of Wernicke's aphasia. In some cases, it must be considered in the explanation of certain abnormalities occurring during reading and writing (see Chapters 5 and 15).

Agnosic disturbances which may impede the comprehension of linguistic messages were previously discussed in the description of Wernicke's aphasia and their occurrence in a pure form will be discussed elsewhere (see Chapter 5). However, there are other varieties of *agnosia* which may be associated with the different clinical forms of Wernicke's aphasia. They are specific disturbances in the recognition of sensory information which, by definition, occur in the absence of elementary sensory deficits or, if such deficits are present, they do not provide an adequate explanation of the patient's behaviour. Various types of agnosia are observed in the neuropsychology clinic: *auditory agnosia* or the inability to recognize meaningful sounds (for example, the noise of a train, a galloping horse, familiar melodies,* etc.), *visual agnosia*, or the

* Amusia.

Insertion 4.3

> Although exceptional, there are certain cases in which the naming disturbance is nearly confined to a single sensory modality (visual or tactile) and also gives rise to errors of a paraphasic type, that is, to errors reflecting conceptual proximity. In such cases, the patient is typically able to draw a correct picture of a stimulus which he has just named incorrectly. Because it is limited to visual or to tactile stimuli, some aphasiologists consider this disturbance to be a particular variety of visual or of tactile agnosia. Because most of the errors cannot be distinguished from the semantic paraphasias produced by aphasics, other aphasiologists consider this disturbance to be a particular form of aphasia (*optic aphasia*[40], *tactile aphasia*). One of us (F.L.) has proposed a physiopathological interpretation of these cases in terms of a disconnection[41, 42].

inability to recognize the meaning of observed objects or pictures; *tactile agnosia*, or the inability to recognize objects through touch (*astereognosis*), or to recognize symbols traced on the skin, particularly on the palm of the hands or on the fingertips (*agraphaesthesia*). Because it affects recognition of stimuli only in a particular sensory modality and is not accompanied by a properly linguistic disturbance, an agnosia can easily be recognized when it is present in a (nearly) pure state. For example, a patient with visual agnosia is unable to name a seen object but can readily identify it if permitted to touch it. However, the assessment of an agnosia becomes much more complex when it coexists with an aphasia in the same patient. Particular difficulty occurs when attempting to interpret the behaviour of certain patients on naming tests. If naming is abnormal for stimuli presented in all sensory modalities but is especially poor for stimuli presented through one particular modality, the presence of an agnosic component can certainly be suspected. The presence of an associated auditory agnosia is particularly likely in Type I Wernicke's aphasia. Although it cannot always be easily demonstrated, it can sometimes be shown that written words can be matched to their corresponding pictures but cannot be matched to their corresponding sounds. The possible association of a visual agnosia with a Wernicke's aphasia can sometimes best be determined through careful attention to the nature of the patient's errors. For example, if a picture of an open umbrella is called a 'mushroom', it may be supposed—on the basis of the similarity in shape between the stimulus object and the object named—that the error is of a *paragnosic* type. On the other hand, if a picture of an open umbrella is named 'rain', it may be supposed—because of the obvious conceptual link between the stimulus and the response—that the error is of the paraphasic type (Insertion 4.3).

Other neuropsychological disorders often coexist with a Wernicke's aphasia, particularly with those forms of Wernicke's aphasia characterized by predominant disturbances of written expression and written language comprehension, and with amnesic aphasia[43] (see Chapter 16). The major types of these disorders are as follows: difficulty in producing and copying drawings, particularly geometric forms, as well as in using blocks and sticks to reproduce bidimensional or tridimensional models, despite the absence of an elementary motor disturbance (*constructional apraxia*); difficulty in carrying out arithmetic operations, even simple ones (*acalculia*); difficulty in discriminating between left and right (*left–right disorientation*); particular difficulty in naming and identifying fingers, from visual or tactile stimulation, either on people or in drawings (*finger agnosia*); an analogous and more general difficulty in recognizing body parts (*autotopoagnosia*), etc. Certain other neuropsychological disorders frequently associated with aphasia will be discussed in the following chapter.

CHILDHOOD APHASIAS

As we have indicated in the introduction, this text is specifically concerned with acquired disorders of articulated language in adults. Thus we shall only mention briefly a few points concerning childhood aphasia. In adult neurology, the term *aphasia* always designates abnormal linguistic behaviour in patients who have generally, through a normal course of learning, acquired the capacity to communicate through language and who exercised this capacity until it was more or less completely disturbed by the onset of a cerebral lesion. In childhood neurology, if one refers to the Anglo-Saxon neuropaediatric literature, the same term designates different conditions. It includes, on one hand, disorders of language acquisition (*aphasias* or *developmental dysphasias*; *developmental dyslexias* and *dysgraphias*) and, on the other hand, acquired disorders which result from cerebral lesions which are often traumatic (see Chapter 9). The latter occur while the brain is still immature and before language learning has approached completion and at a time when the functional specialization of various regions of the brain is not yet fully established (see Chapter 11). These facts are no doubt related to the differences observed between the acquired aphasias of adults and those of children. In terms of clinical features, the childhood aphasias are characterized by the consistent occurrence of the phenomenon of reduction and by the absence, except in the most exceptional—if not doubtful—cases[45], at least until approximately the age of 12 years, of forms of aphasia characterized by a fluent speech flow and, *a fortiori*, of the types of behaviours resembling logorrhoeic jargon[1, 44]. The childhood aphasias also differ from those of adults in the much better recovery which usually occurs in children (see Chapter 11). Nevertheless it is clear, even in certain cases which appear to show an extremely favourable evolution, that the occurrence of an aphasia may have more or less severe repercussions on the child's subsequent mental development (particularly at the time of written language learning).

REFERENCES

1. Alajouanine, Th. (1968) *L'aphasie et le langage pathologique*. Paris: Baillière.
2. Lhermitte, F. (1965) Sémiologie de l'aphasie. *Revue pratique* (Paris), **15**, 1.
3. Lhermitte, F. & Gautier, J.-C. (1969) Aphasia. In *Handbook of Clinical Neurology* (Ed.) Vinken, P.J. & Bruyn, G.W. Vol. 4, p. 84. Amsterdam: North-Holland.
4. Lecours, A.R. (1975) Aphasie. *Encyclopédie médico-chirurgie, 17019 A^{10}*, **7.**
5. Hécaen, H. (1972) Le cerveau et le langage. *La Recherche*, **3,** 829.
6. Geschwind, N. (1971) Medical intelligence—current concepts—aphasia. *New England Journal of Medicine*, **284,** 654.
7 Métellus, J. (1977) La dissociation automatico-volontaire chez les aphasiques. *Rééducation orthophonique*, **15,** 195.
8. Alajouanine, Th. & Lhermitte, F. (1960) Les troubles des activités expressives du langage dans l'aphasie; leurs relations avec les apraxies. *Revue neurologique*, **102,** 66.
9. Goodglass, H. & Kaplan, E. (1972) *The Assessment of Aphasia and Related Disorders*. Philadelphia, PA: Lea and Febiger.
10. Broca, P. (1861) Remarques sur le siège de la faculté du langage articulé, suivies d'une observation d'aphémie (perte de la parole). *Bulletin de la Société d'Anthropologie*, **6,** 330.
11. Jackson, J.H. (1958) *Selected Writing of John Hughlings Jackson*. New York: Basic Books.
12. Lecours, A. R. (1974) Le cerveau et le langage. *Union médicale du Canada*, **103,** 232.
13. Keenan, J.S. (1966) A method for eliciting naming behaviour from aphasic patients. *Journal of Speech Disorders*, **31,** 261.
14. Ali Chérif, A. (1972) *Considérations sur les troubles de l'expression orale et de la compréhension verbale présentés par deux malades aphasiques*. Medical thesis, Marseille.
15. Lordat, J. (1843) Analyse de la parole pour servir à la théorie de divers cas d'alalie et de paralalie que les nosologistes ont mal connus. *Journal de la Société de Médecine pratique de Montpellier*, **7, 8,** 333 and 417, 1.
16. Wernicke, C. (1874) *Der aphasische Symptomencomplex*. Breslau: Cohn et Weigert.
17. Leischner, A. (1969) Agraphias. In *Handbook of Clinical Neurology* (Ed.) Vinken, P. J. & Bruyn, G.W. Vol. 4, p. 141. Amsterdam: North-Holland.
18. Alajouanine, Th., Lhermitte, F. & de Ribaucourt-Ducarne, B. (1960) Les alexies agnosiques et aphasiques. In *Les grandes activités du lobe occipital* (Ed.) Alajouanine, Th. p. 235. Paris: Masson.
19. Lecours, A.R. & Rouillon, F. (1976) Neurolinguistic analysis of jargonaphasia and jargonagraphia. In *Studies in Neurolinguistics* (Ed.) Avakian-Whitaker, H. & Whitaker, H. Vol. II, p. 95. New York: Academic Press.
20. Goodglass, H., Gleason, J.B. & Hyde, M.R. (1970) Some dimensions of auditory language comprehension in aphasia. *Journal of Speech Research*, **13,** 595.

21. Goldstein, K. (1948) *Language and Language Disturbances.* New York: Grune and Stratton.
22. Lecours, A.R. & Lhermitte, F. (1976) The 'pure form' of the phonetic disintegration syndrome (pure anarthria): anatomo-clinical report of a historical case. *Brain and Language*, **3**, 88.
23. Alajouanine, Th., Lhermitte, F., Ledoux, Renaud, D. & Vignolo, L.A. (1964) Les composantes phonémiques et sémantiques de la jargonaphasie. *Revue neurologique*, **110,** 5.
24. Alajouanine, Th. & Lhermitte, F. (1973) The phonemic and semantic components of jargon aphasia. In *Psycholinguistics and Aphasia* (Ed.) Goodglass, H. & Blumstein, S. p. 318. Baltimore, MD: Johns Hopkins.
25. Alajouanine, Th. & Lhermitte, F. (1957) Des anosognosies électives. *Encéphale*, **46,** 505.
26. Alajouanine, Th., Sabouraud, O. & Ribaucourt, B. (de) (1952) Le jargon des aphasiques. *Journal de Psychologie*, **45,** 293.
27. Cyr-Stafford, C. & Boisclair-Papillon, R. (1974) *La dyssyntaxie: essai de définition.* Medical thesis, Montreal.
28. Buckingham, H.N. & Kertesz, A. (1974) A linguistic analysis of fluent aphasia. *Brain and Language*, **1,** 43.
29. Buckingham, H.N. & Kertesz, A. (1976) *Neologistic Jargon Aphasia.* Amsterdam: Swets and Zeitlinger.
30. Lhermitte, F. & Derouesné, J. (1974) Paraphasies et jargonaphasie dans le langage oral avec conservation du langage écrit. *Revue neurologique*, **130,** 21.
31. Lhermitte, F., Lecours, A.R., Ducarne, B. & Escourolle, R. (1974) Unexpected anatomical findings in a case of fluent jargon aphasia. *Cortex*, **10,** 83.
32. Geschwind, N. (1974) *Selected Papers on Language and the Brain.* Dordrecht and Boston: Reidel.
33. Déjerine, J. (1926) *Sémiologie des affections du système nerveux.* Paris: Masson.
34. Derouesné, J. (1970) *Contribution à l'étude des troubles sémantiques chez les aphasiques.* Thesis, Faculté des lettres, Paris.
35. Lhermitte, F., Derouesné, J. & Lecours, A.R. (1971) Contribution à l'étude des troubles sémantiques dans l'aphasie. *Revue neurologique*, **125,** 81.
36. Derouesné, J. & Lecours, A.R. (1972) Two tests for the study of semantic deficits in aphasia. *Internal Journal of Mental Health*, **1,** 14.
37. Lhermitte, F. & Derouesné, J. (1976) L'aphasie amnésique; étude de 25 cas. *Revue neurologique*, **132,** 669.
38. Marie, P. (1926) *Travaux et mémoires.* Vol. I. Paris: Masson.
39. Ajuriaguerra, J. (de) & Hécaen, H. (1960) *Le cortex cérébral.* Paris: Masson.
40. Freund, C.S. (1889) Uber optische Aphasie und Seelenblindheit. *Archiv für Psychiatrie und Nervenkrankheiten*, **20,** 276.
41. Lhermitte, F. & Beauvois, M. F. (1972) Syndrome de dysconnexion entre la perception visuelle et le langage (à propos d'un cas d'aphasie optique et d'agnosie visuelle). *Revue neurologique*, **5,** 563.
42. Lhermitte, F. & Beauvois, M.F. (1973) A visual-speech disconnexion syndrome—report of a case with optic aphasia, agnosic alexia and colour agnosia. *Brain*, **96,** 695.
43. Benton, A.L. (1961) The fiction of the 'Gerstmann Syndrome'. *Journal of Neurology, Neurosurgery and Psychiatry*, **24,** 176.
44. Alajouanine, Th. & Lhermitte, F. (1965) Acquired aphasia in children, *Brain*, **88,** 653.
45. Woods, B.T. & Teuber, H.L. (1978) Changing patterns of childhood aphasia. *Annals of Neurology*, **3,** 273.

BIBLIOGRAPHY

Acevedo, E., Mendilaharsu, S., Mendilaharsu, C. & Berta, M. (1958) Algunas consideraciones sobre la afasia central. *Acta Neurologica Latinoamericana*, **4,** 11.

Ajuriaguerra, J. (de) & Badaracco, J.G. (1955) Contribution à l'étude des désorganisations conjointes de la parole et du mouvement. *Encéphale*, **44,** 297.

Alajouanine, Th. (1968) *L'aphasie et le langage pathologique.* Paris: Baillière.

Alajouanine, Th. & Lhermitte, F. (1963) Activités expressives du langage dans l'aphasie. *Encéphale*, **52,** 5.

Alajouanine, Th. & Lhermitte, F. (1963) Some problems concerning the agnosias, apraxias and aphasia. In *Problems of Dynamic Neurology* (Ed.) Halpern, L. p. 201. Jerusalem: Jerusalem Post Press.

Alajouanine, Th. & Lhermitte, F. (1964) Essai d'introspection sur l'aphasie (l'aphasie vue par les aphasiques). *Revue neurologique*, **110,** 609.

Alajouanine, Th. & Mozziconaci, P. (1947) Aphasie: études sur l'aphasie. *Semaine des Hôpitaux de Paris*, **23,** 1221.

Albert, M.L. (1972) Certains aspects des troubles de la compréhension auditive du langage. *Langages*, **7,** 37.

Alford, L.B. (1940) A simple version of aphasia. *Journal of Mental and Nervous Diseases*, **91,** 190.

Allison, R.S. & Hurwitz, L.J. (1967) On perseveration in aphasics. *Brain*, **90,** 429.

Anastasopoulos, G.K. (1967) Aphasic disorders and verbal hallucinations. *Journal of the Neurological Sciences*, **4,** 83.

Assal, G. (1971) Clinique élémentaire de l'aphasie. *Schweizerische Rundschau für Medizin*, **60,** 272.

Baginsky, A. (1871) Aphasia in folge schwerer Nierenerkrankungen. *Klinische Wochenschrift*, **8,** 428 and 439.

Ballet, G. (1886) *Le langage intérieur et les diverses formes de l'aphasie.* Paris: Alcan.

Barrett, A.M. (1918) Report upon the clinical symptoms and anatomical findings in 3 cases of organic brain diseases showing disturbances of an aphasic and agnostic type. *Journal of the Michigan State Medical Society*, **17,** 330.

Bay, E. (1974) Uber die Beziehungen zwischen der sog. Amnestischen und sensorischen Aphasie. *Deutsche Zeitschrift für Nervenheilkunde*, **177,** 1.

Bay, E. (1951) Neue Wege der Aphasieforschung;

Betrachtungen zu Goldsteins Buch über Sprache und Sprachstörungen. *Nervenartz*, **22,** 302.

Bay, E. (1952) Der gegenwärtige Stand der Aphasieforschung. *Folia Phoniatrica* (Basel), **4,** 9.

Bay, E. (1962) Aphasia and non-verbal disorders of language. *Brain*, **85,** 411.

Bay, E. (1964) Present concepts of aphasia. *Geriatrics*, **19,** 319.

Bay, E. (1973) Der gegenwärtige Stand der Aphasieforschung. *Nervenartz*, **44,** 57.

Bein, E.S. (1964) *Afazia i puti u preodelenia*. Leningrad: Meditina.

Benton, A.L., Smith, K.C. & Lang, M. (1972) Stimulus characteristics and object naming in aphasic patients. *Journal of Communication Disorders*, **5,** 19.

Bernard, D. (1889) *De l'aphasie et ses diverses formes*. Paris: Lecrosnier et Babé.

Berry, M. F. & Eisenson, J. (1956) *Speech Disorders*. New York: Appleton Century Crofts.

Blanchet, P. (1970) Autour de l'aphasie dite motrice. *Nouvelles thérapeutiques*, **34,** 25.

Bleuler, E. (1893) Ein Fall von aphasischen Symptomen, Hemianopsie, amnestischer Farbenblindheit und Seelenlähmung. *Archiv für Psychiatrie und Nervenkrankheiten*, **25,** 32.

Bloomer, H. & Shohara, H. (1952) Speech disorders among European military personnel in World War I. *Journal of Speech Disorders*, **17,** 55.

Boitnott, J.K. (1967) Clinicopathologic conference, case presentation. *Johns Hopkins Medical Journal*, **120,** 275.

Boon, A.A. & Feitscher, P. (1938) Das Zeichen einer Patienten mit totaler Aphasie. *Zentralblatt für die gesamte Neurologie und Psychiatrie*, **163,** 103.

Boone, D.R. (1965) *Adult Aphasia*. Illinois: Interstate Press.

Botez, M.I. (1970) Aphasia: a multidisciplinary approach. *European Neurology*, **3,** 50.

Botez, M.I., Alexandru, S. & Dobrota, I. (1971) *Elemente de neuropsihologie*. Bucharest: Editura stiintifica.

Brain, R. (1961) The neurology of language. *Brain*, **84,** 145.

Bramwell, E. (1898) A remarkable case of aphasia. *Brain*, **21,** 343.

Brissaud, M.E. (1894) Aphasie. In *Traité de médicine* (Ed.) Charcot, J.M., Bouchard, Ch. & Brissaud, M.E. Vol. 6, p. 102. Paris: Masson.

Broadbent, W.H. (1879) A case of peculiar affection of speech, with commentary. *Brain*, **1,** 484.

Brown, J.R. (1960) Some clinical aspects of aphasia. *Transactions of the American Laryngological Association*, **88,** 154.

Bruno, M.S. & Ober, W.B. (1973) Expressive aphasia, elevated enzymes and multisystem involvement. *New York State Journal of Medicine*, **7,** 885.

Buck, M. (1963) The language disorders. *Journal of Rehabilitation*, **29,** 37.

Burr, C.W. (1905) Loss of the sign language in a deaf mute from cerebral tumor and softening. *New York Medical Journal*, **81,** 1106.

Cambier, J., Masson, M., Creissard, P., Dehen, H., Delaporte, P. & Lechevalier, B. (1972) *Abrégé de neurologie*. Paris: Masson.

Caraceni, T. (1962) L'afazia de conduzione. *Revista de patologia nervosa e mentale*, **83,** 531.

Carasco-Zanini, J. (1960) Agnosia, afasia y apracia. *Acta audiologica y foniatrica hispano-americana*, **2,** 189.

Castleman, B. & Kibbee, B.U. (1960) Case records of the Massachusetts general hospital. *New England Journal of Medicine*, **263,** 854.

Chain, F. (1965) Aspects divers de l'aphasie. *Revue pratique* (Paris), **15,** 2295.

Coërs, C. (1967) Aux frontières de l'aphasie. *Acta Neurologica Belgica*, **67,** 1081.

Cohn, R. (1970) Amnestic aphasia and other disturbances in naming. *Archives of Neurology* (Chicago), **22,** 515.

Collignon, R., Hécaen, H. & Angerlergues, R. (1968) A propos de 12 cas d'aphasie acquise chez l'enfant. *Acta Neurologica Belgica*, **68,** 245.

Conrad, K. (1949) Das Problem der gestörten Wortfindung in gestaltthöretischer Betrachtung. *Schweizer Archive für Neurologie und Psychiatrie*, **63,** 141.

Conrad, K. (1954) New problems in aphasia. *Brain*, **77,** 491.

Critchley, M. (1938) Aphasia in a partial deaf-mute. *Brain*, **61,** 163.

Critchley, M. (1942) Aphasic disorders of signalling (constitutional and acquired) occurring in naval signalmen. *Journal of Mount Sinai Hospital*, **9,** 363.

Critchley, M. (1960) Jacksonian ideas and the future with special reference to aphasia. *British Medical Journal*, **1591,** 6.

Critchley, M. (1962) Dr Samuel Johnson's aphasia. *Medical History*, **6,** 27.

Critchley, M. (1964) The drift and dissolution of language. *Proceedings of the Royal Society of Medicine*, **57,** 1189.

Critchley, M. (1970) *Aphasiology and Other Aspects of Language*. London: Arnold.

Curran, F.J. & Schilder, P. (1935) Paraphasic signs in diffuse lesions of the brain. *Journal of Nervous and Mental Diseases*, **82,** 613.

Daujat, C., Gainotti, G. & Tissot, R. (1974) Sur quelques aspects des troubles de la compréhension dans l'aphasie. *Cortex*, **10,** 347.

Delay, J. & Lhermitte, F. (1963) Aphasie. *Encyclopédie médico-chirurgie—système nerveaux, 17019* A^{10}, A^{30} et A^{50}, 1.

Dennis, M. (1976) Dissociated naming and locating of body parts after left anterior temporal lobe resection. *Brain and Language*, **3,** 147.

Doehring, D.G. & Peck-Swisher, L. (1972) Disturbances of connotative meaning in aphasia. *Journal of Communication Disorders*, **5,** 251.

Douglass, E. & Richardson, J.C. (1959) Aphasia in a congenital deaf-mute. *Brain*, **82,** 68.

Ducarne, B. (1976) Sémiologie de l'aphasie. *Revue de Psychologie appliquée*, **26,** 483.

Dyck, E. (van) (1967) Monographie d'un cas d'aphasie. *Le Langage et l'Homme*, **4,** 8.

Eisenson, J. (1963) Aphasic language modifications considered as a disruption of cultural verbal habits. *Journal of the American Speech Association*, **5**, 503.

Eisenson, J. (1963) Aphasic language modifications considered as a disruption of cultural verbal habits. *Folia Phoniatrica* (Basel), **15**, 299.

Eisenson, J. (1973) *Adult Aphasia*. Englewood Cliffs, NJ: Prentice-Hall.

Ewing, A.W.G. (1967) *Aphasia in Children*. New York: Hafner.

Fleming, M. (1957) Relationship between stammering and aphasia. *Journal of the South Africa Logopedic Society*, **4**, 3.

Freund, C.S. (1895) *Labyrinthtaubheit und Sprachtaubheit*. Wiesbaden: Bergmann.

Gainotti, G. & Ibba, R. (1972) La comprensione del significato dei gesti simbolici negli afasici. *Minerva psichiatrica e psicologica*, **13**, 1.

Gainotti, G. & Lemmo, M.A. (1976) Comprehension of symbolic gestures in aphasia. *Brain and Language*, **3**, 451.

Gardner, H. (1973) The contribution of operativity to naming capacity in aphasic patients. *Neuropsychologia*, **11**, 213.

Geets, W. (1972) Le langage perdu ou l'histoire d'un aphasique. *Le Langage et l'Homme*, **18**, 36.

Gerstmann, H.L. (1964) A case of aphasia. *Journal of Speech Disorders*, **29**, 89.

Goldhaimer, H. (1949) Use of language in dreams in analysis of aphasic deficits. *Archives of Neurology and Psychiatry* (Chicago), **62**, 725.

Goldstein, K. (1917) *Die transcortikalen Aphasien*. Jena: Fischer.

Goldstein, K. (1936) Meaning and aphasia. *Journal of Psychology*, **2**, 301–316.

Goldstein, K. & Marmor, J. (1938) A case of aphasia with special reference to the problems of repetition and word-finding. *Journal of Neurology and Psychiatry*, **1**, 329.

Goldstein, L.P. (1964) A case of an edentulous aphasic laryngectomy. *Journal of Speech Disorders*, **29**, 86.

Goodglass, H., Kaplan, E., Weintraub, S. & Ackerman, N. (1976) The 'tip-of-the-tongue' phenomenon in aphasia. *Cortex*, **12**, 145.

Grasset, J. (1896) Aphasie de la main droite chez un sourd-muet. *Progrès médicale* (Paris), **3**, 281.

Guiraud, P. (1936) Analyse du symptôme stéréotypé. *Encéphale*, **31**, 229.

Guttman, E. (1942) Aphasia in children. *Brain*, **65**, 205.

Hall, W.A. (1961) Return from silence; a personal experience. *Journal of Speech Disorders*, **26**, 174.

Halpern, H. (1965) Effects of stimulus variables on dysphasic verbal errors. Effect of stimulus variables on verbal perseveration of dysphasic subjects. *Perceptual and Motor Skills*, **20**, 421; **21**, 291.

Halpern, H. (1971) The differential diagnosis of language in the brain-injured adult. *Journal of Communication Disorders*, **4**, 76.

Heilman, K.M., Scholes, R. & Watson, T.R. (1975) Auditory affective agnosia: disturbed comprehension of affective speech. *Journal of Neurology, Neurosurgery and Psychiatry*, **38**, 69.

Hier, D.B. & Mohr, J.P. (1977) Incongruous oral and written naming. Evidence for a subdivision of the syndrome of Wernicke's aphasia. *Brain and Language*, **4**, 115.

Hirsch, K. (de) (1932) A case of motor aphasia. *British Journal of Children's Diseases*, **29**, 51.

Isserlin, M. (1922) Uber Agrammatismus. *Zeitschrift für die gesamte Neurologie und Psychiatrie*, **75**, 332.

Kertesz, A. & Poole, E. (1974) The aphasia quotient: the taxonomic approach to measurement of aphasic disability. *Canadian Journal of Neurological Sciences*, **1**, 7.

Kinsbourne, M. & Warrington, E. (1963) Jargon aphasia. *Neuropsychologia*, **1**, 27.

Kinsbourne, M. & Warrington, E.K. (1965) A case showing selectively impaired oral spelling. *Journal of Neurology, Neurosurgery and Psychiatry*, **28**, 563.

Kleist, K. (1934) Leitungsaphasie (Nachsprachaphasie). In *Geistesund Nervenkrenkheiten Handbuch der ärztlichen Erfahrungen im Weltkriege 1914–1918* (Ed.) Bonhoeffer, K. Vol. 4, p. 343. Leipzig: Barth.

Kleist, K. (1962) *Sensory Aphasia and Amusia*. Oxford: Pergamon.

Kreindler, A. & Fradis, A. (1967) Les composantes somatiques du comportement verbal dans l'aphasie. *Acta Neurologia Belgica*, **67**, 1003.

Kussmaul, A. (1884) *Les troubles de la parole*. Paris: Baillère.

Kussmaul, A. (1887) Disturbances of speech: an attempt in the pathology of speech. In *Encyclopedia of the Practice of Medicine* (Ed.) Ziemssen, H. p. 581. New York: Wood.

Lecours, A.R. (1974) Le cerveau et le langage. *Union médicale du Canada*, **103**, 232.

Lecours, A.R. (1975) Aphasie. *Encyclopédie médico-chirurgie, 17019 A*^{10}, 7.

Leischner, A. (1943) Die 'Aphasie' der Taubstummen. *Archiv für Psychiatrie und Nervenkrankheiten*, **115**, 469.

Leischner, A. (1948) Uber die Aphasie der Mehsrprachigen. *Archiv für Psychiatrie und Nervenkrankheiten*, **118**, 731.

Leischner, A. (1972) Uber den Verlauf und die Einteilung der aphasischen Syndrome. *Archiv für Psychiatrie und Nervenkrankheiten*, **216**, 219.

Leutenegger, R.R. (1951) Bibliography on aphasia. *Journal of Speech Disorders*, **16**, 280.

Lovell, H.W., Waggoner, R.W. & Kahn, E.A. (1932) Critical study of a case of aphasia. *Archives of Neurology and Psychiatry* (Chicago), **28**, 1178.

Low, A.A. (1931) A case of agrammatism in the English language. *Archives of Neurology and Psychiatry* (Chicago), **25**, 556.

Madonick, M.J. & Stein, J.M. (1953) A case of amnesic aphasia of fifteen years duration. Disturbances in abstract thinking. *Journal of Nervous and Mental Diseases*, **117**, 251.

Mallins, H. (1883) Case of aphasia with right hemiparesis in a girl aged 12 years. *Lancet*, **2**, 895.

Maruszewski, M. (1966) *Afazja*. Varsovie: Panstwowe Wydawn Naukowe.

Mohr, J.P. (1973) Rapid amelioration of motor aphasia. *Archives of Neurology* (Chicago), **28,** 77.

Mohr, J. P. (1976) An unusual case of dyslexia with dysgraphia. *Brain and Language*, **3,** 324.

Mohr, J.P., Sidman, M., Stoddard, L.T., Leicester, J. & Rosenberger, P.R. (1973) Evolution of the deficit in total aphasia. *Neurology*, **23,** 1302.

Monrad-Krohn, G.H. (1947) Dysprosody or altered melody of language. *Brain*, **70,** 405.

Monrad-Krohn, G.H. (1957) The third element of speech: prosody in the neuro-psychiatric clinic. *Journal of Mental Sciences*, **103,** 326.

Moore, N. (1878) Two curious examples of partial aphasia. *St Bartholomew's Hospital Report*, **14,** 159.

Naville, F. (1918) Mémoires d'un médecin aphasique: auto-observation et notes psychologiques du docteur Saloz père. *Archives de Psychologie*, **17,** 65.

Nebes, R.D. (1975) The nature of internal speech in a patient with aphemia. *Brain and Language*, **2,** 489.

Nielsen, J.M. (1963) Speech defects in middle life. *Geriatrics*, **18,** 827.

Nielsen, J.M. & McKeown, M. (1961) Dysprosody: report of two cases. *Bulletin of the Los Angeles Neurological Society*, **26,** 157.

Ombredane, A. (1951) *L'aphasie et l'élaboration de la pensée explicite*. Paris: Presses universitaires de France.

Paget, G.E. (1887) Notes on an exceptional case of aphasia. *British Medical Journal*, **11,** 1258.

Parker, H.L. (1956) *Clinical Studies in Neurology*. Springfield, IL: Thomas.

Riese, W. (1956) Semantic aphasia. *Journal of Nervous and Mental Diseases*, **123,** 18.

Rolnick, M. & Hoops, H.R. (1969) Aphasia as seen by the aphasic. *Journal of Speech Disorders*, **34,** 48.

Rose, R.H. (1948) A physician's account of his own aphasia. *Journal of Speech Disorders*, **13,** 294.

Rusk, H.A. (1955) Aphasia. *Journal of Chronic Diseases*, **2,** 352.

Sarno, J.E., Swisher, L.P. & Sarno, M.T. (1969) Aphasia in a congenitally deaf man. *Cortex*, **5,** 398.

Schuell, H. (1954) Clinical observations on aphasia. *Neurology*, **4,** 179.

Selecki, B.R. & Herron, J.T. (1965) Disturbances of the verbal body image: a particular syndrome of sensory aphasia. *Journal of Nervous and Mental Diseases*, **141,** 42.

Sies, L.F. & Butler, R.A. (1963) A personal account of dysphasia. *Journal of Speech Disorders*, **28,** 261.

Signoret, J.L., Ribadeau-Dumas, J.L. & Poirier, J. (1975) Le cerveau et les activités supérieures; 1re partie: le cerveau—neuropsychologie: introduction; aphasies; agnosies; apraxies. *Cahiers intégrés de médicine*, **150,** 1.

Smith, R.P. (1917–1918) Aphasia in relation to mental disease. *Journal of Mental Science*, **64,** 1.

Spreen, O., Benton, A.L. & van Allen, M.W. (1966) Dissociation of visual and tactile naming in amnesic aphasia. *Neurology*, **16,** 807.

Stengel, E. & Lodge Patch, I.C. (1955) 'Central' aphasia associated with parietal symptoms. *Brain*, **78,** 401.

Stockert, Th. (von) (1974) Aphasia sine aphasia. *Brain and Language*, **1,** 277.

Symonds, C. (1953) Aphasia. *Journal of Neurology, Neurosurgery and Psychiatry*, **16,** 1.

Tureen, L.L., Smolik, E.A. & Tritt, J.H. (1951) Aphasia in a deaf-mute. *Neurology*, **1,** 237.

Weinstein, E.A., Cole, M. & Mitchell, M.S. (1964) Anosognosia and aphasia. *Archives of Neurology* (Chicago), **10,** 376.

Weinstein, E.A. & Kahn, R.L. (1952) Nonaphasic misnaming (paraphasia) in organic brain disease. *Archives of Neurology and Psychiatry* (Chicago), **67,** 72.

Weinstein, E.A. & Kahn, R.L. (1955) *Denial of Illness; Symbolic and Physiological Aspects*. Springfield, IL: Thomas.

Weinstein, E. A. & Lyerly, O.G. (1976) Personality factors in jargon aphasia. *Cortex*, **12,** 122.

Weinstein, E.A., Lyerly, O.G., Cole, M. & Ozer, M.N. (1966) Meaning in jargon aphasia. *Cortex*, **2,** 165.

Wilson, S.A.K. (1920) Discussion on aphasia. *Brain*, **43,** 433.

Wilson, S.A.K. (1926) *Aphasia*. London: Trubner.

Yamadori, A., Osumi, Y., Masuhara, S. & Okubo, M. (1977) Preservation of singing in Broca's aphasia. *Journal of Neurology, Neurosurgery and Psychiatry*, **40,** 221.

5. Word Deafness and Word Blindness

> 'What did you say? That I bargain how? What do you want me to have, exaggeratedly? . . . But there are certain words, nevertheless, which I understand a little. But I can't speak. You see, as soon as I chat a little, like that, of figure, I can all alone. But that's all. It stops there . . . I took care of myself inside and it was impossible for me to hear anything more. And it's not igreeable, I'm telling you. What did I you make some people laugh who made fun of me! I didn't reply to them any more, moreover. But you see, then, I can speak a little all the same. You understand what I understand a little all the same. The proof! I beg you, understand just a little bit what I explain to you.'
>
> (*Conversation with Mrs Que.; December 1968*)

The majority of contemporary aphasiologists acknowledge the existence of *word deafness*, a disturbance in the discrimination and recognition of the auditory features constituting spoken language, and that of *word blindness*, a disturbance in the discrimination and recognition of the visual signs constituting written language. There is, however, fairly general dispute, particularly in regard to word deafness, concerning the occurrence of cases in which one of these disturbances is manifested in a strictly isolated manner (*pure cases*). Moreover, there is relatively little agreement concerning the anatomical localization of the causal lesions. Because of this double uncertainty, the physiopathological interpretation of these two conditions remains controversial.

WORD DEAFNESS

Since the disturbance specifically affects the discrimination and recognition of auditory stimuli constituting spoken language, it is easy to deduce its eventual manifestations in the patient's linguistic behaviour. Not only will the patient have difficulty in understanding spoken linguistic messages, but s/he will also fail on tests of audiophonatory (repetition) and audiomanual (writing to dictation) transposition[1, 2].

Clinical observation confirms that comprehension of spoken language is always severely disturbed, sometimes permanently. Numerous errors occur even during the most elementary tasks such as identifying objects, or pictures of objects, in response to spoken stimuli and carrying out simple commands presented orally (see Chapter 15). Identification tasks involving multiple-choice responses from several pictures whose names are similar in form (e.g., 'fight', 'light', 'right', and 'night') are particularly difficult, as is the identification of spoken words by selection of the appropriate written word from a list of phonemically similar words. The analysis of certain of the patient's behaviours in response to a spoken sentence suggests that a few words were more or less understood and that the patient had then unsuccessfully attempted to deduce the meaning of the entire command from these words. Use of this strategy no doubt also explains how the patient with word deafness is able to carry out certain simple orders. It is typical that the patient's rare successes on word identification tests and in the performance of oral commands occur only after an abnormally long delay.

Oral repetition is very disturbed or even totally impossible. This becomes increasingly obvious as the stimuli to be repeated become longer and more complex, but even repetition of units as simple as a syllable may be grossly abnormal. If it is possible to engage the patient in attempts at repetition, there is often little resemblance between the form of his or her productions and the stimuli presented [(5.1) satisfaction /satisfaksjɔ̃/ →/sɛbne/; (5.2) malentendu /malɑ̃tɑ̃dy/→/pœpʀɑ̃dʀ/; (5.3) hebdomadaire /ɛbdɔmadɛr/→/ɔbytɔba/; (5.4) bibliotheque /biblijɔtɛk/→/piblijɛʀ/]. However, we should point out that recent neurological literature includes reports on subjects with word deafness who were specifically able to discriminate and accurately to repeat vocalic phonemes (vowels) presented in isolation[3,4]. Writing to dictation is totally impossible. In cases where an adequate sample can be obtained, it shows almost no correspondence with the words dictated by the examiner.

PURE WORD DEAFNESS

Pure word deafness is an entity whose existence is theoretically possible, one in which the disturbance of oral language comprehension, repetition, and writing to dictation would not be accompanied by any other neuropsychological abnormality. The disorder would result solely from poor perceptual discrimination of linguistic sounds. Thus the discrimination and recognition of non-verbal sounds would be completely spared, and there would not be the least impairment of language behaviours which do not depend directly on the discrimination of the constituent sounds of language. The patients' discourse would therefore be normally produced even though they would be unable to recognize their own words, and, with the exception of writing to dictation, their written productions would be completely normal and their comprehension of written language would be unaffected. This double dissociation—a disturbance in the reception of spoken language in the absence of any other language impairment and a disturbance in the reception of verbal sounds in the absence of any impairment in the reception of non-verbal sounds—has only very rarely been observed in such an absolute manner[5].

Comprehension of written language was, in fact, reported to be normal in some of the case studies published until now. Similarly, spontaneous writing, sometimes with the exception of a few orthographic deviations (perhaps not more than normal), was also consistent with the theoretical concept of pure word deafness. However, the reports always mention the presence of slight, but undeniable, deficits of oral expression and/or a more or less severe impairment in the recognition of non-verbal sounds[5-7]. If the term 'pure word deafness' has continued to survive in the clinical aphasiological vocabulary, it is because certain patients present a clinical picture in which the manifestations of word deafness are clearly predominant relative to the mildness of associated deficits.

With the exception of the patients' extreme difficulty in repeating the language of others, the disturbance of oral expression is naturally very mild in (quasi) pure word deafness. It affects spontaneous discourse and is limited to the production of a few phonemic paraphasias and slight word-finding difficulty. The latter may be reflected in the occurrence of occasional semantic paraphasias. Perseverative phenomena may sometimes be noted. In typical cases, visuophonatory (oral reading) and visuomanual (copying) transposition are completely normal. Thus patients may be observed to produce some phonemic transformations in conversation but none at all in oral reading. Several points should be noted with regard to hearing for non-verbal sounds. (a) Pure tone audiometry almost always indicates a mild, bilaterally symmetrical, hearing loss with predominant high-frequency involvement[5] (Fig. 16-1). However, this elementary deficit is not sufficient to explain the word deafness because it scarcely affects many of the speech frequencies. Moreover, in certain cases of temporal lobe lesions, more severe hearing losses may be observed in the absence of disturbed comprehension of spoken language. (b) Although such cases are exceptional, certain patients with word deafness can readily identify familiar noises (such as sounds produced by animals, etc.), sometimes even when several noises are presented simultaneously[8,9]. Demonstration of this fact in patients with word-finding difficulty requires, in addition to the use of naming tests, the use of procedures in which the patient identifies each sound by selecting the corresponding picture from a group of matching stimuli. The patient may also be asked to match a stimulus sound with the appropriate sound in a subsequently presented series of sounds. (c) Despite the occurrence of exceptional cases in which the identification of musical sounds remains possible in the presence of word deafness, there is usually some degree of *tone deafness* (difficulty in recognizing the notes of the scale) and/or of *mel-*

odic deafness (difficulty in recognizing familiar melodies).

The behavioural pattern of individual patients presenting (quasi) pure word deafness is quite characteristic. They show no awareness of the errors which slip into their conversation but are very conscious of their auditory disturbance which they typically try to describe. They may report, for example, that they perceive speech as an 'indistinct murmur', 'a buzzing', 'a foreign language', as being 'too soft', 'too loud', 'too remote' or 'too close'. On the other hand, they recognize the voices of familiar speakers although they are unable to understand the words they utter[8, 10, 11]. These patients constantly request information in written form and, moreover, often express themselves in writing. Some of their behaviours are reminiscent of those which may be seen in the hearing-impaired (see Chapter 4, Type I Wernicke's aphasia). They may cup an ear and give great attention to visual information, particularly to that which can be obtained through observation of the speaker's gestures and lip movements. During evolution, some patients thus acquire surprising skill in speech reading[9, 12].

With regard to evolution, two facts should be remembered because of their consistency among typical cases. First, the disturbance of language reception and comprehension is generally refractory. It often shows no tendency towards spontaneous improvement, and attempts to facilitate recovery through therapy usually have little effect (see Chapter 17). Second, and additionally, the disturbance of oral expression slowly and progressively becomes more marked: the number of phonemic transformations increases and the immediately available vocabulary gradually decreases[7]; the patient with word deafness increasingly avoids oral expression whenever circumstances permit written communication.* Because such patients do not perceive their own words any better than those of others, the lack of (verbal) auditory feedback may play a role in this second evolutionary trend. In other words, it may be related to the fact that the individual with word deafness is no longer able to verify the formal and semantic adequacy of his or her language or to reinforce memory traces through the feedback which is continuously available to normal speakers.

CORTICAL DEAFNESS, AUDITORY AGNOSIA AND WORD DEAFNESS

Certain cortical lesions, whose anatomical localization will be specified below, may impair auditory perception, at least temporarily. The disturbance is then called cortical deafness[5, 13]. The hearing loss, which can be demonstrated by audiometric testing[5] and through the study of evoked potentials[14], naturally affects all auditory stimuli whether or not they convey linguistic information. Lack of attention to acoustic signals is obvious and, like individuals with severe peripheral hearing losses, the patient does not react to noise. Moreover, a certain degree of inattention may remain apparent even when the pure tone audiogram indicates improvement to the point where a loss is present only at the higher frequencies. When the audiogram shows improvement, the patient is able to discriminate certain frequencies and intensities but remains unable to discriminate rhythms, even very simple ones[5] (see Chapter 7).

Recognition of auditory information may be impaired in patients whose hearing is unaffected or shows only a high frequency loss which is insufficient to explain the recognition disturbance. The disturbance is then called auditory agnosia. When complete, the clinical picture includes disturbed recognition of non-verbal and non-musical sounds (sound agnosia, auditory agnosia proper for certain aphasiologists), of musical sounds (amusia) and of the acoustic signals constituting spoken language (word deafness). In severe cases, the patient is not only unable to identify familiar noises, musical notes and melodies as well as segments of spoken language, but cannot even say to which of these three categories a stimulus sound belongs. This extreme homogenization of the acoustic environment is particularly clear at the onset of the patient's disease. A patient seen by one of us (F.L.) explained this well in saying '*c'est toujours le même bruit ... lorsque on me parle, j'entends* "aoua aoua aou", *ca roule ... la musique, ça fait tout un brouhaha, un boucan*'. ('It's always the same noise ... when someone talks to me I hear "*aoua aoua aou*", it rolls ... music, it makes a great hubbub, a racket')[5].

It follows from the above that performance on tests of oral language reception and comprehen-

* These anomalies of oral expression might be considered as the fourth bona fide characteristic of word deafness in addition to the disturbances of auditory comprehension, repetition and writing to dictation.

sion is as disturbed in auditory agnosia as in pure word deafness. However, in contrast to patients with pure word deafness, those with auditory agnosia are unable to recognize familiar voices or regional accents or to say whether a conversation which they hear is in their own or in a foreign language.

WORD DEAFNESS AND APHASIA

We have already discussed the possible occurrence of a word-deafness component in Type I Wernicke's aphasia, that is, in Wernicke's aphasia proper (see Chapter 4). In cases where this component is obvious, the comprehension of written language, oral reading and copying are relatively spared whereas the comprehension of spoken language, writing to dictation and repetition are severely disturbed[15]. Oral expression is jargoned: the patient produces all types of paraphasias, with phonemic paraphasias predominating in the most typical cases. As in example (5), an element of dyssyntaxia may be evident:

(5.5) '*Mais alors, je peụx* |pije|, *malgré tout, un tout petit peu. Mais à cause de cela, je suis arrêtée cela. Vous voyez, je ne peux pas↓ je ne* /p/↓ *aucune* /paʀlɔʀ/! *Par exemple, je ne peux écrire personne. Vous ne savez pas. Vous auriez un crayon, je vous VERRAIS↓ vous verriez. Je ne le sais absolument rien écrit dessus. C'est-à-dire que si: je comprends tout ce qu'il écrit vous voyez mais tout cela me* /sut/ *complètement la* /ʀɛ̃pʀimi/ ... *Mais je peux parler. Mais je me rappelle aucune parole. Voilà. Or c'est ça↓ c'est ça qui est* /ɛ̃kɔpʀeɑ̃sif/: *une drôle drôle de voix dans* /tulu/. *Y a pas à DROLE, c'est drôle parce que, autrement, ELLE peut parler un tout petit peu.*'

'But then I can |pije|, despite everything, a little bit. But because of that, I'm stopped that. You see, I can't I /p/ no. /paʀlɔʀ/! For example, I not can write anybody. You don't know, you would have a pencil, I would SEE you↓ you would see. I don't it know absolutely anything written on. That's to say yes: I understand everything that he writes, you see, but all that completely /sut/ me the /ʀɛ̃pʀimi/ ... But I can talk. But I remember no words. And there it is. Then this is it↓ this is what is /ɛ̃kɔpʀeɑ̃sif/: a funny funny voice in /tulu/. There's no FUNNY, it's funny because otherwise SHE can talk a little bit.'

Written expression may be relatively more intact, at least after a certain period of evolution [see (4.27), first and second evaluations]. While no aspect of language, other than articulatory production, is strictly normal in this form of Wernicke's aphasia, those aspects of language which necessarily require the discrimination of the sounds of spoken language are the most obviously, and the most severely, impaired.

LESION LOCALIZATION

The anatomophysiological discussion of both word deafness and word blindness will be integrated into the section of this work dealing with the anatomophysiopathology of aphasia in general (see Chapter 8). Although the theoretical problems raised by these two entities are fairly well defined, it nevertheless seems useful, for those readers who already possess the needed neuroanatomical knowledge, to point out certain aspects within the context of the present chapter. In summary: (a) the unilateral destruction of Heschl's zone does not result in any typical clinical manifestation[5], although it can be detected through the study of evoked potentials[14]; (b) the bilateral destruction of Heschl's zone results in cortical deafness[5, 13]; (c) in right-handers, a left temporal lesion in the neighbourhood of Heschl's zone is necessary for the occurrence of word deafness (pure or in association with other agnosic or aphasic disturbances)[5]; (d) certain left temporal lesions alone can explain the onset of a 'pure' word deafness[5–7]; (e) aphasias resulting from left temporal lesions (significant involvement of Wernicke's area) may include a clear component of word deafness[15]; (f) in most cases where word deafness occurs in the context of a more general auditory agnosia, the causal lesions are bitemporal[5] (Fig. 5-1); (g) certain right temporal lesions in right-handers may result in an agnosia for sounds and amusia without word deafness[16]. The usual aetiology of the lesion or lesions resulting in word deafness is one or more ischaemic embolic accidents (see Chapter 9).

The few anatomical considerations and symptom features discussed above suggest a possible dissociation, in cerebral activity, between the processing of verbal acoustic information and that of non-verbal acoustic information (see Chapter 11). The discrimination of verbal sounds may, in fact, be profoundly impaired while that of non-verbal sounds remains intact and, inversely, impaired discrimination and recognition of non-verbal sounds are not necessarily accompanied by word deafness[5–7, 16]. This dichotomy may even be manifested within the

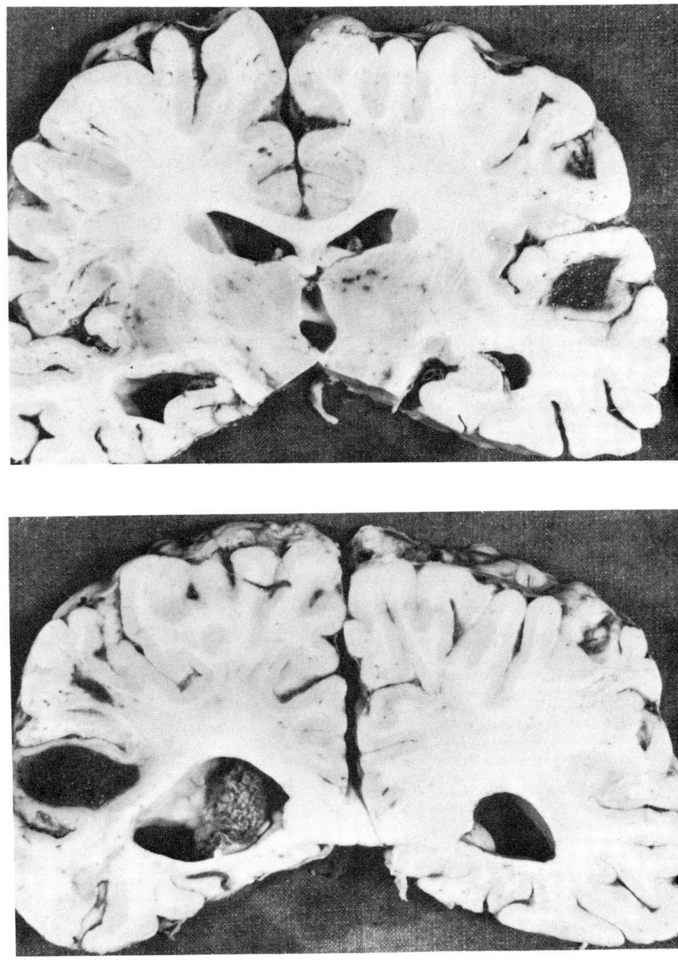

Fig. 5-1 *Bitemporal haemorrhage associated with an aphasia clearly dominated by word deafness. Courtesy of Dr Gérard Boudouresque, C.H.U. de la Timone, Marseille.*

linguistic domain itself, in the purest cases of word deafness, when the *segmental* components of language—formation of *discrete units* of various levels of complexity (see Chapter 2)—are disturbed, whereas the *suprasegmental* components—factors related to prosody, for example tonic accent, regional characteristics, individual vocal characteristics—are recognized normally or almost normally[8, 10, 11]. As suggested by Hécaen[17], after considering the performance of right-handers with left or right temporal lesions on dichotic listening tests (see Chapter 11), it is likely that the two cerebral hemispheres may process various auditory parameters of verbal sounds but that only the left hemisphere can process phonological features (see Chapter 12). This specialized perceptual function for the purely linguistic components of language appears to be primarily ensured by the left temporal cortex adjacent to Heschl's zone, that is, by certain components of Wernicke's area. This appears to be demonstrated by the occurrence of word deafness when these structures are destroyed by a cortical lesion or deprived of afferentation by a subcortical lesion (see Chapter 8).

That word deafness almost never occurs in the absence of other language disturbances (of the Wernicke type) is no doubt related to the fact that the anatomofunctional territory underlying auditory discrimination proper is in immediate physical proximity to the territory which controls other aspects of linguistic functioning. Furthermore, both territories depend on the same blood supply and vascular lesions usually involve both, so that concomitant disorders of both types of linguistic processing are observed.

WORD BLINDNESS

Since the disturbance specifically affects the discrimination and recognition of visual stimuli constituting written language, it is easy to deduce its eventual manifestations in these patients' linguistic behaviour. Not only will they have difficulty in understanding written linguistic messages but they will also fail on tests of visuophonatory (oral reading) and visuomanual (copying) transposition. Word blindness, which is also known as agnosic alexia or alexia without agraphia (see Chapter 10), is a relatively rare syndrome. In general, it has a sudden onset following occlusion of the left posterior cerebral artery (see Fig. 9–1) and is accompanied by a right lateral homonymous hemianopsia (see Chapter 4). Patients with word blindness are completely aware of their alexia and characteristically report that written language has suddenly become incomprehensible. To some patients, writing appears to be scribbling; to others, it seems to be in a foreign language; and, to some others, it appears to be in their own language but cannot be understood.

PURE WORD BLINDNESS

In our opinion, the clinical reality of pure word blindness cannot be contested; the disturbances of reading and of written copying are then unaccompanied by any other neurolinguistic disorder. The reading disturbance disrupts both the comprehension of written language and visuophonatory transposition (oral reading) in a similar fashion. The alexia is usually obvious in the reading of isolated letters, isolated words, sentences and texts. However, the disturbance is typically more severe in word reading (verbal alexia) than in letter reading (literal alexia)[18].This characteristic of agnosic alexia can be contrasted with aphasic alexia, in which difficulty is more obvious in reading isolated letters than in reading isolated words (see Chapter 4).

Literal alexia

The reading of letters presented one at a time in the visual field is almost always disturbed, often to a moderate degree. However, there are cases, especially during the initial phase of evolution, in which the disturbance is so severe that letters are not even recognized as letters. The patient may then report his or her impression of seeing graphic traces having no linguistic significance. More often, at least after a certain period of evolution, the patient can recognize letters as alphabetical signs (although the identification of individual letters is often incorrect) and may sometimes be able to specify certain characteristics (capital or small letters, cursive or printed letters, etc.).

The mistakes and abnormal latencies in letter recognition are, to a certain extent, related to the degree of structural complexity of the individual letters. In general, letters which are relatively simple in form (I, O, L, etc.) elicit fewer errors than letters which are relatively more complex (G, H, F, etc.). Identification errors may also indicate difficulty in discriminating among letters which share many of their constituent graphic features (O and Q, B and R, F and E, etc.). This is particularly clear in the case of letters which have a mirror reversal (b and d, p and q) and/or written signs which correspond to similar phonemes (M and N, P and B, etc.) (see Chapter 2, definition of feature, phoneme and grapheme). Certain visual conditions of stimulus presentation may also influence the patient's performance, namely the lighting, the size of the stimuli, their orientation with respect to the subject, the duration of stimulus exposure, the nature of the background against which letters are exposed, etc.

Some simultaneously presented letters, for example the patient's initials, are often noted to be easily recognized, no doubt because of their particular individual significance. Sometimes it may also be observed that a non-linguistic visual context may permit rapid identification of letters which are otherwise difficult to identify. For example, one of Dejerine's patients could read the letters R and F only when they were presented beside each other and surrounded by drawings of flags, that is, as they are incorporated into the emblem of the Republic of France[19]. One of us observed a similar phenomenon in a patient who could read the words 'Coca-Cola' only when they were written in white on a dark background, that is, as they appear on the bottle. Despite these exceptions, the identification of individual letters (visually) presented in groups or in the context of words or neologisms is generally more difficult than the identification of isolated letters.

Although somewhat unnatural and not based on any systematic learning, the recognition (called blind recognition) of letters presented through non-visual channels is nevertheless normal in patients with word blindness. Passive letter-tracing movements carried out using the patient's index finger as if it were a pencil permits identification of the letters. Similarly, letters traced by the examiner on the palm of the patient's hand are also identified correctly and letters in relief can be recognized through palpitation. The patient can also identify letters when given an adequate verbal description ('a letter like a circle with a little tail at the bottom' = Q; 'a letter formed from two slanting lines which meet at the bottom to form an acute angle' = V; etc.). A letter which cannot be recognized when visually presented to patients with agnosic alexia can be identified correctly if they outline it with a finger (see Chapter 17), and certain patients even learn to identify letters which they see by reproducing the contours through active movements of the head and the eyes. The intactness of 'blind' letter recognition in agnosic alexia is one of the clinical characteristics which distinguishes it from aphasic alexia[18].

Verbal alexia

The reading and comprehension of isolated words is always very disturbed and may be completely impossible in severe cases and early in the course of evolution. The disturbance is particularly obvious in matching tasks involving words with similar literal structures (for example matching the words 'fight', 'light', 'right', 'night', 'sight' to corresponding pictures). Nevertheless the reading of a few words which are very simple in form or are used very frequently often remains possible, even in very severe cases of word blindness. In many patients, there is clearly an almost total loss of the ability to read *globally* whereas attempts at *analytic* reading, letter by letter and syllable by syllable, may prove more or less effective or gradually become so. This dissociation between the loss of global word reading and the relative preservation of analytic reading is one of the pathognomonic features of agnosic alexia[18]. However, it must be emphasized that this partial preservation of analytic decoding abilities seldom constitutes, at least without a period of therapy (see Chapter 17), an effective means of improving reading performance. The effects of the literal alexia are obvious as soon as the segment to be read is increased in length: the patient is unable to give each letter the attention required for its identification while also carrying out the required synthesis of letters into a word; perseverative phenomena may be frequent; etc.

The *verbal paralexias* observed during oral reading tasks are characteristically of the formal type (see Chapter 2). Although there is probably no reason to infer the existence of several essentially different physiopathological mechanisms, the verbal paralexias sometimes appear attributable to the incorrect identification of one or more letters [for example (5.6) *baquet* → '*paquet*' (tub → 'parcel'), (5.7) *plage* → '*place*' (beach → 'place'); (5.8) *terme* → '*terne*' (term → 'dull'); etc.] and sometimes attributable to the incorrect apprehension of the global form of the stimulus word [(5.9) *caravane* → '*cravate*' (trailer → 'tie'); (5.10) *orage* → '*orange*' (storm → 'orange'), (5.11) *souris* → '*soupir*' (mouse → 'sigh'); etc.].* The right hemianopsia, which is almost always present in patients with word blindness, is probably related to the fact that the initial constituents of words are less often and less grossly transformed than are the terminal constituents. An observer sometimes has the impression that, after having somehow managed to read the beginning of a word, the patient then tries to guess the remainder. Perseverative phenomena are frequent in certain cases, especially during the first phase of evolution of the alexia [(5.12) *fleur*→'*fleur*' then *film*→'*fleure*' then *clef*→'*fleur*', etc.]. Whereas formal relationships are usually obvious between the stimulus word and the verbal paralexic response [see examples (6) to (11)], similarity of meaning is unusual and often appears to result by chance. When similarity of meaning is observed it is usually paired with some degree of formal similarity [(5.13) *banane*→'*ananas*' (banana →'pineapple'); (5.14) *cheval*→'*vache*' (horse→ 'cow'); (5.15) *minuit*→'*minute*' (midnight→ 'minute'); etc.].

In certain cases of agnosic alexia, the reading behaviours include the production of transformations which can be named *phonemic paralexias*, *literal paralexias* or *neologisms* depending on the factors considered [(5.16) *maison* (house)→'nouso' /mɛzɔ̃→nuso/; (5.17) *gateau*

* It is noteworthy that certain patients read without error or any hesitation some infrequently used words with a complex alphabetical structure (for example, in French, the words sphinx, wapiti, yacht, etc.) whose principal characteristic seems to be that their literal form bears little or no resemblance to that of any other word in the language.

(cake)→'catévu' /gɑto→katevy/; (5.18) *corbeille* (basket)→'couvile' /kɔʀbɛj→kuvil/; etc.]. An essential feature of these transformations is that the patients are always conscious of their erroneous productions and always indicate when their response does not correspond to an actual word in the language.* During production of such segments the patients' speech typically becomes syllabic and is interspersed with attempts at correction. This appears to indicate that the abnormal productions are related to unsuccessful attempts at analytic reading.

Alexia for written passages (textual alexia)
During the evolution of word blindness there is almost always a period in which the severity of the literal alexia and the verbal alexia is such that it is totally impossible for the patient to understand a written passage or to read it aloud. Depending on the case, this global alexia shows more or less considerable recovery with evolution and with therapy or else it constitutes a permanent state. In cases where the patient reaches a stage in which s/he is willing to attempt the reading of written texts, production of numerous paralexic transformations can be observed. Most of these transformations show an obvious similarity in the form of the replacing and replaced segments (Insertion 5.1).

Alajouanine has pointed out that some patients with word blindness can accurately identify, in a text written in cursives which they are unable to read, the handwriting of certain familiar individuals[18]. This observation is reminiscent of the ability of certain patients with word deafness to identify the individual voices of family members and friends (cf. p. 111). In both cases there is a dissociation between the inability to extract the properly linguistic significance from a language sample and the retained ability to recognize certain paralinguistic visual or auditory features which permit the precise identification of its author, that is, segmental facts are affected while suprasegmental ones are not.

Writing
It is classic to state that patients with pure word blindness write perfectly, except when copying, but are unable to read what they have written. The second proposition is true. The first is generally true but with a few qualifications. Spontaneous writing and writing to dictation often show a few duplications of downstrokes (especially involving 'n', 'm', 'i', 'u', etc.) and of

Insertion 5.1

Some linguistic aspects of the paralexic transformations observed in certain patients deserve mention even though we are uncertain whether they should be attributed to an aphasic disturbance, to an agnosic disturbance, to a defect affecting the right visual hemifield or, as is most probably the case, to a combination of several of these factors.

In these patients, it frequently happens that the first part of singly-presented stimulus words is read correctly, especially if it consists of a lexical moneme, and that the error involves only the second part of the word, especially if it is a suffix and, even more particularly, if it is a morphological marker† (see Chapter 2).

(5.19)	*'jardiner'*	→*'jardin'*	(gardener→garden)
(5.20)	*'rougeaud'*	→*'rougeole'*	(red-faced→measles)
(5.21)	*'individuel'*	→*'indivisible'*	(individual→indivisible)
(5.22)	*'finissait'*	→*'fini'*	(finished→have finished)
(5.23)	*'apparaissant'*	→*'apparaître'*	(appearing→to appear)
(5.24)	*'buffle'*	→*'buffet'*	(buffalo→buffet).

* Similarly, when patients are unable to read a word, they can generally say whether it is an actual word in the language or a neologism (or a word from a foreign language).

† All the examples quoted in Insertion 5.1 were taken from the same patient's file. The authors of this book agree with John Marshall's suggestion that this patient might now be considered to present a deep dyslexia.

However, a fairly large sample usually shows a certain number of errors which involve the initial part of the word. Prefixes may then be particularly susceptible to transformation:

(5.25) *'adroit'* →*'droit'* (skilful→straight or right)

(5.26) *'déambulant'* →*'ambulance'* (strolling→ambulance)

(5.27) *'dérivant'* →*'arriver'* (drifting→to arrive).

When the transformations affect a lexical moneme, the paralexias frequently appear to be of an agnosic type (cf. p. 115), that is, the stimulus and response show similarities in form:

(5.28) *'lieu'* →*'lien'* (place→bond)

(5.29) *'orage'* →*'orange'* (storm→orange)

(5.30) *'indirect'* →*'indiscret'* (indirect→indiscreet)

(5.31) *'cerner'* →*'cerisier'* (to encircle→cherry tree)

(5.32) *'décalerons'* →*'décoller'* (we will shift→to take off)

(5.33) *'roulons'* →*'roucoule'* (let's roll→coo).

In other cases the transformation is clearly of the 'aphasic type' as it is subtended by the existence of a conceptual link between the stimulus and the response:

(5.34) *'créativité'* →*'nativité'* (creativity→nativity)

(5.35) *'grand-oncle'* →*'grand-mère'* (grand-uncle→grandmother)

(5.36) *'géant'* →*'petit'* (giant→small)

(5.37) *'tante'* →*'homosexuel* (pansy→homosexual).

In still other instances, both formal and semantic factors appear to enter into play:

(5.38) *'ensemble'* →*'assemblée'* (whole→assembly)

(5.39) *'mineur'* →*'majeur'* (minor→major)

(5.40) *'pétulant'* →*'pétarade'* (lively→crackling)

(5.41) *'pistonner'* →*'pomper'* (to push→to pump).

On the whole, these verbal paralexias suggest a tendency to replace abstract words by concrete words, rare words by more frequently used words, conjugated verbs by infinitives, adjectives or nouns, and infinitives and adjectives by nouns. In general, they also show that abstract words elicit more reading errors than concrete words, and that rare words elicit more errors than frequently used words. Similarly, conjugated verbs are transformed more often than are infinitives and adjectives which, in turn, are transformed more often than nouns.

In cases where reading of a connected passage is possible, a very clear predominance of paralexic errors involving grammatical words may sometimes be observed.

letters and, less frequently, the omission and repetition of words (particularly of short grammatical words) and, sometimes, of short syntagms. These abnormalities, which are often minimal, are no doubt related to the fact that normal verification of production through feedback generated by concomitant reading is no longer possible in patients with word blindness. Texts written by some patients show an abnormal arrangement within the space of the page. Most often, this takes the form of lines which slope, more or less sharply, towards the bottom right of the page. These particular features of writing in patients with word blindness are reminiscent of those observed in certain blind individuals (acquired blindness) or in normals when writing with the eyes covered.

As mentioned, a copying disturbance which is

usually severe is a characteristic clinical feature of agnosic alexia. The copying of neologisms is always servile, as is that of words and sentences, with the exception of segments correctly identified (read) by the patient.

Oral spelling is normal. Similarly, the identification of words spelled aloud by the examiner is usually normal although it may be slightly disturbed in some patients.

WORD BLINDNESS AND READING OF NON-ALPHABETICAL GRAPHIC SYMBOLS

In agnosic alexia it is not uncommon for the reading of numbers to be less disturbed than that of letters and words. It is even said that the reading of numbers may be completely spared in certain patients. In such cases, this ability generally emerges after a period of evolution. Among other factors which may be related to this dissociation, Benson and Geschwind[20] noted that the numerical system includes only ten elementary graphic symbols and that the learning (in general, particularly extended) of number reading is not based solely on visuo-phonatory transpositions but also involves associations between numbers and sequences of ordered finger movements. It can also be added that the combination of single digits into double- or multidigit numbers is carried out according to fewer and simpler rules than is the combination of letters into words and words into sentences. When the identification of numerical symbols is disturbed in a patient with word blindness, the severity of the disturbance is not necessarily comparable with that of the alexia strictly defined[19]: severe global alexia may coexist with nearly normal ability in the recognition of written numerical symbols and, inversely, a mild alexia may be accompanied by marked difficulty in number identification.

The abnormal productions observed during tests of number reading are analogous to those seen in word reading: numbers can be recognized as being numbers but are not read aloud nor precisely identified; the appearance of difficulty, or increased difficulty, as a function of an increase in the length of the number and/or simultaneous presentation of many stimuli; confusion between numbers which share many of their constituent elements (graphic features for single-digit numbers, for example '6' and '9', '3' and '8', etc., and between individual digits for multidigit numbers, for example '734' and '743'); almost exclusive use of an analytic reading strategy leading to incomplete responses or faulty reconstruction of the stimuli. Confusions may frequently occur between tens and hundreds and between hundreds and thousands.

CORTICAL BLINDNESS, VISUAL AGNOSIA AND WORD BLINDNESS

Certain cortical lesions, whose anatomical localization will be specified below, may impair visual perception. The disturbance is then called cortical blindness. Cortical blindness affects perception of all visual stimuli whether or not they convey linguistic information. On the other hand, the identification of visual information may be disturbed even though the stimuli are normally perceived; a condition which is called visual agnosia. Word blindness is one instance of this type of disorder. It is sometimes unaccompanied by any other type of visual agnosic disturbance and, in this case, is usually quite mild. When it is more severe, as is more often the case, the word blindness is usually accompanied by another form of visual agnosia, namely colour agnosia. As previously employed by one of us (F.L.)[21], the term 'colour agnosia' is used here to designate, without any physiopathological implications, a clinical entity including a disturbance in the naming and identification of colours, in the evocation of colours as object attributes, in the selection of colours during colouring tests and in the recognition of whether or not pictures are conventionally coloured. These deficits cannot be attributed to the slight disturbance of elementary chromatic vision (*pseudodyschromatopsia*) which almost always accompanies them (see Chapter 16). More rarely, and usually in patients whose word blindness is particularly severe, this disturbance and the agnosia for colours may coexist with a visual agnosia for pictures and sometimes even for objects[21]. Whether or not word blindness is associated with other visual agnosic disturbances it is, as a rule which has very few exceptions, accompanied by a right lateral homonymous hemianopsia with or without sparing of the hemimacula.

WORD BLINDNESS AND APHASIA

For purposes of discussion, the relationships between word blindness and aphasia will be divided into two groups of facts, the first concerned with the frequent association of agnosic alexia and word finding difficulty and the second concerned with possible mutual relationships between word blindness and Type III Wernicke's aphasia (see Chapter 4).

Word blindness and naming deficits

A detailed examination of linguistic functioning will permit a demonstration of word-finding difficulty in a large proportion of cases of alexia without agraphia, that is, of agnosic alexia. The word-finding difficulty is often mild, at least in cases where the disturbance results from a thromboembolic accident (see Chapter 9), and is manifested, essentially, during naming tests. No other symptomatic features of aphasia are observed in these patients. Thus certain aphasiologists speak of an association between word blindness and amnesic aphasia (cf. p. 100).

In discussing the problem of disconnection syndromes (cf. p. 26), Geschwind[22] reported an anatomoclinical case study—which he rightfully considered to be of major theoretical importance—associating an alexia without agraphia with a specific naming deficit for colours (colour anomia). Besides a right hemianopsia and alexia without agraphia, Geschwind's patient presented a naming disturbance which affected only colours and was not accompanied by a disturbance of elementary chromatic vision nor by the other clinical anomalies grouped here under the name of colour agnosia. In other words, colour recognition was not disturbed. Geschwind explains this clinical picture, which we consider to be most exceptional, by the presence of a lesion of certain splenial associative fibres which connect right occipital and left temporal regions (cf. Chapter 8).

Word blindness and Wernicke's aphasia

We have discussed elsewhere the fact that written language comprehension may be very disturbed in certain Wernicke's aphasics whereas spoken language comprehension is affected only mildly (see Chapter 4, Type III Wernicke's aphasia). In such cases, oral reading and written expression are both very impaired [see (4.33) to (4.52)], whereas oral expression may be almost normal, with the exception of more or less severe word-finding difficulty. In rare cases, the dissociation between the massive disturbance of the receptive and expressive modalities of written language and the intactness of their oral counterparts is so clear that the clinical picture corresponds to Déjerine's *alexia–agraphia*[23, 24] (see Chapter 10). In many respects, the disturbance of written language comprehension and of oral reading in these patients are similar to those observed in an isolated state in alexia without agraphia. In his book entitled *Sémiologie des affectations du système nerveux*[19] Dejerine designated both of these disorders by the name *word blindness*.

LESION LOCALIZATION

Cortical blindness results from lesions which cause bilateral destruction of the calcarine cortex and/or its afferents. From a review of anatomoclinical case studies reported in the literature[21], it can be concluded that a left occipital lesion is always present in cases of *word blindness* (alexia without agraphia) in right-handers. This lesion involves the calcarine region and/or its optic radiations thus explaining the hemianopsia. It also affects the lingual lobule and the fusiform gyrus and, in some cases, the cuneus as well. The occipital lesion is sometimes accompanied by a lesion of the corpus callosum but more often by involvement of the splenial axonal prolongations within the left cerebral hemisphere. In most cases, the lesions can be attributed to an occlusive accident in the territory of the left posterior cerebral artery (see Chapter 9). In much rarer cases, word blindness appears after trauma or develops gradually in relation to a tumoral or degenerative process. When word blindness is observed after a left occipital lobectomy, it is not accompanied by an agnosia for pictures or visual objects[25] and it regresses more quickly and to a greater degree than in cases where it results from a cerebral vascular accident. The theoretical importance of this fact would be more obvious were it certain—which is not the case—that the procedure which neurosurgeons call an 'occipital lobectomy' usually includes resection of the whole of the lingual lobule and the fusiform gyrus.

After Déjerine[19, 23, 24], Foix and Hillemand[26] (see Chapter 1), Geschwind considers that alexia without agraphia constitutes the prototype of a disconnection syndrome[27]: because of the left occipital lesion, resulting in a right hemianopsia, visual information is received only in the right occipital lobe; because of a splenial lesion, this information cannot be transmitted to the angular gyrus of the left hemisphere which, as one of its roles, carries out the final decoding of written language. Many contemporary researchers do not accept this physiopathological interpretation of word blindness. Rather they consider that it is more appropriately designated by the name of agnosic alexia (see Chapter 10), belongs within the general clinical context of the visual agnosias and is primarily attributable to the cortical lesion. According to them, convincing evidence regarding the last point can be found in the frequency with which, as a result of such lesions, agnosic alexia is associated with disturbed recognition of non-linguistic visual information[21]. If agnosic alexia may occur in an isolated state, it is because the visual symbols constituting written language are particularly complex and are therefore particularly fragile. Because this fragility cannot be readily conceptualized in terms of cerebral functioning, we prefer to consider agnosic alexia as usually being a specific disturbance in the recognition and discrimination of linguistic visual information. This assertion appears to follow from the occurrence of cases in which the linguistic disturbance is strictly isolated: no disturbance is observed in the recognition of visual stimuli other than those of language and, within the domain of written language, these patients show no difficulty in recognizing those aspects which are not properly linguistic. Despite a severe global alexia, one of our patients could, for example, match samples of cursive writing without any hesitation (ten sample pairs presented simultaneously). We do not consider the theoretical importance of such cases to be reduced by their rare occurrence.

Word deafness impedes recognition of spoken language symbols and word blindness impedes recognition of written language symbols. In both cases, one of the two receptive aspects of language is selectively disturbed. Word deafness is usually associated with disturbed recognition of non-linguistic auditory information (non-verbal sounds and music). Similarly, word blindness is frequently associated with disturbed recognition of colours and sometimes of pictures and of visual objects. The occurrence of pure or quasi-pure forms, in which only the strictly linguistic parameters of speech and writing are not recognized whereas their paralinguistic parameters are identified, suggests that the disturbance affects neuronal networks which specifically and exclusively govern the discrimination of linguistic components. It also suggests, as a corollary, that the cerebral processing of suprasegmental features of language is carried out independently from the processing of strictly linguistic, segmental, features.

In cortical deafness, as in cortical blindness, it is the primary sensory area, or its afferents and efferents, which are bilaterally involved. In word deafness, as in word blindness, the disturbance results from a dysfunction of a cortical associative area either because this region itself is lesioned or because a lesion results in its deafferentation. The localization of cerebral regions subtending the processing of paralinguistic parameters (recognition of voices and of handwriting, for example) is not known, at least not on the basis of anatomoclinical evidence. However, it is possible that they are entirely or partially located in the right hemisphere of the brain in right-handers.

An element of word deafness is not uncommonly observed in the context of a Wernicke's aphasia (*auditory aspect*: *versant auditif*). Although perhaps somewhat less frequent, a component of word blindness can also be seen in the context of a Wernicke's aphasia (*visual aspect*: *versant visuel*) (see Chapter 4). On the other hand, (quasi) pure word deafness is much rarer than pure word blindness. These facts can be explained on an anatomical basis: the areas involved in the decoding of spoken language are adjacent to areas subtending other aspects of linguistic functioning and share a common vascular territory (left middle cerebral artery) with them. Certain visual areas involved in the decoding of written language are anatomically more distinct and belong to a different arterial territory (left posterior cerebral artery) (see Chapters 8 and 9).

REFERENCES

1. Sérieux, P. (1893) Sur un cas de surdité verbale pure. *Revue médicale*, **13**, 733.
2. Déjerine, J. & Sérieux, P. (1897) Un cas de surdité verbale pure terminée par aphasie sensorielle, suivie d'autopsie. *Mémoires de la Société de Biologie*, **49**(4), 1074.
3. Studdert-Kennedy, M. & Shankweiler, D.P. (1970) Hemispheric specialization for speech perception. *Journal of the Acoustical Society of America*, **48**, 579.
4. Shankweiler, D.P. & Studdert-Kennedy, M. (1967) Identification of consonants and vowels presented to left and right ears. *Quarterly Journal of Experimental Psychology*, **19**, 59.

5. Lhermitte, F., Chain, F., Escourolle, R., Ducarne, B., Pillon, B. & Chedru, F. (1971) Etudes des troubles perceptifs auditifs dans les lésions temporales bilatérales. A propos de trois observations dont deux anatomo-cliniques. *Revue neurologique*, **124,** 329.
6. Liepmann, H. & Storch, E. (1902) Der mikroskopiche Gehirnbefund bei dem Fall Gorstelle. *Monatschrift für Psychiatrie und Neurologie*, **11,** 115.
7. Schuster, P. & Taterka, H. (1926) Beiträge zur Anatomie und Klinik der reinen Worttaubheit. *Zentralblatt für die gesamte Neurologie und Psychiatrie*, **105,** 494.
8. Klein, R. & Harper, J. (1956) The problem of agnosia in the light of a case of pure word deafness. *Journal of Mental Sciences*, **102,** 112.
9. Hécaen, H., Dubois, J. & Marcie, P. (1968) La désorganisation de la réception des signes verbaux dans l'aphasie sensorielle. *Revue d'Acoustique*, **3-4,** 287.
10. Hemphill, R.E. & Stengel, E. (1940) Study on pure word deafness. *Journal of Neurology, Neurosurgery and Psychiatry*, **3,** 2[illegible]1.
11. Brown, J.W. (1972) *Aphasia, Apraxia and Agnosia: Clinical and Theoretical Aspects*. Springfield, IL: Thomas.
12. Wohlfart, G., Lindgren, A. & Jernelius, B. (1952) Clinical picture and morbid anatomy in a case of 'pure word deafness'. *Journal of Nervous and Mental Diseases*, **116,** 818.
13. Legros Clark, W.E. & Russel, W.R. (1938) Cortical deafness without aphasia. *Brain*, **61,** 375.
14. Peronnet, F. & Michel, F. (1977) The asymmetry of the auditory evoked potentials in normal man and in patients with brain lesions. *Progress in Clinical Neurophysiology*, **2,** 130.
15. Hécaen, H. (1969) Essai de dissociation du syndrome de l'aphasie sensorielle. *Revue neurologique*, **120,** 229.
16. Spreen, O., Benton, A.L. & Fincham, R.W. (1965) Auditory agnosia without aphasia. *Archives of Neurology* (Chicago), **13,** 84.
17. Hécaen, H. (1972) *Introduction à la neuropsychologie*. Paris: Larousse.
18. Alajouanine, Th., Lhermitte, F. & Ribaucourt-Ducarne, B. (de) (1960) Les alexies agnosiques et aphasiques. In *Les grandes activités du lobe occipital* (Ed.) Alajouanine, Th. p. 235. Paris: Masson.
19. Déjerine, J. (1914) *Sémiologie des affections du système nerveux*. Paris: Masson.
20. Benson, D.F. & Geschwind, N. (1969) The alexias. In *Handbook of Clinical Neurology* (Ed.) Vinken, P.J. & Bruyn, G.W. Vol. IV, p. 112. Amsterdam: North-Holland.
21. Lhermitte, F., Chain, F., Aron, D., Leblanc, M. & Souty, O. (1969) Les troubles de la vision des couleurs dans les lésions postérieures du cerveau; à propos de 42 observations. *Revue neurologique*, **121,** 5.
22. Geschwind, N. & Fusillo, M. (1966) Color naming defects in association with alexia. *Archives of Neurology* (Chicago), **15,** 137.
23. Dejerine, J. (1892) Contribution à l'étude anatomo-pathologique et clinique des différentes variétés de cécité verbale. *Mémoires de la Société de Biologie*, **9** (IV), 61.
24. Dejerine, J. & Pélissier, A. (1914) Contribution à l'étude de la cécité verbale pure. *L'encéphale*, **9,** 1.
25. Hécaen, H., Ajuriaguerra, J. (de) & Angelergues, R. (1957) Les troubles de la lecture dans le cadre de la désorganisation des fonctions symboliques. *Psychiatrie und Neurologie* (Basel), **134,** 97.
26. Foix, Ch. & Hillemand, P. (1925) Rôle vraisemblable du splénium dans la pathogénie de l'alexie pure lésion de la cérébrale postérieure. *Bulletin et Mémoires de la Société de Médecine de Paris*, **41,** 393.
27. Geschwind, N. (1965) Disconnexion syndromes in animals and man. *Brain*, **88,** 237 and 585.

BIBLIOGRAPHY

Ajax, E.T. (1967) Dyslexia without agraphia. *Archives of Neurology* (Chicago), **17,** 645.

Alajouanine, Th. (Ed.) (1960) *Les grandes activités du lobe occipital*. Paris: Masson.

Alajouanine, Th., Aubry, M. & Pialoux, P. (1955) Note préliminaire sur l'atteinte auditive dans l'aphasie. In *Les grandes activités du lobe temporal* (Ed.) Alajouanine, Th. p. 203. Paris: Masson.

Albert, M.L. & Bear, D. (1974) Time to understand; a case study of word deafness with reference to the role of time in auditory comprehension. *Brain*, **87,** 373.

Albert, M.L., Sparks, R., Stockert, Th. (von) & Sax, D. (1972) A case study of auditory agnosia: linguistic and non-linguistic processing. *Cortex*, **8,** 427.

Albert, M.L., Yamadori, A., Gardner, H. & Howes, D. (1973) Comprehension in alexia. *Brain*, **96,** 317.

Angelergues, R., Cohen, D. & Gauthier, M. (1967) Sur la notion de surdité verbale dans les troubles aphasiques. *Journal de Psychologie normale et pathologique*, **64,** 189.

Aptman, L., Levin, H. & Senelick, R.C. (1977) Alexia without agraphia in a left-handed patient with prosopagnosia. *Neurology*, **27,** 533.

Arnaud, H. (1887) Contribution à l'étude clinique de la surdité verbale. *Archives de Neurologie*, **13,** 177 and 366.

Assal, G. & Hadj-Djilani, M. (1976) Une nouvelle observation d'alexie pure sans hémianopsie. *Cortéx*, **12,** 169.

Bachman, F. (1927) Uber kongenitale Wortblindheit (angeborene Leseschwache). *Abhandlungen aus der Neurologie, Psychiatrie, Psychologie*, **40,** 1.

Baruk, H. & Dereux, J. (1926) Syndrome occipital avec hallucinose et amnésie verbale et visuelle. *Bulletin et Mémoires de la Société de Médecine de Paris*, **3,** 1463.

Baruk, H. & Hartmann, E. (1927) Un cas d'alexie pure avec agnosie visuelle. *Encéphale*, **22,** 796.

Benson, D.F., Brown, J. & Tomlinson, E.B. (1971) Varieties of alexia. Word and letter blindness. *Neurology*, **21,** 951.

Benton, A.L. (1962) Dyslexia in relation to form perception and directional sense. In *Reading Disability* (Ed.) Money, J. p. 81. Baltimore, MD: Johns Hopkins.

Berlin, C.I., Chase, R.A., Dill, A. & Hagepanos, T. (1965) Auditory findings in temporal lobectomized patients (abstract). *Journal of the American Speech Association*, **7,** 386.

Berlin, C.I., Lowe-Bell, S.S., Jannetta, P.J. & Kline, D.G. (1972) Central auditory deficits after temporal lobectomy. *Archives of Otolaryngology*, **96,** 4.

Botez, M.I., Serbancescu, T. & Vernea, I. (1964) Visual static agnosia with special reference to literal agnosic alexia. *Neurology*, **14,** 1101.

Bramwell, E. (1927) A case of cortical deafness. *Brain*, **50,** 579.

Brisset, C. (1952) Aphasie d'intégration par agnosie auditive congénitale. *Revue neurologique*, **87,** 387.

Chavany, J.A. (1945) Un cas de surdité d'origine corticale. *Progrès médicale* (Paris), **53,** 472.

Cumming, W.J.K., Hurwitz, L.J. & Perl, N.T. (1970) Alexia without agraphia: a case report. *Journal of Neurology, Neurosurgery and Psychiatry*, **33,** 34.

Dattner, B., Davis, V.T. & Smith, C.E. (1952) A case of subcortical visual verbal agnosia. *Journal of Nervous and Mental Diseases*, **116,** 808.

Fincham, R.W., Nibbelink, D.W. & Aschenbrener, C.A. (1975) Alexia with left homonymous hemanopia without agraphia. *Neurology*, **25,** 1164.

Fowler, E.P. (1944) Total monaural deafness for speech, but not for speech frequencies; misleading threshold audiogram. *Laryngoscope*, **54,** 605.

Gazzaniga, M.S., Glass, A.A., Sarno, M.T. & Posner, J.B. (1973) Pure word deafness and hemispheric dynamics: a case history. *Cortex*, **9,** 136.

Gehuchten, A. (van) & Goris, C. (1901) Un cas de surdité verbale pure par abcès du lobe temporal gauche; trépanation, guérison. *Névraxe*, **3,** 65.

Giraudeau, D. (1882) Note sur un cas de surdité cérébrale. *Revue de Médecine* (Paris), **2,** 448.

Goldstein, M.N., Brown, M. & Hollander, J. (1975) Auditory agnosia and cortical deafness; analysis of a case with three-year followup. *Brain and Language*, **2,** 324.

Goldstein, M.N., Joynt, R.J. & Goldblatt, D. (1971) Word blindness with intact central visual fields. *Neurology*, **21,** 873.

Graveleau, D., Baheux, G., Simoneau, F. & Laplane, R. (1964) Alexie agnosique et apraxie constructive régressive chez un enfant de douze ans. *Archives françaises de Pédiatrie*, **21,** 483.

Greenblatt, S.H. (1973) Alexia without agraphia or hemianopsia. *Brain*, **96,** 307.

Greenblatt, S.H. (1976) Subangular alexia without agraphia or hemianopsia. *Brain and Language*, **3,** 229.

Hallgren, B. (1949) Constitutional dyslexia (so-called congenital word blindness); clinical and heredobiologic investigation. *Nordisk Medicin*, **41,** 14.

Hallgren, B. (1950) Specific dyslexia (congenital word blindness): clinical and genetic study. *Acta Psychiatrica Scandinavica* (suppl. 65), 1.

Hécaen, H. (Ed.) (1972) *Neuropsychologie de la perception visuelle*. Paris: Masson.

Hermann, K. (1956) Congenital word-blindness. *Acta Psychiatrica Scandinavica* (suppl. 108), 117.

Hinshelwood, J. (1900) *Letter, Word and Mind-blindness*. London: Lewis.

Hirose, G., Kin, T. & Murakami, E. (1977) Alexia without agraphia associated with right occipital lesion. *Journal of Neurology, Neurosurgery and Psychiatry*, **40,** 225.

Hoff, H., Gloning, I. & Gloning, K. (1954) Uber Alexie. *Wien. Z. Nervenheilk*, **10,** 149.

Holmes, G. (1950) Pure word blindness. *Folia Psychiatrica, Neurologica et Neurochirurgica Neerlandica*, **53,** 279.

Horenstein, S., Lezak, R. &. Pitts, W. (1966) Temporal tone discrimination in auditory agnosia. *Transactions of the American Neurological Association*, **91,** 251.

Jones, J. & Dinolt, R. (1952) Pure word deafness. *Laryngoscope*, **61,** 194.

Kanshepolsky, J., Kelly, J.J. & Waggener, J.D. (1973) A cortical auditory disorder. Clinical, audiologic and pathologic aspects. *Neurology*, **23,** 699.

Karlin, I.W. (1951) Congenital verbal-auditory agnosia. *Pediatrics*, **7,** 60.

Kopeczynski, S. & Zylverblast-Zand (1922) Un cas de surdité verbale pure. *Revue neurologique*, **29,** 1338.

Kreindler, A. & Ionasescu, V. (1961) A case of 'pure' word blindness. *Journal of Neurology, Neurosurgery and Psychiatry*, **24,** 275.

Lühdorf, K. & Paulson, O.B. (1977) Does alexia without agraphia always include hemianopsia? *Acta Psychiatrica Scandinavica*, **55,** 323.

Mahoudeau, D., Lemoyne, J., Dubrisay, J. & Caraes, J. (1957) Etude d'un nouveau cas d'agnosie auditive *Semaine des Hôpitaux de Paris*, **33,** 581.

Maspes, P.E. (1948) Le syndrome expérimental chez l'homme de la section du splénium du corps calleux. *Revue neurologique*, **80,** 100.

Massary, J. (de) (1932) L'alexie. *Encéphale*, **27,** 134.

Money, J. (Ed.) (1962) *Reading Disability*. Baltimore, MD: Johns Hopkins.

Morrison, A.G. (1930) Congenital word-deafness, with some observations on the accompanying idioglossia, *Journal of Neurology and Psychopathology*, **11,** 28, 134.

Mounier-Kuhn, P., Schott, B. & Lafont, J.C. (1960) Diagnostic de l'agnosie auditive et de la surdité corticale. *Revue d'Oto-neuro-ophtalmologie*, **32,** 129.

Penfield, W. & Perot, P. (1963) The brain's record of auditory and visual experience—a final summary and discussion. *Brain*, **86,** 595.

Pershing, H.T. (1897) Auditory aphasia. *Journal of Nervous and Mental Diseases*, **24,** 519.

Reinhold, M. (1950) A case of auditory agnosia. *Brain*, **73,** 203.

Reinhold, M. (1954) Analysis of agnosia. *Neurology*, **4,** 128.

Stachowiak, F.J. & Poeck, K. (1976) Functional disconnection in pure alexia and color naming deficit demonstrated by facilitation methods. *Brain and Language*, **3**, 135.

Vignolo, L.A. (1969) Auditory agnosia: a review and report of recent evidence. In *Contributions to Clinical Neuropsychology* (Ed.) Benton, A.L. p. 172. Chicago: Aldine.

Wechsler, A.F. (1972) Transitory left hemialexia; a clinical and angiographic study. *Neurology*, **22**, 628.

Wolpert, I. (1930) Uber das Wesen der literalen Alexie. *Monatschrift für Psychiatrie und Neurologiè*, **75**, 207.

Ziegler, D.K. (1952) Word deafness and Wernicke's aphasia—report of cases and discussion of the syndrome. *Archives of Neurology and Psychiatry* (Chicago), **67**, 323.

6. Speech and Language in the Frontal Syndrome

[Do you go to university?] I go to university [In which department?] In which department, yes ... [Have you worked before?] Worked. [Did you work in the summer or full time?] Full time. [Do you speak English?] Speak English. [A little bit or ...?] It's awful. [Did you study in French or in English?] In English.* [You're right-handed or left-handed?] Right-handed or left-handed. [Do you have some brothers and sisters?] Brothers and sisters.

(*Conversation with Mr Re.; January 1975*)

We have previously discussed the articulatory disturbances observed in clinical aphasiology (see Chapter 3) as well as the symptomatology of Broca's aphasia and of global aphasia (see Chapter 4). It was mentioned—although a systematic exposition of the problem will be deferred until a later section (see Chapter 8-3)—that the occurrence of these disturbances may be partially or entirely determined by frontal lesions. For example, Broca's aphasia has long been attributed, in right-handers, to a lesion of the pars opercularis and pars triangularis of the left third frontal convolution (see Chapter 11). Despite this localization, neither Broca's aphasia nor anarthria or global aphasia are usually included in the common conception of the *frontal syndrome*. Nevertheless, this syndrome does include abnormalities of speech and language and it is these abnormalities which constitute the principal topic of the present chapter.

The frontal lobe is heterogeneous from the point of view of cerebral anatomy and physiology. Only a few of its constituent structures, as well as the disturbances resulting from lesions of these structures, will be given attention here, namely: (a) the notion of *agraphia* from a lesion of the caudalmost part of the second frontal convolution; certain aspects of this notion, which were discussed in parallel with a disturbance of oral expression (*anarthria*) to which it corresponds on the linguistic level (see Chapter 3), will be briefly reconsidered; (b) speech disturbances which may result from a lesion of the caudal, internal part of the first frontal convolution (*supplementary motor area*) and (c) those which may result from a lesion of the anterior half of the cingulate gyrus will then be discussed; (d) finally and especially, this account will focus on speech and language disturbances in the case of certain less circumscribed lesions affecting the prefrontal region, namely the structures situated rostrally to the caudal thirds of the third, second and first frontal convolutions. These abnormalities belong to the clinical picture of the *frontal syndrome proper* (or the *prefrontal syndrome*). Their nature is such that they must be considered in relation to other, concomitant, neuropsychological disturbances. This last section will close with comments concerning the concept of *dynamic aphasia*, as developed by Luria[1–12] (see Chapter 10).

In this chapter we shall often mention *speech disorders*, using this term to designate various abnormalities in one or more parameters of vocalization (accent, volume, phonation, articulation, etc.). We shall also mention *language disorders*, using this term to refer to abnormalities affecting the mediation of ideas, symbols and signs without regard to the sensorimotor modality. Thus the word *language* implies reference to the conceptual or cognitive aspects of linguistic functioning (or in Saussureian terminol-

* Echolalia: The patient actually studied in French and did not speak English.

ogy, a reference to the *signified* properties of language: *valeurs signifées*) whereas the word *speech* implies reference to the verbal output (or reference to the *signifying* properties of oral language: *valeurs signifiantes*). Our discussion will also refer to the bidimensional nature of language[13–15], a concept which was presented and illustrated elsewhere (see Chapter 2): being a temporally sequenced chain of linguistic events, language requires the constant selection of segments of various complexity from the inventories of available units (*paradigmatic axis*) and the serial integration of the units thus selected (*syntagmatic axis*).

THE PROBLEM OF FRONTAL AGRAPHIA

Towards the end of the last century, Exner's[16] anatomoclinical studies led him to claim that an agraphia may result from a lesion of the caudalmost third of the second frontal convolution in the same way that an aphasia* may result from a lesion of Broca's area. It was then tempting to develop, in parallel with the associationist model of aphasia (see Chapter 1), an associationist model of agraphia. Many such models were devised incorporating, depending on the cases, various dependent or independent relationships between audiophonatory and visuomanual assemblies. The parallelism and the dichotomy are particularly evident in the model proposed by Henschen. It includes two *centres* of written language, one *motor* (caudalmost part of the left second frontal convolution) and the other sensory (left angular gyrus). In addition to the frontal and angular agraphias related to lesions of these *centres*, the model predicts various forms of agraphia related to other cortical lesions, conduction agraphias and even an agraphia resulting from a capsular lesion. Nielsen later specified that an isolated agraphia could result from a lesion of either of the two centres of written language[17].

This conception of agraphia was rejected by the globalists and in particular by Pierre Marie (see Chapter 1). Neither was it accepted without reservation by all the associationists. For example, Wernicke's[18] and Dejerine's[19] writings are quite clear in this respect: a disorganization of language, properly defined, can be manifested only in both the audiophonatory and visuomanual modalities (Insertion 6.1).

The concept of an acquired disturbance

Insertion 6.1

> 'Each time inner language is impaired, an agraphia appears. My research on writing disturbances in motor aphasics of the Broca type also demonstrates ... the presence of agraphia in these patients ... C. Bastien (1898) acknowledged the perfect concordance between the graphic centre and Broca's centre. There is in that, in my view, a complete confusion. The vocal apparatus is an apparatus specialized for speech; writing is only one form of motility of the hand. One can speak only with one's buccopharyngeal–laryngeal apparatus: one can write (Wernicke) with the elbow, the foot, in skating, in short, with any body part provided that it is sufficiently mobile. And there is no difference among these different varieties of writing. If writing with the hand is easier, it is a question of habit and of education ... In summary, clinical observation, pathological anatomy and psychology show that there is no specialized and autonomous graphic centre, which would play for writing the role which Broca's region plays for articulated language.'†
>
> (Excerpts from Dejerine)[19]

* In Exner's conceptual framework, the word *aphasia* refers only to abnormalities of oral language and the word *agraphia* is used in an analogous fashion to refer to the corresponding abnormalities of written language. Thus the meaning of the word *agraphia* is clearly more extensive than the meaning we have given it elsewhere (see Chapter 3) when comparing it with the word *anarthria*.

† Reading Dejerine's papers on aphasia should convince anyone that his reasoning was usually based on much stronger arguments.

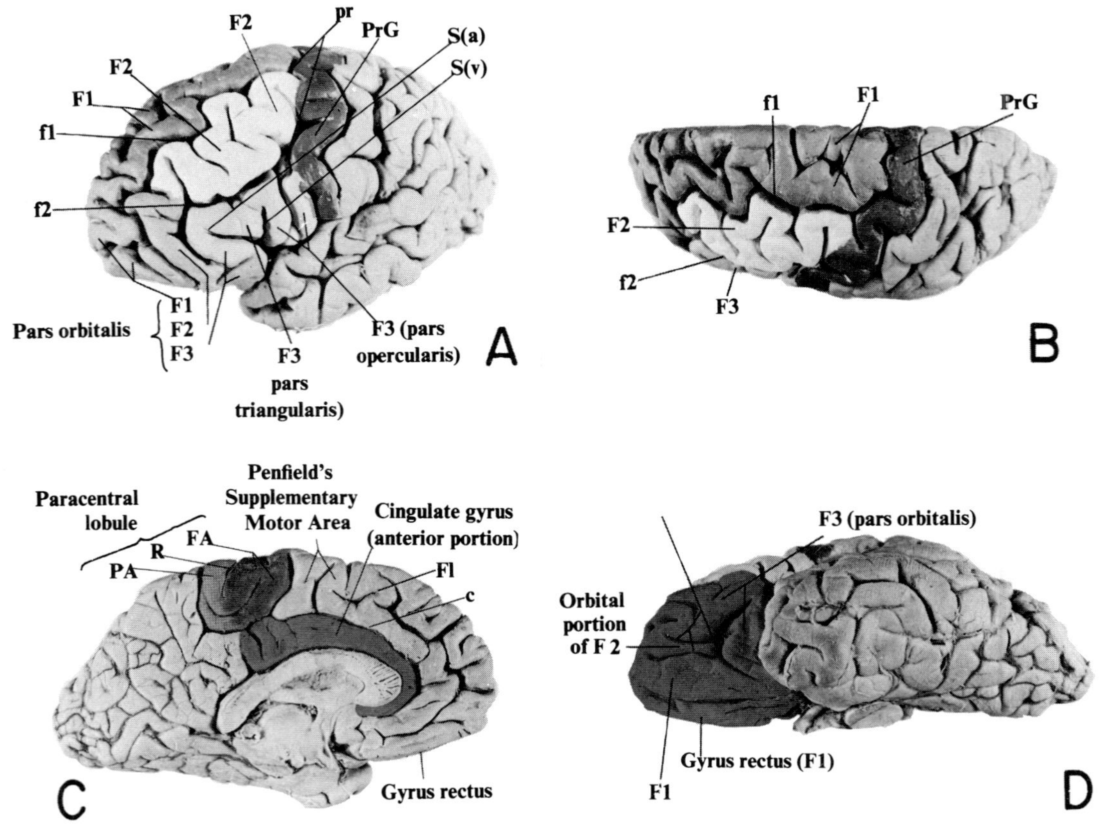

Fig. 6-1 *Left frontal lobe: A = convexity; B = superior surface; C = internal surface; D = orbital surface; F1, F2 and F3 = first, second and third frontal convolutions; PrG = precentral gyrus; PoG = postcentral gyrus; R = fissure of Rolando; S(v) = vertical branch of the fissure of Sylvius; S(a) = anterior branch of the fissure of Sylvius; f1, f2 and f3 = first, second and third frontal sulci; pr = prerolandic sulcus; c = cingulate sulcus.*

disrupting written language in its entirety and occurring in the absence of a concomitant and similar disorganization of oral language is generally not accepted today. On the other hand, contemporary aphasiologists acknowledge the existence of an isolated disturbance affecting only the receptive pole of written language (pure word blindness) (see Chapter 5) as well as the theoretical possibility—or, for some, the actual existence—of an isolated disturbance affecting only the instrumental pole of written language (pure agraphia)[20–22] (see Chapter 3). In our opinion, the very few anatomoclinical case studies reported in the literature might suggest that, in right-handers, there is a causal relationship between lesions of the caudalmost part of the left, second frontal convolution and the onset of an almost exclusive disturbance of written expression. After reviewing the literature and discussing eight cases of their own, Hécaen and Angelergues[21] concluded that there are cases in which the agraphic behaviour very clearly dominates the symptomatology associated with the presence of a frontal lesion. However, the graphic disturbance usually or always appears in the context of an expressive aphasia which is relatively mild and/or in the context of an apraxia (see Chapters 3 and 4). Leischner[22], for his part, maintained that pure agraphia appears only after bilateral frontal lesions in highly literate right-handers but that it may occur after a unilateral lesion in left-handed or ambidexterous individuals or else in minimally literate subjects.

Our own position on the subject of frontal agraphia can (at present) be summarized by the following statements: (a) certain frontal lesions may result in clinical pictures which are clearly dominated by the manifestations of agraphia (Insertion 6.2); (b) a unilateral lesion limited to the caudalmost part of the second frontal convolution of the dominant hemisphere for language (see Chapter 11) very seldom results in long-lasting agraphia;* (c) if a completely *pure* form of frontal agraphia is related to a unilateral lesion, it is rare and transient; (d) in certain cases, the frontal agraphia is primarily apraxic in nature; in other cases it essentially reflects a more elementary disturbance (paralysis, post-paralytic dystonia). When recovery occurs, and particularly at the start of evolution, the apraxia, paresis and dystonia may be manifested in fine manual movements other than those related to writing (Insertion 6.2). In other words, frontal agraphia is similar to pure anarthria (see Chapter 3) in this regard; (e) agraphic behaviour resulting from a frontal lesion is often accompanied by disturbed computation (dyscalculia, acalculia).

			Right hand	Left hand
(chicken)	*POULE*	→	(*PUOLE*)	(*POLE*)
(February)	*FEVRIER*	→	(*FEVRIRE*)	(*FEVIER*)
(work)	*OUVRAGE*	→	(*OUVRURGRU*)	(*AUVALELE*)
(surgery)	*CHIRURGIE*	→	(*GEUEGRUE*)	(*HERURGE*)
(wonder)	*MERVEILLE*	→	(*MERVILLE*)	(*MERVELLLE*)
(equilibrium)	*EQUILIBRE*	→	(*EQUIBLE*)	(*EGUILIBRE*)

Fig. 6–2 *An acquired dysorthographia in a 49-year-old right-hander; cortico-subcortical softening of the left prefrontal convexity, including the caudalmost part of the second frontal convolution. On the fourteenth day after onset of the disease, the spelling disturbance is manifested whether the patient writes with the left hand or with the right (see above); in the latter case, the presence of agraphic disturbance is also observed (see Fig. 3–1 and 4–1, and Insertion 6–2). The sample reproduced here was obtained during a test of writing isolated words to dictation. From Lecours et al.*[23]

Insertion 6.2

The following cases, which we have had the opportunity to observe over the past few years, provide a fairly good illustration of the clinical problem raised by *frontal agraphia*.

A 59-year-old right-handed accountant sustained a critical episode (lasting approximately one hour) during which he was unable to write or carry out arithmetic calculations. A year later, two similar episodes occurred within a week and then a third which was not followed by recovery and was accompanied by a mild right hemiparesis. The agraphia affected all modalities of written expression (composition, writing to dictation, copying). Treatment involved ablation of a benign tumoral lesion (meningioma), compressing the caudalmost thirds of the second and first frontal convolutions of the left hemisphere. Recovery from the agraphia was obvious one month after the surgical intervention (case observed by M. I. Botez).

The patient was a 69-year-old right-handed office employee. His medical history included insidious development, over approximately three years, of a relatively mild disturbance of oral expression (essentially articulatory in nature). In addition, an agraphia, very severe at the time of hospitalization, developed during the last six months of this period. Examination indicated the presence of a slight right hemiparesis as well as a motor disturbance affecting the left side of the body (parkinsonian hemisyndrome). A buccofacial apraxia was also observed. The agraphia was very severe, sparing only servile copying. Written calculation was almost totally impossible. Radiological and electroencephalographic evidence suggested the presence of a slowly progressive disease especially affecting the frontal lobes, more so on the left side (case observed by M. I. Botez).

The patient was a 49-year-old right-handed administrator (with a familial history of left-handedness). The medical history included a sudden recent onset of right hemiparesis, moderate in severity and maximal in the lower limb. After some weeks of evolution, the muscular force of the right upper limb had returned to normal but this limb was not used spontaneously by the

* One of the co-authors of this book, Jean Luc Nespoulous, has observed a case in which such a lesion occurred without the slightest disturbance of written expression.

patient (*aspontaneity*). Some days later, movement was finally obtained in response to repeated and insistent instructions. *Melokinetic apraxic* behaviour was then observed. The patient appeared to concentrate intensely, summing up all his willpower. This was suggested by grunts and facial gestures, comparable with those seen in normal individuals during strong muscular efforts, and by non-specific movements of the trunk and left upper limb. The movement of the right upper limb was then carried out, but slowly, laboriously and awkwardly. Writing with the right hand was totally impossible at onset but gradually recovered. A graphic disturbance was evident only on the right but spelling was impaired regardless of the hand used in writing (Fig. 3-1, 4-1 and 6-2). Oral expression was normal, with the exception of slight word-finding difficulty in conversation. Comprehension of spoken and of written language was also normal. The graphic disturbance regressed and disappeared within a few months. Although gradual improvement occurred, the dysorthographia was still evident a year later. Radiological and electroencephalographic evidence suggested the presence of a superficial, left frontal lesion of vascular origin, centred on the second frontal convolution, including the caudalmost third of this structure. This case was the subject of a published report[23].

The patient was a 46-year-old right-handed film producer (with a left-handed brother) who had hypertension but no neurological antecedents. His referral was prompted by a graphic disturbance and awkwardness in manipulating materials during film editing. These signs had developed over a period of some days (some weeks?) and the patient decided to seek medical attention the day after the appearance of a very mild articulatory disturbance. The examination, carried out by one of us (A.R.L.), revealed a slight right facial paralysis of the central type; Barre's sign was present in the right upper limb; on plantar stimulation, flexion of the great toe was slower on the right than on the left; the fingers of the right hand were less proficient than those of the left in the execution of fine rapidly-alternating movements. The remainder of the sensorimotor examination failed to reveal any other anomalies at the level of the limbs or the trunk. The aphasiological examination did not indicate any articulatory disturbance. Nevertheless, the patient and his family claimed that speech had been slightly impaired (apparently a paretic type of impairment) and that perhaps it still was. Although mild (Fig. 3-2), a graphic disturbance was undeniable when productions were compared with premorbid samples. On the other hand, spelling was not impaired.* The remainder of the aphasiological examination was normal as was the electroencephalographic examination. Tomodensitometric examination revealed the presence of a small, deep subcortical lesion below the left frontal lobe (opposite the frontal horn, probably in the internal capsule): the picture suggested a small area of softening. The favourable evolution (progressive disappearance of the disturbance over a few weeks) confirmed this impression.

The patient was a 59-year-old right-handed financial manager without neurological antecedents. He suddenly presented articulatory and graphic disturbances which increased in severity over a 24-hour period and then stabilized. An examination carried out two days later by one of us (F.L.) revealed the presence of a right facial paralysis of the central type; on protrusion, the tongue deviated slightly towards the right; the plantar reflex showed extension on the right side (presence of Babinski's sign). The remainder of the sensorimotor examination failed to reveal any other anomalies at the level of the limbs or the trunk. In the course of aphasia testing, a significant articulatory disturbance with syllabification was observed; the impairment was primarily related to paretic factors (see Chapter 3). The graphic disturbance was also very obvious, being evident even in the patient's signature and severely limiting his potential for written linguistic expression. Although to a lesser degree, the disturbance also affected non-linguistic graphic productions. Oral spelling was normal. The remainder of the neurological and aphasiological examinations revealed no other abnormalities. The electroencephalograms were normal. The disturbance gradually disappeared over a period of approximately four months. The recorded diagnosis was that of a small, left frontal softening.

* A single literal paragraphia—(anecdote)→('anectode') (!)—in an essay about a film which was under production.

SPEECH DISTURBANCES RELATED TO A LESION OF THE SUPPLEMENTARY MOTOR AREA

In 1940, Brickner[24] published a case study of an epileptic right-hander with a circumscribed left cerebral lesion situated on the internal surface of the caudalmost part of the first frontal convolution, a region which closely corresponds with that known today as *(Penfield's) supplementary motor area*[25–31] (Fig. 6-1). Electrical stimulation of this zone during surgical intervention produced the phenomenon of *palilalia* (progressively more rapid repetition of a syllable, a word or a short phrase) which continued for a few seconds on each occurrence. For example, on stimulation, recitation of the alphabet was interrupted, with palilalia occurring on the last letter uttered, then recitation was resumed as soon as the electrical stimulation was removed. Palilalia, as well as certain vocal behaviours or *arrest of speech* were observed and studied in detail by Penfield and his associates[32] (see Insertion 7.2). It was thus demonstrated that these phenomena may occur during stimulation of the right supplementary motor area as well as during stimulation of the left.

In addition to these particularly conclusive studies employing local electrical stimulation, several clinical studies demonstrated that natural lesions, especially turmoral or vascular lesions (see Chapter 9), may result in palilalia or arrest of speech when they affect the supplementary motor area of the dominant hemisphere[33–37].* It should be noted that this type of speech arrest, when it is not paroxysmal, is often designated by the name of *aphemia*[34, 35], the term used by Broca when referring to the symptom configuration which today bears his name (see Chapters 1 and 10).

On the basis of personal observation and data reported in the literature, Arseni and one of the co-authors of this work (M. I. Botez)[39] differentiated three groups of speech disturbances which may attest to a lesion of the supplementary motor area of the dominant hemisphere (see Chapter 11), namely paroxysmal disturbances, transient disturbances and permanent disturbances.

Paroxysmal disturbances

Included under this heading are critical arrests of speech (brief duration: one to two minutes) and the paroxysmal palilalic phenomena which may accompany them. They probably represent the clinical equivalent of behaviours observed in electrophysiology during stimulation of the supplementary motor area (cf. p. 147). This critical arrest of speech is the most frequent sign of a lesion, particularly of a tumoral lesion, affecting the supplementary motor area of the dominant hemisphere. The arrest of speech may occur as the sole manifestation but it may also precede or accompany a motor epileptic attack limited to the upper limb contralateral to the lesion (*Bravis-Jackson spells*) or constitute the aura of a generalized epileptic attack. During the arrest of speech, the patient characteristically continues to hear and understand the language of others. However, on the expressive level s/he is totally mute or, more often, the speech arrest is soon followed by palilalic phenomena. The speech which is then involuntarily repeated is often the last word uttered voluntarily before the speech arrest or, again, the last syllable of this word (this reminds one of a feature pointed out in Chapter 4 when discussing a different phenomenon, namely the *verbal stereotypes* of certain aphasics). The repeated segment may also be a short syntagm, sometimes a phonemically transformed word, or even a neologism (see Chapter 2). In some instances, the same attack may include brief silences interspersed among several palilalic bursts.

Attacks similar to arrests of speech, which also represent an epileptic phenomenon, may also occur in certain tumoral lesions affecting Broca's area (pars opercularis and pars triangularis of the left third frontal convolution) or Wernicke's area (posterior half of the first or first two

* The right-handed patient who was the subject of a report published by one of the co-authors of this work (M. I. Botez) and Wertheim[38] (arrest of speech by a tumoral lesion affecting the right supplementary motor area) does not constitute a convincing exception given the reported history of familial left-handedness. Thus the effects of a natural lesion appear to differ from those of electrical stimulation in the sense that the same phenomena are observed after electrical stimulation of either the left or the right supplementary motor area.

left temporal convolutions) (see Chapter 8-1).* The attack is then followed by a transient aphasia with a predominant disturbance of expression in the former case and a predominant disturbance of comprehension in the latter (see Insertion 19.1). In contrast, when the critical arrest of speech is related to a lesion of the supplementary motor area, linguistic expression, including articulatory realization, returns to normal as soon as the attack has ended.

Transient disturbances

This heading essentially refers to a relatively long arrest of speech (two to seven days), a type of behaviour which is more and more commonly being designated by the name of *aphemia*[35]. In most cases, it appears after surgical interventions involving the supplementary motor area, or a thrombosis of the anterior cerebral artery (see Chapters 8 and 9). In characteristic cases, motor function is, in general, normal but that of speech is almost abolished; there appears to be a total absence of incentive with regard to articulated production (*manque d'incitation verbale*). However, the mutism is rarely absolute. The patient may occasionally emit a propositional 'yes' or 'no', sometimes even a short sentence ('I'm tired of speaking', said one of Botez's patients), after insistent and repeated interventions by the examiner. Nevertheless, even persistent interventions most often elicit only a shrug of the shoulders. Patients with this type of mutism are aware of their surroundings which they view with evident interest. They carry out elementary routine activities without apparent difficulty: for example, they eat unassisted, using manual gestures to request whatever they might need.

If one selectively considers the absence of speech production, there is obviously no clinical difference between the arrest of speech in aphemia and the initial suppression observed in various clinical forms of aphasia (see Chapter 4). However, when improvement occurs, the evolution of the patient's linguistic behaviours is not the same in both cases: as in the case of critical arrests of speech (cf. p. 129), this aphemia generally disappears without sequelae, whereas improvement from a suppression is accompanied by the emergence of other features of the expressive symptomatology of aphasia (reduction, agrammatism, articulatory difficulty, etc.).

Permanent disturbances

Following a lesion or a resection of the supplementary motor area of the hemisphere dominant for language, behaviour indicative of *word-finding difficulty* (see Chapters 4 and 11) may be observed. Sometimes refractory, it is similar to the word-finding difficulty (*frontal anomia*) which we shall discuss with regard to the frontal syndrome proper (cf. p. 135).

Electrophysiological and clinical data from investigations of the role of the supplementary motor cortex in cerebral activities subserving linguistic functioning suggest that it is probably related to the *starting mechanism* of speech[40, 41]. This hypothesis is supported by findings from recent stereoelectroencephalographic research carried out by Talairach and Bancaud[42]. It can also be reasonably assumed that the transient nature of the aphemia following resection or destruction of the supplementary motor area of the dominant hemisphere for language attests either to contralateral takeover or to termination of inhibitory phenomena related to the acute phase of the lesion (surgical or natural).

SPEECH DISTURBANCES RELATED TO CINGULATE LESIONS, AKINETIC MUTISM AND MUTISM WITHOUT AKINESIS

The syndrome of akinetic mutism was described by Cairns et al[43] in 1941 (Insertion 6.3). The mutism is absolute and is observed in the context of an equally severe general akinesis which, in typical cases, spares only eye movements. Patients are said to show only an *ocular presence* as it is only through their eyes that they are attached to the physical context in which they find themselves, and to the events which there occur. The onset of akinetic mutism may be caused by lesions at different cerebrospinal levels including the brain stem (periaqueductal grey

* Note that Penfield and Roberts[30, 31] demonstrated that there are many points within the classical language areas (those called Broca's and Wernicke's) as well as many points in cortical zones of the left hemisphere which are adjacent or intermediate to the language zone (see Chapter 8) whose stimulation, by an electrical current, may also elicit a critical arrest of speech.

Insertion 6.3

The behaviour of akinetic mutism has long been of interest. Ward[44], in fact, referred to a work published in Switzerland in 1670 under the name of Félix Plater, a professor of medicine at the University of Bâle. It concerned Knight Caspar Benecurtius, the victim of a progressive mental disease which, within two years, rendered him 'incapable of thinking'. He spent the last six years of his life sitting at a table with his head in his hands. He showed almost no reactions to facts and events of the external world. On rare occasions he mumbled a few words conveying little information. Knight Benecurtius died suddenly, and the autopsy, carried out by Plater, revealed the presence of a globular tumour destroying—in modern terms—the anterior portion of the corpus callosum and one of the cingulate gyri.

matter), thalamus, cingulate gyrus (in the anterior half, known as Brodmann's area 24), and the convexity of the frontal lobes[45-51].

Brodmann's area 24[52] consists of the anterior portion of the cingulate gyrus.* It is situated on the internal surface of the hemisphere between the foot of the first frontal convolution and the corpus callosum (Fig. 6-1) (see Chapter 8). The effects of a lesion in Brodmann's area 24 are illustrated in the following summaries of some published anatomoclinical case studies.

Case reported by Neilsen and Jacobs[46]. The patient suddenly presented complete mutism and a general akinesis. State of consciousness appeared unimpaired and the patient's gaze attested to his interest in the external world. The autopsy revealed the presence of two embolic foci (see Chapter 9), one destroying the anterior portion of the left cingulate gyrus and the other the anterior portion of the right cingulate gyrus and of the corpus callosum.

Case reported by Botez and Carp[41]. A 12-year-old left-hander presented complete mutism following a small haematoma of aneurysmal origin (see Chapter 9) located in the anterior portion of the right cingulate gyrus. Motor function in general was fairly intact. The patient had normal understanding of both spoken and written language and quickly learned to respond to questions by use of a binary code (yes: thumb up; no: thumb down).

Case reported by Buge, Escourolle, Rancurel and Poisson[51]. A 43-year-old right-handed male and a 59-year-old right-handed female showed complete mutism with akinesis. In both cases, bilateral cingulate lesions were observed on autopsy (lesions related to surgical intervention: an aneurysm of the anterior communicating artery in the first case, an olfactory meningioma in the second).

These are exemplary cases. In effect, the mutism is typically accompanied by akinesis in the case of bilateral anterior cingulate lesions and is present without akinesis (or with hypokinesis) in

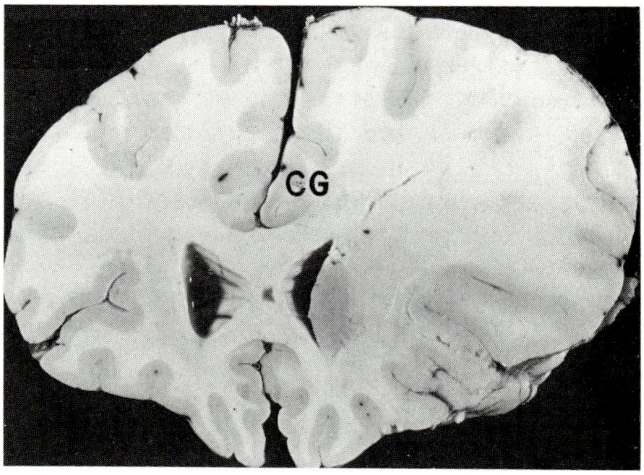

Fig. 6-3 *Cerebral oedema at the level of the right frontal lobe. The right cingulate gyrus (CG) forms a hernia under the* falx cerebri *and compresses the left cingulate gyrus.*

* Functionally, the cingulate gyrus is included in the limbic system (hypothalamus, anterior thalamic nuclei, cingulate gyrus, hippocampic formations and their interconnections) a neuroaxonal network which, since the work of Papez[53], has been considered to play an essential role in the control of so-called emotional behaviours.

unilateral lesions. In the latter case, the mutism may be transient.

Cerebral oedema, mutism and aphasia
It can be assumed that the mutism initially observed in certain cerebral vascular accidents having a sudden onset (see Chapter 9) is related to bilateral involvement of the cingulate gyri. On the side of the lesion, this involvement would be caused by the presence of local oedema (presence of an abnormally large amount of fluid in the intercellular spaces of the cerebral tissue); on the contralateral side it would be due to compression by the oedematous structures (Fig. 6-3). If the patient survives, the mutism disappears with the gradual reduction of the oedema. In the case of a right hemisphere lesion in a right-hander, linguistic functioning then returns to normal; in certain left hemisphere lesions the initial mutism is followed by the emergence of expressive signs of an aphasic syndrome. This mechanism no doubt underlies certain cases of suppression observed during the initial stage of aphasia (see Chapter 4).

SPEECH AND LANGUAGE DISTURBANCES IN THE FRONTAL LOBE SYNDROME

We shall treat this topic under four headings. We shall begin with discussion of the clinical manifestations of the frontal lobe syndrome proper, focusing especially on its linguistic aspects. We shall subsequently raise the issue of *frontal anomia* and then that of frontal lobe *dominance* for language. The chapter will close with comments on Luria's *dynamic* aphasia.

LINGUISTIC SYMPTOMATOLOGY OF THE FRONTAL LOBE SYNDROME

Frontal lobe symptomatology has been studied in various pathological conditions: frontal tumours and trauma, cerebrovascular accidents, surgical resections, etc.[54–75]. Although it is generally agreed that the frontal syndrome may be manifested in various clinical forms, there is less agreement concerning their number. Certain authors have distinguished up to five different forms. In our opinion, this division does not correspond to established anatomoclinical data and we ourselves recognize only two different forms for the time being. In the first, which is usually related to a lesion of the frontal lobe convexity, the patient's behaviour generally attests to a pathological lack of initiative (*lack of drive*, *aspontanéité*, *Antriebsmangel*[62, 67, 69, 71, 74, 75]. In the second form, which is usually related to a lesion of the orbital surface of the frontal lobe, the patient's behaviour generally shows a pathological excitation and euphoria*[62, 67, 68, 71, 75]. We shall here discuss, giving particular attention to their linguistic aspects, only disturbances which result from (certain) lesions of the prefrontal convexity[74, 77].

The frontal lobe syndrome from a lesion of the convexity
The essential characteristic of the clinical picture is a major, and usually global, decrease in physical and intellectual activity. The patient responds only after repeated and insistent interventions by those in his environment. There appears to be a rupture between the patient and the external world and mutual interactions are diminished. The patient rarely responds to events and those responses which do occur are typically delayed and minimal. The term *aspontaneity*,

* In the *frontal lobe syndrome from a lesion of the orbital surface*, linguistic behaviour is particularly notable in terms of its affective tone: the predominant disturbances are in fact those of personality and mood. Patients convey an impression of greatly exaggerated emotional states. They may appear euphoric, excited, unconcerned about present or future events and lacking in self-judgement. They may be irritable, aggressive and show little restraint in controlling their social behaviour. This personality disturbance is naturally reflected in their linguistic behaviour: patients are talkative, even voluble; in certain cases they speak ironically or tell obscene puns. Perseverative phenomena may sometimes be observed in their discourse. In general, this behaviour, which Jastrowitz[76] has designated by the name of *moria* (*μορια*, 'dementia'; morio, 'jester'), is reminiscent of that of certain hypomaniacs. Disturbances of certain instinctual behaviours, boulimia for example, may also be included in the clinical picture. Because the orbital surface has close anatomical and physiological links with the limbic system, it can be supposed that, in such cases, the frontal lesion results in the *release* of inclinations towards primitive instinctual behaviour. It should be noted that, although this syndrome may be observed in the presence of natural lesions, it does not occur as a result of orbital lobectomies.

rather than *akinesis*, is used to refer to those cases in which the psychomotor disturbance can be overcome with repeated stimulation. In its final stage, the disease may lead to indifference (even towards pain), to akinesis and apathy, and to mental deterioration.* The patient may then be totally mute and, as in the case of the cingulate lesions discussed above, this condition can be adequately designated as akinetic mutism. However, in cases which have reached this stage, there has typically been a preceding period where speech and language, like other activities, remained reduced but possible provided that the interlocutor's interventions were insistent and unremitting. This is well illustrated by the following excerpt from a conversation with one of our patients, a right-hander with a malignant tumour of the convexity of the left frontal lobe. (E, examiner's comment; P, patient's response; the figures shown in italics indicate the duration in seconds of the abnormally long latencies):

(6.1) E: Vous me paraissez de bonne humeur ce matin.
P: *(3)*

E. *Etes-vous de bonne humeur?*
P: *Oui.*

E. *Avez-vous passé une bonne nuit?*
P: *(2) Oui*

E. *Avez-vous eu d'autres examens, ce matin?*
P. *Euh (4) non.*

E. *Depuis combien de temps êtes-vous à l'hôpital?*
P: *(6) Quatre jours.*

E: *Est-ce la première fois que vous êtes hospitalisé?*
P: *(3) Quatre jours.*

E: *Dans le passé, avez-vous déjà été hospitalisé?*
P: *(3)*

E: *Avez-vous déjà été malade?*
P: *(2) Non*

E: *Comment votre maladie actuelle a-t-elle débuté?*
P: *(3)*

E: *Qu'est-ce qui s'est passé au début de votre maladie actuelle?*
P: *(19) Oui*

E: *Est-ce difficile à dire?*
P: *(4)*

E: *Est-ce difficile à expliquer?*
P: *(3)*

E: *Quel est le nom de votre médecin?*
P: *(15)*

E: *Est-ce le Docteur Dupont?*
P: *Non.*

E: *Est-ce le Docteur Durand?*
P: *(18)*

E: *Est-ce le Docteur Giscard?*
P: *(10)*

E: *Parlez-moi de votre travail.*
P: *(2)*

E: *Que faisiez-vous comme travail?*
P: *(13) Euh.*

E: *On m'a dit que vous travailliez dans le peinture. Est-ce vrai?*
P: *(5) Oui.*

E: *Pour une compagnie?*
P: *(2) Oui.*

E: *Est-ce que ça fait longtemps?*
P: *(24) Oui.*

E: *Est-ce que vous êtes marié?*
P: *(4) Oui.*

E: *Avez-vous des enfants?*
P: *(6)*

E: *Combien d'enfants avez-vous?*
P: *Quatre.*

E: *Des garçons ou des filles?*
P: *(6) Des filles.*

E: *Quel âge ont-elles?*
P: *(6) Euh (2) dix-sept, dix-huit.*

E: *Pouvez-vous me dire leurs noms?*
P: *Ah oui! (2) Euh (2) Marie (3) Ginette (3) Anne (4) puis Gérard.*

E: *Ah! vous avez un garçon aussi?*
P: *(3)*

E: *C'est le plus jeune, le garçon?*
P: *(5) C'est le plus jeune.*

E: *Est-ce qu'ils vont tous a l'école?*
P: *(4) Oui.*

E: *A Montréal?*
P: *(9) Montréal.*

(6.1) E: You seem to be in a good mood this morning.
P: *(3)*

E: Are you in a good mood?
P: Yes.

* Neurological examination of these patients often reveals pathological reflex reactions similar to those which can be elicited, in normal individuals, during childhood[75].

E: Did you sleep well last night?
P: (*2*) Yes.

E: Did you have some other tests this morning?
P: Uh (*4*) No.

E: How long have you been in the hospital?
P: (*6*) Four days.

E: Is this the first time you've been hospitalized?
P: (*3*) Four days.

E: In the past, were you ever hospitalized?
P: (*3*).

E: Have you ever been sick?
P: (*2*) No.

E: How did your present illness begin?
P: (*3*)

E: What happened at the start of your present illness?
P: (*19*) Yes.

E: Is it hard to say?
P: (*4*)

E: Is it hard to explain?
P: (*3*)

E: What's your Doctor's name?
P: (*15*)

E: Is it Dr Dupont?
P: No.

E: Is it Dr Durand?
P: (*18*)

E: Is it Dr Giscard?
P: (*10*)

E: Tell me about your work.
P: (*2*)

E: What did you do for a living?
P: (*13*) Uh.

E: I've heard that you worked in the paint business. Is that so?
P: (*5*) Yes.

E: For a company?
P: (*2*) Yes.

E: Was that long ago?
P: (*24*) Yes.

E: Are you married?
P: (*4*) Yes.

E: Do you have any children?
P: (*6*)

E: How many children do you have?
P: Four.

E: Boys or girls?
P: (*6*) Girls.

E: How old are they?
P: (*6*) Uh (*2*) sixteen, eighteen.

E: Can you tell me their names?
P: Ah yes! (*2*) Uh (*2*) Marie (*3*) Ginette (*3*) Anne (*4*) then Gérard.*

E: Ah! you have a boy as well?
P: (*3*)

E: Is the boy the youngest?
P: (*5*) He's the youngest.

E: Do they all go to school?
P: (*4*) Yes.

E: In Montreal?
P: (*9*) Montreal.

Although only slightly apparent in the above sample, a tendency towards echolalia (see Chapter 4) and perseveration may be evident in these patients' discourse. In typical cases, repetition and oral reading are almost normal (ignoring the delays which frequently precede responses). Naming tests may or may not elicit grossly abnormal behaviour (cf. p. 135). The lack of incentive is even more obvious in written expression than in oral expression. The understanding of usual conversational language generally appears normal but is nevertheless only partial on relatively complex tests of comprehension (see Chapter 15).

In the vast majority of cases, the linguistic abnormalities resulting from a lesion of the frontal convexity are observed within the context of a disorder which extends far beyond the linguistic domain, a disorder which may be related to a dysfunction of the activating ascending reticular system at the level of its frontal projections. However, this frontal aspontaneity is sometimes partial or is clearly predominant during a particular type of activity (Insertion 6.4). It may have been the occurrence of exceptional cases in which the aspontaneity was thus limited to speech and language behaviours which led certain authors to consider this clinical picture as a form of aphasia (transcortical motor aphasia for Wernicke and Lichteim[78] then Goldstein[79], and dynamic aphasia for Luria[80] (see Chapter 10).

* Note the name of a male although the patient had previously implied his children were all girls.

Insertion 6.4

'I think that lack of incitation to actions which is a common phenomenon in space-occupying lesion of the frontal lobe, may be general and involve all motor activities, or, more or less localized: for example, failure to use the limbs contralateral to the lesion, inadequate initiation of gait (the so-called "frontal apraxia" of gait), and impoverishment of the expressive mechanism of speech of the type peculiar to lesions of the supplementary motor area.' (From Botez[2].)

Other aspects of prefrontal symptomatology

The presence of two predominant easily-recognized clinical features (i.e., euphoria on one hand or aspontaneity on the other) permits the differentiation of two symptomatological pictures related to different sites of lesions. In addition to these predominant features, the prefrontal syndrome may also include intellectual deficits which especially affect attention and memory. They may be more or less evident, depending on the case, but in certain patients are sufficient to convey a global impression of increasingly severe mental confusion. Attempts to identify these abnormalities more precisely lead to the observation that patients are easily distracted from the act in which they are engaged, that they are unable to plan the successive stages of the same activity and that the transition between different activities is not normally accomplished. In certain cases, these facts are sufficiently clear to suggest that the fundamental disturbance is one which impedes the programming of ongoing activities, that is, the anticipation of their execution in the immediate future and of their eventual effects, on the bases of traces ('patterns') formed by previous events[81, 82]. This concept of disrupted programming provides a possible explanation of the results obtained by such patients on various perceptual-motor and psychometric tests (see Chapter 16). In addition, it may also permit better understanding of certain aspects of speech and language behaviour observed in the context of the prefrontal syndrome.

THE PROBLEM OF FRONTAL ANOMIA

It was previously pointed out that word-finding difficulty is included in the symptomatological picture associated with the presence of dominant hemisphere lesions (see Chapter 4). Similarly, the various possible clinical manifestations of word-finding difficulty have already been discussed in detail (see Chapter 4): they vary according to the diffuse or focal nature of the causal lesions, according to lesion localization in the latter case and according to the aetiology of the disease in question[83] (see Chapters 8 and 9).

It is clear that dominant hemisphere lesions limited to the prefrontal convexity, anterior to Broca's area (Fig. 6–1), are to be grouped with those which may be the source of a disturbance in word evocation. After having observed word retrieval behaviours in a hundred patients with an expansive cerebral lesion of known localization, one of the co-authors of this work (Botez[62, 63, 75]) reached the following conclusions on this topic: (a) word-finding difficulty is the first and foremost sign of the presence of an expansive, dominant hemisphere lesion. This is true in the case of prerolandic lesions as well as in the case of retrorolandic lesions; (b) in cases of favourable evolution of the disease (for example, a healed cerebral abscess), word-finding difficulty is generally the last pathological sign to decrease, or, in some cases, to disappear; (c) when a dominant hemisphere tumour is manifested over a long period by isolated or nearly isolated word-finding difficulty, the tumour is usually prerolandic. Although nearly isolated word-finding difficulty may initially be present in the case of tumours in the left temporo-parieto-occipital region (amnesic aphasia), it is a rule that additional linguistic deficits soon appear as the result of an expansion of the lesion into the posterior constituents of the language zone (see Chapters 4 and 8).

Terminological discretion rules out immediate use of the term 'frontal anomia' to designate the expressive behaviour of a patient who has become almost totally mute with the progression of his or her disease. It can nevertheless be assumed, especially in view of the common forms of transition in progressive as well as in recovering diseases, that there is a qualitative relationship between the mutism and the word-finding difficulty (anomia) of prefrontal patients.* In typical cases, frontal anomia is characterized by the following behaviours, of which the first two do not differ from facts observed in amnesic aphasia (see Chapter 4): (a) the word-finding difficulty is more evident when the stimuli eliciting production are less specific and possible responses are numerous and not easily predicted than when the stimuli are very specific and only a single or a very few responses are possible;† (b) when word-finding difficulty is present in naming, it is observed to be present regardless of the modality of stimulus presentation, visual, tactile or auditory; (c) when word-finding difficulty occurs in naming, appropriate responses can often be facilitated by phonetic placement cues; (d) in contrast to the behaviour seen in temporo-parieto-occipital lesions, word-finding difficulty resulting from a prefrontal lesion is manifested by delays and failures to respond, and not by periphrastic productions, circumlocutory comments or paraphasias. If the comparison introduced above between the word-finding difficulty of prefrontal patients and that of aphasics in general is pursued, it could then be added that the behaviour of patients with frontal anomia resembles that of Broca's aphasics far more than the behaviour of amnesic aphasics or other Wernicke's aphasics.

THE PROBLEM OF PREFRONTAL DOMINANCE FOR LANGUAGE

It has been known since the end of the last century that it is lesions of the left cerebral hemisphere which cause, in right-handers, almost all the disturbances observed in clinical aphasiology. We speak, and rightly so, of the dominance of the left hemisphere for language (see Chapter 10). Despite this, it was long acknowledged that the aspontaneity observed in lesions of the prefrontal convexity, including its manifestations in speech and language, was the same regardless of lesion lateralization. It was especially the works of Feutchwanger[55] and those of Kleist[57] which suggested that the linguistic components of the prefrontal syndrome may be more obvious in left than in right hemisphere lesions. This idea was confirmed by several subsequent investigations[62, 63, 75, 84]. Although left hemisphere dominance for linguistic functioning is not as clearly established in the case of the prefrontal region as in the case of the classical language zone (see Chapter 8), it is, at present, generally acknowledged that disturbances of verbal thought, the more or less massive manifestation of aspontaneity in speech and language and, especially, the anomia, are more frequent and quantitatively more significant in lesions of the left frontal convexity (anterior to Broca's area and sparing this area) than in lesions of the homologous parts of the right frontal convexity. This idea is thus consistent with the contemporary conception which holds that the dominant hemisphere (dominant for language and manual dexterity) plays a primary role in relation to *verbal thought* whereas the so-called minor hemisphere plays a predominant role in relation to phenomena which remain ill-defined but are perhaps adequately designated by the term *non-verbal thought*.

LURIA'S DYNAMIC APHASIA

Luria and his student Tsvetkova[5, 9] consider that the language disturbances of patients with prefrontal lesions, like those of patients with lesions of the classical language zone (see Chapters 4 and 8), should be included among the aphasias proper. Following writers of the German school, particularly Kleist[57] and Pick[85], who referred to this verbal behaviour by the name of *adynamia of speech* (*Adynamie der Sprache*), Luria named it *dynamic aphasia*‡[80] (see Chapter 10).

The patient with dynamic aphasia understands usual conversational language. Language repetition is normal or nearly so. Naming of objects or pictured stimuli may be normal or give

* In the same way, the suppression, the reduction and the word-finding difficulty (see Chapter 4) of Broca's aphasia appear to correspond, in certain respects, to different degrees of the same disturbance.

† Examples of the first type include conversation, narration and certain tests of word evocation (e.g., producing as many words as possible which begin with a predetermined letter). A naming test is an example of the second type (see Chapter 15).

‡ Given the nature of these patients' behaviour, both within and beyond the linguistic domain, it is difficult to understand why Luria elected to replace the word *adynamic* by the word *dynamic*.

Insertion 6.5

'Fundamental to this dynamic aphasia is probably a disturbance of inner speech, which, according to Vygotsky ... has a shortened structure, a predicative function, and serves as a fundamental means for the transformation of a foreshortened idea into developed outer speech and for the change of developed speech into a foreshortened scheme of thought. This proposition, as analysis has shown, finds support in the fact that the ability to connect words to simple syntagma, and to perceive directly the grammatical form of a word which allows it to enter into a context with other words, is disturbed in these patients ... The predicative structure of speech is especially damaged in these patients, and, as Svetkova has shown, these patients require five to six times longer to locate verbs than nouns.

All this gives us a foundation for regarding this form of aphasia as a distinctive type of destruction of contextual speech, which leaves the fundamental codes of language relatively well preserved.' (From Luria[80].)

rise to certain abnormalities (failures to respond, delays). The principal symptomatic feature is the aspontaneity in conversational behaviour, a feature which we have described and illustrated in our discussion of the frontal syndrome from a lesion of the convexity [cf pp. 132–133, sample of conversation (6.1)]. Certain additional psycholinguistic considerations led Luria to distinguish three levels of increasing severity, namely: normal evocation of words designating objects but difficulty in evoking words designating actions; difficulty in evoking words designating objects and an inability to evoke words designating actions; an inability to evoke words designating objects as well as those designating actions. In general, the difficulty related to action verbs would be at least four times as great as the difficulty related to object names[5, 9].

For Luria, the fundamental disturbance underlying the occurrence of dynamic aphasia is one which essentially affects *inner language* and the *predicative function*: the initial idea of the action is present but it cannot be incorporated into a linear syntagmatic scheme (see Chapter 1, summary of Jacques Lordat's aphasiological conceptions (Insertion 6.5). This disturbance explains the behaviour observed in conversation (cf. pp. 133–134, frontal syndrome from a lesion of the convexity) and on tests contrasting object names and action verbs; it also results in an impairment of the *regulating role of language*. If we have correctly grasped Luria's thinking, this would at least partially explain the phenomena which we have designated under the name of aspontaneity in non-linguistic behaviour. Whether the direction for action originates within the patient or is provided by the interlocutor, it cannot be followed by the corresponding action whenever the *programme* for this action reaches a certain level of complexity, that is, whenever it is necessary to anticipate a gestural sequence and predict its effects. This state would be similar to that seen in children during the second year of life, when given a verbal instruction.

It cannot be denied that Luria's idea is engaging in many respects. Neither can it be denied that the clinical data on which it is based are rather tenuous. Consequently, it can be suggested that the aspontaneity of frontal patients is manifested in their linguistic behaviour for the same reason that it is manifested in their non-linguistic behaviour and, additionally, that the underlying disturbance of action programming is one which transcends language (i.e., which is not assimilable to *inner language*) and indifferently affects the planning of verbal actions as well as that of non-verbal actions. Depending on one's particular conception of aphasia, the linguistic components of the prefrontal syndrome can then be considered to be, or not to be, a form of aphasia.

REFERENCES

1. Luria, A.R. & Homskaya, E.D. (1963) Le trouble du rôle régulateur du langage au cours des lésions du lobe frontal. *Neuropsychologia*, **1**, 9.
2. Luria, A.R. & Homskaya, E.D. (1964) Disturbances of the regulatory role of speech in frontal lobe lesions. In *The Frontal Granular Cortex and Behavior* (Ed.) Warren, J.M. & Akert, K. p. 353. New York: McGraw-Hill.
3. Luria, A.R., Pribram, K.H. & Homskaya, E.D. (1964) An experimental analysis of the behavioural disturbances produced by a left frontal meningioma. *Neuropsychologia*, **2**, 257.
4. Luria, A.R., Homskaya, E.D., Blinkov, S.M. & Critchley, M. (1967) Impaired selectivity of mental processes in association with lesion of the frontal lobe. *Neuropsychologia*, **5**, 105.
5. Luria, A.R. & Tsvetkova, L.S. (1967) Towards the mechanisms of 'dynamic aphasia'. *Acta Neurologia et Psychiatrica Belgica*, **67**, 1045.
6. Luria, A.R. (1967) Problèmes et faits de la neurolinguistique. *Revue de Science sociale*, **19**, 39.
7. Luria, A.R. (1969) Frontal lobe syndromes. In *Handbook of Clinical Neurology* (Ed.) Vinken, P.J. & Bruyn, G.W. Vol. 2, p. 700. Amsterdam: North-Holland.
8. Luria, A.R. (1970) The functional organization of the brain. *Scientific American*, **222**, 66.
9. Luria, A.R. & Tsvetkova, L.S. (1970) The mechanism of 'dynamic aphasia'. In *Progress in Linguistics* (Ed.) Byerwish, M. & Heidolph, K.E. p. 187. The Hague: Mouton.
10. Luria, A.R. (1973) La afasia reconsiderada. *Acta audiologica y foniatrica hispanoamericana*, **10**, 93.
11. Luria, A.R. (1972) Aphasia reconsidered. *Cortex*, **8**, 34.
12. Luria, A.R. (1974) Language and brain. *Brain and Language*, **1**, 1.
13. Jakobson, R. (1956) Two aspects of language and two types of aphasic disturbances. In *Fundamentals of Language* (Ed.) Jakobson, R. & Halle, M. p. 55. The Hague: Mouton.
14. Sabouraud, O., Gagnepain, J. & Sabouraud, A. (1963) Vers une approche linguistique des problèmes de l'aphasie. *Revue de Neuropsychiatrie de l'Ouest*, **1**, **2**, **3** and **4**, 6, 3, 3 and 3.
15. Lecours, A.R. & Rouillon, F. (1976) Neurolinguistic analysis of jargonaphasia and jargonagraphia. In *Studies in Neurolinguistics* (Ed.) Avakian-Whitaker, H. & Whitaker, H. Vol. 2, p. 95. New York: Academic Press.
16. Exner, S. (1881) *Untersuchungen über die Lokalisation der Funktionen in der Grosshirnrinde des Menschen*. Vienna: Wilhelm Braumuller.
17. Nielsen, J.M. (1962) Agnosias, apraxias, speech and aphasia. In *Clinical Neurology* (Ed.) Baker, A.B. p. 433. New York: Hoeber-Harper.
18. Wernicke, C. (1966) The symptom complex of aphasia. In *Boston Studies in the Philosophy of Science* (Ed.) Cohen, R.S. & Watofsky, M.W. Vol. 4, p. 34. Boston: O. Riedel.
19. Dejerine, J. (1914) *Séméiologie des affections du système nerveux*. Paris: Masson.
20. Ajuriaguerra, J. (de) & Hécaen, H. (1960) *Le cortex cérébral*. Paris: Masson.
21. Hécaen, H. & Angelergues, R. (1966) L'agraphie secondaire aux lésions du lobe frontal. *International Journal of Neurology*, **5**, 381.
22. Leischner, A. (1969) The agraphias. In *Handbook of Clinical Neurology* (Ed.) Vinken, P.J. & Bruyn, G.W. Vol. 4, p. 141. Amsterdam: North-Holland.
23. Lecours, A.R., Bérubé, L., Courtois, G.A. & Lhermitte, F. (1972) Recherches sur le langage des aphasiques: 3. Désorganisation de l'expression orale et désorganisation de l'expression écrite; une étude comparative de deux cas d'aphasie. *Encéphale*, **61**, 208.
24. Brickner, R. (1940) A human cortical area producing repetitive phenomena when stimulated. *Journal of Neurophysiology*, **3**, 128.
25. Penfield, W. (1938) The cerebral cortex in man. *Archives of Neurology and Psychiatry* (Chicago), **40**, 417.
26. Penfield, W. & Rasmussen, T. (1950) *The Cerebral Cortex of Man; a Clinical Study of Localization and Function*. New York: Macmillan.
27. Penfield, W. & Welch, K. (1951) The supplementary motor area of the cerebral cortex. A clinical and experimental study. *Archives of Neurology and Psychiatry* (Chicago), **66**, 289.
28. Penfield, W. (1953) A consideration of the neurophysiological mechanisms of speech. *Proceedings of the American Academy of Arts and Science*, **82**, 199.
29. Penfield, W. & Jasper, H. (1954) *Epilepsy and the Functional Anatomy of the Human Brain*. Boston, MA: Little-Brown.
30. Penfield, W. & Roberts, L. (1959) *Speech and Brain Mechanisms*. Princeton, NJ: Princeton University Press.
31. Penfield, W. & Roberts, L. (1963) *Langage et mécanismes cérébraux*. Paris: Presses universitaires de France (translation by J.-C. Gautier).
32. Penfield, W. & Rasmussen, T. (1949) Vocalization and arrest of speech. *Archives of Neurology and Psychiatry* (Chicago), **61**, 21.
33. Petit-Dutaillis, D., Guiot, G., Messimy, R. & Bourdillon, C. (1954) A propos d'une aphémie par atteinte de la zone motrice supplémentaire de Penfield, au cours de l'évolution d'un anévrisme artério-veineux. Guérison de l'aphémie par ablation de la lésion. *Revue neurologique*, **90**, 95.
34. Barbizet, J., Duizabo, Ph. & Flavigny, R. (1975) Rôle des lobes frontaux dans le langage (une étude neuropsychologique expérimentale). *Revue neurologique*, **131**, 525.
35. Chavany, J.A. & Rougerie, G. (1958) Sur les confins de l'aphasie. L'aphémie post-opératoire transitoire après lobectomie frontale gauche. *Presse médicale*, **66**, 1191.
36. Alajouanine, Th., Castaigne, P., Sabouraud, O. & Contamin, F. (1959) Palilalie paroxystique et vocalisations itératives au cours de crises épileptiques par lésion

intéressant l'aire motrice supplémentaire. *Revue neurologique*, **101**, 585.

37. Castaigne, P. (1964) Vocalisations itératives et crises palilaliques dans les lésions prérolandiques de la face interne du lobe frontal. *Neurologia*, **9**, 39.
38. Botez, M.I. & Wertheim, N. (1959) Expressive aphasia and amusia following right frontal lesion in a right-handed man. *Brain*, **82**, 186.
39. Arseni, C. & Botez, M.I. (1961) Speech disturbances caused by tumors of the supplementary motor area. *Acta Psychiatrica Scandinavica*, **36**, 279.
40. Botez, M.I. (1964) The starting mechanism of speech. *Ldegyogyaszati*, **1**, 13.
41. Botez, M.I. & Carp, N. (1968) Nouvelles données sur le problème du déclenchement de la parole. *Revue roumaine de Neurologie*, **5**, 153.
42. Talairach, J. & Bancaud, J. (1965) The supplementary motor area in man. *International Journal of Neurology*, **5**, 330.
43. Cairns, H., Oldfield, R.C., Pennybacker, J.B. & Whitteridge, D. (1941) Akinetic mutism with an epidermoid cyst of the third ventricule. *Brain*, **64**, 273.
44. Ward, A.A. (1947) The anterior cingulate gyrus and personality. *Research Publications, Association for Research in Nervous and Mental Diseases*, **27**, 438.
45. Poppen, J.L. (1939) Ligation of the left anterior cerebral artery: its hazards and the means of avoidance of its complications. *Archives of Neurology and Psychiatry* (Chicago), **41**, 495.
46. Nielsen, J.M. & Jacobs, L.L. (1951) Bilateral lesions of the anterior cingulate gyri: report of a case. *Bulletin of the Los Angeles Neurological Society*, **16**, 231.
47. Chusid, J., Guterrierez-Mahoney, M. & Margules-Lavergne, A. (1954) Speech disturbances in association with parasagittal frontal lesions. *Journal of Neurosurgery*, **11**, 193.
48. Amyes, E.W. & Nielsen, J.M. (1955) Clinicopathologic study of vascular lesions of the anterior cingulate region. *Bulletin of the Los Angeles Neurological Society*, **20**, 112.
49. Guidetti, B. (1957) Désordres de la parole associés à des lésions de la surface interhémisphérique frontale postérieure. *Revue neurologique*, **97**, 121.
50. Freemon, F.R. (1971) Akinetic mutism and bilateral anterior cerebral artery occlusion. *Journal of Neurology, Neurosurgery and Psychiatry*, **34**, 693.
51. Buge, A., Escourolle, R., Rancurel, G. & Poisson, M. (1975) 'Mutisme akinétique' et ramollissement bicingulaire. *Revue neurologique*, **131**, 121.
52. Ward, A.A. (1948) The cingular gyrus: area 24. *Journal of Neurophysiology*, **11**, 12.
53. Papez, J.W. (1937) A proposed mechanism of emotion. *Archives of Neurology and Psychiatry* (Chicago), **38**, 725.
54. Bianchi, L. (1895) The functions of the frontal lobes. *Brain*, **18**, 497.
55. Feuchtwanger, E. (1923) *Die Funktionen des Stirnhirns, ihre Pathologie und Psychologie*. Berlin: Springer.
56. Baruk, H. (1926) *Les troubles mentaux dans les tumeurs cérébrales*. Paris: Doin.
57. Kleist, K. (1934) *Gehirnpathologie*. Leipzig: Barth.
58. Fulton, J.F. & Jacobsen, C.F. (1935) The functions of the frontal lobes. A comparative study in monkeys, chimpanzee and man. *Abstracts of the 2nd International Neurological Congress*, *p*. 70.
59. Rylander, G. (1939) *Personality Changes after Operation of the Frontal Lobes. A Clinical Study of 32 Cases*. Copenhagen: Munksgaard.
60. Angelergues, R., Hécaen, H. & Ajuriaguerra, J. (de) (1955) Les troubles mentaux au cours des tumeurs du lobe frontal. *Annales médico-psychologiques*, **2**, 577.
61. Hécaen, H. & Ajuriaguerra, J. (de) (1956) *Troubles mentaux au cours des tumeurs intracrâniennes*. Paris: Masson.
62. Botez, M.I. (1960) Clinical contributions to the study of the tumoral frontal syndrome. *Psychiatria et Neurologia*, **140**, 351.
63. Botez, M.I. (1962) *Aphasia and Correlated Syndromes in Intracranial Expanding Processes*. Bucarest. Editura Academici RSR. (In Romanian with an English summary.)
64. Milner, B. (1964) Some effects of frontal lobectomy in man. In *The Frontal Granular Cortex and Behaviour* (Ed. Warren, J.M. & Akert, K. p. 313. New York: McGraw-Hill.
65. Teuber, H.L. (1964) The riddle of the frontal lobe function in man. In *The Frontal Granular Cortex and Behaviour* (Ed.) Warren, J.M. & Akert, K. p. 410. New York: McGraw-Hill.
66. Hécaen, H. (1964) Mental symptoms associated with tumours of the frontal lobe. In *The Frontal Granular Cortex and Behaviour* (Ed.) Warren, J.M. & Akert, K. New York: McGraw-Hill.
67. Ajuriaguerra, J. (de) & Tissot, R. (1965) Le syndrome frontal. In *Encyclopédie méd.-chir.*, 17036 A-10, Paris.
68. Szewczyk, H. (1965) Tumoren des basalen Stirnhirns. In *Die klinische Lokalisation des Hirntumoren in des Kritik der technischen, bioptischen und autoptischen Nachprufung* (Ed.) Leonhard, K. p. 47. Leipzig: J.A. Barth.
69. Muller, T. & Berendt, H. (1965) Tumoren des konvexen Stirnhirns. In *Die klinische Lokalisation des Hirntumoren in des Kritik der technischen, bioptischen und autoptischen Nachprufung* (Ed.) Leonhard, K. p. 29. Leipzig: J.A. Barth.
70. Zangwill, O.L. (1966) Psychological deficits associated with frontal lobe lesions. *International Journal of Neurology*, **5**, 395.
71. Faust, C.L. (1966) Different psychological consequences due to superior frontal and orbitobasal lesions. *International Journal of Neurology*, **5**, 410.
72. Benton, A.L. (1968) Differential behavioral effects in frontal lobe disease. *Neuropsychologia*, **6**, 53.
73. Hécaen, H. (1969) Cerebral localization of mental functions and their disorders. In *Handbook of Clinical Neurology* (Ed.) Vinken, P.J. & Bruyn, G.W. Vol. 3, p. 11. Amsterdam: North-Holland.
74. Lhermitte, F., Derouesné, J. & Signoret, J.L. (1972) Analyse neuropsychologique du syndrome frontal. *Revue neurologique*, **127**, 415.
75. Botez, M.I. (1974) Frontal lobe tumours. In *Handbook of Clinical Neurology* (Ed.) Vinken, P.J. & Bruyn, G.W.

Vol. 17, p. 234. Amsterdam and New York: North-Holland and American Elsevier.
76. Jastrowitz, M. (1897) *Die Geschwülste des Nervensystem.* Berlin.
77. Lecours, A.R. (1975) Aphasie. In *Encyclopédie médico-chirurgicale*, 17019 A-10, 7, Paris.
78. Freud, S. (1891) *Zur Auffasung der Aphasien.* Vienna: Deuticke.
79. Goldstein, K. (1948) *Language and Language Disturbances.* New York: Grune and Stratton.
80. Luria, A.R. (1964) Factors and forms of aphasia. In *Disorders of Language* (Ed.) de Reuck, A.V.S. & O'Connor, M. p. 143. London: Churchill.
81. Luria, A.R. (1966) *The Higher Cortical Functions in Man.* New York: Basic Books.
82. Barbizet, J. (1971) Rôle du lobe frontal dans les conduites mnésiques. *Presse médicale*, **79,** 2033.
83. Geschwind, N. (1967) The varieties of naming errors. *Cortex*, **3,** 97.
84. Ramier, A.M. & Hécaen, H. (1970) Rôle respectif des atteintes frontales et de la latéralisation lésionnelle dans les déficits de la 'fluence verbale'. *Revue neurologique*, **123,** 17.
85. Pick, A. (1973) *Aphasia.* Springfield, IL: Charles C. Thomas. (Originally published in the context of *Handbuch der normalen und pathologischen Physiologie*, Springer-Verlag, Heidelberg, 1931; English translation by Jason Brown.)

BIBLIOGRAPHY

Barbizet, J., Duizabo, Ph. & Flavigny, R. (1975) Rôle des lobes frontaux dans le langage (une étude neuropsychologique expérimentale). *Revue neurologique*, **131,** 525.

Cambier, J., Dehen, H. & Doggui, S. (1975) Syndrome frontal. *Encyclopédie médico-chirurgicale, 17035. B*[10], 1. Paris.

Castaigne, P. (1964) Vocalisations itératives et crises palilaliques dans les lésions prérolandiques de la face interne du lobe frontal. *Neurologia*, **9,** 39.

Critchley, M. (1930) The anterior cerebral artery and its syndromes. *Brain*, **53,** 120.

Erickson, T. & Woolsey C. (1951) Observations on the supplementary motor area of man. *Transactions of the American Neurological Association*, **76,** 50.

Goldstein, K. (1944) Mental changes due to frontal lobe damage. *Journal of Psychology*, **17,** 187.

Hécaen, H., Angelergues, R. & Douzens, J. (1963) Les agraphies. *Neuropsychologia*, **1,** 179.

Lhermitte, F., Derouesné, J. & Signoret, J.-L. (1972) Analyse neuropsychologique du syndrome frontal. *Revue neurologique*, **127,** 415.

Mettler, F.A. (Ed.) (1949) *Selective Partial Ablation of the Frontal Cortex.* New York: Hoeber.

Nielsen, J.M. (1951) Anterior cingulate gyrus and corpus callosum. *Bulletin of the Los Angeles Neurological Society*, **16,** 235.

Ramier, A.M. & Hécaen, H. (1970) Rôle respectif des atteintes frontales et de la latéralisation lésionnelle dans les déficits de la 'fluence verbale'. *Revue neurologique*, **123,** 17.

Robinson, B. (1967) Localization evoked from forebrain in Macaca mulatta. *Physiology and Behavior*, **2,** 345.

Warren, J.M. & Akert, K. (Ed.) (1964) *The Frontal Granular Cortex and Behaviour.* New York: McGraw-Hill.

7. The Thalamus and Linguistic Function*

'Socrates. An ingenious sophist, intervening on the gymnasiums and celebrities and the young disciples running up to the adolestcents' homes on the porches and the academies of Athens. Socrates not taught science, ethics and rhetoric; following the Gorgias, the Protagoras and many others who flocked, served honours and the money, preceded by their famous retinue, bright and prestige. He assured himself, on him, went, common, rustic, approaching the agora to the Pnyx, side to encumber some people and abashed them by the most simple questions and difficult problems. Socrates knew nothing, in appearance.'

(*Written composition by Mr Gu.; January 1967*)

1 ANATOMY OF THE THALAMUS

We have previously considered several clinical forms of aphasia (see Chapters 3 to 6). We were then concerned with symptom complexes which were generally well defined, and easily recognized and labelled on the basis of a systematic evaluation of linguistic behaviour (see Chapter 15). Within the confines of our present knowledge, we also discussed the natural evolution of these disturbances. We shall see that they are, in general, the result of various lesions of the *language zone*, that is, of certain parts of the cortical mantle of the left hemisphere and of the immediately underlying white matter (axonal fibres) (see Chapter 8-1, 8-3, and 8-5). There are other types of acquired language disorders (i.e., other varieties of aphasia) which are much rarer and still remain poorly defined at the critical level. Some of them are probably related to lesions, not of the cerebral cortex and the immediately underlying subcortex, but to a deep neuronal mass, namely the thalamus. The goal of the first section of this chapter is to provide a brief anatomofunctional review of this structure.

ANATOMOFUNCTIONAL REVIEW

The diencephalon corresponds to the highest extremity of the brain stem. It is immediately covered by the telencephalon, that is, by the cerebral hemispheres (see Fig. 8-1). The diencephalon includes, to the right and to the left of the midline, four principal structures, namely the *epithalamus*, the *thalamus*, the *hypothalamus* and the *subthalamus* (or *ventral thalamus*). Situated on either side of the third ventricle, and partially forming its wall, the thalami are ovoid structures chiefly formed of grey matter (nerve and glial cells). They may be linked to each other through a cellular isthmus, the *massa intermedia*. The thalami are surrounded and crossed by various *fasciculi* and *laminae* formed of white matter (axonal prolongations of the nerve cells; fibres). Each thalamus includes a large number of cellular subgroups which are the *thalamic nuclei*. These nuclei are arranged in *groups* which are more or less clearly separated by laminae of white matter.

* Readers who have no knowledge of the anatomical foundations of speech and language are advised to read sections 1 and 3 of Chapter 8 before reading the present chapter.

From a functional point of view, most of the thalamic nuclei, including all those of interest here, belong to one or another of three groups 1–4:

Specific relay nuclei [R]: those of interest here are the nuclei which receive input from the large, pre-thalamic sensory pathways (optic, acoustic, somaesthetic) and which exchange projection fibres (post-thalamic pathways) with the ipsilateral primary cortex for each sensory modality. Also of interest are the nuclei which exchange projection fibres with the ipsilateral primary motor cortex involved in activities of the phono-articulatory apparatus and of the dominant hand (see Chapter 8–1, 8–2, 8–5 and 11; Fig. 8–4, 8–11, 8–32 and 9–1).

Association nuclei [A]: the principal characteristic of the association nuclei is that they have important intra-thalamic connections and also share projection fibres with the cortical association areas (including, in certain cases, those cortical association areas which constitute the classical language zone) (see Chapter 8–1; Fig. 8–5). As far as is known, the projections are exclusively ipsilateral in man.

Subcortical projection nuclei [SC] share all or most of their connections with other subcortical structures.

It is far beyond the aims of this book to present a detailed discussion of the anatomy of the thalamus (which is, on the whole, very complex and not very well known). Furthermore, only certain nuclei are of particular interest here. We shall first place them within the context of a general classification of thalamic nuclei and then briefly mention the principal anatomofunctional characteristics of each one.

In the classification below, which is that of Truex and Carpenter[1, 2], we have listed in bold-face type the names of those thalamic nuclei which appear of potential interest in relation to speech and language behaviours. This classification includes nine headings:

(a) The *anterior nuclear group* comprises the anteroventral (AV) [R] and anterodorsal (AD) [R], and anteromedial (AM) [?] nuclei.
(b) The *medial nuclear group* has, as its principal constituent (and only constituent according to some) the **dorsomedial nucleus** (DM). It includes a parvocellular portion [A] and a magnocellular portion [SC].
(c) The *lateral nuclear group* comprises the lateral dorsal nucleus (LD) [A], the **lateral posterior nucleus** (LP) [A] and the **pulvinar** (P) [A]. The pulvinar is subdivided into three portions: medial, lateral and inferior.
(d) The *ventral nuclear group* comprises the ventral anterior nucleus (VA), the **ventral lateral nucleus** (VL) [R] and the ventral posterior nuclei (VP) [R]. The ventral anterior nucleus includes a parvocellular portion [R] and a magnocellular portion [SC]. The ventral lateral nucleus is subdivided into three parts, oral, caudal and medial. There are three ventral posterior nuclei (VP), namely the ventral posterolateral nucleus (VPL), subdivided into two parts (oral and caudal), the **ventral posteromedial nucleus** (VPM) and the ventral postero-inferior (VPI) nucleus.
(e) The *intralaminar nuclear group* comprises five nuclei [SC]: the centromedian (CM), which is the most important of the group, the parafascicular, the paracentral, the central lateral and the central medial.
(f) The *midline nuclear group* comprises four nuclei [?]: the paratenial, the paraventricular, the reuniens and the rhomboid.
(g) The *metathalamus* comprises the **medial geniculate** (MG) **body** or **nucleus**, divided into a parvocellular part [R] and a magnocellular part, as well as the **lateral geniculate** (LG) **body** or **nucleus**, divided into a dorsal part [R] and a ventral part.
(h) The *reticular thalamic nucleus* is a neuronal sheet rather than a nucleus, and encases the lateral and anterior portions of the dorsal thalamus.
(i) The *unclassified group of nuclei* (which are then classified on this basis) comprises the submedial, the suprageniculate and the limitans.

The diagrams accompanying this classification illustrate the reciprocal relations of the principal thalamic nuclei and their cortical projection territories (Fig. 7–1 and 7–2).

Some anatomical features of the thalamus[1–3] should be discussed in slightly greater detail, at least if a theoretical point of view is to be assumed. They are as follows:

The pre-thalamic acoustic pathway terminates in the parvocellular (dorsal) part of the **medial**

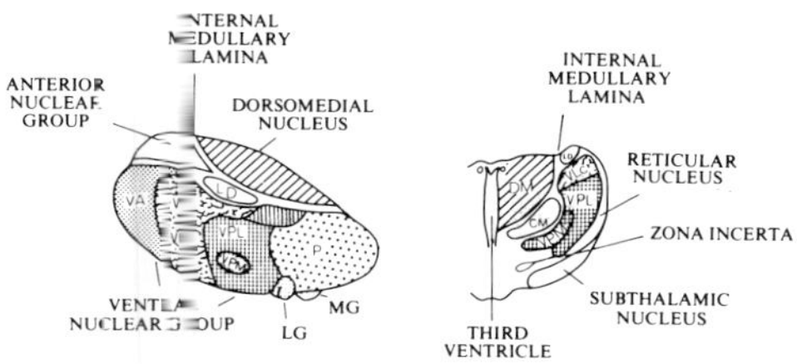

Fig. 7-1 *Mutual connections among the thalamic nuclei. Schematic laterodorsal view and schematic frontal section of the thalamus. LG = lateral geniculate body; MG = medial geniculate body. Adapted from Carpenter*[2].

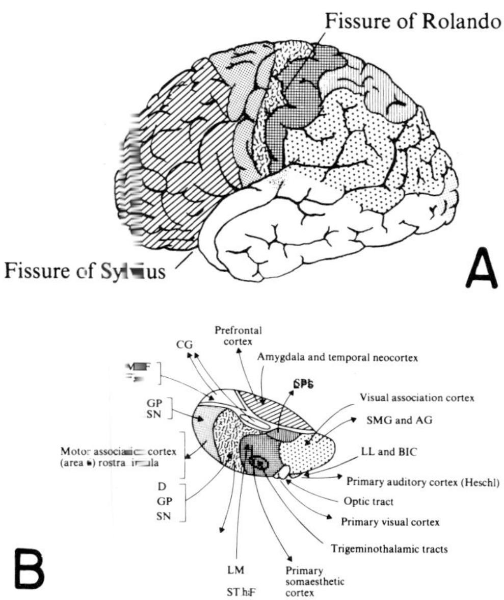

Fig. 7-2 *Mutual connections of the thalamic nuclei and the cortex of the cerebral hemispheres. (A) Schematic view of the convexity of the left hemisphere and (B) schematic laterodorsal view of the thalamus. SPL = superior parietal lobule; SMG = supramarginal gyrus (inferior parietal lobule); AG = angular gyrus (inferior parietal lobule); LL = lateral lemniscus; BIC = brachium of the inferior colliculus; ML = medial lemniscus; SThF = spinothalamic fasciculus; D = dentate nucleus of the cerebellum; GP = globus pallidus; SN = substantia nigra; MTF = mamillothalamic fasciculus; Fx = fornix; CG = cingulate gyrus. Adapted from Carpenter*[2].

geniculate body (MG); its principal efferents constitute the acoustic radiations (geniculotemporal radiations) which terminate in Heschl's region (primary auditory cortex), that is, in the left hemisphere, immediately in front of Wernicke's area (Fig 7-1, 7-2, 8-14, 8-16, 8-32 and 11-1); some of these efferents join the pulvinar directly. The magnocellular part of the MG is associated with the contralateral MG through Meynert's commissure* (supra-optic commissure).

The pre-thalamic optic pathway terminates in the dorsal part of the **lateral geniculate body** (LG); its principal efferents constitute the optic radiations (geniculocalcarine radiations; Gratiolet's radiations) which terminate in the calcarine cortex of the occipital lobe (primary visual cortex) (Fig. 7-1, 7-2, 8-16, 8-21 and 8-32); some of these efferents join the pulvinar directly.

The pre-thalamic somaesthetic pathway, which conveys exteroceptive and proprioceptive information from several muscular–cutaneous structures of the head and neck (including the buccophonatory apparatus), terminates in the **ventral posteromedial nucleus** (VPM); its principal efferents are distributed in the inferior third of the postcentral gyrus[5,6] and probably also in the corresponding part of the precentral gyrus[7] (Fig. 7-1, 7-2, 8-2 and 8-4); some of its efferents link it to (LP).

The **ventral lateral nucleus** (VL) receives composite afferents. Those principally related to our interests come from the cerebellum (oral portion of the VL) and from the globus pallidus, one of the central grey nuclei (oral and medial portions of VL). The oral and caudal parts exchange projection fibres with the precentral gyrus. In the case of the oral part, the cells giving rise to these projections are arranged in a somatotopic organization which corresponds to that of Penfield's homunculus (it is the medial section of the oral portion which exchanges projections with the inferior third of the precentral gyrus, the zone in which the buccophonatory apparatus is represented)[1,2,5,6] (Fig. 7-1, 7-2, 8-2 and 8-4). The possibility cannot be excluded that VL also shares projection fibres with certain parts of the prefrontal convexity, including, in the left hemisphere, parts of Broca's area[8–10] (Fig. 7-3); if so, VL must be considered to be both of type [R] and type [A] (cf. p. 142).

The **dorsomedial nucleus** (DM) receives many fibres which originate subcortically, particularly from other thalamic nuclei and from the central grey nuclei. Only its parvocellular portion is type

* Commissure: group of axonal fibres crossing the midline and establishing connections between left and right homologues.

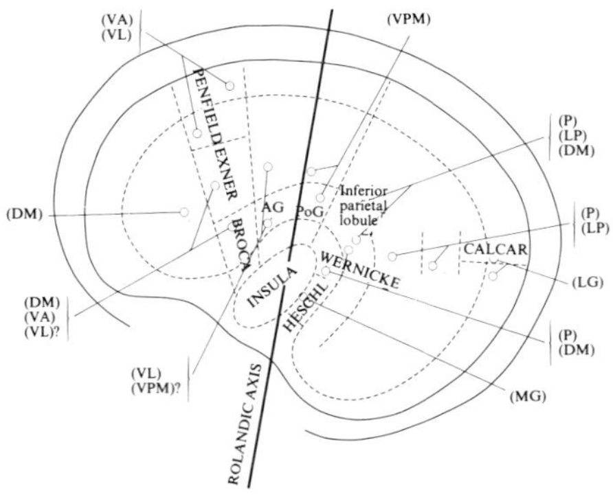

Fig. 7-3 *Mutual connections of the thalamic nuclei and the language zone of the cortex. The left hemisphere is represented here in a Mercator projection (see also Fig. 8-32). VA, VL and VPM = ventral anterior, ventral lateral and ventral postero-medial nuclei of the thalamus; LP = lateral posterior nucleus of the thalamus; DM = dorsomedial nucleus of the thalamus; P = pulvinar; LG = lateral geniculate body; MG = medial geniculate body; PrG = precentral gyrus; PoG = postcentral gyrus; Calcar = axis of the calcarine fissure.*

[A]: it shares important contingents of projection fibres with the prefrontal convexity (through the *anterior thalamic radiations*) and with the temporal operculum. Although there is not complete agreement on this matter[8, 11], the projection zone of the parvocellular part of DM may comprise, in the left hemisphere, parts of the caudal halves of the third (Broca's area) and second frontal convolutions, Wernicke's area proper, and parts of the supramarginal gyrus[3, 5, 6] (Fig. 7-3, 8-2 and 8-32).

The **lateral posterior nucleus** (LP) receives most of its afferents from the adjacent [R] nuclei, in particular the VP nuclei including VPM[12]. It exchanges projection fibres with the superior parietal lobule and probably also with the inferior parietal lobule (which, in the left hemisphere, belongs to the classical language zone) and the neighbouring occipital convexity[5, 6, 13] (Fig. 7-1, 7-2, 8-2 and 8-5).

The **pulvinar** (P) also receives its principal afferents from [R] nuclei, in particular from the MG and LG and perhaps also from the VP nuclei. The lateral and medial portions of P exchange their principal contingents of projection fibres with the association cortex of the temporo-parieto-occipital convexity[5, 6, 13–15]; as for the inferior portion of P, it especially exchanges fibres with the immediately pericalcarine cortex (Brodmann's area 18)[16]. Thus, the pulvinar's projection zone includes, in the left hemisphere, all the retrorolandic components of the classical language zone (Fig. 7-1, 7-2 and 8-5).

Penfield, Roberts and Jasper[17–19] consider that the thalamocortical projections play a predominant role in linguistic function: in their opinion, *speech elaboration* depends more on these projection fibres than on the association fibres of the classical language zone (cf. Chapter 8; Fig. 7-4). The major argument which these investigators put forward in support of their hypothesis is that the number of thalamocortical and corticothalamic axons linked to Broca's area, to Wernicke's area and to the left inferior parietal lobule would appear to be much greater than the number of long cortico-cortical axons linking the first of these regions to the other two (through the superior longitudinal and arcuate fasciculi).

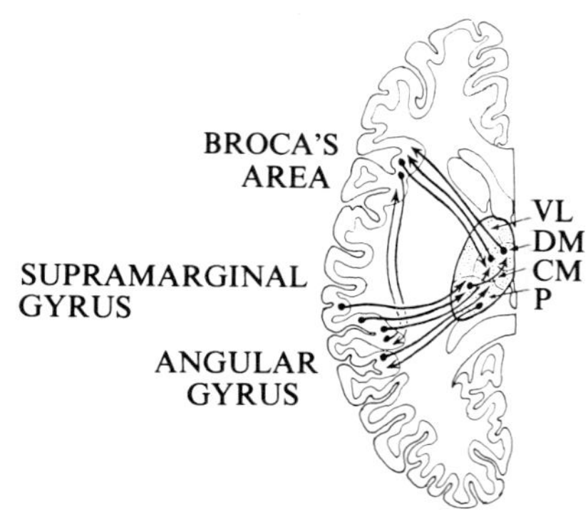

Fig. 7-4 *Mutual connections between the thalamus and the language zone according to Penfield and Roberts. VL, DM, CM and P = ventral lateral, dorsomedial, centromedial and pulvinar nuclei. Adapted from Penfield and Roberts*[18].

2 ELECTRICAL STIMULATION OF THE THALAMUS AND THE CORTEX

Knowledge of the mutual relations between the classical *language zone* (Fig. 8-5) and language behaviour has been almost entirely accumulated through the anatomoclinical method. Various disturbances acquired as a result of natural lesions [particularly cerebral softenings and traumas (see Chapter 9)] were described in detail and, after study of the corresponding autopsy specimens, the role of different parts of the telencephalon in speech and language behaviours was deduced at best (see Chapter 8-1, 8-3 and 8-4). This has not been the case with respect to presently available knowledge of the mutual relations between the thalamus and linguistic behaviours. Although some knowledge has been accumulated through studies of the effects of natural lesions (see Chapter 7-3), most has been acquired through studies of the effects of electrical stimulation of the thalamus or of (therapeutic) surgical destruction of different parts of this structure. The goal of the second part of the present chapter is to discuss the effects, on speech and language behaviours, of electrical stimulation applied to various points of the cortex and the thalamus.

Certain neurosurgical interventions are carried out only after preliminary applications of electrical stimulation at various points of the brain. Among these interventions, two different types have been of primary importance in leading to the accumulation of data which we shall now discuss. The first type of intervention involves the surgical excision of different parts of the cortical mantle, sometimes carried out in the treatment of epilepsy. Preliminary study of the effects of superficial electrical stimulation then permits the delineation and, as far as possible, the conservation of cortical areas judged essential to linguistic functioning. The second type of intervention involves the destruction of different subcortical (grey) structures, in particular, certain thalamic nuclei, which is carried out with the aim of controlling various sensory or motor anomalies, for example Parkinson's disease. Preliminary study of the effects of deep electrical stimulation then permits delineation of the target structures and as far as possible, restriction of the destruction.

Basing our discussion on studies carried out by different investigators, we shall consider three aspects of the mutual relations between the thalamus and linguistic function. We shall first discuss the various types of oral production elicited by stimulation of different points of the cortex and the thalamus (investigations by Penfield, Roberts, Jasper, Guiot, Schaltenbrand, Fedio, van Buren, and their collaborators[17–28]). We shall then review a study by Fedio and van Buren[29] comparing naming and matching-to-sample behaviours during electrical stimulation of the pulvinar and posterior parietal subcortex. Finally, we shall consider an experiment by Ojemann[30] examining naming behaviour and recall in relation to electrical stimulation applied to the ventral lateral nucleus of the thalamus. Because thalamic stimulation has often been studied in patients with Parkinson's disease[31–34], it should be considered that the clinical picture may include a disturbance of articulatory production [hypokinetic dysarthria (cf. p. 67)].

ORAL PRODUCTIONS

The forms of expressive behaviour which will be considered in relation to superficial and deep electrical stimulation are as follows:

Vocalizations: unarticulated vocalic productions sustained during a few seconds (they are vocal noises rather than articulated linguistic entities);

Tachylalia: acceleration of the speech flow, in this case temporary, sometimes to the extent that speech is slurred;

Palilalia: rapid repetition of the same segment—which is usually a syllable but is sometimes more complex—during a few seconds [for example, before naming the stimulus (tulip) the patient articulates /tu/ - /tu/ - /tu/ - /tu/ - /tu/ - /tu/ ... for as long as the stimulation is continued (see Chapter 6)]; associated articulatory distortions may also occur;

Arrest: a temporary inability to achieve any oral production (see Chapter 6);

Hesitation: obvious difficulty in initiating oral production;

Anomia: lack of adequate production during a naming test (in the absence of an arrest);*

Perseveration:repeated production of the same word in response to several different stimuli during a naming test;

Verbal paraphasia: production of an erroneous word during a naming test (with or without formal or conceptual relations between the target word and the uttered word; without perseverative phenomena).

One or another of these forms of oral behaviour have been observed during electrical stimulation of the following points of the left and right

* The patient says 'It's a ...' and then fails to complete the utterance.

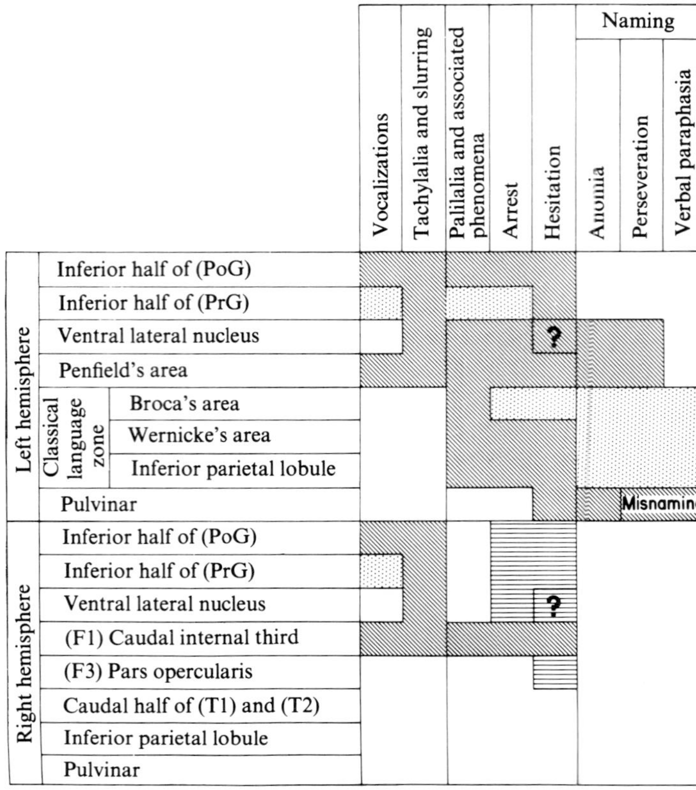

Fig. 7-5 *Electrical stimulation: cortical results and thalamic results summarized from the literature. From greater to lesser intensity of observed phenomena: dots, oblique lines, horizontal lines.*

cerebral hemispheres: inferior half of the precentral gyrus (PrG); inferior half of the postcentral gyrus (PoG); ventral lateral nucleus of the thalamus (see Fig. 7-1); Penfield's supplementary motor area (SMA) [internal surface of the caudalmost third of the first frontal convolution (Fig. 6-1)], pars opercularis of the third frontal convolution (F3); caudal half of the first and second temporal convolutions (T1 and T2); inferior parietal lobule; pulvinar; posterior parietal subcortex (Insertion 7-1). These accumulated data have been summarized schematically* in Fig. 7-5. This summary does not include mention of the anomalies of writing and oral reading, nor of the difficulties in counting, which may occur during electrical stimulation of the cortical components of the classical language zone (see Fig. 8-5).

When discussing electrical stimulation of the cortex, Penfield and Roberts[17] distinguish between its *positive* and its *negative* effects on speech and language behaviour. They consider that the *positive* effect corresponds to vocalization phenomena whereas the *negative* effect corresponds to all inappropriate productions (i.e., to all other observed phenomena). The *positive* effect, which we think should not be likened to articulated language behaviour, is observed during stimulation of the lower rolandic region and of the caudalmost internal third of F1 (supplementary motor area) without significant lateral predominance. Penfield and Roberts[17] interpret the *negative* effect in terms of a disturbance of the *motor mechanisms of language* if it does not include impaired naming (especially the rolandic region) and in terms of a disturbance of *ideational language* if naming is impaired [especially the classical language zone and, in a less obvious manner, the caudalmost internal third of F1, on the left side (Penfield's area)].

In considering the schematic summary presented here (Fig. 7-5), it can be seen that certain phenomena (vocalization, tachylalia) occur without lateral predominance, that others occur with relative left hemisphere predominance, and

* It should be noted that some of the subjects included in the thalamic stimulation studies already had surgical lesions of the thalamus prior to the study.

Insertion 7.1

After the current reaches a certain intensity, electrical stimulation of the brain, and particularly of the thalamus, may often elicit unpleasant, dysaesthesic phenomena. This rules out continued experimentation related to speech and language behaviour as the maximum current applied must consequently be fixed below the threshold of dysaesthesia. As a result, the major investigations which are pertinent to the topic of the present chapter have, until now, been limited to the effects of thalamic stimulation involving the ventral lateral nucleus and the pulvinar. The form of behaviour then observed depends, to a certain extent, on the intensity of the applied electrical stimulation. The following data (average current intensity) relevant to stimulation of the left VL were provided by Ojemann[27, 28, 30]: 4.5 mA for arrest of speech; 5.5 mA for palilalia; 8 mA for anomia; 9.5 mA for perseveration. He specified that stimulation of the left VL of less than 6 mA never elicited anomalies. The intensity of the electrical current required to elicit a particular behaviour may also vary depending on the structure stimulated: thus anomia may be observed when a 5 mA stimulation is applied to Wernicke's area proper or to the left inferior parietal lobule.

that still others (impaired naming) attest to a quasi-absolute association with the left hemisphere. Since the data obtained from these investigations were often fragmentary and the writings of different authors are often difficult to compare, the summary does not permit definitive conclusions. Nevertheless, the following assertions can be proposed:

(a) Vocalization, tachylalia and slurring occur without clear lateral predominance. They occur upon stimulation of the lower rolandic region and of the caudalmost internal third of F1. An acceleration of the speech flow may also occur during stimulation of the VL nuclei of the thalamus. Vocalization phenomena (the *positive* effect of Penfield and Roberts[17]) are particularly frequent as a result of electrical stimulation of the inferior half of the precentral gyrus (this predominance is slightly clearer on the left than on the right). It should also be noted that these phenomena, the only behaviours observed which do not correspond to a requested activity, were not observed during stimulation of either the left or right VL nuclei.

(b) Palilalia, arrest and hesitation generally occur with relative left predominance. On this side, they occur upon stimulation of the lower rolandic region, the VL nucleus of the thalamus, Penfield's area and the three components of the classical language zone (Fig. 8–5); hesitation phenomena have also been observed following stimulation of the left pulvinar.* The phenomena of arrest and hesitation also occur, although less frequently than on the left, during stimulation of the right lower rolandic region and the right VL nucleus. Results obtained during stimulation of the caudalmost third of F1 on the left and on the right are approximately the same in terms of palilalia, arrest and hesitation. The last two phenomena occur more frequently upon stimulation of Broca's area than during stimulation of any other region. Similarly, palilalia and arrest are particularly frequent during stimulation of the inferior half of the left PrG. Finally, it should be noted that stimulation of pars opercularis of F3, on the right, sometimes gives rise to hesitation phenomena. This might be an effect of indirect (transcallosal) stimulation of Broca's area, a zone which is

*And following parasplenial stimulation applied within the depths the left posterior parietal subcortex (Fedio and van Buren[29]).

particularly sensitive in this respect* (Fig. 7-5). With the exception of this area, the stimulation of cortical surfaces of the right hemisphere which are symmetrical to the classical language zone, as well as stimulation of the right pulvinar, almost never elicits palilalia, arrest or hesitation phenomena.

(c) The observed disturbances in naming suggest nearly absolute left dominance in relation to this behaviour.† The disturbances are particularly clear during stimulation of the three components of the classical language zone (Fig. 8-5). Anomia and perseveration may also occur, to a lesser degree, during stimulation of Penfield's area, the left VL nucleus, the left pulvinar or the left posterior parietal subcortex. We think it important to point out that production of verbal paraphasias clearly exceeding that occurring in normal discourse (see Chapter 14) was observed only during stimulation of the three components of the classical language zone (Broca's area, Wernicke's area proper, left inferior parietal lobule) and, perhaps, of the left pulvinar.

(d) Certain observed behaviours, such as tachylalia, can be considered primarily to involve *speech*, whereas others, such as the production of verbal paraphasias, primarily involve *language* (see Chapter 12). While the former may occur when stimulation is applied to several points of the cortical mantle, particularly on the left side (Fig. 8-32), the latter occur in a clear fashion only when stimulation is applied to the classical language zone (Fig. 8-5). With regard to the dichotomy between *speech* and *language*, it should be noted that certain observed behaviours—particularly the phenomena of arrest and hesitation, and perhaps even anomia in certain cases—cannot be specifically attributed, with absolute certainty, to the instrumental pole (*speech*) rather than to the ideational pole (*language*), or vice versa. These behaviours are, in fact, as commonly observed upon stimulation of various points located outside the classical language zone as upon stimulation within this zone. The high frequency of arrests and hesitations in stimulation of Broca's area may be related to the double role it appears to play—if one reasons from the clinical picture presented in Broca's aphasia (see Chapters 4 and 8-3)—in the control of both *speech* behaviours and *language* behaviours.

(e) With the exception of the *quantitative* difference observed, in regard to arrest and hesitation phenomena, during stimulation of Broca's area, the behaviours observed upon stimulation of various points of the classical language zone are qualitatively and quantitatively the same, whether the stimulation is applied to Broca's area, Wernicke's area proper, or the left inferior parietal lobule. If the quantitative differences (anomia and perseveration) and qualitative differences (paraphasia) observed in naming behaviour are ignored, one may add, like Penfield and Roberts[17], the left supplementary motor area (caudalmost internal third of F1 on this side) to the three components of the classical language zone (see Chapter 8-1). According to Penfield and Roberts[17, 18], the reason for this lack of difference may be that these three regions‡ are integrated into a single system by both transcortical pathways [associative fibres (see Chapter 8-1)] and subcortical pathways [cortex↔thalamus↔thalamus↔cortex (Fig. 7-2 to 7-4)]: an electrical disturbance set up in any one part of the system may disrupt the functioning of the entire system.

(f) The stimulation of the VL nucleus of the left thalamus may elicit most of the phenomena observed during cortical stimulation of the same side, including anomia and hesitation behaviours during naming tests. This is undoubtedly significant if it is considered that the VL nucleus shares reciprocal projections with the PrG and perhaps also with the pars opercularis of F3 (Fig. 7-

* The data of Penfield and Roberts[17] show that hesitation phenomena are four times more frequent upon stimulation of Broca's area than upon stimulation of its right-hemisphere counterpart.

† Fedio and van Buren[29] point out the occasional occurrence of anomic behaviour during parasplenial stimulations applied within the depths of the right, posterior parietal subcortex. They logically suggest that it may result from transcallosal inactivation of the temporoparietal components of the classical language zone.

‡ The three regions are: (a) Wernicke's area proper, and the inferior parietal lobule; (b) Broca's area; (c) Penfield's area.

3). Certain phenomena, no doubt related to *speech* rather than to *language*, are also observed during stimulation of the right VL nucleus. In this respect, it may be appropriate to recall Pierre Marie's[35] doctrine according to which *anarthria* could result from right subcortical lesions as well as from left subcortical lesions (see Chapter 1).*

(g) Stimulation of the pulvinar may result in hesitations, anomia and, according to Fedio and van Buren[29], in *misnaming* (perseveration? paraphasia?). This is undoubtedly significant if it is considered that this structure shares reciprocal connections with the retrorolandic components of the classical language zone (Fig. 7-2 and 7-4). Like the left VL nucleus, the left pulvinar thus becomes a prime candidate within the context of an eventual tridimensional conception of the language zone (see Chapter 8-5). Implicit in Penfield's teachings[17], this conclusion was recently re-acknowledged by Ojemann[30]: 'Left thalamus appears to be related to language processes. This is suggested by the ability to evoke the same types of object naming errors from left thalamus as can be evoked from the cortex concerned with language. Indeed, only portions of the left thalamus, including anterior superior pulvinar, and medial central ventrolateral nucleus may be thus related to language.'†

NAMING AND MATCHING (OF PICTURES)

In a study of the effects of electrical stimulation of the pulvinar and the paracallosal white matter deep within the parietal lobes (in right-handed subjects), Fedio and van Buren[29] compared subjects' performance during a naming task and a task requiring the matching of complex, non-meaningful visual patterns. The results of this study are shown here as a percentage of errors occurring on each task during electrical stimulation at each location (Fig. 7-6). Abnormalities observed on the naming test are grouped under two headings, *absence of naming* and *naming errors*, while those on the matching task are categorized as *absence of matching* or *matching errors*. The results of this study are interesting in several respects:

		Naming	Matching
Left hemisphere	Pulvinar	28.2%	26.8%
	Posterior parietal subcortex	26.4%	26.7%
Right hemisphere	Pulvinar	0%	28%
	Posterior parietal subcortex	14.4%	29.9%

Fig. 7-6 *Percentage of errors in naming pictures of common objects and in matching random, non-verbal patterns during electrical stimulation of the pulvinar and posterior parietal subcortex in the right and in the left hemisphere. Commentary in the text. The results obtained in naming during pulvinar stimulation confirm the specialization of the left hemisphere for language production in right-handers. This specialization is, however, more relative at the thalamic level than at the cortical level. Data excerpted from Fedio and van Buren*[29].

(a) The error rates for left hemisphere and right hemisphere stimulations are approximately equal on the matching task.‡ This lack of difference suggests that the role of the left and the right pulvinar is approximately

* In this matter, we have not used Pierre Marie's terminology in the present work. Without denying the occasional occurrence of transient articulatory disturbances in right-handers following a right hemisphere lesion (see Chapter 3), we have in fact reserved the term *anarthria* for phonetic disturbances occurring in right-handers either in a nearly isolated fashion or in a more complex symptomatological context (for example, in *Broca's aphasia*) after certain left hemisphere lesions (see Chapters 3 and 4).

† It is perhaps significant that all previous data on naming during electrical stimulation of the thalamus were obtained using visual stimuli. It would be interesting to know, for example, what would occur if stimuli for the naming tasks consisted of various tape-recorded sounds.

‡ Given these results and their implications, it would be interesting to observe the effects of stimulation of the left and right inferior parietal lobules on the same naming and matching tasks.

equivalent on this task which has few linguistic connotations.

(b) The results obtained in naming during stimulation of the left and the right pulvinar confirm the clear specialization of the left hemisphere of right-handers for language production (see Chapter 11). They suggest, as previously mentioned, that the left pulvinar will find its place in a tridimensional conception of the language zone (see Chapter 8-5).

(c) The observed similarity between error rates in naming and in matching during stimulation on the left side could no doubt be expected to be found in a study of the effects of natural lesions of those parts of the retrorolandic cortical mantle which receive pulvinar projections.

(d) It would be interesting to be able to compare the effects of stimulation of the left and the right pulvinar on naming versus identification-by-pointing tasks. If predictions were to be made in this regard, it should be considered that, in right-handers, a certain elementary level of comprehension (see Insertions 11.1 and 11.2) can be mediated by the right hemisphere. It should also be considered that a dissociation between naming and pointing, in favour of the latter, is also usual in natural retrorolandic lesions of the left hemisphere.

(e) Although almost twice as infrequent as in left stimulations, the naming errors observed during electrical stimulations deep within the right posterior parietal subcortex (Fig. 7-6) are unexpected. The interpretation proposed by Fedio and van Buren[29] has already been mentioned (retrograde stimulation of the language zone).

(f) Compared with errors involving an absence of response (omission), substitution-type errors were relatively frequent only in relation to left pulvinar stimulations. The significance of this finding remains unclear. In our opinion it may reflect—at least in regard to naming behaviour*—a more direct influence of the left pulvinar on the classical language zone (which appears essential for most articulated linguistic productions, even deviant ones).

NAMING AND RECALL

In order to study the eventual effects of electrical stimulation of the VL nucleus of the thalamus on (short-term) recall of verbal production, Ojemann[30] used a test involving a three-phase procedure on each trial:

(a) *Naming phase*: (oral) verbal identification of a visual stimulus (picture of a familiar object) is requested of the subject.

(b) *Distraction phase*: the subject engages in mental arithmetic for six seconds.

(c) *Recall phase*: the subject is asked to name the stimulus presented during the first phase.

Subjects completed the test under five different experimental conditions, four of them involving electrical stimulation of the VL nucleus of the thalamus. The stimulation was below the threshold current for object naming errors (see Insertion 7-1). The observed data were as follows:

(a) *Trials without electrical stimulation* were control trials. The number of failures in recall on these trials provided a basis for comparison with results obtained under other conditions.

(b) *Stimulation of the VL during the naming phase* resulted in a significant improvement of recall scores in 11 of the 13 subjects stimulated on the left. This systematic trend was not observed when stimulation was applied to the right VL (in this case seven subjects showed improved recall and seven showed decreased recall).

(c) *Stimulation of the VL during the recall phase* resulted in a significant reduction of recall accuracy (compared with the control condition) in the 13 subjects stimulated on the left. This systematic trend was not observed when stimulation was applied to the right VL (eight subjects showed decreased recall and six showed improved recall).

(d) *Stimulation of the left VL and of the right VL during the naming phase and the recall phase* resulted in performance comparable with that observed during trials without electrical stimulation.

(e) *Stimulation of the left VL and of the right*

* Of the errors, 42 per cent occurred during stimulation of the left pulvinar while approximately 10 per cent occurred during subcortical stimulation in the depths of the left and right parietal lobes (Fedio and van Buren[29]).

> *VL during the distraction phase* resulted in performance comparable with that observed during trials without electrical stimulation.

The data obtained during stimulation of the right VL have few obvious implications. However, those obtained during stimulation of the left VL led Ojemann[30] to formulate a hypothesis as ingenious as his experimental design. He proposed that stimulation of the left VL evokes a '*specific alerting response*' which directs the subject's attention to external information. In the experimental condition in which such stimulation is applied during the naming phase, the subject's attention to the stimulus is increased and retrieval during the recall phase would be superior to that observed in the control condition. Conversely, in the condition in which stimulation is applied during the recall phase, the subject's attention is inappropriately directed to the external environment and retrieval is impeded, so that recall would be inferior to that in the control condition. The favourable effects are cancelled by the unfavourable effects in the condition in which stimulation is applied to the VL during both the naming and recall phases so that recall scores are, not surprisingly, similar to those of the control condition. In support of Ojemann's hypothesis, it is interesting to note that while stimulation of the VL during the distraction phase did not affect either naming or recall, it did hamper performance on the mental arithmetic task (cf. p. 150). It can be assumed that this reflects the effect of turning attention towards the external environment.

We have previously discussed certain aspects of a study (Fig. 7-6) by Fedio and van Buren[29]. In the context of this investigation, these authors noted that stimulation of the left pulvinar during the recall phase hindered recall of stimuli from the naming test whereas stimulation of the right pulvinar during the recall* phase hindered recall of stimuli from the matching task. Ojemann's hypothesis (of a specific alerting response) concerning the ventral lateral nucleus may thus be applicable to the pulvinar. In the case of the latter, it would be related to certain linguistic behaviours for the left thalamus and to certain non-linguistic behaviours for the right thalamus.

3 THALAMIC LESIONS AND SPEECH AND LANGUAGE BEHAVIOURS

Lesions limited to the thalamus, particularly natural lesions, often do not disturb linguistic behaviour[36]. Nevertheless, certain thalamic lesions, particularly those of surgical origin, may cause disturbances—which are generally transient—of speech or even language. These disturbances are the topic of the last section of this chapter. We shall first discuss the effects of surgical lesions and then those of natural lesions of the thalamus.

SURGICAL LESIONS

In the aim of reducing the tremor and rigidity of parkinsonian patients, or else of reducing the abnormal movements, spasticity or pain occurring in other neurological diseases, contemporary neurosurgeons sometimes carry out procedures involving the destruction of various parts of the central grey nuclei and/or of the thalamus. These interventions are usually carried out at the expense of zones which are themselves individually healthy (Insertion 7-2) but which form part of networks involved in diseases whose control is attempted through modification of their functions. The surgical lesions thus created are small, very circumscribed and limited to a fraction of the nuclei whose functioning is to be altered. Besides the desired therapeutic effect, these lesions may also result in various neurological disturbances which sometimes include vocal abnormalities (reduced intensity of the voice) or articulatory disturbances (see Chapter 3) and no doubt certain phenomena which can be likened to other features of aphasic symptomatology. When these anomalies occur, they are mild and transient in the great majority of cases. According to Riklan and Cooper[37], the transient nature of the disturbances can be explained (in referring to the concepts of *plasticity* and functional *equipotentiality*) by the fact that they result from limited destruction within a relatively much larger functional territory: the uninvolved parts

* The procedure was analogous to that described in regard to Ojemann's experiment[14].

of this territory are themselves sufficient to ensure a return to the preoperative functional level eventually. The same reasoning could readily be extended to certain limited lesions of the classical language zone (see Fig. 8–5) whose effects on linguistic behaviour, particularly in younger subjects (see Fig. 11–2), are also transient. It can thus be further suggested that, in both cases, the regressive clinical anomalies result from a transient functional disturbance in the neighbourhood of the lesion (caused, for example, by oedema) rather than from the lesion itself.

During recent years, specialized journals have included several articles concerning speech and language disturbances which may occur following therapeutic interventions on the central grey nuclei and on the thalamus[20, 23, 33, 34, 38–47]. With the exception of the finding that such disturbances may indeed occur, a fact that we consider of primary importance (see Chapter 8–5), it is very difficult to draw precise conclusions from these reports. This is partly because methods of studying the observed disturbances are not standardized and partly because the terminology used to designate the disturbances is usually imprecise and often varies among different publications. This being stated, guarded consideration can nevertheless be given to the following statements:

(a) The 'lesions' generally involve the globus pallidus, the VL nucleus of the thalamus or else the pulvinar, and only destroy a part of the target nucleus.
(b) The 'lesions' may be unilateral left, unilateral right or bilateral.
(c) Regardless of the structure involved, no lesion invariably results in the appearance of a speech or language disturbance. In fact, such disturbances are relatively rare and their occurrence depends on the laterality of surgical lesions, their extent, and the preoperative neuropsychological status of the patients[34, 37]. This last factor may or may not be related to a pre-existing lesion which may be natural or surgical, cortical-subcortical or deep subcortical.
(d) The observed disturbances are usually transient (cf. p. 151).
(e) Most authors appear to distinguish among three types of phenomena: vocal impairments (decreased vocal intensity), speech disturbances (*speech deficits*, *speech impairments*, *transient speech abnormality*, *dysarthria*, *slurring and stuttering in the absence of true aphasia*, *changes in patterns of rate and rhythm*, etc.; and language disturbances (*language disturbances*, *aphasic difficulties*, *transient dysphasia*, *true disorder of language*, *disorders of expression similar to cortically-produced aphasia*, etc.[20, 23, 33, 34, 38–47]).*
(f) *Vocal* anomalies and *speech* disturbances may occur following unilateral or bilateral lesions. They occur more frequently and are more severe and of longer duration in the latter case.† They are perhaps more frequent following lesions of the VL nucleus of the thalamus and/or of the globus pallidus. In the case of unilateral lesions, the side of the lesion (*left* or *right*) does not appear to play an important role in the origin of the disturbances.
(g) Language disturbances may appear following unilateral or bilateral lesions. They occur more frequently and are more severe and of longer duration in the latter case. In the case of unilateral lesions (in a right-handed subject) it is almost always the *left* or *dominant* hemisphere which is involved.

Language evaluations in surgical lesions of the thalamus

Very few investigators have considered the results of a detailed evaluation of speech and language behaviours (see Chapter 15) carried out before and after surgical lesions of the thalamus. A recent study by Darley, Brown and Swenson[40] has presented several interesting findings. They carried out an aphasia assessment, pre- and post-operatively, on 123 subjects (mostly with parkinsonism). The evaluation included several subtests: naming, identification of auditory stimuli

* In the days following onset of a surgically-induced lesion of the left VL nucleus in right-handers, Riklan and Cooper[37] observed alterations of fluency and the occurrence of hesitations and blockings. They considered that 'these changes cannot be distinguished from dysphasia frequently described following left-sided cortical lesions'.

† Bilateral lesions may result in articulatory behaviour similar to *pseudobulbar dysarthria* (see Chapter 3) and sometimes in transient *mutism*.

Insertion 7.2

While the subcortical (thalamic and other) surgical lesions induced during treatment of Parkinson's disease and other neurological disorders generally involve healthy nervous tissue, the same is not true of cortical excisions carried out within the language zone (see Chapter 8-1) in certain cases of epilepsy which resist all other forms of treatment. In this regard, Penfield and Roberts[17, 18] have discussed excisions, sometimes complete, of one or another of the following portions of the cortical mantle (in right-handed subjects): caudalmost third of F1 on the left side (external and internal surfaces); Broca's area; inferior half of the precentral gyrus and the postcentral gyrus; inferior parietal lobule; Wernicke's area proper. Most, if not all, of these cases have the following common characteristics:

(a) Except at its edge, the excised cortical zone consisted of pathological tissue (usually cicatricial); in most cases, the pathology was long standing, often dating since early childhood (see Chapter 11).
(b) In general, excision did not cause immediate changes in speech and language behaviours. This strongly suggests that, in these patients, the excised (pathological) zones did not play an important role in the control of their linguistic behaviours.
(c) After one to four days, and for periods extending from one to several weeks, signs of aphasia followed the initial asymptomatic period. Most often transient in nature and in the vast majority of cases, these manifestations of aphasia no doubt reflected oedema of neighbouring tissue and the effects of *diaschisis* (see Chapter 1). In certain respects they were related to the location, not of the excised zones, but of immediately neighbouring zones.
(d) There was usually a return to the preoperative functional level (as far as could be determined from limited evaluations carried out pre- and postoperatively).

According to Penfield and Roberts[17, 18] these observations suggest that no single constituent of the cortical language zone is absolutely essential for the control of linguistic functioning.* Without prejudging the validity of this hypothesis (which could, moreover, be readily applied to the thalamus), it seems clear that the facts on which it is based are extremely tenuous: how, in fact, is it possible to make generalizations about normal brains on the basis of phenomena observed after surgical interventions on brains which have long been abnormal? Given the data discussed by Penfield and Roberts, we would consider it more logical to suggest that: an early lesion of the language zone may be followed by a functional rearrangement such that linguistic behaviour would eventually not be grossly affected (see Chapter 11); the zones which are immediately adjacent to such lesions probably play an important role in this functional rearrangement; in these subjects the 'language zone' could not be considered in the same (anatomical) terms as in subjects having a normal brain; and, despite its great interest, the observation of the effects of excision of an area of abnormal cortex, situated for example at the caudalmost part of the left, third frontal convolution, does not permit prediction of the effects which would result from the excision of Broca's area in a neurologically healthy right-hander.

(single or multiple), matching (written words and pictures), repetition, word definitions, comprehension of written sentences, comprehension of a spoken passage and of a written passage, explanation of proverbs. Findings from this study can be summarized as follows: approximately one-quarter of the subjects presented a disturbance postoperatively; rather than on the easier subtests (naming, identification, matching), it was on the more complex subtests (comprehension of a passage, accurate definitions, etc.) that the disturbances were apparent ('impairments were predominantly of higher language functions'); although no site of lesion was completely without effects on speech or language, the frequency and severity of observed disturbances

* In the opinion of these investigators, the temporoparietal components play a more important role than Broca's area which in turn plays a more important role than the left supplementary motor area.

was clearly greater after left thalamotomy,* after multiple thalamotomies and after mixed pallidectomy–thalamotomy. Psychometric testing was carried out on 13 subjects and the obtained results suggested that the observed linguistic disturbances were not a reflection of a generalized intellectual impairment (see Chapter 16).

Psychometric evaluations in surgical lesions of the thalamus

Riklan, Levita, Cooper and their collaborators[34, 37, 42, 44, 45–47] presented different psychometric tests to patients treated by surgical lesions of the thalamus (ventral lateral nucleus or pulvinar). They were particularly interested in comparing results obtained (pre- and post-operatively) on the 'verbal' and 'non-verbal' subtests of the *Wechsler Adult Intelligence Scale* [WAIS] (see Chapter 16). The principal finding was a transient decrease in the verbal intelligence quotient following lesions of the left VL nucleus (nine cases: average decrease 8.7 points) or of the left pulvinar (16 cases: average decrease of 10.2 points)[37]. Based on these and other findings, Riklan and Cooper[37] consider that the thalamic nuclei, and in particular the VL nucleus and the pulvinar, play a role in linguistic functioning, a role which is especially related to the *fluency* of verbal production. While the left thalamus tends to be dominant in this respect, the difference between the left and right appears to be quantitative rather than qualitative ('more in the nature of a continuum than a dichotomy') (see Chapter 11).

NATURAL LESIONS

Softenings

Much of the knowledge accumulated on the mutual relationships between language and the brain has been acquired through clinical and anatomical study of thromboembolic softenings affecting different parts of the superficial irrigation territory of the left, middle cerebral artery. In contrast, and with the exclusion of a few very exceptional cases (to which we shall return), the study of thromboembolic softenings of the thalamus has, until now, provided little (positive) information which can be considered in developing a biological conception of language. Among the syndromes which have been described is the *syndrome of the thalamo-perforating arteries* (or *posterior thalamic syndrome*), assumed to be related to the occlusion of those branches of the posterior cerebral artery whose irrigation territory includes the VL, DM and CM thalamic nuclei. Its recognized effects are, however, limited to motor involvement of the contralateral side of the body (tremor, choreic movements, rigidity). A *syndrome of the thalamo-geniculate arteries* has also been described and assumed to be related to the occlusion of those branches of the posterior cerebral artery whose irrigation territory includes the pulvinar and the MG, LG and VP thalamic nuclei. Here again, there are no recognized effects on linguistic functioning (rather the effects are limited to the contralateral side of the body: transient paresis, sensory disturbances and 'thalamic pain' (*Dejerine–Roussy syndrome*))[49]. If it is presumed that left thalamic structures such as the pulvinar and VL nucleus were in fact the site of important lesions in some of the previously studied thalamo-perforating and thalamo-geniculate softenings, can it be concluded, given the absence of any recognized linguistic symptomatology, that these structures play no role in the control of speech and language? Such a conclusion would doubtless be too hasty. It is, in fact, almost certain that the destruction of a structure playing a subordinate (and limited) role in normal linguistic behaviour may sometimes escape notice because the function in question is taken over by other ipsilateral or contralateral structures. Furthermore, it is clear that tests which are commonly used to assess the integrity of linguistic behaviour are not well adapted to the demonstration of relatively subtle disturbances, so that their presence can easily remain undetected (especially when a dramatic sensorimotor disturbance and a serious medical condition direct attention elsewhere).

The exceptional case studies referred to above can be summarized as follows:

Two of these case studies were carried out in Bucharest by Sager, Mares and Nestianu[50]. Botez and Barbeau[51] considered these studies when formulating their hypotheses about the role of the thalamus in relation to linguistic behaviours: 'The first patient was a 62-year-old right-handed male who presented receptive dysphasia, alexia, alcalculia and amnesic aphasia following a cerebral vascular accident. He died two weeks later.

* The site of the thalamic lesions was not specified: it was probably the VL nucleus in most of the cases.

The autopsy revealed the presence of a haemorrhagic softening in the posterior part of the (left) thalamus. The cortex did not present either macroscopic or microscopic lesions. The other patient, a 55-year-old right-handed male, presented alexia and receptive dysphasia following a cerebral vascular accident. He died seven days later. The neuropathological examination revealed the presence of two haemorrhagic softenings, one situated in the LP nucleus of the left thalamus and the other in the pulvinar on the same side. The cortex was intact.' The clinical features attributed to a left thalamic lesion are so surprising in these two cases, especially the alexia and acalculia, that one would wish to study the anatomical specimens in detail.

Elghozi[52] recently reported, but without necropsic verification, a case of left thalamic softening presumably involving the pulvinar and the ventral posterior nuclei. This author described the neuropsychological status of his patient as follows: 'Increased verbal output; absence of articulatory deficits; presence of paraphasias; anomia;* impaired ideoverbal control; disturbed oral comprehension in keeping with an impairment in the short-term memorization of verbal messages.'

In a study of 28 anatomoclinical cases of paramedial thalamic infarcts observed at la Salpêtrière, Lyon-Caen[36] discussed four patients who had presented naming difficulties within the context of a global reduction of intellectual functions. He also reported a case of agraphia with impaired spelling in the absence of an oral language disturbance: in this case the paramedial thalamic lesion was bilateral, extending behind the pulvinar and not associated with any cortical lesion.

Thalamic structures have also been considered in other anatomoclinical studies of thromboembolic softenings. For example, in a study of two anatomoclinical cases in which the symptomatology was dominated by a major element of cortical deafness (see Chapter 5), one of us (F.L.)[53] observed that the lesions were bitemporal in both cases and affected the acoustic radiations; that the MG nuclei of the thalami were spared; that the patients were able to discriminate paired sounds differing in intensity or in frequency but could not recognize rhythms nor appreciate the duration of sounds. Emphasis can thus be placed on 'the role of the internal geniculate bodies (MG) in the discrimination of frequency and intensity and [on] the essential role of the cortical structures in the processes of temporal integration of the message and of analysis of the components of complex sounds.'

Van Buren[13] carried out a detailed study of an anatomical specimen from the *Yakovlev collection* [aphasia—global at onset with evolution towards a Wernicke's aphasia with an auditory aspect (see Chapters 4 and 5)—from a putamino-insulo-temporal thromboembolic softening with caudal extension of the subcortical part of the lesion]. Although this study scarcely clarified the role of the thalamus in linguistic functioning, it did contribute to knowledge of the reciprocal projections linking the retrorolandic components of the language zone and certain thalamic structures including the pulvinar as well as the LP and MG nuclei.

Tumours

Generally speaking, the study of thalamic tumours has not shed additional light on the problem of the reciprocal relations between the thalamus and language in adults. In the context of research carried out in different neurosurgery departments, the presence of 'aphasia' or 'dysphasia' has nevertheless been pointed out, without further specification, in certain patients with a thalamic tumour. McKissock and Paine[54] reported that two of their 24 patients were 'aphasic' and specified that the tumour was situated in the 'left thalamus' in both cases, and that it extended towards the frontal and temporal regions of the hemisphere. Cheek and Taveras[55], for their part, observed 'dysphasia' in 11 of 50 subjects with thalamic tumours. Other series of patients have been the topic of other published reports. No mention was made in any cases of the clinical characteristics of the linguistic disturbances, nor of the localization of the lesions within the thalamus (sometimes not even of their laterality), nor of the localization or extent of eventual invasion into neighbouring regions. Moreover, even if these data were available, it would be impossible in most cases to distinguish between signs of thalamic localization and signs of intracranial hypertension with compression of various components of the classical speech areas.

* 'Word-finding difficulty.'

Haemorrhages

The study of thalamic haemorrhages* has proved relatively more gratifying, in relation to our interests, than has that of thromboembolic softenings and thalamic tumours. In a discussion on this topic, Mohr and his collaborators at the Massachusetts General Hospital considered the following cases:

Case 1 (Mohr, Walters and Duncan)[57]: hypertensive cerebral haemorrhage (see Chapter 9) in a 72-year-old right-handed female. A sensorimotor hemideficit was present on the right. Significant fluctuations in the state of consciousness were observed. The patient was 'present' for brief intervals during which she was tested on a wide range of tasks. During these brief periods, she responded sensibly to simple questions and her conversation did not include any deviations. Similarly, she could name objects and pictures, repeat words and neologisms having a complex phonemic structure, spell words and read sentences. At other moments, all these activities were impossible and the patient engaged in logorrhoeic, paraphasic discourse which included elements of perseveration, dyssyntaxia and muttering. The logorrhoeic utterances often ended with a progressive decrease in vocal intensity followed by silence. Articulation was not disturbed. Computerized tomography showed the haemorrhage to involve the entire left thalamus and to extend towards the insula on this side. Total recovery occurred in two months and the patient had no memory of her aphasia.

Case 2 (Mohr, Walters and Duncan)[57]: hypertensive cerebral haemorrhage in a 74-year-old right-handed male. The patient was agitated, lethargic and disoriented. A sensorimotor hemideficit was present on the right. Logorrhoeic, paraphasic jargon with marked echolalia and perseveration were observed. Again, in this case the logorrhoeic utterances often ended with a progressive decrease in vocal intensity followed by silence. Vigorous stimulation from the examiner was then required to reinitiate the patient's jargoned production. Repetition of words and phonemically complex neologisms remained impossible but other tasks elicited many errors which were not noticed by the patient (no attempt at correction). Articulation was not disturbed. Computerized tomography showed the lesion to involve the anterior part of the left thalamus as well as the caudate nucleus and the putamen on this side.

Case 3 (Massachusetts General Hospital archives)[57]: hypertensive cerebral haemorrhage in a 57-year-old right-handed male. Right hemiparesis was observed as well as hemihypo-aesthesia and a (probable) hemianopsia on the same side. Despite an articulatory disturbance, the output was abundant and characterized by intermittent utterances which included many paraphasic deviations and neologisms ('jargon in bursts intermixed with true speech . . . typical jargon though performance is variable'). Presentation of a naming test permitted observation of word-finding difficulty; repetition and oral reading tests were not presented. Oral comprehension was sufficient only to permit correct performance of simple commands. Progressive recovery from the aphasia occurred during the following weeks but the patient died just over two months later following a cerebellar haemorrhage. In addition to the latter, the autopsy revealed the presence of a less recent thalamic haemorrhage which involved the left pulvinar and the DM, LP and VP nuclei of the left thalamus.

Case 4 (Massachusetts General Hospital archives)[57]: hypertensive cerebral haemorrhage in a 46-year-old right-handed male. A right hemiparesis was present but the sensory examination was normal in all respects. With the exception of an articulatory disturbance ('slurred speech'), linguistic functioning was normal. The patient died just over ten months later from myocardial infarction. The autopsy revealed traces of a haemorrhage deep within the left cerebral hemisphere; it involved the VL and the CM nuclei of the thalamus and the adjacent part of the anterior limb of the internal capsule.

Case 5 (Bugiani, Conforto and Sacco)[58]: hypertensive cerebral haemorrhage in a 74-year-old man. A right hemiparesis was present without hemihypo-aesthesia. Spontaneous speech included paraphasias, dyssyntactic transformations and preferred segments. Articulation was normal but vocal intensity was reduced. Word repetition remained intact but comprehension was disturbed ('poor comprehension'). The patient died 13 days later. The autopsy revealed

* With regard to thalamic haemorrhages, Fisher et al[56] wrote, as early as 1962, that: 'Dysphasia may be present with lesions of the dominant side and apractognosia [with lesions of] the nondominant.'

the presence of a haemorrhage destroying the entire left thalamus. The pathological characteristics were such that the following evolution of the disease can be suggested: there was first a haemorrhage limited to the anterior part of the thalamus—and it was this lesion which caused the aphasia—then, on the thirteenth day, there was massive bleeding with extension of the lesion to the rest of the thalamus.

Case 6 (Ciemins)[59]: hypertensive cerebral haemorrhage in a 53-year-old male. Onset of the disease was accompanied by confusion and somnolence. Testing carried out five days later showed a reduction and word-finding difficulty in spontaneous speech and perseverative phenomena during naming and writing tasks. Word repetition remained intact. Oral comprehension was normal only for simple commands but written comprehension was abolished. The patient died after 22 days. The autopsy revealed the presence of several small softenings (right thalamus, left occipital cortex, left supramarginal gyrus) and a more recent haemorrhage limited to the entire left thalamus.*

Case 7 (Ciemins)[59]: hypertensive cerebral haemorrhage in a 58-year-old female. A right sensorimotor hemideficit was noted, as was a 'slight expressive aphasia' which no doubt included an articulatory parameter ('thick speech'). The autopsy, carried out three years later, revealed the presence of a cavitated lesion involving the pulvinar as well as the VP and LP nuclei of the left thalamus.†

In discussing these cases, Mohr[57] emphasizes two points which appear to be important. First, there may be an alternation (see Case 1) between short periods during which, under the influence of continued stimulation, the patient's linguistic behaviour approaches normalcy in many respects, and longer periods during which the patient either shows jargonaphasia and lack of attention or is somnolent. This dissociation alone may be sufficient to permit a clinical distinction between aphasia resulting from a thalamic haemorrhage and certain aphasias resulting from lesions of the temporoparietal components of the classical language zone. In this regard, the phenomenon of decreased vocal intensity at the end of jargoned utterances followed by a crepuscular state appears to us as even more characteristic of a thalamic haemorrhage. The second point concerns the apparently usual intactness of (word) repetition (Cases 1, 2, 5 and 6). According to Mohr, such would probably not be the case if the observed linguistic disturbances were the result of compression of the classical language zone rather than the result of the thalamic lesion itself. Indeed, the supramarginal subcortex, which is thought to be important in repetition behaviour (see Chapter 8-1), is certainly among the structures which would be most susceptible to compression by a thalamic haemorrhage.

DISCUSSION

Even without considering the known effects of thalamic stimulation and lesions, the established and presumed anatomical facts (mutual axonal exchanges between the thalamus and the language zone[2, 3, 6, 14, 17, 18, 61–63] (Fig. 7-1 to 7-4, 8-5 and 8-32) are themselves sufficient to suggest the hypothesis of thalamic participation in the cerebral substratum of linguistic behaviour. Many of the questions which can be raised in this regard exceed the answers or quasi-answers which could be expected from even the most rigorous application of the anatomoclinical method (see Chapter 8-4) or from electrophysiological experiments. For example, what would be the effects of bilateral lesions of the MG nuclei of the thalamus? A disturbance similar to deafness from a lesion below the thalamus? A disturbance similar to cortical deafness[53]? Or perhaps confinement to a distressing dysacoustic world? To our knowledge, there is at present no definitive answer to these questions. Similarly, might not a lesion of the VPM result, at least in a transient manner, in speech abnormalities analogous to those which Luria[64] attributes, in his *afferent motor aphasia*, to a disturbance in proprioceptive feedback from the buccophonatory apparatus (see Chapter 10)? Here again, the

---

* Given the left supramarginal lesion and the nature of the linguistic deficits, this case scarcely permits conclusions concerning the mutual relationships between the thalamus and language.

† Other cases have been reported in the literature which are similar to the seven which served as the basis for Mohr's discussion. Fazio, Sacco and Bugiani[60] also reported a case of a haemorrhage involving the entire left thalamus in which there was no evident disturbance of speech and language.

question remains unanswered. It can nevertheless be suggested that certain articulatory disturbances observed after natural or surgical lesions of the thalamus are related to such a mechanism. Finally, the DM nucleus shares, on the left, reciprocal fibres with several components of the classical language zone (Broca's area, Wernicke's area proper, supramarginal gyrus) and it also shares fibres with the prefrontal convexity (Fig. 6–1, 7–3 and 7–4), so that it could be asked whether a lesion of this nucleus would not, in some way or another, interfere with linguistic functioning? This is another question which cannot be answered at present, except perhaps by suggesting that certain cases of *akinetic mutism*, observed after thalamic lesions, might possibly be related to a dysfunction involving participation of the DM nuclei.*

While it would thus be possible to add to these examples, this would no doubt lead, given the present state of knowledge, to the same conclusion: if anatomoclinical and electrophysiological data are used as a basis, only the VL and P nuclei, particularly those of the left thalamus in right-handers, can presently be considered in respect of the anatomical foundations of speech and language.

The thalamus is postulated to play a role in linguistic functioning on the basis of the following facts: both on the left and on the right, its stimulation or partial surgical destruction may cause a transient *speech* disturbance; on the left (especially), its stimulation or partial destruction may cause a transient *language* disturbance; it shares mutual connections with the lower part of the precentral gyrus and perhaps also with the pars opercularis of the third frontal convolution. The pulvinar (particularly the left pulvinar)† is postulated to play a role in linguistic functioning on the basis of the following facts: its stimulation or partial surgical destruction sometimes causes transient disturbances which can be interpreted as *language* impairments, it shares mutual connections with the posterior half of T1 and T2 and with the inferior parietal lobule. While not providing uncontestable confirmation, the clinical pictures observed after certain thalamic lesions, particularly after thalamic haemorrhages, are compatible with these postulates. Although there is not a clear-cut dichotomy, it seems that these clinical pictures (which can clearly be likened to aphasia—mixed or Wernicke's—in some cases) are more likely to include an articulatory disturbance if the VL nucleus is involved and more likely not to include such a disturbance if the lesion is limited to the left pulvinar. On the other hand, Ojemann's[30] experiments and those of Fedio and van Buren[29] (see Chapter 7–2), as well as Mohr's[57] case studies and the work of Riklan and Levita[34], support the suggestion that the ventral lateral nucleus, the pulvinar, and perhaps other thalamic nuclei play, with regard to linguistic functioning, the same activating role directed towards various cortical structures.

With regard to the phenomena considered to involve *speech* (cf. p. 148), whether observed during electrophysiological experiments or in conjunction with thalamic lesions (surgical or natural), there does not appear to be a clear dominance of one thalamus over the other. In a certain manner, this conclusion was already implicit in the teachings of Pierre Marie[35] [who attributed *anarthria* to deep subcortical lesions of either hemisphere (see Chapter 1)]. At least in adults, the thalamus differs in this respect from the cortical mantle where the effects of stimulation and lesions (*phonetic disintegration*) suggest a left hemisphere dominance in right-handers (see Chapters 3, 4, 8 and 11). Regarding the phenomena considered to involve *language*, whether observed during electrophysiological experiments or in conjunction with thalamic lesions (surgical or natural), it seems pertinent to suggest the presence of left thalamic dominance in right-handers. Nevertheless, it appears that this dominance should be conceived of in even more relative terms than is the case for the cortical mantle (see Chapter 11). Riklan's and Cooper's[37] distinction between dominance viewed in terms of a *continuum* versus a *dichotomy* (cf. p. 154) is probably entirely justified.

The linguistic anomalies observed during electrical stimulation of the thalamus are transient. Although persisting for a longer period, those resulting from natural or surgical thalamic lesions are usually transient as well (except in the

* Marinesco et al[65], on the one hand, and Kreindler et al[66] on the other have reported two cases of bithalamic softening with mutism. The lesion directly involved the (left) DM nucleus in the first of these cases but not in the second.

† Rather than speaking of the left pulvinar alone, one may, as several investigators have done, speak of the LP–pulvinar complex of the left hemisphere.

case of inexorably progressive diseases, particularly tumours[54, 55, 67] (see Chapter 9). In hypertensive haemorrhages, this fact is unsurprising (when the patient survives) and is not necessarily related to the site of lesion (see Chapter 9). In the case of surgical lesions, the transient nature of the deficits can probably be explained, as we have already emphasized, by the fact that functional territories are only partially destroyed and that their remaining, intact portions—ipsilateral and perhaps contralateral—may eventually ensure almost normal functioning.

In this regard, the facts commonly observed in clinical aphasiology appear to indicate that cortical representations are less diffuse and less plastic than thalamic representations. It would, however, be wrong to present this view as an indubitable fact. With the exception of cases in which the impairments result from inexorable progressive diseases, aphasic disturbances resulting from lesions of the classical language zone do in fact show, especially in younger subjects[68] (see Fig. 11-2) a clear tendency towards at least partial improvement, a tendency which in many cases can be accelerated and accentuated through a well-directed programme of aphasia therapy (see Chapter 17). Even when incomplete, such improvement can be explained, as in the case of thalamic lesions, only by the hypothesis of progressive recovery from a transient dysfunction in the neighbourhood of the lesion and/or by recourse to the idea of a lesion limited to only a part of a functional territory, or to the concepts of equipotentiality, plasticity or ipsi- or contralateral functional participation (see Chapters 8 and 11; Insertion 7-2).

It is sometimes claimed that the effects of natural lesions of the thalamus (haemorrhages and tumours) on linguistic behaviour reflect the compression exerted by these lesions on the classical language zone, rather than dysfunction of the thalamus itself.* While this interpretation is no doubt valid in certain cases, we consider the opposing arguments presented by Mohr[57] (cf. p. 157) to be equally valid in other cases. Moreover, the argument of compression effects is inapplicable to certain important case studies, for example those of Sager[50, 51] and Elghozi[52] (cf. p. 155).

The exact nature of the role played by the thalamus in linguistic activities remains to be determined. Since solid anatomoclinical case studies are as yet exceptional, this topic remains a matter of conjecture. For our part, we could easily conceive that certain parts of the thalamus, particularly the left pulvinar, normally function as a modulator of certain activities of the classical language zone, particularly of its retrorolandic constituents (see Chapter 8-1 and Fig. 8-5): the aphasic disturbances observed in certain thalamic lesions would then reflect an indirect disruption of the functioning of the language zone. There would therefore be no reason for surprise at the few qualitative differences between linguistic deviations attributable to certain thalamic lesions and those observed in certain cortical lesions.

REFERENCES

1. Truex, R. & Carpenter, M.B. (1969) *Human neuroanatomy*. Baltimore: Williams and Wilkins.
2. Carpenter, M.B. (1973) *Core Text of Neuroanatomy*. Baltimore: Williams and Wilkins.
3. Crosby, E.C., Humphrey, T. & Laver, E.W. (1962) *Correlative Anatomy of the Nervous System*. New York: Macmillan.
4. Percheron, G., Castaigne, P. & Escourolle, R. (1970) Présentation d'un modèle de division et d'une nomenclature raisonnée pour le thalamus de l'homme et des autres simioïdes. In *La journée du thalamus* (Ed.) Percheron, G. p. 7. Paris: Drop.
5. Yakovlev, P.I. (1969) Localization of lesions of the thalamus. In *Bing's Local Diagnosis in Neurological Diseases* (Ed.) Haymaker, W. p. 441. St Louis: Mosby.
6. Yakovlev, P.I. (1972) Localisation des lésions du thalamus. In *Diagnostic des localisations en neurologie* (Ed.) Haymaker, W. p. 529. Paris: Maloine.
7. Yakovlev, P.I. & Lecours, A.R. (1967) The myelogenetic cycles of regional maturation of the brain. In *Regional Development of the Brain in Early Life* (Ed.) Minkowski, A. p. 3. Oxford: Blackwell.
8. Fulton, J.F. (1949) *Functional Localization in the Frontal Lobes and Cerebellum*. Oxford: Clarendon Press.

---

* In our opinion, negative observations are of neither greater nor lesser importance in relation to thalamic lesions than in relation to cortical lesions. In both cases they may reflect exceptional occurrences, incomplete examinations, or shared dominance.

9. Bonin, G. (von) (1949) The cytoarchitecture of the precentral motor cortex. In *The Precentral Motor Cortex* (Ed.) Bucy, P.C. p. 7. Urbana, IL: University of Illinois Press.
10. Vogt, C. & Vogt, O. (1904) Die Markreifung des Kindergehirns während der ersten vier Lebensmonate und ihre methodogische Bedeutung. In *Neurobiologische Arbeiten* (Erster Serie, Erster Band) (Ed.) Vogt, O. Iéna: Fischer.
11. Meyer, A. Beck, E. & McLardy, T. (1947) Prefrontal leucotomy: a neuro-anatomical report. *Brain*, **70**, 18.
12. Walker, A.E. (1966) The thalamus. In *Internal Structure and Afferent-efferent Relations of the Thalamus* (Ed.) Purpura, D. & Yahr, M. p. 1. New York: Columbia University Press.
13. Buren, J.M. (van) (1975) The question of thalamic participation in speech mechanisms. *Brain and Language*, **2**, 31.
14. Simpson, D. (1952) The projection of the pulvinar to the temporal lobe. *Journal of Anatomy* (London), **86**, 20.
15. Walker, A.E. (1959) Normal and pathological physiology of the thalamus. In *Introduction to Stereotaxis with an Atlas of the Human Brain* (Ed.) Schaltenbrand, G. & Bailey, P. Vol I, p. 291. Stuttgart: Thieme.
16. Hassler, R. (1959) Anatomy of the thalamus. In *Introduction to Stereotaxis with an Atlas of the Human Brain* (Ed.) Schaltenbrand, G. & Bailey, P. Vol I, p. 230. Stuttgart: Thieme.
17. Penfield, W. & Roberts, L. (1959) *Speech and Brain Mechanisms*. (Ed.) Schaltenbrand, G. & Bailey, P. Princeton, NJ: Princeton University Press.
18. Penfield, W. & Roberts, L. (1963) *Langage et mécanismes cérébraux*. Paris: Presses Universitaires de France. (French translation by J.C. Gautier.)
19. Penfield, W. & Jasper, H.H. (1954) *Epilepsy and the Functional Anatomy of the Human Brain*. Boston: Little and Brown.
20. Guiot, G., Hertzog, E., Rondot, P & Molina, P. (1961) Arrest or acceleration of speech evoked by thalamic stimulation in the course of stereotaxic procedures for parkinsonism. *Brain*, **84**, 363.
21. Schaltenbrand, G. & Woolsey, C.N. (1964) *Cerebral Localization and Organization*. Wisconsin: University of Wisconsin Press.
22. Schaltenbrand, G. (1965) The effects of stereotactic electrical stimulation in the depth of the brain. *Brain*, **88**, 835.
23. Schaltenbrand, G. (1975) The effects on speech and language of stereotactical stimulation in thalamus and corpus callosum. *Brain and Language*, **2**, 70.
24. Fedio, P. & Buren, J.M. (van) (1974) Memory deficits during electrical stimulation of the speech cortex in conscious man. *Brain and Language*, **1**, 29.
25. Ojemann, G.A., Fedio, P. & Buren, J.M. (van) (1968) Anomia from pulvinar and subcortical parietal stimulation. *Brain*, **91**, 99.
26. Ojemann, G.A., Blick, K.I. & Ward, A.A. (1971) Improvement and disturbance of short-term verbal memory with human ventrolateral thalamic stimulation. *Brain*, **94**, 225.
27. Ojemann, G.A., Hoyenga, K. & Ward, A. (1971) Prediction of short-term verbal memory disturbance after ventrolateral thalamotomy. *Journal of Neurosurgery*, **35**, 203.
28. Ojemann, G.A. & Ward, A.A. (1971) Speech representation in ventrolateral thalamus. *Brain*, **94**, 669.
29. Fedio, P. & Buren, J.M. (van) (1975) Memory and perceptual deficits during electrical stimulation in the left and right thalamus and parietal subcortex. *Brain and Language*, **2**, 78.
30. Ojemann, G.A. (1975) Language and the thalamus: object naming and recall during and after thalamic stimulation. *Brain and Language*, **2**, 101.
31. Laitinen, L. (1966) Thalamic targets in the stereotaxic treatment of Parkinson's disease. *Journal of Neurosurgery*, **24**, 82.
32. Samra, K., Riklan, M., Levita, E., Zimmerman, J., Waltz, J.M., Bergmann, L. & Cooper, I.S. (1969) Language and speech correlates of anatomically verified lesions in thalamic surgery for parkinsonism. *Journal of Speech Research*, **12**, 510.
33. Riklan, M., Levita, E., Zimmerman, J. & Cooper, I.S. (1969) Thalamic correlates of language and speech. *Journal of the Neurological Sciences*, **8**, 307.
34. Riklan, M. & Levita, E. (1969) *Subcortical Correlates of Human Behavior: a Psychological Study of Thalamus and Basal Ganglia Surgery*. Baltimore, MD: Williams and Wilkins.
35. Marie, P. (1906) Révision de la question de l'aphasie: la troisième circonvolution frontale ne joue aucun rôle spécial dans la fonction du langage. *Semaine médicale* (Paris), **26**, 241.
36. Lyon-Caen, O. (1977) *Contribution à l'étude des infarctus paramédians et pédonculaires (territoire du pédicule rétromamillaire): 28 observations*. Medical thesis, Paris.
37. Riklan, M. & Cooper, I.S. (1975) Psychometric studies of verbal functions following thalamic lesions in humans. *Brain and Language*, **2**, 45.
38. Allan, C.M., Turner, J.W. & Gadea-Ciria, M. (1966) Investigation into speech disturbances following stereotaxic surgery for parkinsonism. *British Journal of Communication Disorders*, **1**, 55.
39. Cooper, I.S., Amin, I., Chandra, R. & Waltz, J.M. (1973). A surgical investigation of the clinical physiology of the LP-pulvinar complex in man. *Journal of the Neurological Sciences*, **18**, 89.
40. Darley, F.L., Brown, J.R. & Swenson, W.M. (1975) Language changes after neurosurgery for parkinsonism. *Brain and Language*, **2**, 65.
41. Krayenbühl, H., Siegfried, J., Kohenof, M. & Yasargil, G.M. (1965) Is there a dominant thalamus? *Confinia Neurologica* (Basel), **26**, 246.
42. Levita, E. & Riklan, M. (1965) Laterality of subcortical involvement and cognitive performance: a factor analysis. *Perceptual and Motor Skills*, **20**, 151.
43. Levita, E. & Riklan, M. (1973) On subcortical correlates of verbal functions in parkinsonism: critical considera-

tions. *Journal of General Psychology*, **89**, 3.

44. Levita, E., Riklan, M. & Cooper, I.S. (1964) Verbal and perceptual functions after surgery of subcortical structures. *Perceptual and Motor Skills*, **18**, 195.
45. Levita, E., Riklan, M. & Cooper, I.S. (1967) A psychological comparison of unilateral and bilateral thalamic surgery: a preliminary report. *Journal of Abnormal Psychology*, **72**, 251.
46. Riklan, M. & Levita, E. (1970) Psychological studies of thalamic lesions in humans. *Journal of Nervous and Mental Diseases*, **150**, 251.
47. Riklan, M., Weissman, D. & Cooper, I.S. (1974) Psychological functions following pulvinectomy in man. In *The Pulvinar-LP Complex* (Ed.) Cooper, A., Riklan, M. & Rakic, R. p. 138. Springfield, IL: Thomas.
48. Wechsler, D. (1955) *Wechsler Adult Intelligence Scale Manual*. New York: Psychological Corporation.
49. Dejerine, J. (1914) *Séméiologie des affections du système nerveux*. Paris: Masson.
50. Sager, O., Mares, A. & Nestianu, V. (1965) *Formatia reticulata*. Bucharest: Editions Académiques RSR. (In Romanian.)
51. Botez, M.I. & Barbeau, A. (1971) Role of subcortical structures and particularly of the thalamus, in the mechanisms of speech and language. *International Journal of Neurology*, **8**, 300.
52. Elghozi, D. (1977) *Discussion sur le rôle du thalamus dans l'activité du langage*. Medical thesis, Paris.
53. Lhermitte, F., Chain, F., Escourolle, R., Ducarne, B., Pillon, B. & Chedru, F. (1971) Etude des troubles perceptifs auditifs dans les lésions temporales bilatérales. A propos de trois observations dont deux anatomo-cliniques. *Revue neurologique*, **124**, 329.
54. McKissock, W. & Paine, K.W.E. (1958) Primary tumors of the thalamus. *Brain*, **81**, 41.
55. Cheek, W.R. & Traveras, J.M. (1966) Thalamic tumors. *Journal of Neurosurgery*, **24**, 505.
56. Miller Fisher, C., Dalal, P.M. & Adams, R.D. (1962) Cerebrovascular disease and the stroke syndrome. In *Principles of Internal Medicine* (Ed.) Harrison, T.R. p. 1746. New York: McGraw-Hill.
57. Mohr, J.P., Watters, W.C. & Duncan, G.W. (1975) Thalamic hemorrhage and aphasia. *Brain and Language*, **2**, 3.
58. Bugiani, O., Conforto, C. & Sacco, G. (1969) Aphasia in thalamic haemorrhage. *Lancet*, **24**, 1052.
59. Ciemins, V.A. (1970) Localized thalamic hemorrhage: a cause of aphasia. *Neurology*, **20**, 776.
60. Fazio, C., Sacco, G. & Bugiani, O. (1973) The thalamic haemorrhage. An anatomo-clinical study. *European Neurology*, **9**, 30.
61. Buren, J.M. (van) & Borke, R.C. (1969) Alterations in speech and the pulvinar. *Brain*, **92**, 255.
62. Brown, J.W. (1974) Language, cognition and the thalamus. *Confinia Neurologica* (Basel), **36**, 33.
63. Brown, J.W. (1975) On the neural organization of language: thalamic and cortical relationships. *Brain and Language*, **2**, 18.
64. Luria, A.R. (1964) Factors and forms of aphasia. In *Disorders of Language* (Ed.) de Reuck, A.V.S. & O'Connor, M. p. 143. London: Churchill.
65. Marinesco, G., Nicolesco, J. & Nicolesco, M. (1935) Lésions bilatérales du thalamus. *Encéphale*, **30**, 153.
66. Kreindler, A., Nereantiu, F. & Botez, M.I. (1962) Tulburari de constünta intr-un caz de ramolisment talamic bilateral. *Neurologia*, **7**, 121. (In Romanian.)
67. Smythe, G.E. & Stern, K. (1938) Tumors of the thalamus. *Brain*, **61**, 339.
68. Teuber, H.L. (1975) Recovery of function after brain injury in man. Ciba Foundation, *Outcome of Severe Damage to the Central Nervous System*, p. 159. Amsterdam: North-Holland.

BIBLIOGRAPHY

Almgren, P.E. Andreson, A.L. & Kullberg, G. (1972) Long-term effects on verbally expressed cognition following left and right ventrolateral thalamotomy. *Confinia neurologica* (Basel), **34**, 162.

Andrea, F. (d') Morello, G. & Todeschi, G. (1964) Linguaggio e lesioni talamiche stereotassiche. *Acta Neurologica*, **19**, 749.

Bell, D.S. (1968) Speech functions of the thalamus inferred from the effects of thalamotomy. *Brain*, **91**, 619.

Bravo, G.J., Parera, C. & Seiquer, G. (1966) Neurological side-effects in a series of operations on the basal ganglia. *Journal of Neurosurgery*, **24**, 640.

Brown, J.W., Riklan, M., Waltz, J., Jackson, S. & Cooper, I.S. (1971) Preliminary studies of language and cognition following surgical lesions of the pulvinar in man. *Journal of Neurology*, **8**, 276.

Buck, J.F. & Cooper, I.S. (1956) Speech problems in parkinsonian patients undergoing anterior choroidal artery occlusion or chemopallidectomy. *Journal of the American Geriatric Society*, **4**, 1285.

Canter, G.J. (1965) Speech characteristics of Parkinson's disease: III, articulation, diadochokinesis and overall speech adequacy. *Journal of Speech Disorders*, **30**, 217.

Ciemins, V.A. (1968) Aphasia with thalamic disorders. *Neurology*, **18**, 307.

Crosby, E.C., Humphrey, T. & Lauer, E.W. (1962) *Correlative Anatomy of the Nervous System*. New York. Macmillan.

Hermann, K., Turner, J.W., Gillingham, F.J. & Gaze, R.M. (1966) The effects of destructive lesions and stimulation of the basal ganglia on speech mechanisms. *Confinia Neurologica* (Basel), **27**, 197.

McAdam, D.W. & Whitaker, H.A. (1971) Language production: electrophysiological localization in the normal human brain. *Science*, **172**, 499.

Moruzzi, G., Fessard, A. & Jasper, H.H. (Ed.) (1963). *Progress in Brain Research*. Amsterdam: Elsevier.

Ojemann, G.A. & Whitaker, H.A. (1978) Language localization and variability. *Brain and Language*, **6**, 239.

Papez, J. (1939) Connections of the pulvinar. *Archives of Neurology and Psychiatry*, **41,** 277.

Penfield, W. & Roberts, L. (1963) *Langage et mécanismes cérébraux*. Paris: Presses Universitaires de France. (French translation by J.-C. Gautier.)

Petras, J. (1971) Connections of the parietal lobe, *Journal of Psychiatric Research*, **8,** 189.

Reynolds, A.F., Turner, P.T. Harris, A.B., Ojemann, G.A. & Davis, L.E. (1979) Left thalamic hemorrhage with dysphasia: a report of five cases. *Brain and Language*, **7,** 62.

Roberts, L. (1949) *A Study of Certain Alterations in Speech during Stimulation of Specific Cortical Regions*. Thesis, McGill university, Montreal.

Roberts, L. (1952) *Alterations in Speech Produced by Cerebral Stimulation and Excision*. Thesis, McGill university, Montreal.

Smith, W.K. (1945) The functional significance of the rostral cingular cortex as revealed by its responses to electrical excitation. *Journal of Neurophysiology*, **8,** 240.

Truex, R. & Carpenter, M.B. (1969) *Human Neuroananatomy*. Baltimore, MD: Williams and Wilkins.

Vilki, J. & Laitinen, L.V. (1974) Differential effects of left and right ventrolateral thalamotomy on receptive and expressive verbal performances and face-matching. *Neuropsychologia*, **12,** 11.

Yakovlev, P.I. (1972) Localisation des lésions du thalamus. In *Diagnostic des localisations en neurologie* (Ed.) Haymaker, W. p. 529. Paris: Maloine.

8. Biology of Speech and Language

'That's it. On June 18 1966 I go to Saumur to get to Angers to do a swimming championship. But 30 kilometers from Angers, I caught an accident ... Yes, a automobile. It's a jeep. But me, all alone in the car. It's a storm which surprised me on an road, but the road straight. And me, lost the /trum/ ... consciousness and then, after, me to wake up in ss ... in the hospital of Tour ... The of ... the doctor operated on my ... the ... the ... the head, on the left side ... Because the brains remained on the jeep ... on the mm ... the car.'

(*Conversation with Mr Le.; November 1966*)

1 THE ANATOMICAL SUBSTRATUM OF SPEECH AND LANGUAGE

By means of receptor organs which provide information and effector organs which exert control, man's central nervous system permits him to perceive, to learn, to understand and to produce speech and language. The number of nervous structures participating in these activities is certainly very high but they are not all of equal importance in linguistic functioning. In nearly all dextrals and in a significant proportion of ambidextrals and left-handers as well, certain structures of the left half of the brain play a predominant role (see Chapters 1 and 11). Aphasiology appears much less interesting to those who are unfamiliar with their names, their localization and their principal relations to other cerebral structures.

The first section of this chapter is especially intended for the reader with very little knowledge of neuroanatomy. Its only goal is to present the basic concepts and vocabulary necessary for an understanding of a fundamental approach to aphasiology, namely the anatomoclinical method. In other words, the present discussion will be concerned only with general facts. Several texts on neuroanatomy are available to provide the interested reader with more detailed information[1–7].

GENERAL CONFIGURATION OF THE NERVOUS SYSTEM

With the exception of its supporting tissue (the *glia*) and its vascular system (see Fig. 9–1), the human brain is composed of at least ten billion nerve cells (*neurones*). Through their centrifugal or centripetal prolongations, each of them establishes up to ten thousand contacts with other neurones. It is these contacts (*synapses*) which permit the integration of central nervous system functioning.

The *cerebral hemispheres* form the most rostral and the largest part of the central nervous system. Situated below the hemispheres are large cellular masses, the major ones being the *central grey nuclei*, the *thalamus* (see Chapter 7) and the *hypothalamus*. The great majority of central nervous system neurones belong to these higher-placed structures. A large proportion of these neurones establish contacts only with each other. In other words, only a relatively small proportion of these neurones establish, through centrifugal prolongations (*axons*) issuing from or reaching them, direct contacts with structures located lower in the central nervous system. These lower structures are the *brain stem*, including the *cerebellum*, and the *spinal cord*. Besides the long axons issuing from or directed towards the higher parts of the brain, they include neuronal masses, called *nuclei*. Of the many prolongations which leave or arrive at these nuclei, a large proportion are related to a localized activity. Most of the *cranial nerves*[8] leave or join certain of these nuclei at the level of the brain stem. The exchange of information between the central nervous system and the receptor and effector organs of speech begins and ends with the

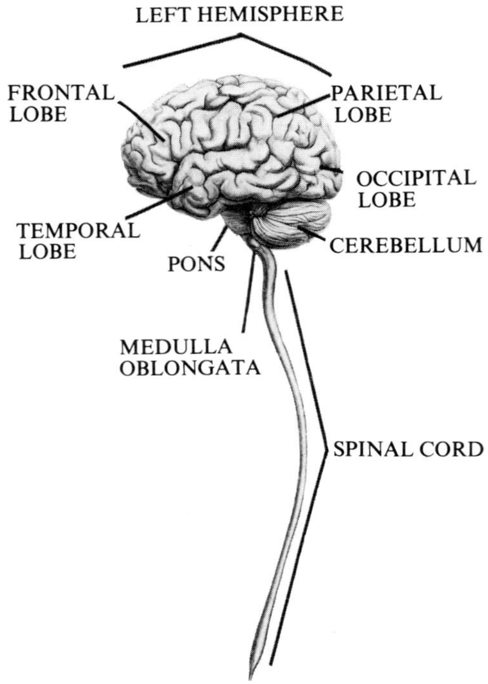

Fig. 8-1 *Left lateral view of the brain and the spinal cord. Adapted from Woerdeman*[82].

cranial nerves. The *spinal nerves* leave or join the central nervous system at the level of the spinal cord (Fig. 8-1).

The cerebral hemispheres. The cerebral hemispheres cover the brain-stem. On the phylogenetic scale, they reach their maximal functional development in man. They are generally considered to be the principal physical substratum of higher mental functions, and thus of language. The surface of the cerebral hemispheres, namely the *cortex*, is composed of several layers of neurones, or more precisely, of their cell bodies and their shortest prolongations. Like the cellular masses situated elsewhere in the central nervous system, this superficial cellular layer is called *grey matter*. Only a small proportion can actually be seen on direct inspection of the hemispheres because most of the cortex is, in fact, buried in grooves of varying depth which furrow the brain's surface. Under the cortical *grey matter* of the hemispheres is found the *white matter*. It is mainly composed of axonal prolongations which leave or enter the cortex. Some of these prolongations provide connections, in both directions, between the cortex and lower structures whereas others provide connections among various cortical zones, either within the same hemisphere or across hemispheres. Those fibres which thus pass from one hemisphere to the other constitute the *commissures*, of which the most important is the *corpus callosum*. In a medial sagittal section, the corpus callosum has more or less the shape of a bow with a superior convexity (see Fig. 8-2). The corpus callosum plays a major role in the interhemispheric exchange of information.

Lobes, convolutions, fissures and sulci. In a lateral view, each hemisphere is seen to have four territories called *lobes*: the *frontal lobe*, *parietal lobe*, *occipital lobe* and *temporal lobe*. They are separated by particularly deep grooves in the cortex called *fissures*: the *fissure of Rolando*, *fissure of Sylvius*, *parieto-occipital fissure*, *calcarine fissure*. Each lobe includes several *convolutions*

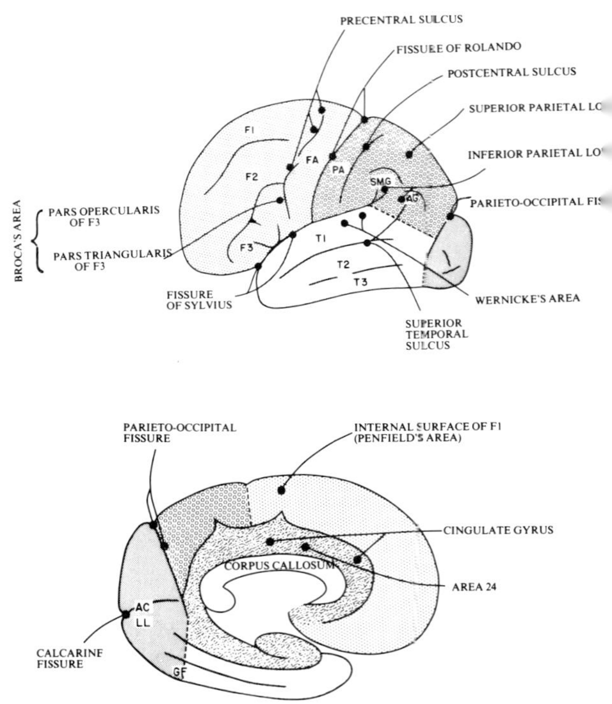

Fig. 8-2 *Lobes and convolutions; fissures and sulci. Left cerebral hemisphere: schematic lateral and internal views. F1, F2 and F3 = first, second and third frontal convolutions; T1, T2 and T3 = first, second and third temporal convolutions; PrG = precentral gyrus; PoG = postcentral gyrus; SMG and AG = supramarginal gyrus and angular gyrus (inferior parietal lobule); FG = fusiform gyrus; LL = lingual lobule; CA = calcarine area.*

(or *gyri*) delineated by relatively shallower grooves called *sulci* (Fig. 8-2).

Larger than the others, the frontal lobe occupies nearly all of the anterior half of the cranium. It is bounded ventrally by the sylvian sulcus and rostrally by the rolandic fissure. Between the latter and the precentral sulcus is the precentral gyrus (PrG) The orientation of the *third, second* and *first* frontal convolutions (F3, F2, F1) is more or less perpendicular to that of the PrG. The precentral sulcus marks the caudal limit of each of these convolutions. The third frontal convolution comprises three parts known—from back to front—as *pars opercularis* (foot), *pars triangularis* (cape) and *pars orbitalis*. The first frontal convolution constitutes the superior edge of the lobe; hence it can be seen on inspection of both the external and internal surfaces of the hemisphere. At the level of its internal surface, the caudal third of the first frontal convolution includes *Penfield's supplementary motor area*. Between this area and the corpus callosum, on the internal surface, the rostral third of the cingulate gyrus is visible, that is, Brodmann's area 24 (Fig. 6-1 and 8-2) (see Chapter 6).

The parietal lobe is retrorolandic and suprasylvian. Its caudal limit is marked by the parieto-occipital fissure. Approximately parallel to the PrG and situated between the fissure of Rolando and the postcentral sulcus is the postcentral gyrus (PoG). Behind it, the external surface of the parietal lobe is composed (on both sides of the interparietal sulcus) of the *superior parietal lobule* and the *inferior parietal lobule*. The latter has two major components, namely the *supramarginal gyrus* (SMG) and the *angular gyrus* (AG).

When viewed laterally, the temporal lobe includes three horizontal convolutions (T1, T2, T3). On its external surface, the *first temporal convolution* (or *superior temporal gyrus*) is bounded by the fissure of Sylvius and the *superior temporal sulcus*. The superior surface of T1, which is buried within the fissure of Sylvius, is known in its posterior third as the *planum temporale*. The cortex immediately rostral to the planum is formed of one or two small convolutions called the *transverse gyri of Heschl*. In right-handers, the surface of the planum temporale may be noticeably larger on the left than on the right (see Fig. 8-5). The supramarginal gyrus curves around the posterior extremity of the sylvian fissure and the angular gyrus curves around that of the superior temporal sulcus. The *first and second temporal convolutions* terminate, posteriorly in the inferior parietal lobe to which they are thus closely linked (the macroscopic border between these temporal and parietal structures is very imprecise).

The edges of the fissure of Sylvius are often designated by the following names, depending on the region considered: the *frontal operculum*,* *parietal operculum*, or *temporal operculum*. At the bottom of the fissure, and hidden from view if the edges are not retracted, lies a considerable cortical surface called the *insula* or the *insular lobe* (see Fig. 8-32).

The lateral surface of the occipital lobe is formed of three small convolutions (O1, O2, O3) rather poorly delineated by sulci. The first of these convolutions is situated immediately behind AG and T2. The inferior external edge of the temporal and occipital lobes constitute the *temporo-occipital convolution* (or *fusiform gyrus*) (*FG*). The inferior internal edge of the occipital lobe constitutes the *lingual lobule* (LL). On the internal surface of the occipital lobe, the *calcarine area* (CA) spreads out on both sides of the calcarine fissure; it extends externally to the tip of the occipital pole.

Primary and association cortices, long and short association fibres. Despite the macroscopic similarity of their surfaces, the cortices of the different convolutions whose location was described differ in both their microscopic structure and function. Those zones which first receive incoming sensory information from the periphery, or which constitute the point of departure for motor commands in response to this information, are called *primary cortical areas*. The *primary visual cortex* is that of the calcarine area; with the possible exception of information coming from the fixation point, all information coming from the right visual field directly reaches only the left calcarine area and all information from the left visual field directly reaches only the right calcarine area. The *primary auditory cortex* is that of the transverse gyri of Heschl; although there are certain phenomena of lateral dominance which will be discussed elsewhere in this book (see Chapter 11), the arrangement of the auditory pathways is such that both the left and right primary auditory cortex receive information on all auditory events, whether this

* Operculum: a covering[9]. The opercula cover the insular lobe.

information comes from the right or from the left ear (see Fig. 11-1). The *primary somaesthetic cortex* is that of the postcentral gyrus; somaesthetic information coming from the right side of the body arrives at the PoG of the left hemisphere and vice versa. The *primary motor cortex* is located in the precentral gyrus; motor commands governing the right side of the body depart from the left PrG and vice versa. The axial musculature of the body, which includes the buccophonatory apparatus, may nevertheless respond to commands coming from either hemisphere. Each muscular area of the body corresponds to a particular area of the motor cortex (the cortical representation is thus said to be *somatotopic*). The buccophonatory apparatus is represented on the opercular third of the PrG, that is, on the part immediately adjacent to the pars opercularis of F3[10] (see Fig. 8-4). The primary sensory cortices are arranged in an analogous fashion; for example, various points of the calcarine cortex correspond to various, precise points of the visual fields.

According to *Flechsig's law*[11], there are no direct connections between the different primary cortical zones.* However, each primary cortex includes *short association fibres* (called U-fibres because these axons are immediately subcortical and their path follows the contour of the convolutions) which link it directly to an adjacent area. This immediately adjacent area is said to be of the *specific association type* because it receives no direct information from the periphery and receives information only from a particular primary cortex. The *specific visual association cortex* almost completely surrounds the calcarine area on the external, inferior and internal surfaces of the occipital lobe. The posterior half of he first temporal convolution, including the planum, belongs to the *specific auditory association cortex*. The specific *somaesthetic association cortex* is situated immediately behind the corresponding primary cortex. The *specific motor association cortex* is situated immediately in front of the corresponding primary cortex; thus, for example, the pars opercularis of F3 constitutes a part of the specific association cortex corresponding to the opercular third of the precentral gyrus (which governs the buccophonatory apparatus).

In addition to *short association fibres* which connect them to immediately adjacent cortical zones, the specific association cortices also possess *long association fibres* (Fig. 8-3). These long fibres provide connections between the different specific association cortices: for example, the specific auditory association cortex and the specific motor association cortex are linked by long axons which curve around the extremity of the fissure of Sylvius and then travel within the depths of the parietal operculum; these axons belong to the *arcuate fasciculus* (see Fig. 8-6), which is, in turn, a part of a larger structure called the *superior longitudinal fasciculus*[1]. The long association fibres also link, through the callosal pathway, each specific association cortex to association areas in the contralateral hemisphere and, in particular, to its contralateral counterpart.

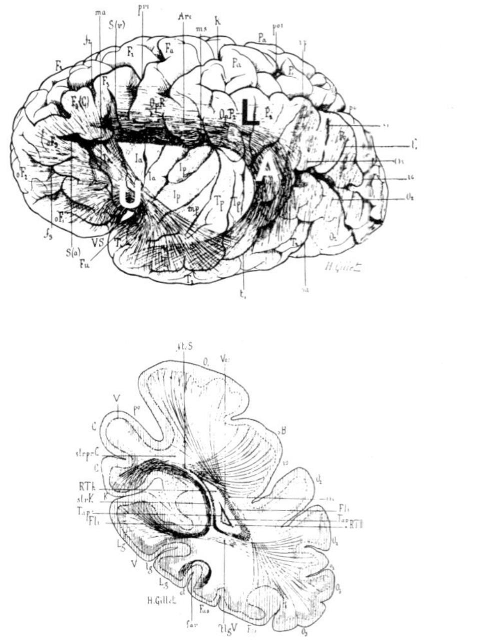

Fig. 8-3 *Long association axons. Upper drawing: the convexity of the left cerebral hemisphere; the opercula have been retracted to show the insula; the uncinate (U), arcuate (A), superior longitudinal (L) and vertical occipital (O) fasciculi are shown by transparency. Lower drawing: coronal section of the left occipital lobe; association fibres of the occipital lobe. From Dejerine*[1].

Certain cortical areas are situated at the junc-

* An exception should be pointed out: within each hemisphere, the primary somaesthetic and primary motor cortices are directly connected by short, U-shaped fibres. Moreover, it is possible that the parts of each of the primary cortices first receive input from the midline or that control in axial musculature is directly linked, through a small contingent of (long) callosal fibres, with the symmetrical portion of the contralateral hemisphere[12, 13].

tion zone of the specific association cortices. These areas are interconnected, ipsilaterally and contralaterally, by long association axons and are also directly linked to the specific association cortices. On the other hand, these areas have no direct connections to the primary cortical zones and, for this reason, their cortical covering is said to be of the *non-specific association* type. The two non-specific association areas which are of particular interest in the context of this work are the inferior parietal lobule (supramarginal gyrus and angular gyrus) and the prefrontal convexity (Fig. 8-2).

Afferent and efferent fibres. Each primary sensory cortex receives, via its own afferent system, a type of information related to a given sensory modality. For example, the reception of auditory stimuli begins at the level of the ear. Incoming sounds cause vibration of the *tympanic membrane* and then of the middle ear *ossicles*. These vibrations are transmitted to the *endolymph*, a fluid contained in the inner ear which is set into motion. This movement affects the sensory apparatus situated in the *cochlea* of the inner ear and called the *organ of Corti*. It gives rise to nerve fibres which constitute the *cochlear branch* of the auditory nerve. Thus acoustic stimuli are transformed into a neural influx. After at least one synapse, and often after several, the acoustic influx reaches the *medial geniculate* body of the thalamus (*prethalamic acoustic pathway*) (see Chapter 7-1); from there, the *acoustic radiations* convey the information to the transverse gyri of Heschl (post-thalamic acoustic pathway) (see Fig. 8-14 to 8-16). Because of the partially crossed structure of the prethalamic acoustic pathway (*acoustic decussation*), each hemisphere receives direct information of the auditory events detected at each ear (see Fig. 11-1). Likewise the reception of visual stimuli begins at the level of the eyes. The visual stimuli affect the photoreceptors of the retina (*rods and cones*) and, by the action of specialized retinal neurones (*bipolar* and *ganglion cells*), are transformed into a neural influx which reaches the *optic nerve* and then the *lateral geniculate body* of the thalamus (*prethalamic optic pathway*) (see Chapter 7-1); from there, the *optic radiations* or *geniculocalcarine fibres* convey the information to the calcarine area (*post-thalamic optic pathway*). Because of the crossed structure of the optical pathway for information from the *nasal hemifields* (*optic chiasm*), only the left hemisphere is directly informed about the right visual field and only the left hemisphere is directly informed about the left visual field (see Fig. 8-21). The somaesthetic receptors (*exteroceptive and proprioceptive*) are located in the skin, the tendons, the muscles. The stimuli are transformed into a neural influx which is transmitted by the sensory nerves; they merge at different levels to form the sensory components of the spinal nerves and of certain cranial nerves. Some of the latter, for example the *glossopharyngeal nerve*, thus convey influxes which inform the brain of the activity of the buccophonatory apparatus. Through the *prethalamic somaesthetic pathway*, information coming from one side of the body reaches certain thalamic nuclei of the opposite side (cf. pp. 142–144; VP nuclei); from there, most of this information is transmitted to the cortex of the postcentral gyrus by the *post-thalamic somaesthetic pathway*. The structure of the somaesthetic pathways is therefore such that each hemisphere is only directly and totally informed about the contralateral half of the body.

The *efferent pathway*, that is, the one which permits the transmission of *voluntary* commands from the brain to the periphery, has its origin in neurones of the primary motor cortex (precentral gyrus). We have already mentioned its somatotopic arrangement[10] (Fig. 8-4). After having passed through the *internal capsule*, in the depths of the hemispheres, a significant proportion of the axons of this long executive pathway terminate in the motor nuclei of the brainstem. The cranial nerves involved in the activities of the buccophonatory apparatus, in particular the *facial nerve* and the *hypoglossal* nerve, originate in certain of these nuclei. As in the case of other structures participating in the control of an axial activity, they receive, although lateralized, instructions coming from each of the two hemispheres. As for voluntary movement of the limbs, it is ensured by the very long axons of the efferent pathway which terminate, after decussation, at different levels of the spinal cord; from there, commands are transmitted through the motor components of the spinal nerves, and then through their various motor branches, to the muscular effectors. In the case of the limbs, motor control is thus almost exclusively contralateral.

The specific and non-specific association cortices also share large contingents of mutual *projection fibres* with various thalamic nuclei; those of particular interest in relation to linguistic

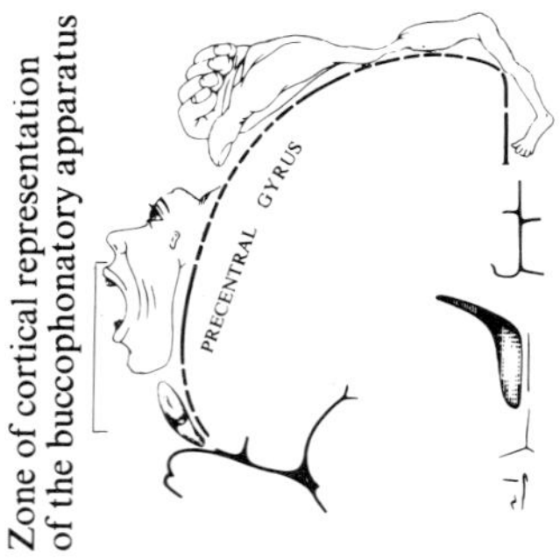

Fig. 8-4 *Penfield's homunculus, left hemisphere. Adapted from Penfield and Rasmussen*[10].

functioning[14] (fibres to and from the pulvinar and ventral lateral nucleus) have been described elsewhere (see Chapter 7, Fig. 7-1 to 7-4).

CLASSICAL CONCEPTION OF THE LANGUAGE ZONE

Since the work of Marc Dax[15] and Paul Broca[16], and then of Carl Wernicke[17] (see Chapter 1), there has been little doubt that certain portions of the cortex of the left hemisphere play a predominant role, at least in nearly all right-handers and in a fair proportion of left-handers and ambidextrals as well (see Chapter 11), as the biological substratum of linguistic behaviours. These cortical areas are commonly designated by the collective name of the *language zone* or *speech area*. The lateralization of this zone reflects the phenomenon of hemispheric specialization, that is, *cerebral dominance* for language (Insertion 8.1). The biological foundations of this functional asymmetry are not well known. There are, nevertheless, reasons to believe that certain anatomical asymmetries are involved: among them, the most clearly demonstrated is that of the planum temporale, whose surface is usually larger in the left than in the right hemisphere[18–27] (see Chapter 11) (Fig. 1-1 and 8-5).

According to the classical view, the language zone, which is situated in the left hemisphere, is considered to be composed of two specific association areas, called *Broca's* area and *Wernicke's* area, plus a non-specific association area, the inferior parietal lobule (Fig. 8-5):

(a) *Broca's area* is composed of the pars opercularis and pars triangularis of the left, third frontal convolution: it lies in the inferior external third of the specific motor association cortex. It is thus situated just in front of that part of the precentral gyrus which controls, in the final instance, the action of the buccophonatory apparatus. Broca's area is thought to be related to the learning and control of movement patterns—involving the lips, tongue, velum, pharynx, larynx—

Insertion 8.1

The dominance of the left hemisphere for language appears to be even more universal than its dominance for manual dexterity. On one hand, right-handers constitute approximately 90 per cent of the general population and the left hemisphere is dominant for language in approximately 99 per cent of this group. On the other hand, left-handers constitute approximately 10 per cent of the population and the left hemisphere is dominant for language in over 50 per cent of this group as well. Thus individuals with right hemisphere dominance for language would constitute only 4 to 5 per cent of the human species. While these figures, cited by Geschwind[28] undoubtedly reflect a general truth, they are nevertheless subject to certain reservations. They effectively suggest that left-handers and right-handers constitute completely homogeneous populations. However, it is now known that many individuals do not show the extremes of either absolute right-handedness nor that of absolute left-handedness: the monograph by Hécaen and Ajuriaguerra[29], as well as Subirana's publications[30–32], are very explicit on this matter. For example, Subirana concludes that only 25 per cent of the human race are absolute right-handers and 40 per cent are preferred right-handers (see Chapter 11). Absolute left-handedness is exceptional. Although numerous facts suggest that linguistic dominance is primarily left-sided in 95 per cent of the population, the proportion in which it is exclusively left-sided may well be much smaller (see Chapter 11).

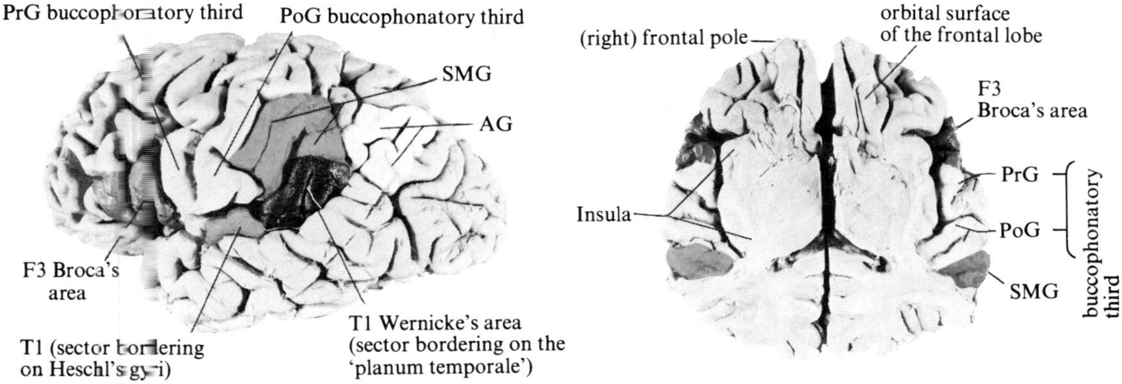

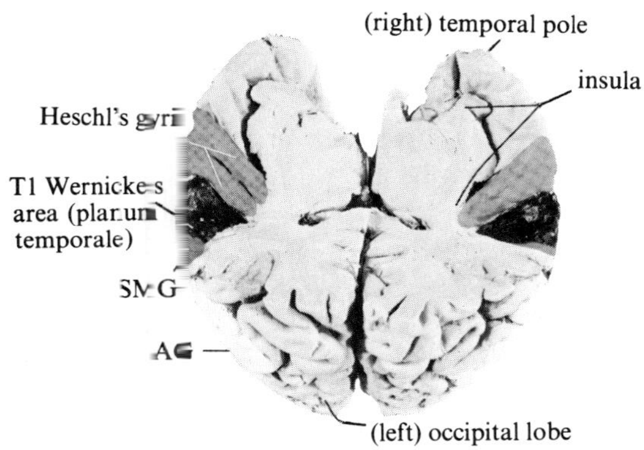

Fig. 8-5 *Classical conception of the language zone (Broca's area, Wernicke's area proper, left inferior parietal lobule): (A) external surface; (B) temporal opercular surface; (C) fronto-parietal opercular surface. F3 = third frontal convolution; PrG = precentral gyrus; PoG = postcentral gyrus; SMG = supramarginal gyrus (inferior parietal lobule); AG = angular gyrus (inferior parietal lobule); T1 = first temporal convolution.*

which correspond to the constituent sounds of language.

(b) *Wernicke's area* (proper)* is composed of the posterior half or third of the left, first temporal convolution, including the *planum temporale*; certain aphasiologists also include the adjacent portion of the second temporal convolution. Wernicke's area lies in the specific auditory association cortex and is situated immediately behind and below the primary auditory cortex (Heschl's zone on the left side). It is generally thought that Wernicke's area plays a major role in the decoding of auditory stimuli, particularly in the decoding of auditory stimuli which convey linguistic information.

(c) The *inferior parietal lobe* of the left hemisphere is also included in the classical language zone (Fig. 8-5). For the most part, it is a non-specific association cortical zone whose principal components are the supramarginal gyrus and the angular gyrus. The inferior parietal lobule is situated at the crossroads of the three principal (sensory) specific association zones of the left hemisphere, namely the auditory, the visual and the somaesthetic. It shares large contingents of associative axons with these zones as well as with other ipsilateral and contralateral associative cortices. Through this particularly extensive associative network, the inferior parietal lobule has access to traces of previous learning as well as to information (presently) processed by the specific association cortices. This region is thought to be of prime importance for numerous cognitive processes and, in particular, for language comprehension (spoken and written). According to Geschwind[28], it is the comparative analysis—at the level of the inferior parietal lobule—of present linguistic information (usually of auditory or visual origin) with traces of previous linguistic and non-linguistic events which, in the final analysis, ensures language comprehension.

Limits of the language zone. The term 'language zone' has classically been reserved for a small

* In the French literature the term *Wernicke's area, zone* or *territory* often includes Wernicke's area (proper) as defined here, and the left inferior parietal lobule.

Insertion 8.2

Concerning aphasia resulting from a left temporal lesion: comprehension of written or printed symbols is a completely different matter. This will be dependent or independent of the presence of auditory word images, according to the patient's educational level. The person with little practice in reading understands the written word only when he hears himself say it. [On the other hand], the scholarly person, familiar with reading since childhood, quickly glances over a page and understands its meaning without even being aware of the individual words. [After a temporal lesion], the former presents symptoms of alexia as well as those of aphasia whereas the latter, in striking contrast to his inability to understand spoken language, shows normal comprehension of all written material. Nevertheless, in oral reading, [the second patient] will be as aphasic as in conversation. [Translated from Wernicke[17].]

number of well-defined cortical areas, one said to be *anterior* (Broca's area) and the two others said to be *posterior* (Wernicke's area and the inferior parietal lobule). Without suggesting changes in a term which is convenient because it is widely used, we shall devote a later section of this text to the notion of the *language zone* and discuss the merits of a less restrictive conception than that outlined here (see Section 8–5).

Connections of the language zone. The language zone is generally envisaged in terms of cortical

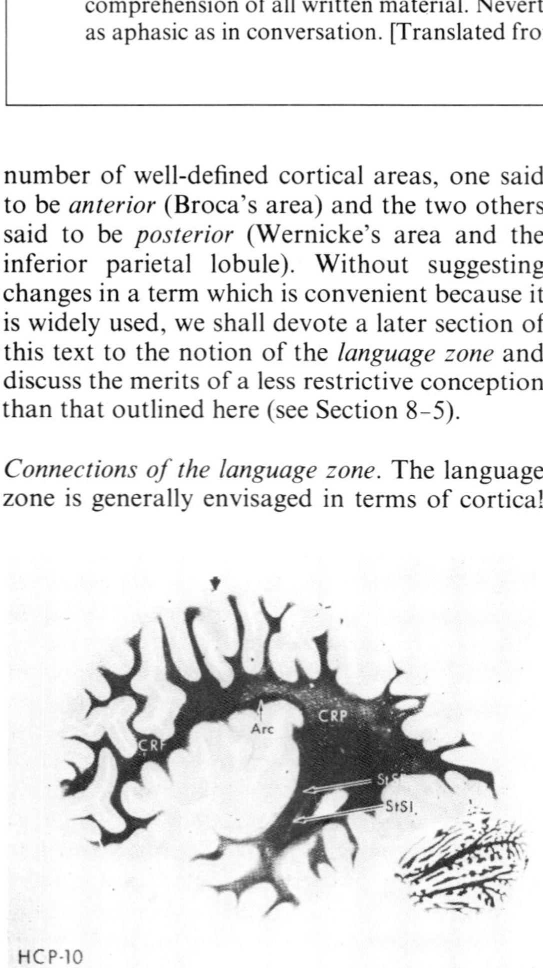

Fig. 8–6 *Sagittal section of the brain of a nine-year-old child; Loyez staining (from Bertrand[58]); myelinogenetics delay related to a rubella syndrome. The arcuate fasciculus (Arc) is clearly delineated by the abnormal pallor of the fibres of the parietal sector of the corona radiata (CRP). StSI = stratum sagittale internum; StSE = stratum sagittale externum; CRF = frontal section of the corona radiata. Specimen HCP-10 of the Yakovlev collection (now at the Armed Forces Institute of Pathology, Washington, DC, USA). From Kemper et al[36].*

surfaces. It is nevertheless obvious that consideration must be given to the networks or associative axons which connect its different components to each other and to the rest of the brain. Since the time of Wernicke's[17] postulate concerning conduction aphasia (see Chapters 1 and 4), there has been, for example, much emphasis on the importance of the associative network of the fibres of the arcuate fasciculus (Fig. 8–6) which connects, among other structures, Wernicke's area to Broca's area: it is reasonable to suppose that these fibres play a role in numerous forms of linguistic behaviour (repetition, which is based on audiophonatory transposition, is the most obvious example). Similarly, it can be assumed that other contingents of long axons, no doubt belonging to the superior longitudinal fasciculus and linking the visual association cortex and the angular region to the anterior component of the language zone, play a role in visuophonatory transposition activities (oral reading). Likewise, normal performance of audiomanual transposition activities (writing to dictation) and visuomanual transposition (copying of writing) no doubt also requires the integrity of certain long posterior–anterior association fibres[1].

Other associative axonal contingents doubtless play a major role in the activities of the language zone. The transfer of auditory linguistic data from Wernicke's area to the inferior parietal lobule probably occurs through one of them. As for visual linguistic data (which are initially processed in the occipital regions), it appears—on the basis of anatomoclinical observations—that they are transferred directly to the inferior parietal lobule in some individuals whereas they reach this area only after a relay to

Wernicke's area in other individuals[33]. The former may be the case for individuals who have undergone prolonged learning of written language and who use it frequently whereas the latter may be the case for individuals who, after a relatively brief education, have only very sporadic encounters with written language (cf. pp. 199–204) (Insertion 8.2).

The associative axons entering or leaving the non-specific association cortex of the left inferior parietal lobule give this structure access to information initially sent (ipsilaterally and contralaterally) to the specific association cortices, or stored at this level. Hence, these associative axons are no doubt essential for linguistic functioning and particularly for language comprehension. The role of the afferents and efferents of the left frontal convexity is not well known in regard to language: it can be assumed, however, that the axonal fibres entering or leaving this other non-specific association cortical zone, especially those which link it to Broca's area, are of considerable importance for verbal expression (see Chapter 5).

ACQUISITION OF AN OBJECT'S NAME

According to the associationist hypotheses adopted by Geschwind[28], the acquisition of the name of an object first requires the establishment of an associative bond between a visual stimulus, the object, and a corresponding auditory stimulus, the word which is heard. (The word 'bond' here refers to an anatomical fact as much as to a psychological one without, of course, implying a one-to-one relationship.) This bond would be established between the specific visual association cortex and the specific auditory association cortex, namely Wernicke's area proper, through the medium of the non-specific association cortex of the inferior parietal lobule and the axons uniting it to each of the two cortical areas involved. Other information, for example, somaesthetic information (from palpation of the object) may be integrated into the learning experience through an analogous process. Once the learning is completed, the name may be 'understood' when it is later heard in the absence of the object: the auditory data then transmitted from Wernicke's area to the inferior parietal lobule would permit 'comprehension' on the basis of the access which the inferior parietal lobule has to information stored elsewhere in the cortical mantle.

Oral production of the object's name, again according to Geschwind[28], requires the initial establishment—occurring through echolalic repetition (see Section 8-2)—of an associative bond between a pattern of articulatory movements and the corresponding auditory pattern. This bond would have its anatomical substratum in the specific motor and auditory association cortices of Broca's and Wernicke's areas, regions which are interrelated through associative axons belonging to the arcuate fasciculus (Fig. 8-6). Once this learning has been completed, spontaneous production of the name (i.e., other than in the context of repetition) becomes possible: the motor command, which comes from Broca's area, is transmitted to a more peripheral, executive functional area (the primary motor cortex of the precentral gyrus), and from there, through the common efferent pathway, to the motor nuclei of the cranial nerves and then from the nuclei to the buccophonatory apparatus. During articulatory production, proprioceptive afferents would keep the brain constantly informed of the dynamics of the buccophonatory apparatus.

Comprehension of the written word corresponding to an object is generally acquired only when its oral equivalent is mastered or nearly mastered. In most cases (and in contrast to what occurs for spoken language), this new learning is not based on the formation of an associative bond between the written word and the attributes (visual, tactile, auditory, olfactory) of the object itself, but rather on the formation of an associative bond between the written word and its oral counterpart. As a result, in almost all normal speakers and during a variable period which depends upon the intensity of written language learning and its later use (Insertion 8.2), the comprehension of visual (written) names would depend on associative assemblies whose original role was to ensure comprehension of their auditory (oral) names.

2 CEREBRAL MATURATION AND LANGUAGE ACQUISITION

In the preceding section, we discussed, in somewhat simplistic terms, the fact that the principal structures subtending language production and comprehension differ in terms of the type of anatomical relations which they establish with each other and, to a large extent, in terms of their functions (see Section 8–1). While we shall later return to these considerations (see Sections 8–3 to 8–5), we shall presently show how these structures and neuroaxonal networks also differ in terms of the chronology of their biological maturation. We shall, in fact, attempt to establish parallels between various periods of cerebral maturation and various stages in the normal development of speech and language.

In mammals, the process of cerebral maturation begins during the embryonic stage of gastrulation, that is, during one of the earliest stages of intrauterine life[34]. In the human species, this process of cerebral maturation is undoubtedly not completed before adolescence; there are even reasons to believe that it continues, at least in regard to certain neocortical structures, until the age of 40 years and perhaps beyond[35]. All types of biological changes, chemical, electrical, anatomical, etc., occur at different periods during the maturation of the brain. Present knowledge of these biological changes, and especially of their significance, is in fact uncertain and fragmentary. Among the best known—and this is not necessarily a truism—are those which are most accessible to observations carried out without great technical efforts. This is generally the case for the morphological changes which will now be considered with the aim of matching them, when this is plausible, with behaviours observed during the course of maternal language acquisition in normal children.

The study of some of the morphological parameters of cerebral maturation, for example encephalometric measures such as the cranial circumference or the weight of the brain, yield only global measures. Consequently, they permit only general correlations concerning the foundations of different behaviours. On the other hand, other parameters are defined through reference to specifically identified cerebral regions or neuroaxonal networks. Such is the case, for example, for several myelinogenetic and corticogenetic parameters which we shall presently consider. The study of this type of parameter has shown that the morphological maturation of the brain occurs, at least in certain aspects, according to temporal patterns which are characteristic of various animal species. It has also shown that the temporal patterns are quite variable, within the same species, from one cerebral region to another and from one neuroaxonal system to another, with each one having its own characteristic maturation cycle[34]. It can be reasonably supposed that these cycles of morphological maturation reflect, at least to a certain extent, the functional maturation of the brain. It can thus be hypothesized that they are related to the emergence and progressive differentiation of specific behavioural patterns such as, in man for example, locomotion in a vertical position, the manipulation of tools, expression by means of articulated language, etc. Conclusive demonstration of the validity of this hypothesis is obviously impossible. It is, however, consistent with common sense and can be supported by the occurrence of well-documented cases in which a delay or arrest in the morphological development of the brain was accompanied by a delay or arrest in behavioural development[36]. It remains to be seen whether present knowledge of the stages of cerebral maturation and of language acquisition is sufficiently precise to permit obvious conclusions concerning certain mutual relationships.

ENCEPHALOMETRIC DATA

From the start of embryogenesis until the end of the first year of postnatal life, the weight of the human brain increases in a regular and extraordinarily rapid manner (Fig. 8–7). Weighing approximately 50 g at the middle of the gestation period, the cerebral weight reaches 200 g towards the thirtieth week of gestation, around 400 g at full-term birth and around 1000 g at the age of one year. The rate of gain subsequently decreases gradually until puberty, when the brain weighs about 1250 g in girls and about 1375 g in boys. Events follow a similar course in regard to the circumference of the cranium: it increases from approximately 34 cm at the time of full-term birth, to approximately 46 cm at the age of one year (i.e., an increase of 1 cm per month); the rate of increase subsequently decreases, the cranial circumference reaching approximately 54 cm at puberty (i.e., an annual increase of approxi-

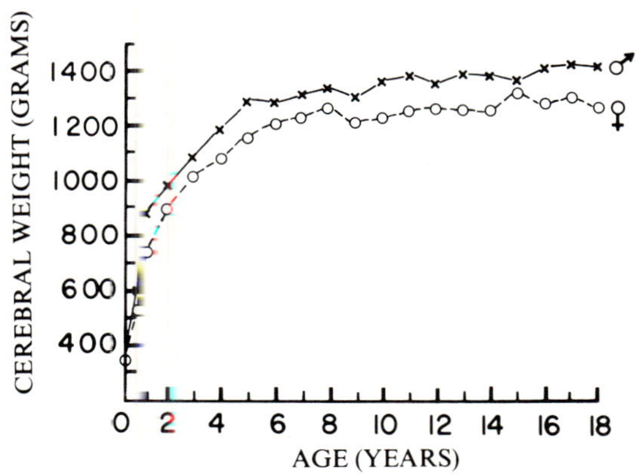

Fig. 8-7 *Weight increase of the brain, in boys (♂) and girls (♀), from birth to 18 years. Adapted from Boyd, in Altman and Dittmar*[37].

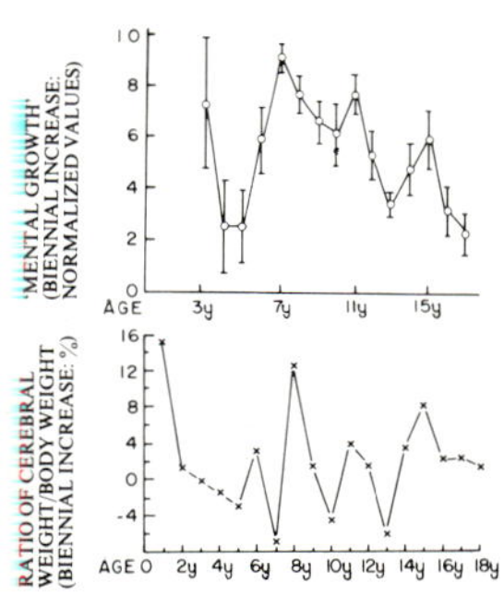

Fig. 8-8 *'Mental growth' and growth of the cerebral weight/body weight ratio. Epstein suggests there is a gross positive correlation between periods in which the increase in brain weight is relatively more advanced than that of body weight and periods in which there is relatively greater potential for behavioural development. He discusses this phenomenon under the astonishing name 'phrenoblysis'. Adapted from Epstein*[42].

mately 0.5 cm between the ages of two and ten years).

What can be said about these encephalometric data[34, 37–40] in relation to language acquisition? Knowing that serious anomalies of the latter may occur in the absence of the slightest encephalometric anomaly, one hesitates to engage in speculation which could readily become too risky. It can certainly be noted that language acquisition begins during a period of rapid encephalometric growth and that it continues during a period of much slower encephalometric growth. Furthermore, there is nothing which permits the biphasic nature of these morphological parameters to be related to any overall discontinuity in the development of articulated language. Is it nevertheless possible to advance beyond these truisms? The answer may be yes, according to work by Epstein[41, 42] (Fig. 8-8) who, in fact, approached a related problem in a different fashion. He first considered a graph representing the relative increases in cerebral and body weights. He thus observed that there are some periods during which the weight increase of the brain is in advance of that of the body and other periods during which the reverse occurs. He next prepared a graph representing, in a global manner, various behavioural acquisitions as measured by use of different perceptual-motor and psychometric tests (see Chapter 15). He observed that this graph also showed highs and lows between the ages of 3 and 17 years. When comparing the two graphs, Epstein suggested that there is a gross positive correlation between periods in which cerebral growth exceeds body growth and periods of relatively greater potential for behavioural development.

Knowing that, in certain respects, language development also proceeds by leaps and gradations, one may be tempted to extrapolate from Epstein's hypothesis to language. Consideration of the specific case of language acquisition raises the following question: if there are periods when the growth of the brain is relatively more rapid than that of the body, is it conceivable that these periods—or rather certain of these periods—are particularly auspicious for language learning? Given our present state of knowledge, we can do no more than raise the question.

CONFIGURATION OF THE EXTERNAL SURFACE OF THE BRAIN

Telencephalon impar, telencephalon semipar and telencephalon totopar

In the human embryo of about four weeks, the rostral extremity of the neural tube has the form of a medial holosphere: it represents the *anlage* of the rhinic structures of the adult brain. A pair of paramedial vesicles develops lateral to this sphere around the eighth week of embryonic life: these vesicles represent the *anlage* of the limbic structures of the adult brain. At about the eleventh or twelfth week, a second pair of evaginations, this time dorsolateral, begin to appear: they represent the *anlage* of the supralimbic structures of the adult brain. It was on these embryological facts that Yakovlev[43–47] founded his anatomofunctional theory of the 'cerebral hemispheres' (Fig. 8-9). He divided them into three zones, of which only one is functionally lateralized to a maximal extent. Yakovlev distinguishes:

(a) A *telencephalon impar*, or rhinic lobe, which is mainly related to endokinesis, that is, to visceral mobility such as that of the heart, digestive tube, etc.: it is thus a medial structure which first governs the mobility of organs without functional lateralization.
(b) A *telencephalon semipar*, or limbic lobe, which is especially related to ereismokinesis, that is, to emotive motility (*ex-motion*) and is manifested through vocalizations, certain gestures, etc.: in Yakovlev's terms, these movements are directed towards the body itself (*body-bound movements*).
(c) A *telencephalon totopar*, or supralimbic lobe, especially related to telokinesis, that is, to effective mobility which is expressed through the manipulation of tools, through propositional linguistic productions, etc. These movements are thus directed towards the external world (*object-bound movements*), and it is only for this behavioural domain that there is strong functional lateralization of the brain; the hemispheric structures which govern this type of behaviour are those whose anatomical lateralization is most obvious.

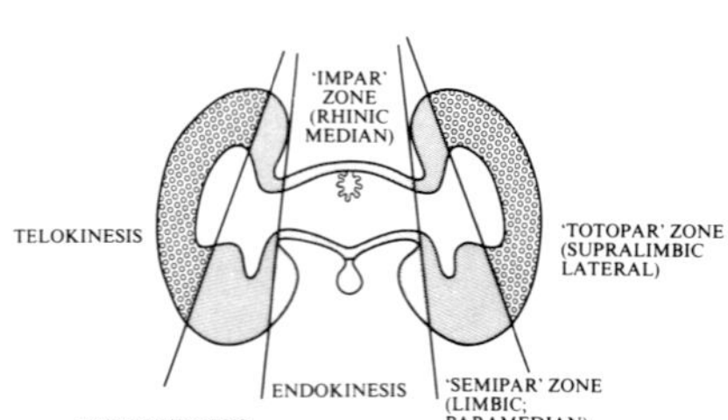

Fig. 8-9 *Paul Ivan Yakovlev's telencephalon impar (rhinic, median), telencephalon semipar (limbic, paramedian) and telencephalon totopar (supralimbic, lateral). Commentary in the text. Adapted from Yakovlev*[45].

The behavioural facts of interest to us—those concerning language acquisition—are especially related to mobility directed towards the external world. Although Yakovlev's impar and semipar telencephalic compartments no doubt participate, their organization is primarily ensured by the totopar compartment, namely, by the compartment having the clearest functional and anatomical lateralization. In terms of its superficial configuration, the principal developmental characteristics of this compartment can be summarized as follows[34]: (a) its *anlage* is the last to appear at around the end of the third month of fetal life; (b) once its development has begun, this structure quickly gains a huge quantitative preponderance over the other two: in fact, the supralimbic structures very soon push the rhinic and limbic structures to the midline and the edge of the hemisphere; (c) the totopar compartment is the one whose definitive formal characteristics are the last to develop; (d) according to Yakovlev[34], the totopar compartment is also the last to be affected by the involutional changes of normal senescence.

Fissures and sulci of the telencephalon totopar

We shall now consider the appearance of the primary, secondary and tertiary sulci of the totopar compartment. With regard to the fissures, or primary sulci, we shall refer to Larroche's[38] exemplary work which indicates that the parieto-occipital and calcarine fissures are already traced at the end of the fifth (lunar) month of gestation, with a delay of four to six weeks relative to the hippocampic fissure. The sylvian and rolandic fissures appear and deepen towards the end of the sixth month and during the seventh. As for the secondary sulci, the first ones to appear, around the end of the seventh month and during the eighth, are the superior frontal, the precentral, the postcentral, the second temporal and the cingulate (see Fig. 1-1). The last six weeks of gestation are marked by rapid progress in the formation of the other secondary sulci. Still open at its rostral extremity at the time of birth, the sylvian fissure becomes completely closed about one month later: the opercularization of the insula is then complete. The primary and secondary fissures continue to deepen long after birth (during at least six months and probably much longer). There are very few tertiary sulci—those which have no name—on the cerebral surface of the newborn; in fact a large number are not seen before the age of two years and new ones appear until adulthood. The tertiary sulci differ from one hemisphere to the other and are as characteristic of each individual as are fingerprints[34]. In the human species, approximately two-thirds of the adult's cortical mantle is buried within the depths of the sulci.

Asymmetries in the surface configuration of the cerebral hemispheres

Only attentive consideration of a human brain is required to note that the supralimbic surface asymmetry, which is often more apparent in the prefrontal regions and at the temporo-parieto-occipital junctions, does not involve tertiary sulci only. Although this is not always reported in contemporary teaching, it has in fact long been known (see Chapters 1, 8 and 11) (Fig. 1-1 and 8-5). Given our concerns, it is of particular interest to note that the surface of the *planum temporale* is often larger on the left than on the right (a phenomenon observed by Wada[25] after the twenty-ninth week of gestation)* (Fig. 8-5).

The supralimbic configuration and the acquisition of language

The macroscopic study of the external configuration of the brain during its course of development has, itself, a certain intrinsic interest. This is fortunate because the parallels which can be established between these morphological facts and the acquisition of language are hardly sufficient to suggest very precise conclusions. In summary:

(a) The postnatal period during which morphological rearrangement of the brain's surface continues to occur is also a critical period for the acquisition of speech and language.

(b) It is probable that anomalies of language acquisition may occur while morphological surface maturation follows an apparently normal course.

(c) The quantitative preponderance of the supralimbic surfaces, which is maximal in man among all the mammals, appears to be related to an undeniable linguistic superiority[49];

(d) The recognized phenomenon of lateralized functional specialization with regard to speech and language is perhaps partially subtended by the formal asymmetries of the supralimbic structures[22, 24, 25]. If so, it must be recognized that these asymmetries appear well before the start of the language learning process[25, 48].

CALLOSOGENESIS

In collaboration with Rakič, Yakovlev[50] also studied the morphological maturation of the large interhemispheric commissures. Some of their observations concerning the corpus callosum are of interest in relation to the preceding discussion of the supralimbic cortical mantle:

(a) As could be anticipated from the chronological appearance of the respective *anlagen* of the rhinic, limbic and supralimbic structures, the fibres of the anterior commissure begin to cross the midline before those of the corpus callosum (the tenth versus the thirteenth week in the human embryo).

(b) As could be anticipated from the relative development of the supralimbic mantle, the fibres of the corpus callosum rapidly acquire a huge, quantitative preponderance over those of the other commissures.

(c) During fetal life, the growth of the *genu* of the corpus callosum is relatively more rapid than that of the *splenium* (Fig. 8-10). After birth, the opposite is true and the rate of growth of the splenium then exceeds that of the genu.

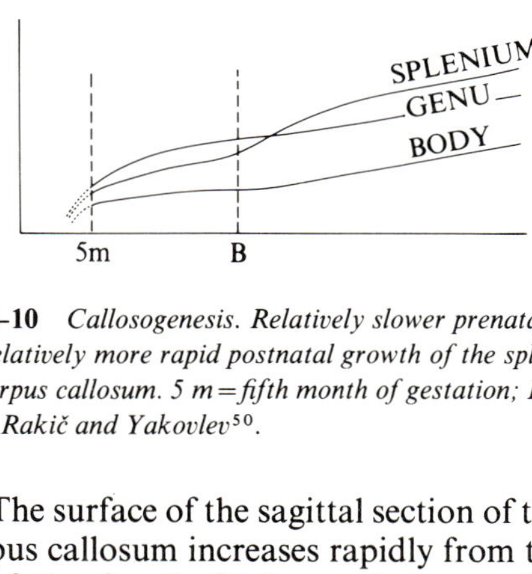

Fig. 8-10 *Callosogenesis. Relatively slower prenatal growth and relatively more rapid postnatal growth of the splenium of the corpus callosum. 5 m = fifth month of gestation; B = birth. From Rakič and Yakovlev[50].*

(d) The surface of the sagittal section of the corpus callosum increases rapidly from the end of the fourth fetal month (approximately 23 mm^2), to birth (approximately 67 mm^2), then from birth until the age of two years (approximately 148 mm^2); after this, it continues to increase at a slower rate until adulthood (approximately 345 mm^2). Thus

* Although not specifically mentioning the *planum temporale*, Gratiolet[48] nevertheless considered, as early as 1854, asymmetries which he had observed on the surface of the human brain at the same period of gestation. Recent research led by Albert Galaburda in Boston has documented, with regard to Wernicke's area and Broca's area, the existence of microscopic (cytoarchitectonic) as well as macroscopic asymmetries in favour of the left hemisphere.

a biphasic type cycle is observed, analogous to that already described with regard to encephalometric data (see Fig. 8-7). More direct comparison of these two types of measures shows that while the cerebral weight increases by approximately 35 per cent between the age of two years and adolescence, the sagittal surface of the corpus callosum increases by over 100 per cent during the same period. The difference between these two figures is striking and even more intriguing since they would both seem, at first glance, to provide nearly proportional indices of supralimbic growth.

This being said, can the facts of callogenesis observed by Rakič and Yakovlev somehow be related to language acquisition? Here again, it is clear that any parallels can only be remote, imprecise and tentative. Despite this, we shall risk the following three comments:

(a) The first, which is almost trivial, is that, both phylogenetically and ontogenetically, the growth of the callosal mass is contemporaneous with an increasing capacity for complex learning; in man this culminates in, among others, a linguistic learning ability which is apparently not present in other animal species. This parallel resembles that already pointed out with regard to the supralimbic covering and is quite unsurprising since the majority of callosal axons doubtless arise from the supralimbic mantle.

(b) The second comment concerns the relative splenial preponderance observed after birth. Does this involve the simple mechanical effect of a formal rearrangement? Or is there perhaps a postnatal spurt of growth which affects certain interparietal and interoccipital contingents more than others? If so, it may be tempting to consider this fact first in relation to the passage from a world of darkness to a world which is often illuminated and, second, in relation to the subsequent beginning and continuation of an entirely postnatal learning process, namely that of acquiring articulated language[51]. In regard to the latter, there can be little doubt about the importance of the long interparietal and interoccipital associations (see Chapter 8-1 and 8-5).

(c) The third comment no doubt falls within the realm of heedless neurophilosophy. It concerns the observed difference, after the age of two years, between the increase of brain weight and that of the surface of the sagittal section of the corpus callosum. Is it totally impossible that this difference might be partially explained by the fact that new interhemispheric collaterals continue to cross the midline in the years after birth? If so, it could be postulated that this phenomenon also occurs in the case of the long intrahemispheric associative axons. In these circumstances, the maturation of certain regions playing a predominant role in regard to the most prolonged stages of language acquisition—consider the left inferior parietal lobule, for example—would be completed, in terms of their long associations, only as the years go by (and perhaps, as needs arise)[51].

Numerous objections can be raised in reply to this third comment, and some may be sufficient to demolish it completely. Nevertheless, the conclusion should be borne in mind because other arguments, this time based on data concerning myelinogenetic maturation, will lead us to return to it.

MYELINOGENESIS

As we have already indicated, the process of brain maturation is expressed by numerous chemical, histological and anatomical changes, some of which are accessible to direct observation. One of them, namely *myelinogenesis* (i.e., the development of the *myelin sheaths* which wrap most of the axons of the central nervous system) has been the subject of numerous investigations. During the first half of the present century, epoch-making work, was carried out by Flechsig[11, 52, 53], Kaes[35], Vogt and Vogt[54, 55] and Langworthy[56]. More recently, a further study was carried out by Yakovlev and one of us (A.R.L.).[57] and led to the concept of *myelinogenetic cycles*.

Myelinogenetic cycles

Many of the data on myelinogenetic maturation which will now be considered were obtained from the last investigation cited above[57]. The aim of this research was to identify the beginning, the progression and the end of the *myelinogenetic cycles* of different neuroaxonal networks and of different regions of the human brain. It involved the study of over 250 fetal, infantile and adult brains cut in whole-brain gapless serial sections.

The concept of a myelinogenetic cycle had been predefined as being the period extending from the appearance, in the region or the network considered, of some myelin sheaths stainable by Loyez's method[58], to the age at which the tinctorial sheaths are no longer discernible by comparison with the same region or the same network as seen in the normal brain of a 28-year-old adult arbitrarily chosen as the standard of reference[57]. According to Yakovlev, the myelinogenetic maturity of an axonal system indicates that, henceforth, nervous conduction within the system will be space-committed. Consequently, a system which has completed its myelinogenetic cycle might be presumed to have reached functional maturity.

Length of the myelinogenetic cycles

The rate of myelinogenesis varies greatly from one axonal system to another. Let us consider the following examples (Fig. 8-11):

(a) In the trapezoid body and lateral lemniscus, myelinogenesis essentially occurs between the fifth and ninth months of gestation. Hence the cycle is very brief and entirely prenatal.

(b) In the optic radiations of the thalamus, the myelinogenetic cycle begins shortly before full-term birth and is completed around the fifth month after birth. Here again the cycle is very brief but, unlike the preceding one, it is almost entirely postnatal.

(c) In the somaesthetic radiations of the thalamus, the cycle begins during the ninth or tenth month of gestation and ends at about the age of one year. Thus the cycle is again predominantly postnatal but, in this case, it is of an intermediate length.

(d) In the acoustic radiations of the thalamus the myelinogenetic cycle begins at birth or around this time and does not reach completion before the age of at least three years. Thus this cycle is entirely postnatal and is approximately three times longer than the preceding one.

(e) In the non-specific radiations of the thalamus, the cycle begins at about the third month of postnatal life and continues for at least five or six years. Thus myelinogenesis begins later than in the preceding case and the cycle is markedly more prolonged.

(f) The longest of the myelinogenetic cycles are no doubt those of the short tangential fibres of the intracortical neuropil, particularly in the non-specific association areas of the supralimbic mantle. As shown by Kaes' work[35] at the beginning of the century, these cycles begin more than a year after birth and continue through several decades. The illustration presented here (Fig. 8-12) is borrowed from Kaes[35]: it shows sections perpendicular to the cortex, at the ages of three months, one year, and 5, 15, 30, 45 and 60, made in the inferior parietal lobule and in the prefrontal convexity.

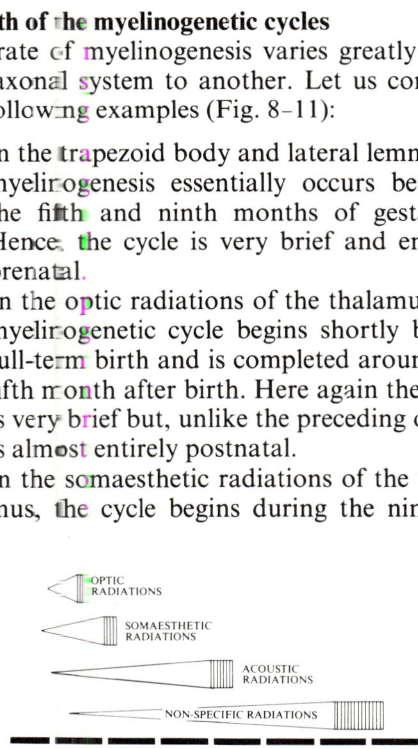

Fig. 8-11 *Myelinogenetic cycles of the thalamic radiations. The cycle of the optic radiations is very short, that of the somaesthetic radiations is relatively short, that of the acoustic radiations is relatively long and that of the non-specific thalamic radiations is very long. As in Fig. 8-15, 8-17 and 8-18, the apex of each triangular graph marks the start of the myelinogenetic cycle; the growth in the number of myelinated fibres and their tinctorial intensity is indicated by the progressive divergence of the sides of the triangle; the vertical lines extending from the base of the triangle mark the approximate end of the cycle. B = birth; 1Y, 2Y, etc. = one, two, three years, etc. From Lecours*[51].

Myelinogenesis of the cerebral hemispheres

Of Yakovlev's three telencephalons[45], the *totopar* (i.e., the one which comprises the supralimbic structures) is the last to begin its myelination and is, by far, the last to complete it (if, in fact, it is ever completed). On the whole, the supralimbic axonal systems linked to primary cortices begin and end their myelinogenetic cycles before those linked to the specific association cortices. The latter, in turn, begin and end their myelinogenetic cycles before those linked to the non-specific association cortices. Such, at least, are the conclusions suggested by the study of Flechsig's myelinogenetic maps[11, 34, 59]. We shall now consider these maps, focusing attention on those zones which are important in the control of speech and language (Fig. 8-13). In Flechsig's maps:

(a) The precentral and postcentral gyri, the calcarine area and Heschl's gyri belong to the *primordial myelinogenetic field.*

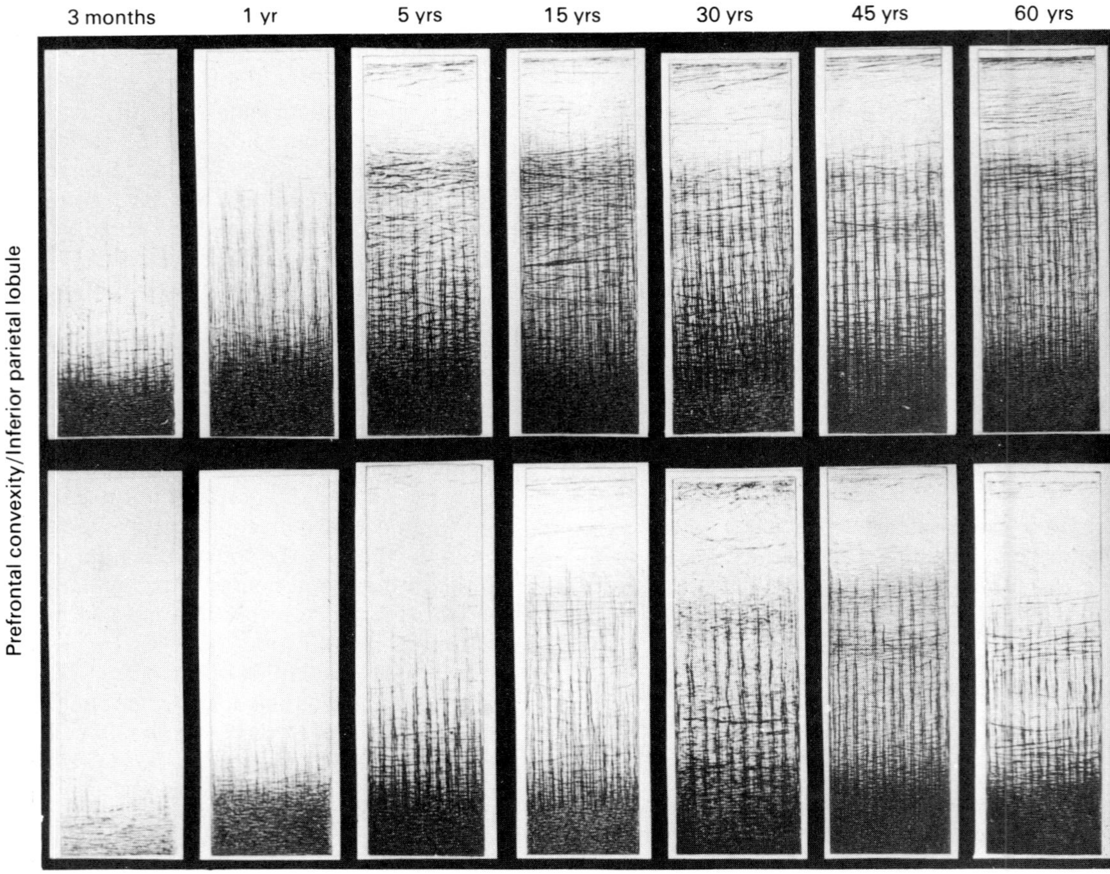

Fig. 8-12 *The nerve fibres having the longest myelinogenetic cycle are the tangential axons of the intracortical neuropil in the non-specific association cortices. This can be seen above at the level of the inferior parietal lobule and of the prefrontal convexity. From Kaes*[35].

(b) The caudal part of the third frontal convolution and that of the second, the caudal part of the first temporal convolution and the occipital areas adjacent to the primary visual cortex belong to the *intermediate myelinogenetic fields.*

(c) The supramarginal gyrus and the angular gyrus, as well as a substantial portion of the prefrontal convexity, belong to the *terminal myelinogenetic fields.*

The role of certain association fibres in the acquisition and use of language has been recognized since the time of Wernicke's[60] work in the last century (see Chapters 1, 8-1, and 8-5). The myelination of these particular fibres can be summarized as follows:

(a) During the first four to eight weeks of postnatal life, the only supralimbic association systems having myelin sheaths which can be stained with haematoxylin are the short U-fibres: the vast majority of these fibres link one of the primary cortices to its immediately adjacent specific association cortex.

(b) Among the long association fibres, those which join the specific association cortices to each other, as for example the fibres of the arcuate fasciculus (see Fig. 8-6), begin and complete their myelinogenetic cycles before those fibres which reach the non-specific association cortices or arise from them.

Myelinogenetic cycles and behaviour

We have, until now, scarcely felt confident in our attempts to establish certain parallels between features of morphological maturation and events related to language acquisition. Without, of course, implying any causal links, a somewhat bolder stance can probably be taken with regard to the relationships between myelinogenesis and behaviour. To illustrate this point, let us consider one of Yakovlev's favourite arguments[57] which

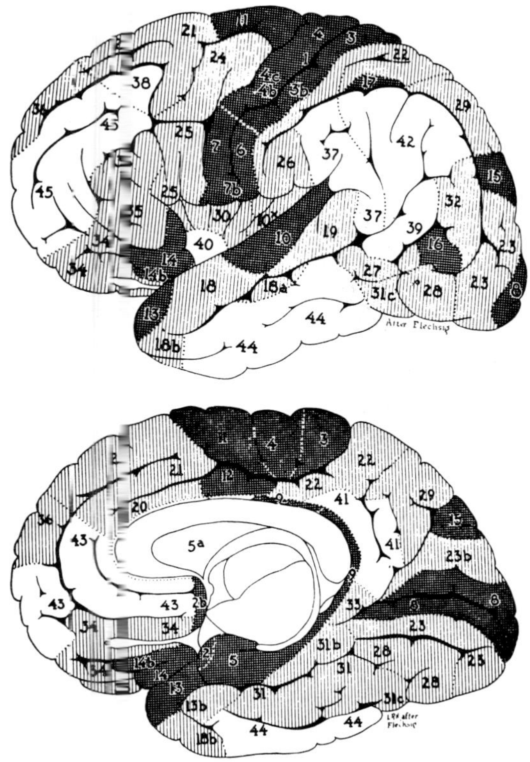

Fig. 8-13 *Paul Flechsig's myelinogenetic maps: primary or primordial (black), intermediate (lined) and terminal (white) myelinogenetic fields. Commentary in text. Adapted from Bailey and von Bonin*[59].

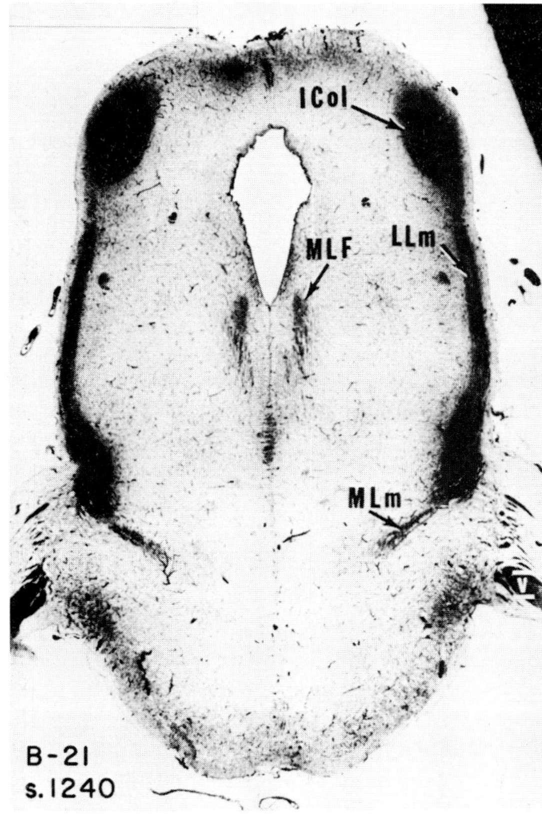

Fig. 8-14 *Coronal section of the brain stem of a premature infant; Loyez staining. In the pre-thalamic acoustic pathway, the myelinogenetic cycle is essentially complete after 29 days of gestation and eight days of postnatal life. ICol = inferior colliculus; LLm = lateral lemniscus; MLm = medial lemniscus; MLF = medial longitudinal fasciculus; V = roots of the trigeminal nerve (the fibres which are already myelinated are those of the motor root of the trigeminal). Specimen from the Yakovlev Collection. From Yakovlev and Lecours*[57].

is based on a comparison between the myelinogenetic cycle of the acoustic pathway and that of the visual pathway. From the semicircular canals to the medial geniculate bodies, the myelinogenesis of the prethalamic acoustic fibres is very brief, beginning towards the middle of gestation and reaching completion around three months after birth. As can be seen in the illustration (Fig. 8-14), myelinogenesis of the lateral lemniscus is complete in an eight-day-old premature born after 29 weeks of gestation. On the other hand (Fig. 8-15), as we have previously mentioned, the myelinogenesis of the post-thalamic acoustic fibres begins only at birth and lasts at least three years. This differs from the case of the optic pathways whose myelinogenetic cycle is very short for both the pre-thalamic and the post-thalamic pathways and extends from the eighth fetal month to the fifth postnatal month. In summary:

(a) The cycle of the auditory pathways is biphasic: short and primarily prenatal for the helicogeniculate (pre-thalamic) component; long and entirely postnatal for the geniculotemporal (post-thalamic) component.
(b) The cycle of the visual pathways is monophasic: short and perinatal for both the retinogeniculate (pre-thalamic) and the geniculocalcarine (post-thalamic) components.

We shall now attempt to match this series of facts concerning morphological maturation with the chronological sequence in which different modalities of sensory information successively enter into play in the origin of fetal and infantile behaviours.

During gestation, the fetus is exposed to gravitational (vestibular) stimuli generated primarily

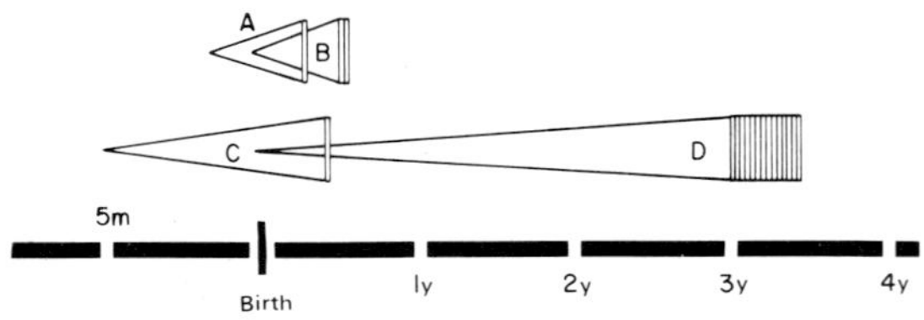

Fig. 8-15 *The monophasic cycle, brief and perinatal, of the optic pathway, pre-thalamic as well as post-thalamic. The biphasic cycle of the acoustic pathway (see Fig. 11-1): very brief and essentially prenatal in the pre-thalamic component; long and postnatal in the post-thalamic component. A = pre-thalamic optic pathway; B = post-thalamic optic pathway; C = pre-thalamic acoustic pathway; D = post-thalamic acoustic pathway; 5m = fifth month of gestation; 1Y, 2Y, etc. = one year, two years, etc. (see Fig. 8-11 for the meaning of the graphic shapes).*

by its own body movements. It is also exposed to acoustic (cochlear) stimuli—sounds coming from the external world, sounds of the maternal life (heart beats, respiration, intestinal rumblings,* etc.)—transmitted through the maternal walls and the amniotic sac which, on the other hand, remain impermeable to photic stimuli. Considering the precociousness and brevity of the myelinogenetic cycle of the pathway linking the internal ear to the inferior colliculi and to the thalamus, it may be assumed that the central apparatus ensuring the integration of such cochlear and vestibular stimuli is located principally at the level of the tegmentum of the brain stem (see Fig. 8-1).

At the end of gestation, and as a result of birth itself, there is an abrupt change in the types of imputs which reach the central nervous system. (a) Visual stimuli, which were previously nonexistent, suddenly become one of the key factors of behavioural development. If the brevity of the myelinogenetic cycle of all the optic pathways—a cycle which is perinatal for both the pre- and post-thalamic components—provides a relevant index, it may then be supposed that visual information rapidly assumes a role which, in certain respects, remains unchanged after early infancy. (b) On the other hand, the relative importance of stimuli of vestibular and cochlear origin decreases considerably, and the latter soon assume a completely new role since they constitute one of the primordial foundations of the acquisition of articulated language. In this regard it should be pointed out, once again without implying a causal link, that there is a temporal correspondence between the long period during which language is progressively acquired and the entirely postnatal and relatively prolonged myelinogenetic cycle of the post-thalamic component of the acoustic pathways. The contrast between this prolonged cycle and that of the post-thalamic component of the optic pathways is very clear in the illustration presented here (Fig. 8-16) showing a sagittal section of the sublenticular portion of the internal capsule. It can be seen that in the six-week-old infant, and still in the one-year-old infant, the myelinogenetic maturation of the optic radiations of the thalamus is far more advanced than that of its acoustic radiations.

Myelinogenetic correlates of speech and language acquisition

In the context of a monograph edited by Eric Lenneberg shortly before his death, one of us (A.R.L.)[61] recently attempted to establish a parallel between various aspects of human myelinogenetic maturation and the traditional categories of behaviours observed during the acquisition of speech and language[62-68] (Insertion 8.3). We shall now present a summary of this attempt.

Babbling consists of non-specific phonatory responses to non-specific stimuli which may be visceral and somatic as well as auditory and visual. The sounds initially produced are mainly vocalic, including both closer and more distant approximations to the vowels produced by adults in the child's linguistic community, but the babbled productions soon include more or less clearly articulated consonants. Non-specific feedback possibly has a role in babbling but, regardless of the stimuli eliciting or maintaining this behaviour, it appears to constitute, in terms of speech development, the infant's global initiation to the motor use of his buccal, lingual, velar, pharyngeal and laryngeal muscles. At the time when babbling first occurs [*A*],† relatively few neural structures have achieved an advanced degree of myelinogenetic maturity. On the one hand, the motor roots of the cranial nerves related to sound production have completed their cycle [*8*] and myelinogenesis of several brain stem

* Borborygmi.

† In the next several paragraphs, the letters and figures which appear in italics and parentheses refer to the different graphs in Figure 8-17.

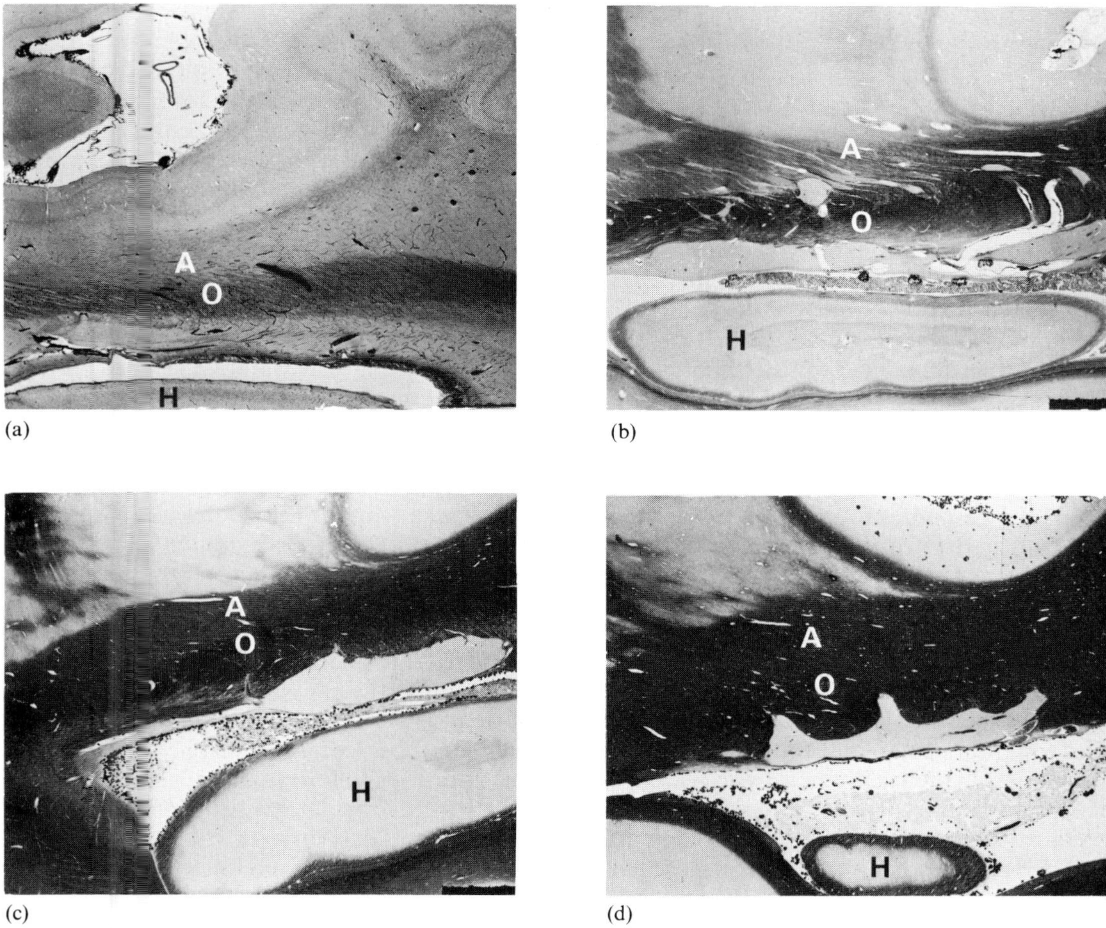

Fig. 8-16 *Sagittal sections of the sublenticular portion of the internal capsule at six weeks (a), 11 months (b), four years (c), and 16 (d); Loyez staining. At six weeks, the myelinogenetic cycle of the optic radiations (O) is already well advanced whereas that of the acoustic radiations (A) has hardly begun. The difference between the staining of the post-thalamic optical and acoustic fibres is still visible at 11 months and has only completely disappeared at four years. The four specimens are from the Yakovlev Collection (a = case B-152, section 700R, 6 ×; b = case B-132, section 700L, 5 ×; c = case MU-108, section 610L, 5 ×; d = case MU-87, section 570L, 5 ×). From Lecours[61].*

Insertion 8.3

Those who, through their knowledge of the neurological literature of the last 30 years, are familiar with the work of Paul Ivan Yakovlev will have undoubtedly recognized, in these pages, the influence of his ideas about the relations between different spatiotemporal stages of morphological brain maturation, including myelinogenetic cycles, and also about the emergence and subsequent progressive organization of man's behavioural patterns. We have attempted here to present myelinogenesis in a dynamic perspective, one which is summarized by the concept of myelinogenetic cycles. This concept is entirely the fruit of Yakovlev's experience and reflection. During lengthy discussions with one of us (A.R.L.), Yakovlev also argued, much more clearly than we have been able to do so, that there is an undeniable parallel between myelinogenesis of the optic and acoustic pathways and certain contemporaneous behavioural features (related to language development).

structures, including the pre-thalamic pathways for all sensory modalities, is not far from completion [*1*, *3* and *5*]; on the other hand, the corticobulbar pathway [*7*], the associative fasciculi [*9*] and, with the exception of the geniculocalcarine radiations [*4*], the thalamocortical projections [*2* and *6*], are only beginning their respective myelinogenetic cycles. It therefore follows that if babbling is entirely or partially governed at cortical levels, this is done through cortico-subcortical connections which are still very immature. On the other hand, it is also possible that babbling is essentially governed at subcortical levels, that is, by structures which have already attained a certain degree of anatomical maturation.

Echolalia [*B*] consists of specific imitative phonatory responses to specific acoustic stimuli. It is usually the prosodic aspects of speech (i.e., the melody of speech) which the baby first tries to imitate; initial attempts to reproduce certain articulated segments generally occur during the final months of the first year. Phonatory imitation clearly requires a relatively complex sensorimotor apparatus: the infant hears sounds; s/he tries to reproduce them through the medium of phono-articulatory activity; this activity in turn generates auditory and proprioceptive feedback which allows the infant to evaluate and, if necessary, correct his/her production. At the time when echolalia [*B*] becomes a dominant form of speech behaviour (generally during the second year of life) all the neural pathways which are presumably involved in its production have reached a certain degree of myelination but not all of them have completed their cycle. Although continuing since birth, myelinogenesis of the geniculotemporal auditory fibres, through which the specific inputs for echolalic imitation presumably reach the auditory cortex, is not yet complete [*2*]. Myelination of the U-fibres (cf. p. 166) linking each primary cortex to its immediately adjacent specific association cortex is probably almost complete. The cycles of the long association fibres linking the different specific association cortices, including that of the arcuate fasciculus (see Fig. 8-6) through which auditory information is presumably transmitted from temporal to frontal areas in order to permit echolalic repetition, are quite advanced although not yet complete [*9*]. Finally, myelinogenesis is terminated or nearly terminated in the efferent pathways [*7*], whose motoric role is probably the same in repetition as in other forms of speech production, and in the afferent proprioceptive pathways [*5* and *6*] which, together with the acoustic afferences, appear to allow the brain to control and correct the echolalic imitation. If the circuit thus defined does in fact constitute the anatomical substratum of echolalic behaviour, this activity begins—and is at first very approximate—when the degree of anatomical maturation of its underlying structures has attained a certain, obvious functional sufficiency but is not yet maximal. In the usual course of chronological maturation, the young child's speech imitation later shows progressive improvement as the anatomical maturation of its substratum approaches its term (Fig. 8-17).

A limited role could probably be attributed to babbling, and certainly a primordial one to echolalia, in the learning of the motor patterns of speech, that is, in the formation of links between specific sounds and their corresponding buccophonatory movements. In other words, echolalia is one of the essential factors which lead the child to differentiate and master the phonemic inventory of his or her linguistic community. In the course of this process, the child first acquires the ability to recognize individual phonemes (in context) and then, following an order of increasing difficulty in articulatory production, to utter them appropriately (in context). During the early phases, the articulatory productions are approximate. Certain individual phonemes are not entirely consistent with the model and, regardless of their consistency, some phonemes are displaced or added. Omissions are observed, especially in the context of consonant clusters. Even more frequently, certain pairs of similar phonemes (see Chapter 2) are at first produced one for the other with or without preferential usage of one of them. It is through successive trials, errors and corrections that echolalic imitations gradually approach the forms accepted by the linguistic community. For example, interphonemic confusions decrease in frequency and the child learns to discriminate and contrast the units of the phonemic stock which s/he will later use. During the same period, s/he gradually acquires a completely operative although unconscious knowledge of the rules governing the linear associations between the units of this phonemic stock. In learning to utter individual phonemes correctly (in context), the young child gains mastery of a community-accepted phonetic convention; in learning to select and contrast phonemes and to utter them in structurally acceptable

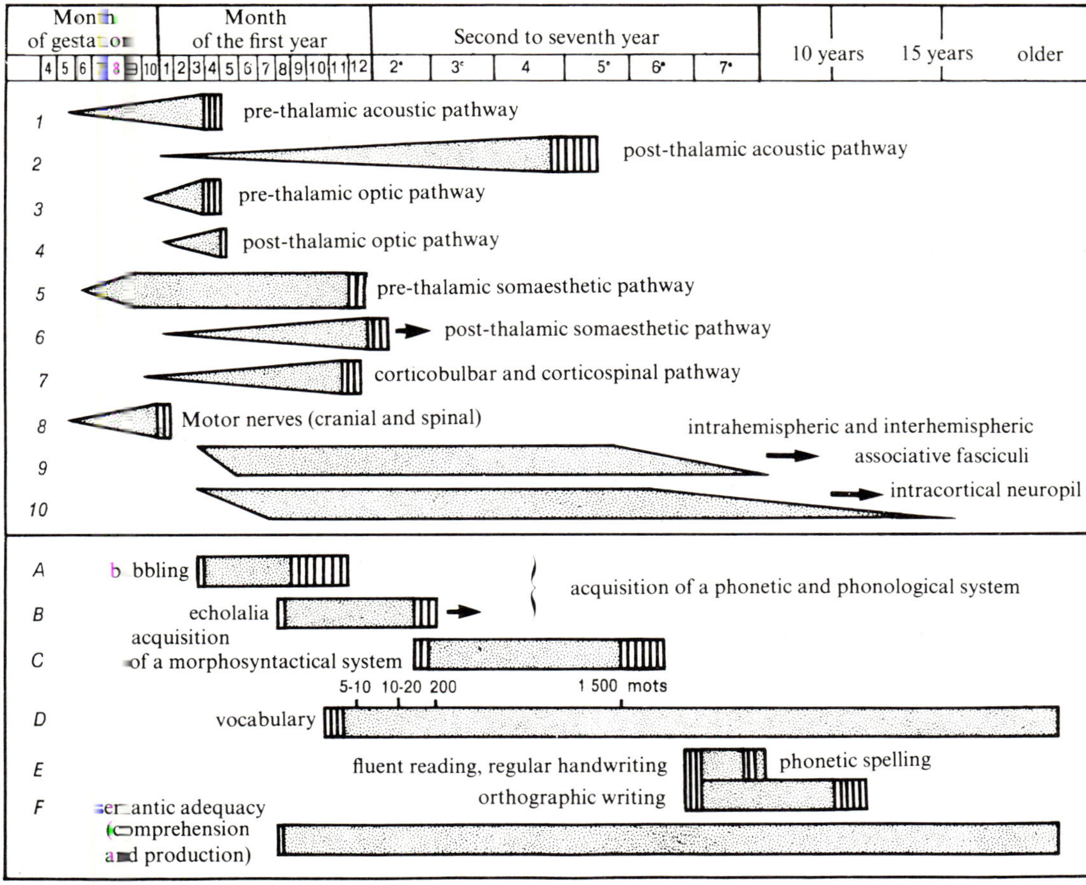

Fig. 8–17 *Myelinogenesis and language acquisition. Comparative cycles.*

linear sequences, s/he gains mastery of a community-accepted phonemic (or phonological) convention. With perhaps a certain lag of the latter, these two intricately intermingled processes have generally reached a fairly advanced stage by the age of 30 to 36 months. Nevertheless, occasional phonetic distortions and phonemic transformations still occur in the speech of normal five- or six-year-old children, or even older ones, under the effects of fatigue, distraction, emotional stress, etc. (as they sometimes occur, with a lower frequency, in the speech of normal adults[69] (see Chapter 14). It is not surprising that more recently acquired words and/or more complex phonemic structures are particularly susceptible to such deviations.

Before the age of 18 to 24 months, and sometimes even later, most of a child's utterances are unitary in terms of their form and meaning. In other words, they correspond to single and (syntactically) associated selections whether or not they can be described as including several words according to adult standards. Thus it is generally around the age of 18 to 24 months that the child begins a course of learning which will lead to a certain mastery of a community-accepted morphosyntactical convention, that is, s/he begins to acquire operative knowledge of the rule system governing associations between units of the first linguistic phase (see Chapter 2). During the first year of this learning process, a (decreasing) majority of the strings of words produced will conform to relatively simple rules which are more or less specific to infantile language and will be gradually abandoned at a later stage. During this period, the child's use of language is largely oriented towards the expression of his or her needs, desires, satisfaction or unhappiness. Between the third and the fourth year, or sometimes earlier, when the child begins to transcend this unilateral expressive mode and increasingly participates in linguistic exchanges with an interlocutor, s/he produces a progressively larger number of sentences which are syntactically adequate according to adult standards. The child learns to construct, with recently acquired words, sentences which s/he has presumably never heard nor uttered before. If (almost) perfect mastery of the morphosyntactical convention is to be attained, it will only be after several more years [*C*] and the child's progress will be more or less closely related to a scale of difficulties particularly to this system (see Chapters 12 and 17). Although the sentences produced by normal five- to six-year-old speakers are generally syntactical, this is not always the case, and 'errors' of morphology or syntax are not uncommon in the language productions of normal children between the ages of five and ten years, nor are they later in life for that matter.

The lengthy process of learning the meanings conventionally associated with sounds begins very early. Such learning is protracted well beyond the ill-defined limits of adulthood [*F*] and its complete cessation may, in fact, be a sign of disease or senility. Although significant interindividual variation must be considered, it appears that the ability to apprehend and acquire linguistic meanings does not generally reach its maximum before the age of 15 years. During the initial phases of this learning process, children recognize sounds and associate them with diffuse semantic values, which are more or less closely related to their conventional meanings, several weeks or months before they attempt to utter them themselves. From a psychological point of view, to learn the meanings of words initially corresponds to forming associations between (heard) sounds and (seen, touched, heard) objects perceived as distinct from their environment, between sounds and the attributes of these objects or their mutual relationships, and between sounds and actions or events observed in the environment[70]. The semantic values of the language segments heard and used by the children are progressively defined through the gradual enrichment of their experiences in relation to specific speech segments, that is, through the repetition and increase in the number of associations to each particular segment. Because word meanings are modified through their linear relations to other words, certain aspects of this process merge with the acquisition of syntactical rules, namely with the combination rules of the first linguistic phase. Thus the development of a more precise semantic system parallels and depends upon the development of a more elaborate syntactic system since sentences—and not isolated words or phrases—are the ultimate meaningful linguistic units which children must learn to understand and produce. Although they begin to emerge somewhat later, these complex types of linguistic learning cannot be clearly distinguished from those which underlie cognitive organization[71–75], that is, *intellectual* development (see Chapter 19).

A 12-month-old child may have acquired five to ten words which are more or less correctly uttered but whose meanings are often overgeneralized or imprecise. Six months later, his/her vocabulary will generally be twice as large and by the age of two years it may include some 200 words. A five-year-old child may have acquired up to 1500 words whose meanings are known quite precisely and which s/he can arrange—with occasional confusions between words which are semantically or syntactically related—in sentences which follow the rules of a relatively simple syntactic system. The number of adults who have scarcely progressed beyond this stage is not negligible. Their conversation attests to the availability of a slightly more elaborate syntactical system and a vocabulary of approximately 2000 words. On the other hand, in comparison with a five-year-old child, their ability to understand abstract language usually shows a marked increase [*D*].

The anatomophysiological substratum of the semantic aspects of language comprehension and production is not precisely known. It can nevertheless be suggested, primarily on the basis of anatomoclinical evidence, that certain specific and non-specific association areas of the cortex, as well as the axonal connections linking them together, play a major role. Among these structures, it appears to be the left inferior parietal lobule which, because of its location at the borders of the principal ipsilateral specific association areas and its universal connections, ensures functional control in right-handers (see Sections 8-1 and 8-5). In permitting the formation, through learning, of a highly complex associative network, these structures become the biological foundation of available memory traces, traces which ensure the semantic adequacy of language comprehension and production. It can therefore be emphasized that the lengthy period of concurrent syntactic and semantic learning is more or less contemporaneous with the myelinogenetic cycles, not only of the post-thalamic acoustic fibres[35] (see Fig. 8–15), but also of the long intra- and interhemispheric association fasciculi [*9*], especially those leaving or entering the non-specific association cortices. In addition, this period of linguistic acquisition is also contemporaneous with the myelinogenetic cycle of the intracortical neuropil (a short fibre network parallel to the hemispheric surface and located between the cellular layers of the cortex), and especially of the neuropil of the non-specific association cortices [*10*]. In this respect, the contemporaneity (and the lengthy duration) of learning leading to *semantic maturity* and of the myelinogenetic cycle of the inferior parietal lobule [*F* and *10*] (see Fig. 8–12) may well be of particular significance.*

For almost all individuals who learn to read and to write,† this learning is (nowadays) part of their formal education [*E*]. Thus it generally does not begin before the child is five or six years old. In most cases learning to read will mean establishing associations between visual signs (letters, written words and groups of written words) and acoustic signs whose meanings are usually familiar, that is, the acoustic signs have already acquired a definite symbolic value. Thus the seen written words become linked with their acoustic counterparts and with the corresponding phonatory-kinaesthetic patterns. Moreover, in learning to write, movements of the hand permit the reproduction of seen visual signs; this early phase in the development of written speech corresponds to echolalia in the development of spoken speech (cf. p. 182). Since, as pointed out by Brain and Walton[70], one reads as one writes in the same way that one hears as one talks, links are also established between written visual signs, which are integrated into an already rich associative network, and their corresponding manual kinaesthetic patterns.

As a general rule, the first year of schooling provides the child with rather extensive experience of the written symbolic code which s/he then endeavours to superimpose on the already well-practised oral code. By the end of the first year of school, the average pupil can read and understand written passages provided that s/he is, on the whole, familiar with their lexical components. Nevertheless, reading will be slow and sometimes syllabic and may include substitutions between words which are similar in form and/or in meaning. Similarly, handwriting will still be slow but, over a period of a few months, graphism will have reached a stage of regular and well-differentiated production. With the exception of some confusions between similarly-shaped letters or between graphemes corresponding to identical or similar phonemes (see Chapter 2), the child will have at least reached a stage where s/he can write *phonetically*. However, this is not the case for orthographic writing whose mastery, if it will in fact ever be fully acquired, will be attained only much later. The time required will depend, among other factors, on teaching methods and, even more in our opinion, on the extent of one-to-one correspondence between the phonemic and graphic codes of a particular language. By the age of 10 or 11 years, contemporary French-speaking school children—who have had to learn, for instance, more than 25 written equivalents of the single phoneme /ã/ and to acquire some operative knowledge of the rules governing the choice of one rather than another (see Insertion 17.4)—still usually make a sizeable number of *orthographic errors* which are compounded by errors related to the syntactical oddities of the language. One to three years later, their written productions are usually markedly closer to the norm.

If learning to read involved the formation of direct associations between seen objects, their attributes and their mutual relations, etc., on the one hand, and written visual signs, on the other hand, such learning could likely begin very early, perhaps in the last six months of the first post-natal year. Since myelinogenesis of the U-fibres is more precocious than that of the longer association fibres [*9*], the formation of associations between seen objects and visual signs could conceivably begin earlier than the formation of associations between seen objects and acoustic signs. As for the acquisition of linguistic expression through a written code, it could, in such circumstances, conceivably begin as soon as sufficient control of the upper limbs has been achieved [*5* to *8*]. However, the oral code is

---

* We are not implying a causal relationship between these features of myelinogenesis and *semantic maturity*. The former is only one of the parameters of the latter and there is no doubt that myelinogenesis may be completed in the absence of functional development.

† All comments on written language refer only to the use of non-ideographic codes.

immediately more convenient than the written code and the acquisition of linguistic communication very rarely occurs according to the above alternative or one based primarily on somaesthetic information. Thus written language is normally learned, at least in the initial stages (which are never surpassed by many normal speakers), through reference to the oral code rather than through direct reference to objects and events. This fundamental difference between the acquisition of the oral and written codes probably explains and perhaps justifies the generally accepted notion that the degree of brain maturation necessary for optimal learning of the written code is not attained before the age of five or six years [*E*]. It is indeed likely that several structures having protracted myelinogenetic cycles, including the long associative bundles as well as the intracortical neuropil [*9* and *10*], play a role in the acquisition of a symbolic code (at least partially) used to represent another symbolic code.

Although this type of speculation cannot be readily extended, a final question merits consideration before turning attention to more general aspects of our comparison between myelinogenetic maturation and language development. Are there, in fact, differences between the myelinogenetic cycles of the various components of the language zone (see Fig. 8-5) and their right-hemisphere counterparts? We do not know the answer to this question but if such differences exist they have not, to our knowledge, been reported nor even investigated. They could, moreover, be very subtle and of short duration.

Temporal patterns in language acquisition and myelinogenetic maturation

The learning of many behaviours, including language, does not progress with a constant rhythm. A graphic representation of language acquisition, considered either globally or in terms of particular aspects, would no doubt show (more or less regular) plateaus or even temporary dips, phenomena which we have already mentioned in discussing Epstein's hypotheses[41, 42]. The question which we shall now consider is whether these interruptions or slowings in the course of learning (linguistic or other) correspond to observable biological facts[61]. Our proposed, and tentative, answer will be formulated in several steps.

We shall first reconsider the myelinogenesis of the acoustic pathways (see Fig. 8-15) which we described as 'biphasic' when comparing it with the myelinogenetic cycle of the optic pathways. Our intention was then to emphasize the contrast between the short duration (and precocity) of the myelinogenesis of the pre-thalamic acoustic fibres and the long duration of the myelinogenesis of the post-thalamic acoustic pathways. When viewed in a different perspective, the myelinogenetic cycle of the acoustic pathways could also be said to be 'polyphasic'. As illustrated in Fig. 8-18, myelinogenesis actually occurs in a centripetal manner, with some overlappings, from the auditory nerve to the trapezoid body and to the lateral lemniscus, then to the brachium of the inferior colliculus then—with certain differences in the rate of maturation—to the

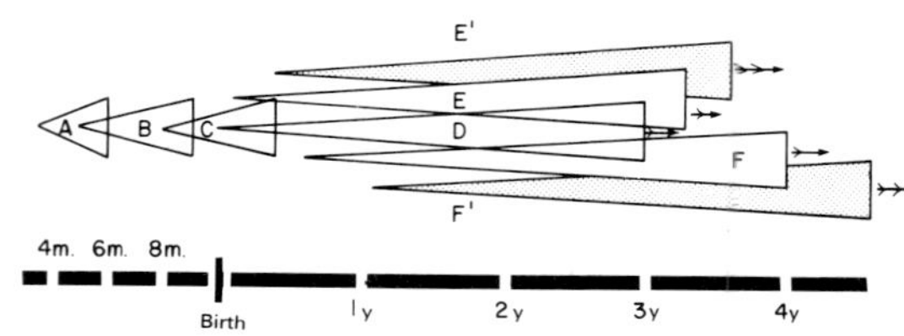

Fig. 8-18 *Polyphasic myelinogenesis of the acoustic path ways (see Fig. 8-11 for the meaning of the graphic shapes). Myelinogenetic cycles of: A = the auditory nerve; B = the trapezoid body and lateral lemniscus; C = the bracchium of the inferior colliculus; D = the geniculotemporal (acoustic) radiations of the thalamus; E = the short association fibres linked to the primary auditory and specific association cortices: E' = the long association fibres linked to the specific auditory association cortex; F = the intracortical neuropil of the primary auditory cortex; F' = the intracortical neuropil of the specific auditory association cortex. 4m, etc. = fourth month of gestation, etc.; 1Y, 2Y, etc. = one year, two years, etc. From Lecours*[51].

acoustic radiations, to the association fibres connecting Heschl's gyri to the neighbouring temporal cortex, and finally to the tangential plexuses of the neuropil of Heschl's gyri and then of the neighbouring temporal cortex.

This being said, we shall now reconsider babbling and echolalia. Having previously intended only to suggest the possibility of executive mechanisms operating at different levels of integration, these behaviours were considered as if they were completely homogeneous and independent of each other. However, babbling and echolalia can be considered—and this perspective is probably more realistic—as a behavioural continuum gradually leading the child to mastery of a phonetic and phonological convention (motoric exercises, then prosodic imitation, then progressively more accurate production of vowel sounds, of consonant sounds, of phonemic sequences). This learning is probably polyphasic as well in the sense that its progress is irregular (periods of rapid gains, slowings, plateaus).

The above considerations raise the question of a possible parallel. Is there some type of relationship between the *polyphasic nature* of the myelinogenetic cycle of the acoustic pathways and that of the babbling-echolalia behavioural continuum? Considered more generally, is the polyphasic nature of certain aspects of morphological maturation somehow related to the polyphasic nature of certain aspects of learning (including certain of those leading to language acquisition)? In other words, could certain plateaus in learning curves be a possible reflection of temporal differences in the morphological, physiological and chemical maturation of the brain? If so, it can be assumed that certain plateaus correspond to periods during which the brain would be waiting, so to speak, until a particular axonal contingent or neuronal region reaches the degree of maturity necessary for a given course of learning to be resumed and to progress to qualitatively and/or quantitatively more complex stages.

In pursuing this parallel further, we shall use the term *vertical polyphasic nature* to refer to the successive stages in the myelinogenetic cycle of a given neural pathway (Fig. 8–18). This choice of terminology obviously raises the question of what would correspond to the notion of a *horizontal polyphasic nature*. In our opinion, this term would appropriately include the eventual interactions between the various stages of myelinogenetic maturation of axonal contingents from the same 'functional level', for example, that of the specific thalamic radiations—optic, somaesthetic (exteroceptive and proprioceptive), acoustic—and the non-specific thalamic radiations (see Fig. 8–11). For instance, in regard to the babbling-echolalia continuum, it would then be possible to take into consideration the different temporal patterns of maturation at various levels of the acoustic, proprioceptive and corticobulbar pathways. When considering language acquisition more generally, one of the most interesting of the 'functional levels' would certainly be that of the subcortical and intracortical associative contingents. We have not attempted a schematic representation of the (hypothetical) differences in the temporal patterns of the myelinogenetic cycles of these structures. Those who might be tempted to do so should remember the following facts:

(a) The myelinogenesis of the U-shaped association fibres is more precocious and of shorter duration than that of the longer association fibres[11, 52, 53].
(b) Myelinogenesis begins later and is more protracted in the subcortical axonal networks linked to the non-specific association cortices than in those linked to the specific association cortices, and it begins later and is more protracted in the latter than in those linked to the primary cortices[11, 52, 53].
(c) The myelinogenesis of the intracortical neuropil, especially that of its tangential plexuses, is particularly late in beginning and particularly protracted (see Fig. 8–12); it starts first in the primary cortices, then in the specific association cortices and then in the non-specific association cortices[54, 59].
(d) The temporal pattern of myelinogenetic maturation no doubt differs among the various contingents of the same associative 'functional level': at least, such differences are suggested by the numbering in Flechsig's myelinogenetic maps[11, 34, 59] (see Fig. 8–13).
(e) Finally, individual variations are possible and would be unsurprising given that which is commonly observed in individual learning abilities as a function of age.

Given the complexity of these facts of anatomical maturation, one might wish, if this appears pertinent, to refer to the notion of a *horizontal polyphasic nature* when interpreting the plateaus observed in the most complex and latest learning curves such as those leading to the acquisition of written language.

CORTICAL NEURONOGENESIS

As shown by the work of Brodmann[76], Bailey and Von Bonin[59, 77] and Conel[78], the tectogenesis of the human brain extends over a lengthy pre- and postnatal period (Fig. 8–19). According to Yakovlev[34], there is a fairly clear temporal relationship between the rate of neurogenesis and that of myelinogenesis as summarized by Flechsig's primary and terminal myelinogenetic fields but such a relationship is less evident in the case of the intermediate myelinogenetic fields. However this may be, it is clear that language acquisition, including its latest stages, is contemporaneous with the neuronogenetic maturation

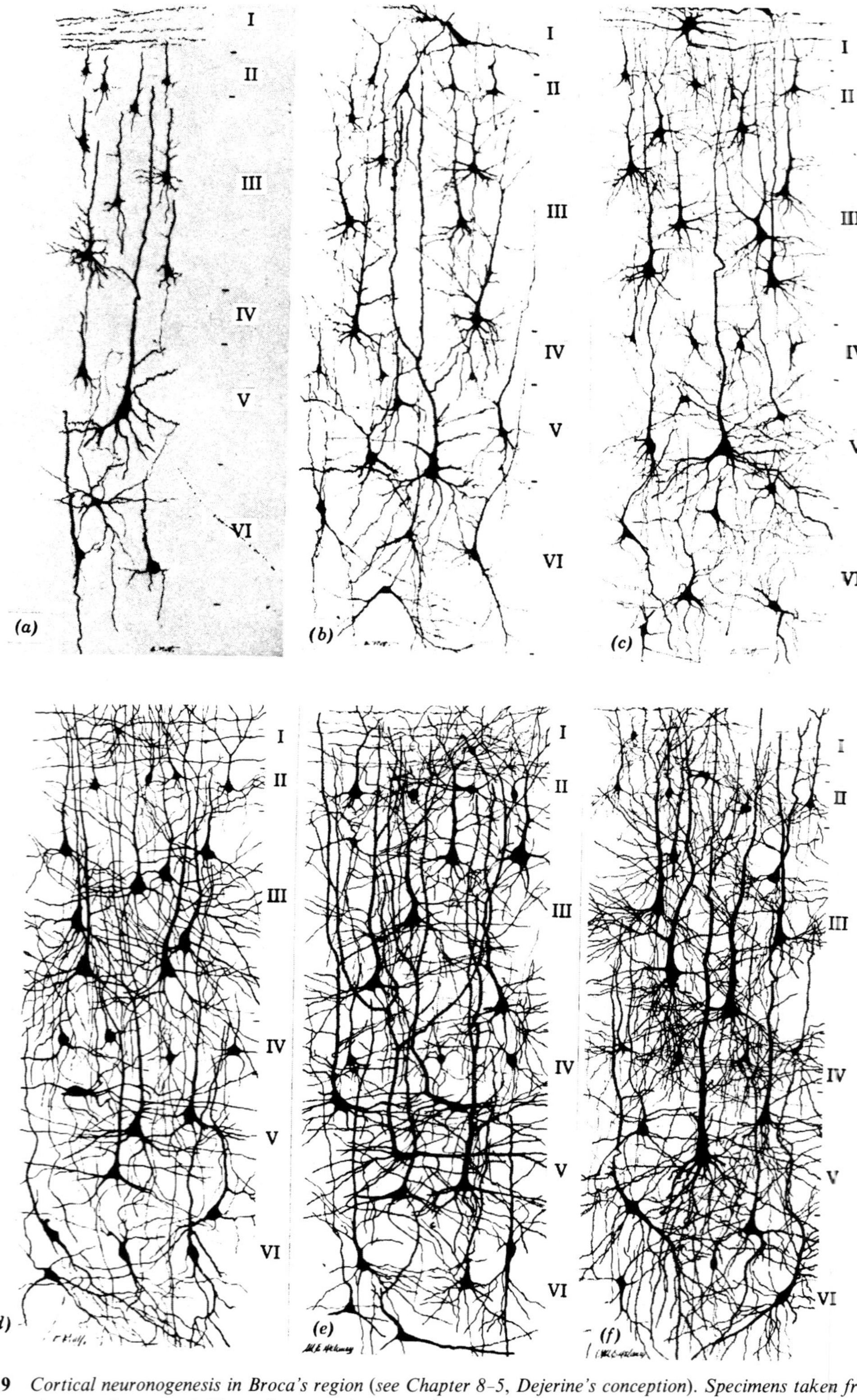

Fig. 8-19 *Cortical neuronogenesis in Broca's region (see Chapter 8-5, Dejerine's conception). Specimens taken from a newborn (a), at the age of one month (b), at three months (c), six months (d), 15 months (e) and two years (f). The density of the neuropil increases progressively. From Conel[78].*

of the cortical mantle. Here again, it may be assumed that the most complex learning can take place only at a time when a certain degree of neuronogenetic maturity has been attained in the non-specific association cortices.

SYNAPTOGENESIS

During the last decades, fragmentary data have been obtained on synaptogenetic maturation in the brain of cats, rabbits, chickens, etc. It is now known that the development of axodendritic synapses generally precedes that of axosomatic synapses. It is also known that the number of synapses continues to increase during periods of variable duration in the different cerebral structures of different animals[79–81]. Since their linguistic abilities are at best very limited, these data provide little information on the biological foundations of human language. It can nevertheless be supposed that a sizeable team of particularly compulsive morphologists will one day prepare regional maps of the synaptogenesis of the human brain. Since the latter includes several billion synaptic contacts, such a study could lead to the identification of rather intricate synaptogenetic cycles. They could then be investigated as possible morphological correlates of the various stages of speech and language development.

If the established facts permitted a detailed and integrated conception of cerebral maturation, it would no doubt be possible to attempt the identification of causal relationships between various biological states of the brain and various language learning abilities. However, such knowledge is likely to remain unavailable in the near future. Thus at present it is possible to adopt only one of the following attitudes: either to assert that the brain and language are somehow related, perhaps even suggesting that brain maturation and language acquisition are somehow related, and then hastily abandon the problem; or else consider, for want of anything better, partial and sometimes uncertain data and formulate probable hypotheses. Taking the latter approach, we have suggested that certain morphological events, and particularly certain features of myelinogenesis, are perhaps the indicators, rather than the causes, of certain events which characterize the acquisition of speech and language by man.

3 PHYSIOPATHOLOGY AND LOCALIZATION OF CEREBRAL LESIONS CAUSING APHASIA

The disputes between the associationists and globalists concerning the notion of cerebral localization and its significance in regard to modes of brain functioning were discussed elsewhere (see Chapter 1). Although we shall not return to this topic here, it should be recalled that, with the exception of Pierre Marie[83, 84] and even then only to a certain extent, the most fervent globalists never denied that the site of a cerebral lesion causing aphasia could often be more or less precisely deduced from the clinical study of the resulting disturbances. In other words, while there was much disagreement about the physiological concept of a *centre as a site of function*, there was little dispute concerning the physiopathological concept of a *centre as a site of lesion*[85] (cf. p. 18 and Chapter 8-5). At present, as during the period of intense polemics, the facts which are universally recognized and taught with regard to the anatomoclinical correlates of aphasia are neither particularly numerous nor particularly precise. They can, in fact, be summarized in three statements: in right-handers, aphasia is almost always the result of certain lesions of the left hemisphere of the brain (see Chapter 11) and particularly of its external surface and/or its connections; aphasias in which the clinical picture is dominated by an articulatory disturbance, a qualitative and quantitative reduction, a laborious speech flow and the absence of a marked comprehension disturbance are related to the presence of central and prerolandic lesions; aphasias in which the clinical picture is dominated by an abundance of paraphasic and/or neologistic productions, fluent speech, the absence of an articulatory disturbance and the presence of an obvious comprehension disturbance are related to retrorolandic lesions. These statements are not very specific but many clinicians and pathologists go well beyond these generalities when attempting to predict the localization of an aphasia-producing lesion. Although aware of the risk of possible error (which is increased when the predicted localization is more exclusive and more precise and is decreased when left hemispheric dominance is well documented), aphasiologists are generally fond of anatomoclinical exercises in which identified clinical disorders (see Chapters 3 to 7) are attributed to specific sites of lesions within the prerolandic and retrorolandic regions.

Two fundamental considerations always guide the analysis of abnormal behaviours and provide the basis for anatomoclinical prediction in aphasiology. First, these behaviours should be viewed as the result, not only of the non-functioning of a totally destroyed cerebral zone but also of the abnormal functioning of partially damaged structures and of the functional adaptation of the rest of the brain to the presence of the lesions. Second, the structure of the brain and the usual distribution of aphasia-causing lesions, particularly in cerebral vascular accidents (see Chapter 9), are such that cortical-subcortical injuries are more frequent than purely subcortical injuries and the latter are, in turn, much more frequent than (almost) pure cortical injuries.

Although certitude is often lacking in this domain, the anatomoclinical predictions which can thus be formulated prove to be accurate in a large enough proportion of cases that consideration should be given to the notions on which they are based. They are summarized below.

PREROLANDIC LESIONS

Broca's aphasia

The common form of Broca's aphasia most often results from a cerebral vascular accident (see Chapter 9). It is thought to be related, in most cases, to a cortical-subcortical lesion of Broca's area[86], that is, to a lesion of the caudal third of the left, third frontal convolution (see Fig. 8-5). Besides destroying a portion of the specific motor association cortex, this lesion would undoubtedly affect the functioning of other structures having direct axonal connections to Broca's area, for instance the adjacent primary motor cortex (opercular third of the precentral gyrus), the prefrontal convexity and certain retrorolandic components of the language zone (see Fig 8-4 and 8-5). These considerations are totally applicable in only a fairly limited number of cases because the lesion is commonly not restricted to Broca's area but extends to other superficial and/or deep structures in the same vascular territory (see Fig. 9-1). It is these concomitant lesions which result in the neurological disorders generally associated with Broca's aphasia, particularly a right hemiparesis and, less frequently, an apraxia of the left limbs.

The fundamental disorder resulting from a lesion of Broca's area is classically interpreted as being an inability to transform the sounds of language into articulatory patterns: such a disorder would result from the fact that Broca's area is no longer able to control, through the medium of its association fibres, the ipsilateral and contralateral primary association cortices. There is undoubtedly some truth in this interpretation—which we present because we know of no better one—but it clearly does not account for all the symptomatological components of Broca's aphasia (see Chapter 4). While it provides, for example, a reasonable explanation of the occurrence of phonetic deviations, and even of certain aspects of the impaired sequential chaining of elementary linguistic units, this interpretation certainly does not explain why there is generally a transformation, rather than an absence, of linguistic production, nor does it provide any explanation of the linguistic characteristics of this transformation or of the nature of its usual evolution (see Chapter 3). In addition, this interpretation does not explain why the articulatory disturbance is often more evident in conversation than in repetition; it does not explain the eventual occurrence of paraphasias and paragraphias, nor, when it occurs, the evolution towards agrammatism. Finally, it does not explain instances of automatic-voluntary dissociation. The frequency of these dissociation phenomena, when considered with respect to the results of particularly relevant anatomoclinical case studies, suggests that the motoric role of Broca's area is especially important in the production of propositional language[87] (see Chapter 8-4).

(Quasi) pure anarthria

The selective impairment of the third linguistic phase of spoken language which, since Pierre Marie's work, is often designated by the name of pure anarthria (see Chapters 1 and 3) may appear following various lesions affecting the most peripheral of the hemispheric structures commanding articulatory production. For example, in the fourth section of this chapter we shall discuss a case of pure anarthria in which the lesion destroyed the cortex and subcortex of the inferior two-thirds of the left precentral gyrus[88]. Dejerine's work showed that a circumscribed left-subcortical lesion, involving the association fibres linking Broca's area to the inferior third of the precentral gyrus, could result in the appearance of a nearly isolated articulatory disorder[89, 90]. It can thus be logically supposed that the disturbed articulation of many Broca's aphasics also results from such a lesion (common, of course, in cases where the cortex of Broca's area is destroyed[91]). Various lesions of the lenticular region (Fig. 8-20), no doubt involving fibres coming from the precentral gyrus, may also cause

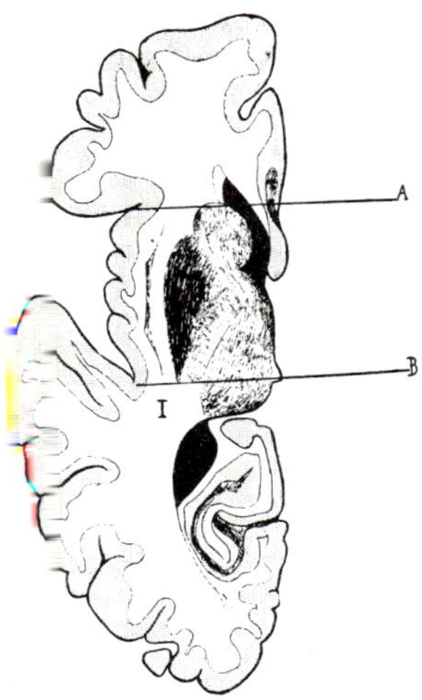

Fig. 8-20 *Pierre Marie's quadrilateral. From Pierre Marie[83]. See also, on this topic, Dejerine's address to the meeting of the Société Neurologique de Paris, 9 July 1908[124].*

anarthria[92], and it is possible that its linguistic (phonetic) characteristics may then not be entirely the same as those of disturbances related to cortical and immediately subcortical lesions. Finally, it is probable that certain lesions of the postcentral gyrus may be the source of an articulatory disturbance because of the deficits which they cause in disrupting the proprioceptive feedback generated by buccophonatory activity[93] (see Chapter 10, Luria's *afferent motor aphasia*). Because the buccophonatory apparatus is bilaterally innervated, the primary motor cortex of the right hemisphere and its connections can be presumed to play a role in the evolution, which is often favourable, of articulatory disturbances (be it 'pure' anarthria or the articulatory disturbance of a Broca's aphasic). In any case, it has been demonstrated that certain right hemisphere lesions may cause a transient articulatory disturbance in right-handers.*

Other speech and language disturbances resulting from prerolandic lesions

The anatomoclinical correlates and the physiopathology of other speech and language disturbances resulting from prerolandic lesions were discussed elsewhere (see Chapter 6). The disturbances included critical arrests of speech and aphemia (lesion of the left or right supplementary motor area), certain forms of akinetic mutism (lesion of the anterior portion of the left or right cingulate gyrus), the behaviour of *linguistic aspontaneity* which is often referred to as transcortical motor aphasia or as dynamic aphasia (see Chapter 10) (lesion of the left prefrontal convexity), and frontal agraphia (lesion of the foot of the left, second frontal convolution).

RETROROLANDIC LESIONS

Conduction aphasia

Since the publication of Wernicke's monograph on aphasia in 1874[17] (see Chapter 1), it has generally been taught that a lesion of the fibres linking the first temporal convolution to the third frontal convolution is the only cause of conduction aphasia. Although the majority of these fibres belong to the arcuate fasciculus (which is itself a component of the superior longitudinal fasciculus) (Fig. 8-6 and 8-22), it is nevertheless possible that some may have a subinsular course. The disturbed repetition[94-96] which is characteristic of conduction aphasia (see Chapter 4) when it is not, at onset, associated with a disturbance of spoken language comprehension,† would thus be explained by a disruption in the transfer of information between two specific association cortices (auditory and motor) of the left hemisphere: the anomalies observed during oral reading, and which occur despite normal comprehension of written language, would be explained in an analogous manner, that is, in terms of an accompanying involvement of certain occipito-

---

* In the terminology of the French school, this would be called dysarthria rather than anarthria (see Chapter 3).

† We shall later discuss cases in which the clinical picture of conduction aphasia gradually emerges from the more complex one of Type I Wernicke's aphasia.

Insertion 8.4

The structure of phonemic paraphasias[102] was previously discussed and illustrated (see Chapter 2) when defining the concepts of a *selection error* and a *sequencing error* [see examples (2–67) to (2–77)]. We then suggested that both types of errors could be related to a disorder which selectively impaired paradigmatic functioning (according to Jakobson's meaning of this term[103], that is, to an anomaly in the selection of the constituent phonemes [LPUs] of more complex segments [HPUs]. While the validity of this hypothesis cannot be conclusively demonstrated, its probable accuracy was indicated through simulation experiments carried out using a computer. In these experiments, conducted in collaboration with Deloche[104], the electronic simulator was given the general instructions to respect the phonological code of the language (as do conduction aphasics[105]) and to produce phonemic omissions and additions at random. The random probability of these two basic operations was weighted according to the extent of similarity between the units of the stimuli and those of the phonemic inventory of the language, and also according to the degrees of similarity and proximity existing among the different units of the stimuli. The degree of similarity was judged in terms of the number of features which were common to any two phonemes being compared and the degree of proximity was equal to the number of phonemes interspersed between any two units being compared. It is interesting to note that under these conditions, the simulator's output included not only sequences which were similar to the phonemic paraphasias of conduction aphasics [(8.1) /pʀɔʒɛktil→piʀɔʒekil/; (8.2) /motosiklɛt→otoskilɛp/] but also a certain number of sequences which resembled formal verbal paraphasias [(8.3) economy (*économie*/ekɔnɔmi/)→economical (*économique*/ekɔnɔmik/); (8.4) experience (*expérience*/ɛksperjãs)→hope (*espérance*/ɛspeʀãs/); (8.5) elephant (*éléphant* /elefã/)→moose (*élan*/elã/)]. Since these two forms of paraphasias are commonly associated in conduction aphasia[97], it can then be suggested that they result from a single dysfunction.

frontal fibres also belonging to the superior longitudinal fasciculus and linking the specific visual and motor association cortices.

While no doubt valid in certain respects, this exclusively associationistic interpretation of conduction aphasia would appear more convincing if the characteristic disturbances of audiophonatory and visuophonatory transposition were manifested by an inability to repeat or read aloud, that is, by an absence of production. This is not, however, what is generally observed[97]. Rather, in the most typical cases, the patient does in fact repeat and read aloud but his productions then include, as does his spontaneous language, a greater or lesser number of phonemic transformations (see Chapter 2). Repetition is more disturbed than reading[98]; the productions are sometimes normal, sometimes transformed; the transformations increase in frequency with an increase in stimulus length; stimuli including numerous grammatical monemes are more difficult to repeat and to read than are those whose syntactic structure is simpler, etc. Many features of this symptomatology, particularly those which emerge from a linguistic description of the transformed segments (Insertion 8.4), seem to us to be more compatible with a lesion which directly affects the cortical analyser than with a lesion which is confined only to the white matter[99]. It also appears significant that, in most cases, (a) the lesion involves the cortex of the supramarginal* gyrus and (b) affects the arcuate fasciculus at a particular point in its course, that is, in the most caudal part of the left parietal operculum, beneath the supramarginal gyrus.

Wernicke's aphasia proper (Type I Wernicke's aphasia)

Most authors agree that Wernicke's aphasia proper is usually due to a lesion of Wernicke's area,

* This is not, however, an absolute rule. For example, Benson et al[96] have reported an anatomoclinical case study of a patient whose lesion, located beneath the supramarginal gyrus, was confined to the white matter. Because death rapidly ensued, a detailed linguistic study of the patient's abnormal productions could not be carried out. On the other hand, Whitaker[100] reported a case of conduction asphasia whose left supramarginal lesion was almost entirely cortical.

that is, of the caudal part of the left, first temporal convolution[17, 101] (see Fig. 8-5). Such a lesion would disturb spoken language comprehension because auditory information could no longer be transmitted to the inferior parietal lobule. Thus the comparison of auditory information with traces stored elsewhere in the cortex, which underlies the process of oral language comprehension, could no longer occur in a normal manner[94]. The lesion of the fibres of the arcuate fasciculus at their point of origin would explain the repetition disturbance. It persists in some patients who show a gradual improvement in comprehension (conceivably because of some form of functional takeover by the right temporal regions) and the clinical picture then evolves towards that of conduction aphasia. It can be assumed that the comprehension of written language would be more or less disturbed (see Chapter 4) depending on whether it is accomplished through axonal assemblies involving direct links or indirect links (through the medium of an occipitotemporal connection) between the specific visual association cortex and the inferior parietal lobule[17] (see Insertion 8.2). The logorrhoea, which is frequently observed at onset, is attributed to a liberation of frontal lobe activities, that is, to the functioning of Broca's area which remains intact but is no longer subject to control by Wernicke's area.

Although satisfying in certain respects, this physiopathological interpretation nevertheless fails to explain the production of verbal paraphasic and paragraphic deviations (for example, why are semantically related words often substituted for each other?) or the production of neologisms. More generally, this interpretation does not explain the linguistic characteristics of jargonaphasia and jargonagraphia[105] (see Chapters 2 and 4).

Type II Wernicke's aphasia

This clinical picture, called *isolation of the speech area* by some[106] and *transcortical sensory aphasia* by others[99], is essentially characterized by a comprehension disturbance, which affects oral language as much as written language, and by the preservation of audiophonatory transposition. Geschwind[94] teaches that this form of aphasia corresponds to the following physiopathology: repetition remains normal because the lesion spares Wernicke's area proper, the arcuate fasciculus and Broca's area. On the other hand, the left inferior parietal lobe is lesioned or else it is intact but the structures surrounding it are lesioned. In either case, the effect is the same: contacts between the angular region and the rest of the brain are no longer possible and language comprehension is impaired.

Type III Wernicke's aphasia

Little is known about the anatomophysiological foundations of this form of Wernicke's aphasia which is characterized by predominant disturbances in the expression and comprehension of written language[97] (see Chapter 4). The question raised by this form of aphasia is even more complicated because the clinical picture most often emerges during the course of favourable evolution from a more complex symptom constellation. Dejerine maintained that the usual cause is a partial lesion of the angular gyrus[107–109] and, more recently, this position has been adopted by Geschwind[94]. Reasoning by analogy from Type I Wernicke's aphasia would logically suggest that Type III could result from lesions destroying (and/or isolating from the classical language zone) those parts of the specific visual association cortex adjacent to the left angular region (see Fig. 8-32).

Amnesic aphasia

Considered by itself, word-finding difficulty has no localizing significance (except as a left hemisphere indicator in right-handers and even this is not absolute). In other words, word-finding difficulty—and this fact merits emphasis—may be related to different physiopathological mechanisms[110–113] (see Chapter 4). As we have mentioned elsewhere, certain left prefrontal lesions, which are tumoral in most cases (see Chapter 9), may sometimes cause the gradual onset of a disturbance almost limited to anomia[114] (see Chapter 4). As for the clinical picture which we have discussed under the name of (Pitres') amnesic aphasia (see Chapter 4), certain aphasiologists believe that it is usually related to a left temporal lesion and attribute it to a functional impairment of the auditory memory traces for words[93, 115]; the presence of this clinical picture then includes an aetiological indication [tumour, haematoma, abscess, degenerative disease (see Chapter 9)]. For other aphasiologists, a 'pure' amnesic aphasia is most frequently a manifestation of the presence of a circumscribed lesion of the left angular gyrus[116] (Insertion 8.5).

(Quasi) pure word deafness

As previously stated, a unilateral lesion limited to the primary auditory cortex (Heschl's zone) may not be evident clinically[117] although its presence can be detected through certain paraclinical procedures[118] (see Chapter 5). On the other hand, bilateral destruction of Heschl's cortex results in cortical deafness[117]. These facts are easily explained when the arrangement of the pre-thalamic and post-thalamic acoustic pathways (see Fig. 11-1) is considered. The lesion resulting in (quasi) pure word deafness is such that it disrupts the connection between the left and right primary auditory cortices on the one hand and Wernicke's area on the other. This condition is created* by certain left temporal lesions and by certain bitemporal lesions: the destruction may be subcortical or else affect the cortex and the immediate subcortex (it is then located at the middle part of the left, first temporal convolution, probably affecting the rostral margin of Wernicke's area)[117]. Other facts concerning the anatomopathology and physiopathology of pure word deafness have been discussed elsewhere (see Chapter 5).

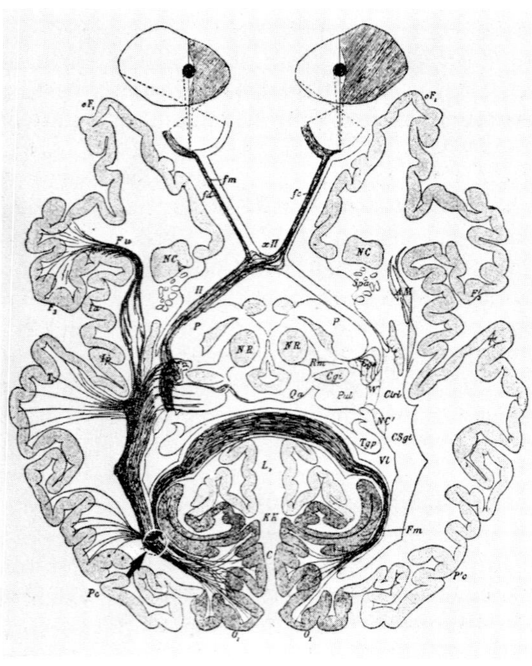

Fig. 8-21 *The left hemisphere lesion (arrow) resulting in pure word blindness and collectively involving, according to Dejerine, the occipito-angular association fibres, the visual radiations, and the occipito-occipital splenial contingent. From Dejerine*[125].

Pure word blindness

Eighteen anatomoclinical case studies of agnosic alexia were recently collected by Bouche[119]. His study confirmed that the lesion causing this disorder is located in the left occipital lobe, almost always involving the lingual gyrus but never confined only to this area. The lesion usually involves the fusiform gyrus and very often includes the ventral fibres of the splenium of the corpus callosum as well as the optic radiations and the axons of the inferior longitudinal fasciculus. The calcarine cortex itself is affected in many cases. On the other hand, involvement of the cuneus is rare (although less so in cases of agnosia for forms). Whatever the case, the lesion which causes pure word blindness (see Chapter 5) is such that the visual information necessary for reading no longer reaches the (intact) temporo-parietal components of the language zone. The associationists' hypotheses on this subject are well known. According to Dejerine[107–109] for example, the necessary and sufficient lesion affects the white matter of the left occipital lobe (Fig. 8-21) and is localized in such a way that it collectively involves the left visual radiations, the long association fibres of the callosal pathway (*forceps major*) and the left occipito-angular association fibres. For Geschwind[94, 120], *alexia without agraphia* also constitutes the prototype of a *disconnection syndrome*: a left occipital lesion results in a right hemianopsia; because of accompanying involvement of the splenium, the visual information which is now received only at the level of the right occipital regions can no longer be transmitted to the language zone. Reference to the literature[119, 121] suggests that this interpretation, solely in terms of disconnection, is completely valid in only a small number of cases: thus pure word blindness may be produced in the absence of a midline callosal lesion. On the other hand, certain cortical–subcortical lesions (lingual and fusiform gyrus) are, as we have just mentioned, almost always present. It could per-

* Explanation of the extreme rarity of pure word deafness should no doubt be sought in the immediate anatomical juxtaposition of the cortical–subcortical networks of auditory perception and of language and, additionally, in the fact that these networks are within the same vascular territory. Thus a lesion of one is almost always accompanied by a lesion of the other.

Insertion 8.5

A rather impressive number of neuropsychological disorders has been attributed to left posterior parietal lesions, particularly to those of the inferior parietal lobule. Among the most important are various types of apraxia, including constructional apraxia (see Chapter 16), acalculia, right-left orientation, autotopoagnosia and finger agnosia, and spatial disorientation. If we add to this list the agraphia which some consider to be part of the so-called Gerstmann's syndrome[122, 123] as well as the various forms of aphasia which we have discussed in relation to the left inferior parietal lobule (conduction aphasia, Type II and Type III Wernicke's aphasia, Pitres amnesic aphasia), one wonders about the factors which determine the appearance, in a given patient, of one particular symptom constellation rather than another. It can, of course, be assumed that it all depends on the precise location of the lesion within the cortex and the non-specific association networks of the left parietal lobe and, in addition, that this localization is determined by aetiological factors (see Chapter 9). It is nevertheless possible that this assertion constitutes only a partial explanation. In our opinion, individual variation may also be a factor, especially in cases where a particular symptom constellation only emerges after a certain period of evolution. Such variation may be related, for example, to the types and intensity of previous learning or to the age at which learning occurred. It could also be related, for a given individual, to the more or less absolute nature of his or her functional lateralizations, and thus to the potential for substitution by the contralateral hemisphere (see Chapter 11), as well as to age.

haps be logically suggested that these lesions result in a disconnection, elsewhere than in the splenium itself, between the language zone and the visual areas of the right hemisphere. Nevertheless, it appears to us that certain aspects of the symptomatology of word blindness (see Chapter 5) are more compatible with damage of the cortical analyser itself than with a pure and simple lesion of interhemispheric association axons[121]. Other facts concerning the anatomopathology and physiopathology of pure word blindness have been discussed elsewhere (see Chapter 5).

MASSIVE LESIONS OF THE LANGUAGE ZONE (GLOBAL APHASIA)

A massive lesion may be formed, usually following an acute disorder affecting the circulation of blood to the entire cerebral territory nourished by the left sylvian artery (see Chapter 9), which involves both the prerolandic and retrorolandic components of the language zone. The patient then presents a global aphasia (see Chapter 4): the characteristics of linguistic expression are those of the most severe forms of Broca's aphasia, and language comprehension, at least during the early stages of evolution, is disturbed in the same way as in the most severe forms of Wernicke's aphasia. The precise localization or the limits of the smallest lesion which can result in global aphasia are not known.

THALAMIC LESIONS

The effects of natural and surgical thalamic lesions on speech and language behaviours were discussed elsewhere (see Chapter 7) with particular attention given to the effects of lesions of the left ventral lateral nucleus and the left pulvinar.

4 THE ANATOMOCLINICAL METHOD

Most of the anatomoclinical notions previously discussed (see Chapters 3, 5, 6, 7, 8-1 and 8-3) were acquired through the application of the anatomoclinical method. We shall now illustrate this approach through discussion of three cases observed in the Language Centre of the *Hôpital de la Salpêtrière*. Each case involved a right-handed individual who had become aphasic following a cerebral vascular accident (see Chapter 9) and whose brain was examined after cardiac death. Each case study will be presented according to the following plan: clinical history; orthodox predictions concerning lesion sites; anatomopathological examination; and discussion of the predictions with respect to the observed findings.

WERNICKE'S APHASIA WITH RAPID EVOLUTION TOWARDS THE CLINICAL PICTURE OF CONDUCTION APHASIA

The first case is that of Mr W. Spo., a right-handed journalist and radio broadcaster with no familial history of left-handedness or ambidexterity. After a routine medical examination carried out when Mr Spo. was 33 years of age, he was informed that he had hypertension. In October 1968, at the age of 42 years, he presented an episode of vertical diplopia of sudden onset. His arterial tension was then 200/100 mmHg; the electrocardiogram showed a tachyarythmia with auricular fibrillation. The neurological disturbance completely regressed in three days. Shortly after leaving the hospital, the patient interrupted his prescribed treatment (digitalis and anticoagulotherapy).

As was his habit, Mr Spo. called a taxi to take him to work on the morning of 5 February 1969. The driver was astonished by his client's language which he could not understand. Perplexed about this, Mr Spo. decided to take the subway and thus arrived, without any difficulty, at the broadcasting studio where he worked. It was then his colleagues' turn to be astonished and Mr Spo.'s hospitalization followed shortly thereafter. In the hospital, a Type I Wernicke's aphasia (see Chapter 4) with disturbed comprehension, jargonaphasia and anosognosia was observed, as well as the presence of a right lateral homonymous hemianopsia. The arterial tension was then 200/120 mmHg and cardiac tachyarythmia was present. Appropriate treatment was instituted. The vascular status being under control and the aphasia having improved considerably, the patient was transferred to the *Salpêtrière* Language Centre, for aphasia therapy, early in March 1969. At this time, the hemianopsia was no longer present and the observed linguistic disturbance corresponded exactly to the clinical picture of conduction aphasia (see Chapter 4).

The comprehension of both spoken and written language was almost completely normal (Marie's Three Papers Test was carried out with no hesitation and written sentences were rapidly matched to their corresponding pictures in a set of sequential pictures [see Fig. 15–5]). No articulatory disturbance was present. Severe word-finding difficulty was manifested in conversation by hesitations, aborted sentences, repetition of determiners, prepositions, etc. All forms of oral production included an abnormally large number of phonemic approximations and transformations [see Chapter 14 and example (2–24)]. The following sample was excerpted from a conversation recorded on March 8, 1969 (see also Insertions 15.1 and 17.1).

(8.6) *'C'est-à-dire que ça consiste à présenter des* |anime|↓ des↓ des↓ des /eni/↓ des /emize/↓ des /emis/↓ *Ça consiste à présenter des* /emise/↓ *des émissions—ça y est —à la↓ à la radio . . . C'est une* /spesjazi/↓ *une spécialité qu'on m'a donnée, si j'ose dire . . . C'est une↓ un jeu qui se joue par téléphone. Les* /kɑ̃di/↓ *les candidats, les↓ par* /kɔ̃/↓ *c'est-à-dire↓ par conséquent les↓ les* /odida/↓ *les auditeurs téléphonent . . . D'apres les dix jours, il me semble qu'il y a un* /pϕ/↓ *un* |pʀɔʒɛ|↓ *un* |pʀɔsɛ↓*—non, pas un* /pʀɔsɛ|↓*—un pro-grès, euh c'est plutôt encourageant.*'

'That's to say that it involves the presentation of some |anime|/↓ some↓ some↓ some /eni/↓ some /emize/↓ some /emis/↓ It involves the presentation of some /emise/↓ some programs—that's it—on the↓ on the radio . . . It's a /spesjazi/↓ a specialty which was given to me, if I dare say so . . . It's an↓ a game which is played by telephone. The /kɑ̃di/↓ the candidates, the↓ by /kɔ̃/↓ that's to say↓ consequently the↓ the /odida/↓ the listeners telephone . . . From the ten days, it seems to me that there is a /pϕ/↓ a |prɔʒɛ|↓ a /prɔsɛ|↓—no, not a /prɔsɛ|—a pro-gress, uh, it's rather encouraging.'

As is usual in these cases[105], the serial integration of the words of a sentence sometimes shows errors which are analogous to those characterizing the serial integration of the phonemes or letters of a word [see examples (2–73) to (2–77)]. Thus the patient defined a 'fork' in the following terms:

(8.7) '*C'est une petite fourche avec quatre manches . . . quatre dents et, au bout, un manche.*'

'It's a small pitchfork with four handles . . . four prongs and, at the end, a handle.'

Numerous phonemic deviations were produced during repetition:

(8.8) /spɛktakl→spɛktatʀ/

(8.9) /kɔ̃stitysjɔ→kɔ̃styty/

(8.10) '*Le central Alésia ne fonctionne plus*'→"*le* /se/↓ *central* /as/↓ /ase/↓ /ale/↓ /asela/ *ne fonctionne plus*".'

'The Alesia Center is no longer functioning'→"The / as/↕ /ase/↕ /ale/↕ /asela/ /se/↕ center is no longer functioning".'

Although less disturbed[126], oral reading nevertheless gave rise to the same type of deviations:

(8.11) '*On déplore des dégâts importants*'→'*On déplore des* /gede↓ /greda/ |abɔdɑ̃|.'

'*They regret the extensive damage*'→'*They regret the* /gede↓ /greda/ |abɔdɑ̃|.'

Copying was almost normal, but other types of written production included numerous deviations, almost all in the form of literal paragraphias. This was the case for writing to dictation:

(8.12) '*Malmenés par la tempête, les voiliers dispersés ont finalement tous sombré.*'→'*Ne Màlmenés par la tempête, les voiliers disperessés ont (fait) fl filen finalement tous sombrés.*'

'*Mauled by the storm, the scattered sailboats all finally sank*'→'Not mauled *by the storm the* scattered sailboats all *(fait) fl filen finally* sank.'

This was also the case, perhaps to a lesser degree, for spontaneous written expression (also of 8 March, 1969).

(8.13) '*Le dernier en date constituant en un concours donnant aux (audi.) auditeurs la (possibol) (i) possibilité de gagner des sommes importantes ... Chaque concurrent pose une question qui tend a (defirnit) definir l'usage du verbe recherché ... constituée par les primes publicitaires proposées par les firmes qui (pra) (patroni) patronent cette emission.*'

'*The latest one constituting a competition giving the (audit) listeners the (possibol) (i) possibility to win large sums ... Each contestant asks a question which tends to (defirnit) define the use of the verb to be found ... constituted by the publicity subsidies deposited by the firms which (pra) (patroni) patronize this programme.*'

Oral spelling was often faulty for relatively long words [e.g., (8.14) /spɛktakylɛʀ/ (*spectaculaire*) → (S-P-E-S-T-A-C-A-L-U-S-R-E)]. The naming of pictures and objects was generally normal in terms of word selection but abnormal in terms of their phonemic production:

(8.15) (clock) *horloge*→/ɔʀlɔʒ/

(8.16) (thermometer) *thermomètre*→/tɛʀmɔlɔʒ/

(8.17) (anvil) *enclum*→/emelo/↓ /ekly/↓ /ɑ̃klym/

(8.18) (globe) *globe terrestre*→/mapʀɔ̃d/

During the same period, Mr Spo. obtained an IQ equivalent of 124 on the (purely verbal) Binois-Pichot Vocabulary Test and his score on the Standard Progressive Matrices (PM-38) (see Chapter 16) was above the 90th percentile. The Complex Figure of Rey was normally reproduced. The electroencephalogram showed left temporal abnormalities.

Seven weeks after the onset of his aphasia, the patient presented a brief episode of intense sudation and vertigo accompanied by an 'impression of having a veil in front of my eyes'. A second episode occurred the following day during a language therapy session. During this second episode, Mr Spo. said to his clinician 'But, Miss, what's happening to me? I no longer recognize you!' Following this episode, the patient's neurological status was greatly altered: he presented a left superior quadranopsia, an agnosia for pictures (particularly obvious when identifying photographs of Parisian monuments: for example, the Madeleine was confused with the Chamber of Deputies and the Pantheon with the Invalides), a spectacular prosopagnosia[127] (although he no longer recognized people by face, Mr Spo. easily identified them by their voice), a colour agnosia, and a slight agnosic alexia. The electroencephalogram showed left temporo-parieto-occipital anomalies. Mr Spo. died on 5 May 1969 as the result of myocardial infarction.

Anatomoclinical predictions

Given the facts observed in this case, the following predictions can be made concerning the lesions causing the patient's disturbances:

(a) Because the episode of diplopia was brief and followed by complete recovery, no anatomical trace would likely be found.
(b) Immediately after the cerebral vascular accident of 5 February 1969 the aphasiological picture was that of a Wernicke's aphasia, strictly defined; it was, however, rapidly modified and became a conduction aphasia. There could be a partial lesion of Wernicke's area (in its most caudal part) or, more likely, given the complete and rapid regression of the initial comprehension disturbance, a cortical-subcortical lesion destroying a part

of the supramarginal gyrus and the fibres located beneath it.* In the latter case, the observed performance on the Progressive Matrices and on the Complex Figure of Rey would suggest that the parietal lesion is small and limited to the supramarginal gyrus.

(c) Given the left quadranopsia, there was certainly a right-sided lesion resulting from the last cerebral vascular accident; an additional left lesion, no doubt involving some part of Brodmann's[76] areas 18 and 19, is no less certain, given the visual agnosia (for pictures), the colour agnosia and the electroencephalographic signs. The presence of the prosopagnosia strongly suggests bilateral lesions[119], probably involving the infero-internal surfaces of the occipital lobes. The agnosic alexia was too mild to risk a firm prediction in this regard (Fig. 8-21).

Anatomopathological examination

Examination of the brain revealed softenings of different ages which involved the territory of the supramarginal branch of the left sylvian artery and those of the two posterior cerebral arteries (Fig. 8-22). The brain stem and cerebellum were normal.

Left hemisphere. There was a relatively old lesion of the supramarginal gyrus as well as a more recent lesion of the fusiform gyrus and the optic radiations.

As shown by a coronal section passing through the lateral geniculate bodies (Fig. 8-22a), Wernicke's area proper was intact (including the *planum*). The only anomaly observed at this level was a certain pallor of the optic radiations (demyelination). Furthermore, there were no lesions rostral to this section.

The oldest lesion is shown in a section immediately caudal to the extremity of the fissure of Sylvius (Fig. 8-22c). The cortex and the subcortex of the left supramarginal gyrus were partially destroyed at this level and the lesion no doubt involved the fibres of the arcuate fasciculus.

There was also a more recent cortical-subcortical softening which especially affected the fusiform gyrus (Fig. 8-22c and e) and extended beneath to the optic radiations and, probably, also to the fibres travelling from or to the lingual gyrus.

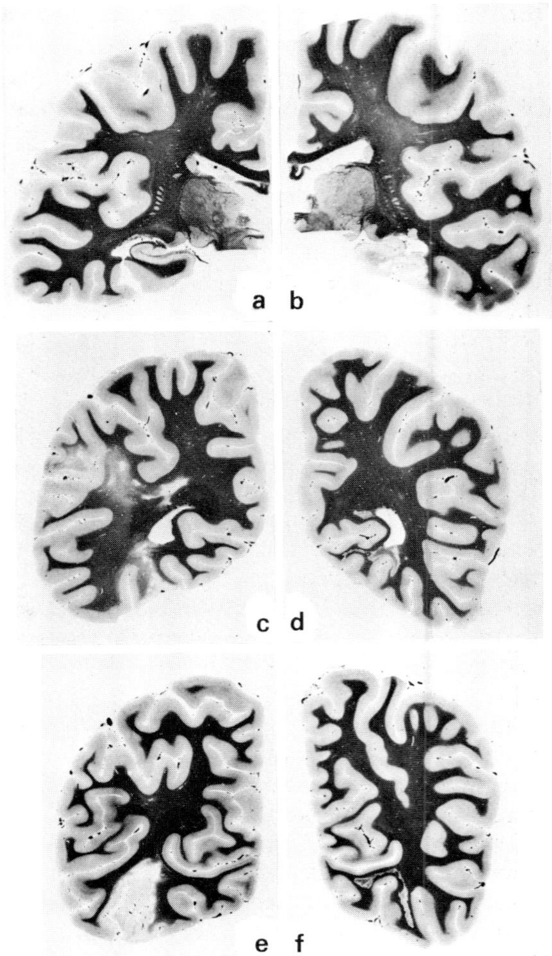

Fig. 8-22 *Case W. Spo. Wernicke's aphasia with rapid evolution towards the clinical picture of conduction aphasia; pathological anatomy; coronal sections of the left (a, c, e) and right (b, d, f) cerebral hemispheres; Loyez staining. Detailed description in the text. Wernicke's area proper is intact (a). The cortical-subcortical lesion which caused the conduction aphasia damaged the supramarginal gyrus and no doubt the arcuate fasciculus (see Fig. 8-6) located beneath it. The more recent bilateral lesions, which caused the prosopagnosia, involved the lingual and fusiform gyri: they are cortical-subcortical on the left (e) and essentially subcortical on the right (d, f). c, d, e and f from Lhermitte et al[127].*

Right hemisphere. The right hemisphere lesion, which was contemporaneous with the left fusiform lesion, extended from the caudal portion of the hippocampal and parahippocampal gyri, in

* Some would no doubt suggest that the lesion could be strictly confined to the subcortex of the left posterior parietal operculum (see Chapter 8-3).

the front, to the posterior third of the lingual and fusiform gyri in the rear.

The most rostral portion of this lesion is seen in the section crossing the lateral geniculate bodies (Fig. 8–22b). It damaged the cortex and subcortex of the hippocampal and parahippocampal gyri as well as the most internal portion of the fourth temporal convolution.

Further behind, as can be seen in the section crossing the occipital horn (Fig. 8–22d) and in the section caudal to it (Fig. 8–22e), the lesion was entirely subcortical, involving the axes of the lingual and fusiform gyri. The most caudal portion of this lesion involved a part of the optic radiations.

Discussion

The anatomoclinical predictions proved to be generally accurate in this case. The lesion responsible for the aphasia occupied part of the classical language zone (see Chapter 8–1, Fig. 8–5): it was located at the level of the supramarginal gyrus and spared both Broca's area and Wernicke's area. Although this case could be cited in support of the hypothesis that conduction aphasia results from damage to the arcuate fasciculus[94], it could also be cited in support of the hypothesis that the cortical analyser is damaged in this clinical form of aphasia[89] (see Chapter 8–1). On the other hand, this case also shows that conduction aphasia (*Goldstein's central aphasia*) may occur in the absence of insular involvement (see Chapter 10). The bilaterality of the occipital lesions responsible for the prosopagnosia was confirmed[119, 127].

UNEXPECTED LESIONS IN A CASE OF JARGONAPHASIA

The second case[87] is that of Mr J. Com. (1915–1968), a right-handed pharmacist with no familial history of left-handedness or ambidexterity. At the age of 15 years, he had scarlatina and then presented an acute episode of rheumatic fever: he was since known to have mitral stenosis. At the age of 37 he had a transient episode of hemiparesis with aphasia; this lasted only a few hours. The symptoms which characterized the first aphasic episode are not known.

In November 1959, at the age of 43 years, the patient suddenly developed Wernicke's aphasia and was rapidly admitted to the *Hôpital de la Salpêtrière*. Examination revealed the presence of a tachyarythmia and a mild right hemiparesis. Visual fields were normal (on confrontation) and no buccofacial, constructional, indeomotor or ideational apraxia was present. The right hemiparesis regressed after a few hours but the aphasia persisted. The patient was considered to have suffered an embolus in the left sylvian territory (see Chapter 9), with temporal softening; the integrity of the visual fields suggested that the lesion was relatively superficial.

Mr Com.'s aphasia was very closely observed from November 1959 until April 1963. The initial picture was that of fluent jargonaphasia. Production was normal in terms of articulation. Conversation, narration and picture description included many aborted sentences and ready-made expressions but few lexical words. As indicated by the following excerpt from a conversation recorded a few days after the onset of Mr Com.'s aphasia, neologisms were common.

(8.19) '*Ça a dû m'arriver le huit-neuf et non pas le sept-dix du mois de* /kɔ̃dene/. *Oui, c'était dans un* /liktye/ *pour* /lekonise/ *un* /pʀɔbile/ *spécial, pour dépasser les trains et tous leurs éléments. C'est pour* /opye/ *des* /pʀesisasɑ̃/. *Je ne sais pas si vous m'avez compris.*'

'That must have happened to me on the eight-nine and not the seven-ten of the month of /kɔ̃dene/. Yes, it was in a /liktye/ for /lekonise/ a special /pʀɔbile/ to go beyond the trains and all their elements. It's to /opye/ some /pʀesisasɑ̃/. I don't know if you have understood me.'

Many neologisms were also noted in attempts at naming [(20 to (24)], repetition [(25) to (29)] and oral reading. These deviant segments included a large number of apical consonants:

	Naming			Repetition
(8.20)	(pencil)	*crayon* →/dɔndœlin/	**(8.25)**	/kafe → dele/
(8.21)	(blotter)	*buvard* →/desɑ̃tʀɑ̃de/	**(8.26)**	/klima → lede/
(8.22)	(ink-well)	*encrier* →/delovelɛʀnale/	**(8.27)**	/pʀɔfi → lepʀonele/
(8.23)	(flowers)	*fleurs* →/ɔtalɔpe/	**(8.28)**	/pyni → dɔdile/
(8.24)	(flowers)	*fleurs* →/dʀenedene/	**(8.29)**	/ʒefɛ̃ → dene/.

Just as articulation was normal in all forms of oral expression, the purely graphic aspects of writing were normal in all forms of written expression. With the exception of copying, which included only a few orthographic deviations, for example,

(8.30)

'*La bibliothéque est fermée*'	→	'*La bibliotheque est ferme.*'
'*The library is closed*'	→	'*The* library *is* close.'

written expression was jargonagraphic. The following example of (spontaneous) writing was obtained a few days after onset of the patient's illness:

(4.27) '*Ma dumorale, ferdant donc une pouette de péa près. Mes pelits beaubpoud persent des blassisseuses.*'

'My *dumorale*, thus *ferding a pouette* of *péa* near. My *pelits beaubpoud persent* of the *blassisseuses*.'

Neologisms are seen to replace lexical words and the selection of grammatical words appears to be adequate. In the original production, *pelits* was crossed out and *persent* was inserted as if it were a correction. Comprehension of spoken language was impaired on even the simplest tasks, that is, on word identification by pointing tasks (see Chapter 15) and the patient's anosognosia of his comprehension difficulties was more evident than that of his spoken jargon [see the last sentence of example (8.19) above]. On the other hand, comprehension of written language was normal or nearly so from the very first days of Mr Com.'s aphasia, when he had no difficulty in matching relatively complex written sentences to their corresponding pictures in a set of sequential pictures (see Fig. 15-5).

The patient was unable to recognize the melodies of popular songs. His copy of the Complex Figure of Rey was normal. In January 1960, his IQ, as calculated from his results on the Cattel Culture Free Test ('G' factor), was 140. An electroencephalogram obtained on November 1959 showed evidence of left temporal softening.

During the next three and a half years, while Mr Com. followed an intensive programme of aphasia therapy (see Chapter 17), comprehension of spoken language improved considerably. He came to understand relatively complex sentences provided that they were spoken fairly slowly and dealt with concrete matters. Naming gradually improved but repetition and oral reading remained very impaired. The production of neologistic segments in spontaneous discourse continued for some time (the examiners noted the presence of a preferred neologism, namely /tʀefwɛlg/, as well as the less frequent production of certain variants, for example /fʀɛlg/, /ɛnfɛlg/, /fefɛlg/, /defɛld/), but later decreased and then disappeared. Written language comprehension remained excellent and greatly facilitated the course of language therapy. Written expression improved markedly as a means of effective communication but the dyssyntaxia gradually became more apparent. The types of sentences which Mr Com. could write in 1962 are exemplified below:

(8.31) '*Bonjour Madame. Je donne des hommages à vous.*'
'*Good day Madame. I give you my regards.*'

(8.32) '*J'ai* (langage→) *languege.*'
'*I have* language.'

(8.33) '*J'ai à perdu des mots.* (Analphabète→) *Anaphèle.*'
'*I've to lost some words.* Illiterate.'

(8.34) '*Alors, j'espère la santé d'un cerveau.*'
'*So, I hope the health of a brain.*'

(8.35) '*Le matin de l'élever à 9h ou 10 h. De plus de faire de lits au ménage et pour manger.*'
'*The morning of the to rise at 9 or 10 o'clock. Moreover to make some beds do the housekeeping and in order to eat.*'

(8.36) '*Lundi et Mardi je travaille souvenir des mots et* (plutôt→) *plustot des verbes.*'
'*Monday and Tuesday I work memory of the words and* rather *of the verbs.*'

(8.37) '*La situation mettre la complexion.*'
'*The situation to put the constitution.*'

As can be observed in (32) and (33) above, a certain number of literal paragraphias [(2.54) to (2.59)] could be definitely identified at that time. It is noteworthy that their production remained limited in this patient whose writing was solidly based on extended learning and experience.

Throughout these years Mr Com. remained the fervent and formidable chess player he had been in the past. He also continued to sketch, having been particularly gifted in this form of expression, and one day drew a satirical cartoon of another patient whom he frequently met at the *Salpêtrière* Language Centre (Fig. 8-23). In the fall of 1962, Mr Com.'s scores on the Wechsler-Bellevue Intelligence Scale (see Chapter 16) were as follows: verbal IQ = 117; performance IQ = 132; full-scale IQ = 124. An electroencephalogram, carried out near the same time, was within normal limits.

During the two years which followed Mr Com.'s second cerebral vascular accident, his conversational behaviour underwent profound modification. After a period of relative anosognosia and neologistic jargon, a certain quantitative reduction became evident. Such a phenomenon is commonly observed in cases of jargonaphasia with a favourable evolution[105] (see Chapter 4). A less common phenomenon, or at least a less commonly recognized one, was the progressive emergence, after some months of language therapy, of a second pattern of oral production. Mr Com.'s conversation then included two types of utterances: certain segments were normal in terms of fluency, articulation and prosody but conveyed little or no information because they were primarily composed of ready-made expressions or aborted syntagms or even occasional neologisms: in contrast, other segments were uttered in a slow, laborious and syllabic manner, resembled agrammatism in

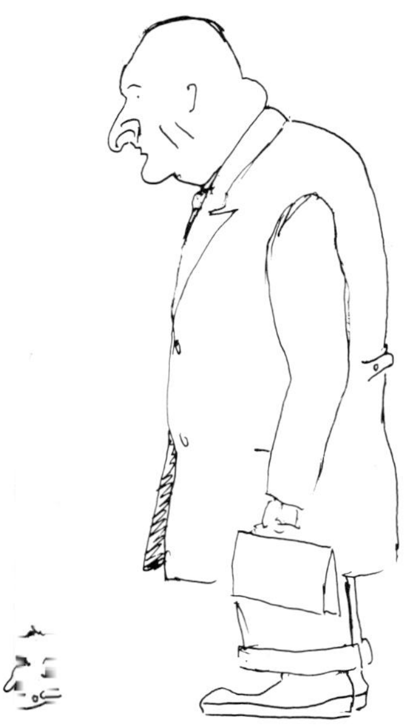

Fig. 8-23 *Cartoon drawn by a patient who presented Wernicke's aphasia proper (case J. Com.; see text). From Lhermitte et al.*[7].

their usual reduction to lexical constituents and, as in the case of agrammatism, were frequently effective in terms of conveyed information. The articulatory difficulty which was obvious during this second type of production resembled that of the dystonic phase of phonetic disintegration[128, 129] (see Chapter 3). It should be noted that both of these two productive patterns could be observed within the context of a single conversational exchange. This is illustrated in the following example (38) where the dystonic productions are indicated by underlining and the symbol □ is used to indicate momentary interruption of the utterance.

(8.38) '*Maintenant, j'étais ... □ Le □ jar □ din. □ On était bien, là. Je faisais un petit peu ... □ Lis. □ Je □ lis. Et puis, un peu des ... C'est tout. □ Si □ es □ te.*'

'Now, I was ... □ The □ gar□den. □ It was comfortable there. I was doing a bit ... □ Read. □ I □ read. And then, a bit of ... That's all. □ Si□es□ta.'

After the first two years of evolution, the principal changes observed in Mr Com.'s linguistic behaviour mainly reflected a progressive lexical enrichment. As a consequence, his conversation showed an increase in the number of segments which were laboriously articulated but effective in communication. The lexical enrichment was also evident in written expression so that the written dyssyntaxia became even more apparent[105]; example (2.82), cited elsewhere in this work, was taken from Mr Com.'s file. Repetition and oral reading remained severely disturbed during these years of evolution. In March 1963, the patient obtained an IQ equivalent of 139 on the Binois–Pichot Vocabulary Test: his semantic competence was thus astonishingly well preserved provided that it proceeded from written stimuli.

Between the summer of 1963 and the spring of 1968, Mr Com.'s visits to *la Salpêtrière* became less regular and less frequent (although never less than twice a year) until his last visit around April 1968. During this period, it was observed that the patient was either sad or depressed, or else that his habitual impulsiveness had changed to overt aggressiveness and violence. These behavioural changes were primarily attributed to the particularly intricate social and family context in which the patient now lived.* No noticeable changes occurred in Mr Com.'s aphasia during these last five years.

On 19 June 1968, the patient suffered his third and final cerebral vascular accident. Following a convulsive episode, he developed left hemiparesis and global aphasia. After two days, mobility of the left limbs had nearly returned to normal but the aphasia was to show no subsequent improvement. Oral expression was limited to the repetitive production of a few mumbled and undifferentiated sounds, and oral comprehension was impaired for even the most simple stimuli. It was impossible to assess residual abilities—if any—in the production and comprehension of written language. The patient died of heart

* 'Which is typically Parisian' (Boris Vian, *Bourrée de complexes*).

failure five and a half weeks later, that is, on 28 July 1968 at the age of 53 years.

Anatomoclinical predictions

Given Mr Com.'s neurological history, anatomoclinical predictions can be easily formulated if based on orthodox reasoning:

Because of its brevity, his first cerebral vascular accident, sustained at the age of 37 years should not have left any important anatomical traces and, in any case, they could scarcely be expected to be distinct from those of the second episode.

The second accident produced a linguistic disturbance dominated by jargonaphasia (with normal fluency but all sorts of deviations) and a severe disturbance of oral comprehension; it could therefore be predicted that there would be a substantial lesion involving Wernicke's area proper and perhaps Heschl's gyri but sparing Broca's area because normal articulation would have otherwise been impossible.

The normal comprehension of written language and the relative recovery of written expression (Insertion 8.2), as well as the results of psychometric testing, particularly on the Complex Figure of Rey (see Chapter 16), suggest that there would be no significant parietal lesion.

Given the left hemiparesis, there would undoubtedly be a right hemisphere lesion associated with the third vascular accident. The transient nature of this hemiparesis suggests that there would be no substantial anterior damage. The extreme severity of the accompanying aphasia has two possible explanations. If Mr Com.'s substantial linguistic recovery after his second vascular accident was mediated by right hemisphere activity, then recent retrorolandic right-hemisphere lesions would be expected to be found, probably in the temporoparietal region. On the other hand, there may have been bilateral lesions at the time of the third episode with the worsening of the aphasia resulting from new left-hemisphere lesions. In this case it would be difficult to predict the exact location of these lesions but the absence of right hemiparesis and the severity of the comprehension disturbance suggest particular involvement of the retrorolandic components of the language zone.

Anatomopathological examination

Anatomopathological examination revealed the presence of cystic areas of ancient softening in both frontal lobes and in the left temporal and left parietal lobes (Fig. 8-24 and 8-25a, b and c). There was also recent haemorrhagic infarction of the right temporoparietal region (Fig. 8-25d).

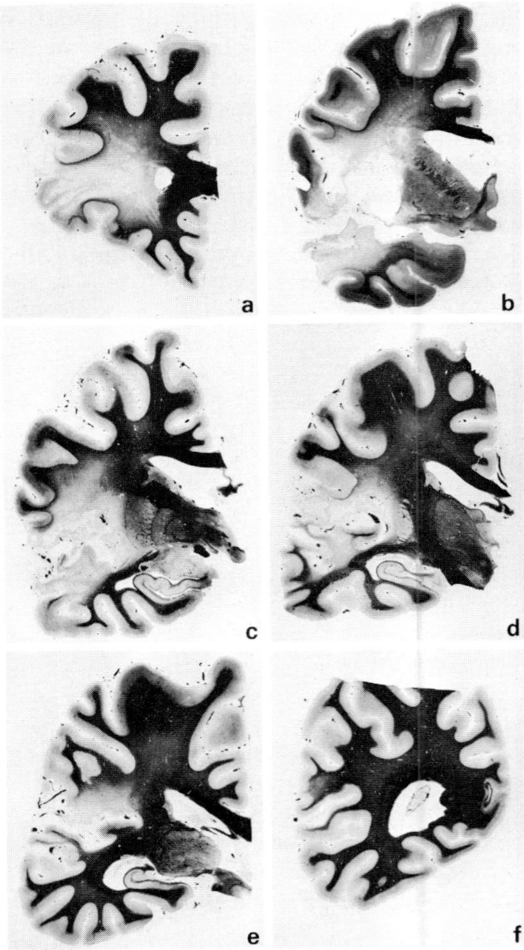

Fig. 8-24 *Case J. Com. Wernicke's aphasia proper; pathological anatomy; coronal sections through the left hemisphere; Loyez staining. Detailed description in the text. Although the cortical-subcortical lesions damaged the prefrontal convexity (a) and destroyed Broca's area (b), the opercular third of the precentral and postcentral gyri (c, d) as well as Heschl's gyri and Wernicke's area proper (c, d), the clinical picture was that of Wernicke's aphasia proper with a marked auditory aspect* (versant auditif) *(see Chapters 4 and 10). Note that the inferior parietal lobule is relatively spared (e, f). From Lhermitte et al*[87].

Left hemisphere. The old left hemisphere infarct was cortical-subcortical, spreading without interruption from the third frontal convolution to the anterior portion of the inferior parietal lobule (Fig. 8-24). It had almost totally destroyed the *pars triangularis* and *pars opercularis* of F3, the opercular third of the precentral gyrus and postcentral gyrus, the insula, Heschl's gyri and Wernicke's area proper. In its rostral half, it completely sectioned the superior longitudinal fasciculus including its arcuate component.

In a coronal section through the genu of the corpus callosum (Fig. 8-24a), in front of Broca's area, the lesion was cystic and destroyed almost the entire cortex and subcortex of the *pars triangularis* of F3. With the exception of a relative sparing of the U-fibres, myelin pallor extended to the axes of F2 and adjacent orbital convolutions and, deep to the core of the lesion, reached the lateral wall of the frontal horn.

In a section showing the head of the caudate and the rostralmost part of the putamen (Fig. 8-24b), the cystic appearance of the left lesion was even clearer. At this level it destroyed almost all of the cortex and subcortex of Broca's area. Beneath the latter it also destroyed the anterior part of the insula, the claustrum and the extreme and internal capsules. The softening extended to the striatum but hardly encroached upon it. On the other hand it interrupted the fibres of the superior longitudinal fasciculus and its arcuate component. Marked pallor was noted in the fibres of the superior occipitofrontal fasciculus and in the dorsalmost fibres of the anterior limb of the internal capsule. There was cortical-subcortical involvement of the rostralmost part of T1 and myelin pallor was observed deep below T1, F2, F1 and the cingulate gyrus.

More caudal sections through the insula (Fig. 8-24 c and d) show involvement of this structure and of both opercula. The opercular third of both the precentral gyrus and postcentral gyrus was destroyed as were the insula and underlying structures (including the superior longitudinal fasciculus and its arcuate component but excluding the striatum and pallidum). At this level, almost nothing remained of Heschl's gyri nor of Wernicke's area. Above the softening, myelin pallor spared little besides the U-fibres; beneath it, the damage to T2 was less obvious.

A section through the rostral part of the supramarginal gyrus (Fig. 8-24e) shows partial involvement of the cortex and subcortex of this structure; the caudalmost part of the planum is less affected at this level.

The caudal limit of the left softening is seen in a section through the juxta-angular part of the supramarginal gyrus (Fig. 8-24f). At this level there was only a small area of cortical-subcortical damage.

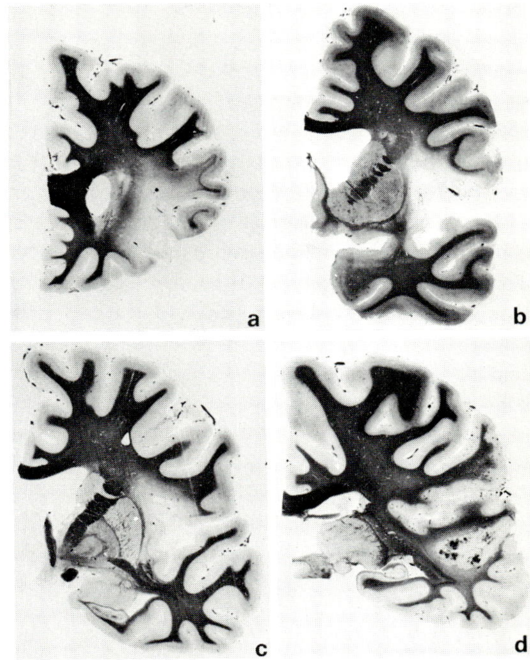

Fig. 8-25 *Case J. Com. Wernicke's aphasia proper; pathological anatomy; coronal sections through the right hemisphere; Loyez staining. Detailed description in the text. Old cortical-subcortical lesions partially destroyed the* pars triangularis (*a*) *and* pars opercularis (*b*) *of the third frontal convolution; they caused only slight damage to the opercular portion of the precentral gyrus* (*c*) *and spared the postcentral gyrus; more caudal sections* (*d*) *show numerous small haemorrhagic infarcts, especially in the first temporal convolution and the inferior parietal lobule. From Lhermitte et al*[87].

Right hemisphere. Two zones of softening were found in the right hemisphere, an old fronto-insular one (Fig. 8-25a, b, c) and a recent insulo-temporo-parietal one (Fig. 8-25d). Neither of them damaged the grey nuclei or the thalamus.

As shown in a coronal section through the callosal genu (Fig. 8-25a), the lesion of the *pars triangularis* of F3 was similar to that observed in the left hemisphere.

A section through the head of the caudate and the rostralmost part of the putamen (Fig. 8-25b) shows that the *pars opercularis* of F3 was considerably less damaged than the corresponding area of the left hemisphere. At this level, the rostral damage to the insula, the claustrum, the extreme and internal capsules and the superior longitudinal and arcuate fasciculi is comparable to that in the left hemisphere. As on the left, the striatum was spared.

The caudalmost portion of the old right hemisphere softening destroyed a small part of the precentral operculum (Fig. 8–25c). The postcentral operculum was spared.

More caudal sections (Fig. 8–25d), behind the old lesion and separated from it by a zone of healthy tissue, showed numerous small haemorrhagic infarcts (many of them microscopic) within the caudal third of the insula, the anterior part of the inferior parietal lobule and the first two temporal convolutions (including the *planum temporale*).

Discussion

It is not possible, through anatomopathological examination, to assert that all the old cerebral lesions observed in Mr Com.'s case were in fact constituted at the same time. Given the patient's clinical history, it is nevertheless reasonable to consider that they may have all been formed at the time of the thromboembolic accident (see Chapter 9) of November 1969. In any case, it can definitely be concluded that they were all present at a time when the patient's performance was well above average on several psychometric tests and when his language was characterized by abundant, normally articulated oral production, relatively good, although abnormal, spoken language comprehension, dyssyntactic but informative and graphically normal written production, and normal written language comprehension. This case is therefore surprising in some respects and interesting in several others.

Because the old, right hemisphere lesion was almost restricted to the *pars triangularis* and *pars opercularis* of F3, the rostral third of the insula and only a part of the precentral operculum, it is not so surprising that its presence was not suspected during Mr Com.'s lifetime.

On the other hand, the destruction of Broca's area and of the adjacent part of the precentral and postcentral gyri is totally unexpected in a case of jargonaphasia. It is even more unexpected when, as in the present case, possible substitution by the right hemisphere counterpart of Broca's area is ruled out because this area was itself destroyed. It is tempting to compare these neuropathological observations with the evolution of the patient's spontaneous oral expression (coexistence of two speech patterns: one normally articulated and conveying little information, the other 'dysarthric' and informative) [see (38)]. It could then be suggested that Broca's area is essential only for the production of propositional language and, additionally, that normal articulation of 'automatized' utterances remains possible under the exclusive control of other structures[87]. In this regard it should be stressed that, in Mr Com.'s case, the central grey nuclei and the thalamus (see Chapter 7) were preserved and it must be concluded that a bidimensional view of the language zone does not facilitate the explanation of such cases in terms of cerebral pathology[130] (see Chapter 8–1 and 8–5).

The initial conservation of written language and the rapid recovery of written expression despite complete destruction of the left, first temporal convolution, confirm Wernicke's thoughts on this matter[17] (see Insertion 8.2).

The permanent nature of the disturbance in repetition and in oral reading is readily explained when it is considered that the superior longitudinal fasciculus, including its arcuate component, was bilaterally sectioned by the lesions.

The psychometric test results can no doubt be related to the integrity of the parietal lobes[131].

The effects of the recent right hemisphere lesion on the patient's linguistic behaviour suggest that his right hemisphere played a major role in the recovery observed after the embolic accident of November 1959.

'PURE' APHASIA FROM A LESION 'OUTSIDE' THE LANGUAGE ZONE

Mr E. Fri. (1884–1957) was born in France of an English mother and a French father[88, 132]. Although both parents spoke French and English fluently, the latter was used almost exclusively in linguistic exchanges among the family. Thus Mr Fri. spoke mainly English until the age of four. When he entered primary school at the age of six, his knowledge of French was, at best, rudimentary. He attended French schools from 1890 to 1900 and rapidly achieved native-like mastery of the French language. He obtained a *Certificate d'Etudes Primaires* at the age of 12 years and a *Brevet Elémentaire* at the age of 16. At that time, the latter diploma required higher than average proficiency in both spoken and written French. Mr Fri worked as a commercial agent and always lived in France but his social, familial and occupational relationships were such that he continued to speak English as well as French. He was, in his own opinion and in that of his family, 'completely bilingual' and could speak both languages 'without accent'. Mr

Fri. was right-handed, as were all members of his immediate family.

On 10 December 1947, Mr Fri., who was then 63 years old, was admitted at the Cardiology Department of the *Hôpital Lariboisière* in Paris for study and treatment of a long-standing cardiac ailment (approximately 10 years) manifested by episodes of paroxystic tachycardia. On 12 December, while walking in a hospital corridor, the patient suddenly fell to the floor. Immediate examination indicated a normal state of consciousness and the presence of right hemiplegia and right hemihypo-aesthesia. Speech was suppressed (all attempts at speech resulted in the production of a raucous and undifferentiated sound) but, as far as could be determined, language comprehension was normal. The right sensorimotor deficit regressed rapidly; on 13 December the patient could move his right arm and leg and by the end of the month he could walk unassisted. Speech remained suppressed until the beginning of January 1948. Rapid improvement occurred over the next four weeks and, by the end of January, Mr Fri. was able to communicate through speech although it remained laborious, syllabic, almost totally aprosodic and poorly articulated. In other words, he presented an isolated case of phonetic disintegration, that is, *pure anarthria*[132]. Right-handed writing was indeed normal and showed no evidence of a graphic disturbance. Thus he wrote the following letter during the month of January:

(8.39) *'Docteur*

Je vais essayer de vous expliquer la raison que j'ai de syllaber. A l'état normal la pensée s'exprime, par la parole, automatiquement. On ne s'occupe pas ou peu de l'articulation; par la force de l'habitude l'articulation devient 'machinale'' ...

Il y a 4 semaines tout ce qui me sortait de la bouche quand je voulais dire un mot, c'était un son rauque. Je suis arrivé un jour à prononcer A, I, ensuite A, E, I, O, U. Les jours suivants je réussis certaines syllabes et des mots commençant par des voyelles. Il y a seulement une dizaine de jours que je sais dire Oui. Depuis que je suis ici j'ai à peu près vaincu les J, G, L. Il ya a trois jours, je ne pouvais arriver à dire le nom de mon fils Jean; je ne pouvais pas dire "le", "la", "les". Il me faut syllaber parce que l'articulation est paresseuse, elle n'est plus automatique mais doit être commandée, dirigée. Je dois penser au mot que je vais dire et à la façon de le dire, de l'articuler. Si je veux dire Bonjour, l'habitude ne joue plus, ce n'est plus automatique, si je ne fais très attention, je vais dire Beuseu. Si je veux dire Le, La en ne faisant pas très attention, je dirais De, Da. En raison de cela il faut que j'articule chaque voyelle, chaque consonne, en somme chaque syllabe.'

'Doctor

I shall try to explain to you the reason why I have to speak syllabically. In the normal state, thought is expressed, through speech, automatically. One pays little or no attention to articulation; through the force of habit articulation becomes "mechanical" ...

Four weeks ago, all that came out of my mouth when I wanted to say a word was a raucous sound. One day I managed to pronounce A, I, and later A, E, I, O, U. In the following days I managed certain syllables and words beginning with a vowel. It was only about ten days ago that I was able to say "yes". Since I've been here I have pretty well mastered J, G, L. Three days ago I was unable to say my son's name, "Jean"; I could not say "le", "la", "les".

I have to speak syllabically because my articulation is lazy, it is no longer automatic but has to be commanded, directed. I have to think of the word I am going to say and how to say it, to articulate it. If I want to say Bonjour, habit no longer takes over, it is no longer automatic, if I don't pay strict attention, I'll say Beuseu. If I want to say Le, La without paying attention, I'll say De, Da. Because of that, I must articulate each vowel, each consonant, in short, each syllable.'

On 24 January 1948 Mr Fri. was transferred to the *Salpêtrière* Language Centre to begin a programme of aphasia therapy. At that time he presented a mild residual right hemiparesis with brisker osteotendinous reflexes on the right and a right Babinski sign. On the other hand, no evidence of buccofacial apraxia was obvious[133] (the possible presence of this sign had not been previously explored). Although at a slower rate than during the previous four weeks, the anarthria continued to regress until the middle of February. Subsequent gains were minimal and primarily involved an increase in conversational fluency.

Results of assessment carried out at *la Salpêtrière* in January and February can be summarized as follows:

Oral expression: spontaneous conversation showed a striking dissociation between lexical, semantic and syntactic adequacy on the one hand and a severe articulatory disturbance on the other (phonetic disintegration in the dystonic phase[88, 128, 132]). The speech flow remained laboured and syllabic with marked anomalies of scansion and rhythm. There were numerous hesitations, often in the form of repetitions of initial phonemes[134, 135]. In order to gain an idea of the patient's speech, the reader should try to read example (4.4) aloud, slowly and syllabically, exaggerating the force and amplitude of bucco-

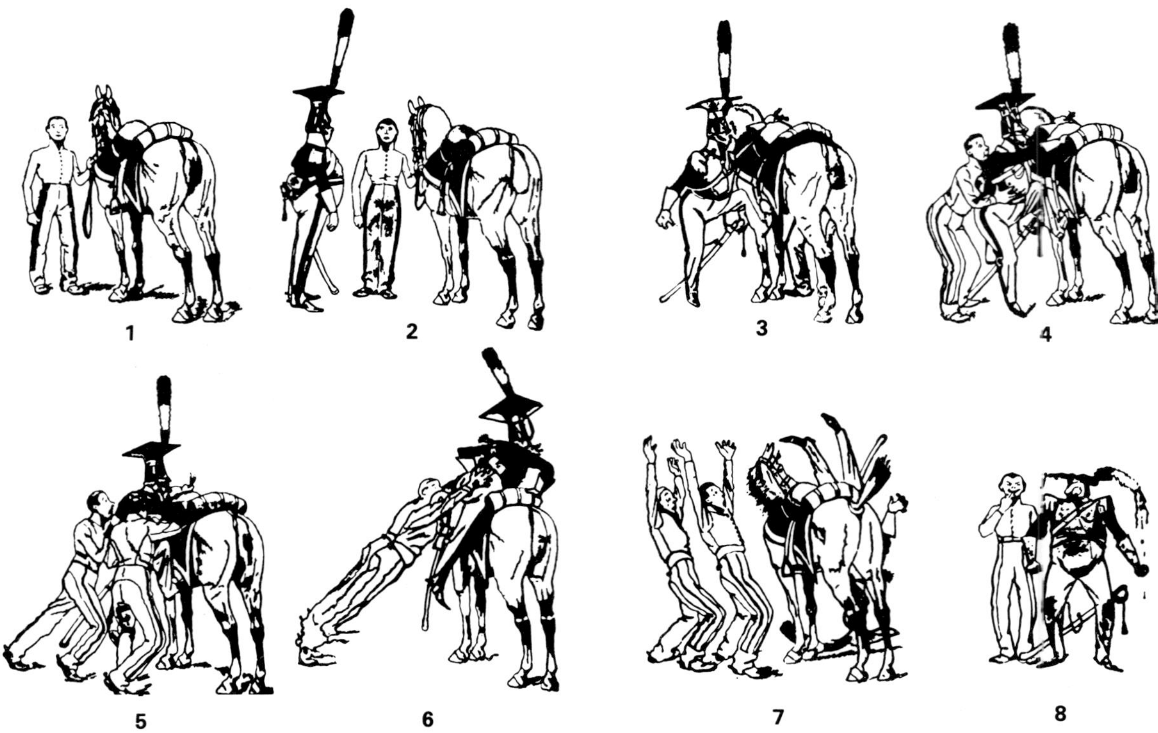

Fig. 8-26 *A story without words by Caran d'Ache* (Depart for the review). *From Ombredane*[141].

phonatory movements, particularly in the case of plosive consonants (exaggerated bursts). The patient is answering a question about his work.

(4.4) '/mɔ/↓ /mɔm/↓ *Momentanément, je* /sʃ/↓ /sʃ/↓ *je suis* / Rœ/↓ /Rœ/↓ *représentant en vins. C'est*↓ *ce*↓ *ce n'est pas mon métier en temps normal. Mais*↓ *mais*↓ *J'*/eti/↓ *j'étais représentant, mais de*↓ *de* /li/↓ /le/↓ *linoléums.* /ɑ̃/↓ /ɑ̃/↓ *Avant* /li/↓ *la guerre, j'étais agent d'une* /y/↓ /y/↓ *usine de . . . d'une* /pa/↓ /pafi/↓ /fabikœ/ *de linoléums et* /twa/ *cirées.*'

'/mɔ/↓ /mɔm/↓ Momentarily, I /sʃ/↓ /sʃ/↓ I'm a /Rœ/ ↓ /Rœ/↓ representative for wines. It's↓ it↓ It's not my work in usual times. But↓ But↓ I /eti/↓ I was a representative, but of↓ of ↓ /li/↓ /le/↓ linoleums. /ɑ̃/↓ /ɑ̃/↓ Before /li/↓ the war, I was an agent for a /y/↓ /y/↓ factory of . . . of a /pa/↓ /pafi/↓ /fabikœ/ of linoleums and waxed /twa/.'

Phonetic disintegration was also evident in repetition and in oral reading. While the articulatory disturbance was observed in both French and English utterances, it was considered to be less obvious in English.*

Written expression: written composition was slower than expected, probably as a result of the residual right hemiparesis. Written language was otherwise normal, including its properly graphic aspects. In January 1948, Mr Fri. wrote the following passage (40) in 19 minutes. It describes one of Caran d'Ache's stories without words (Fig. 8-26). The few deviations which appear in his text are less frequent than those which can be observed in the written compositions of many normal subjects (see Chapter 14):

(8.40) '*Un officier de hussard a manifesté le désir de se rendre à la revue, monté, je veux dire à cheval. Depuis des années il n'avait pas fait d'équitation et avait pris un embonpoint remarquable. Son désir (est) exaucé, c'est-a-dire qu'on lui amène un superbe pur-sang en vue de l'exaucer. Mais pour monter à cheval, c'est une affaire qui s'avère impossible sans le secours d'un aide. L'aide qui avait (amené) le cheval est à proximité. L'officier l'appelle, mais malgré tous ses efforts, c'est en vain que l'opération est tentée. Il se trouve à passer un camarade de notre homme de corvée, il l'appelle, et tous deux au prix d'efforts considérables, arrivent à mettre l'officier sur le cheval. Mais patatras, le bel officier pique une tête et son uniforme de grande tenue, le plumet, le casque qui lui est descendu plus bas que les oreilles, son bedon a fait éclater sa veste, ses*

* It was this particular dissociation which was emphasized in the clinical study of Mr Fri.'s case, published by Alajouanine, Pichot and Durand[132].

genoux qui ont marqué sur la culotte. Le rêve n'est plus réalisable. Le bel officier est ramené par le jeune homme de corvée, à qui l'aventure provoque une hilarité bien compréhensive.'

'A hussard officer expressed the desire to go to the review, mounted, I mean on a horse. He had not been horseback riding for years and had become remarkably stout. His desire (is) granted, that is, he is given a superb thoroughbred in order to grant it. But mounting a horse turns out to be an impossible venture without the succour of an aide-de-camp. The aide-de-camp who had (brought) the horse is nearby. The officer calls him, but in spite of all his efforts, it is in vain that the operation is attempted. It so happens that a comrade of our chore man passes by, he calls him, and the both of them at the expense of considerable effort succeed in getting the officer on the horse. But bang, the handsome officer falls on his head and his ceremonial uniform, the plume, the helmet that has fallen below his ears, his belly had made his jacket burst, his knees that have stamped on the breeches. The dream is no longer possible. The handsome officer is brought back by the chore man to whom the adventure was the cause of very understandable hilarity.'

Comprehension: both spoken and written language comprehension were normal. In January 1948, Mr Fri. had no difficulty in following the 25 progressively more complex orders on the Weisenberg and McBride test[136–138].

Psychological evaluation: during the first trimester of 1948, Mr Fri. completed an extensive battery of psychological tests (see Chapter 16). All results were found to be within normal limits, including those obtained on the Standard Progressive Matrices (PM-38) (90th percentile), the Weigl-Goldstein-Scheerer Colour Form Sorting Test and the Trist-Hargreaves Progressive Shapes Test (thus there was no disturbance, in Goldstein's terms[99], of abstract attitude [see Insertion 10.2]), the Bender Motor Gestalt Test; the Complex Figure of Rey; the Thurstone S Factor Test and W Factor Test; and the Binois-Pichot Vocabulary Test (90th percentile). Very similar results were obtained during the first trimester of 1949.

Mr Fri. was followed at *la Salpêtrière* until 1952. In later years, he complained that his memory was declining. Although his speech became slightly more rapid, his articulatory disturbance never disappeared completely. He died of cardiac disease in 1957. An autopsy was performed and the brain was kept in formalin. In 1963 the specimen was brought to *la Salpêtrière* where a neuropathological description was made by Professor Jean-Claude Gautier.

Anatomoclinical predictions

Mr Fri.'s case could not be more classical as it very clearly demonstrates the three characteristic dissociations of isolated anarthria (see Insertion 3.1). Consequently, one speaks of a 'pure' form of aphasia; and one does not hesitate to attribute it to a lesion 'outside' the language zone. This lesion could be small and subcortical, disconnecting Broca's area from the adjacent portion of the precentral gyrus; it could destroy this structure itself or be limited, perhaps in depth, to the axons leaving it; it could destroy other structures of Pierre Marie's quadrilateral[83, 139] (see Fig. 8-20); or it could involve a combination of all these different possibilities (see Chapter 8-3). Furthermore, it would not be surprising to find, in addition, a partial lesion of Broca's area (perhaps only such a lesion?), or again a partial lesion of the inferior portion of the left postcentral gyrus[93].

Anatomoclinical examination

The specimen was artefactually flattened in its dorsoventral aspect. Surface inspection showed

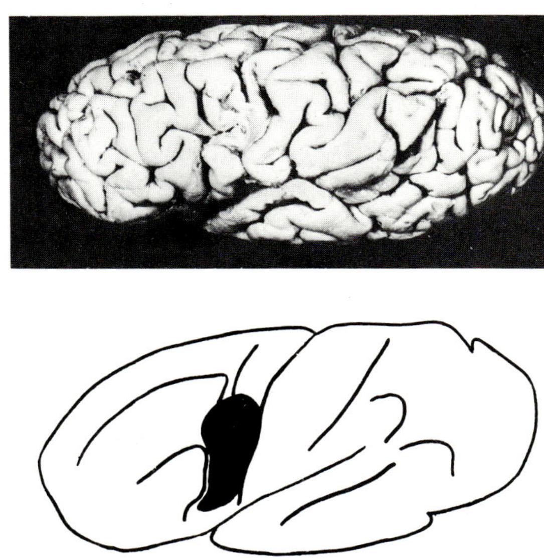

Fig. 8-27 *Case E. Fri. Pure anarthria (clinical picture described in Alajouanine, Pichot and Durand[132]). Above, macroscopic pathological anatomy: lateral surface of the left hemisphere and superficial location of the infarct according to a sketch made at the time of autopsy by Professor Jean-Claude Gautier* (Hôpital de la Salpêtrière). *On the surface, the infarct is confined to the lower half of the precentral gyrus. From Lecours and Lhermitte[88].*

an old softening of the inferior half of the left precentral gyrus. It spared the *pars opercularis* of F3 but slightly encroached upon the corresponding part of F2 (Fig. 8–27).

Brain sections revealed the presence of a very small cortical–subcortical lesion (old infarct) in the depths of the left cingulate sulcus (Fig. 8–28a, arrow). Coronal sections through and in front of Broca's area (Fig. 8–28a and b) showed no macroscopic or microscopic evidence of a lesion. On the other hand, the lesion destroyed the caudalmost few millimetres of the caudalmost part of F2 (Fig. 8–27b). A section through the left precentral gyrus (Fig. 8–28c) showed an ischaemic necrotic cortical–subcortical lesion of its inferior half. It destroyed, with the exception of a very narrow opercular fringe, the cortex of the precentral gyrus and the subjacent fibres including the U-fibres linking the precentral gyrus to F3, F2 and the postcentral gyrus. The cortex of the anterior part of the insula was damaged (Fig. 8–28c and d) but the underlying structures were spared. The temporoparietal structures were undamaged (Fig. 8–28d, e and f). Moderate neuronal rarefaction was observed throughout the entire cortical mantle.

Discussion

In this case, the lesions observed at autopsy were located in the expected sites, that is, outside the classical language zone (see Fig. 8–5). They are completely consistent with the articulatory disturbance observed after Mr Fri.'s cerebral vascular accident of December 1947. Considering the lesions observed in this patient and in the two

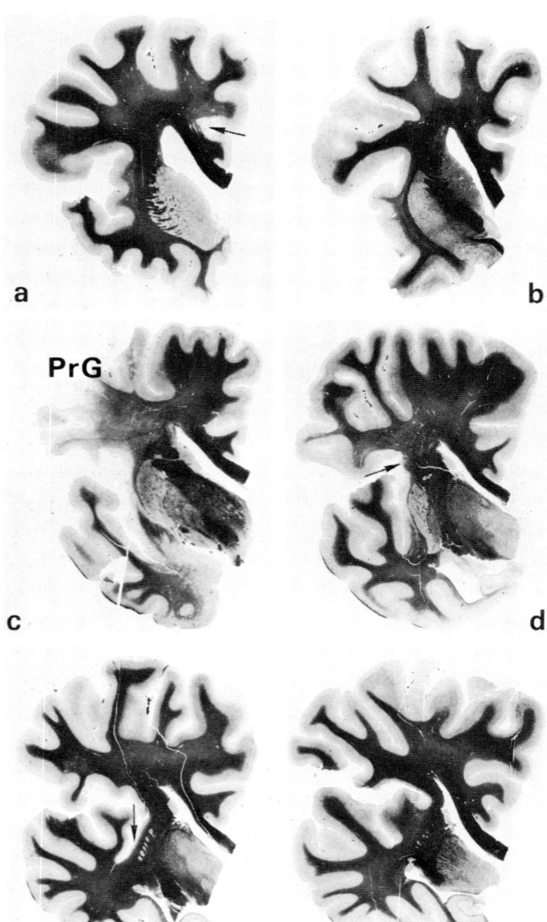

Fig. 8–28 *Case E. Fri. Pure anarthria (clinical picture described in Alajouanine, Pichot and Durand[132]). Above, pathological anatomy: coronal sections of the left cerebral hemisphere; Loyez staining. Detailed description in the text. The principal lesion involved the cortex and subcortex of the inferior half of the precentral gyrus (PrG in c) but spared Broca's area. There were also small cortical lesions of the insula (c, d, e: arrows) as well as a small infarct in the depth of the left cingulate sulcus (a: arrow). From Lecours and Lhermitte[88].*

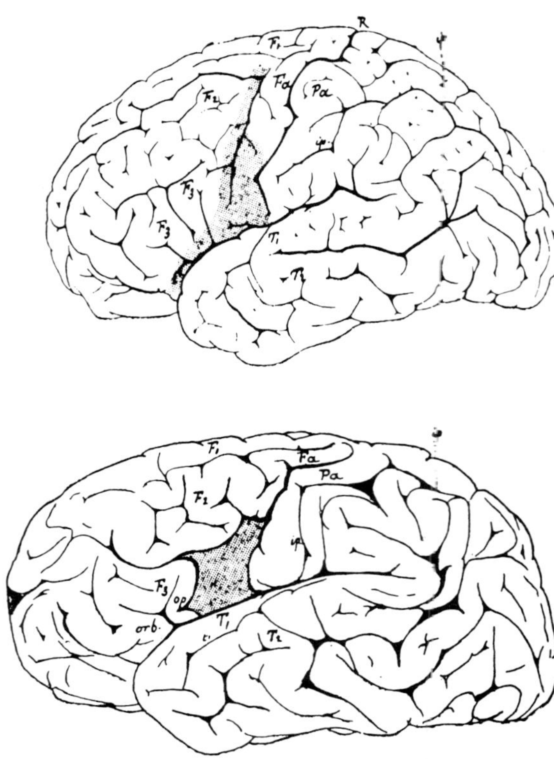

Fig. 8–29 *Bernheim's (upper) and Ladame's (lower) cases, the latter after Von Monakow. Commentary in the text. From Dejerine[90].*

cases on which Dejerine[90] based his theory of *motor aphasia* (the Ladame and Bernheim cases; Fig. 8-29), it can be suggested that damage to the precentral gyrus is more frequently involved in the origin of the articulatory disturbance in Broca's aphasia[140] than is usually thought. It can also be suggested that partial or complete regression of the articulatory disturbance—as may be the case for any sign of aphasia—results from a functional rearrangement, which is possible when there is only a relatively restricted lesion of a relatively vast functional territory (see Chapters 7-3 and 8-3).

We have presented three anatomoclinical case studies intended to illustrate an unquestionably valuable method of investigation. Each case was discussed with reference to the classical 'language zone': in the first case, the aphasia resulted from a predicted lesion within the 'language zone'; in the second case, the 'language zone' was also involved but the lesions were not entirely predictable and the case could not be readily explained within a bidimensional conceptual framework of the neural structures responsible for the control of linguistic behaviours; in the third case, the aphasia resulted from a lesion whose localization was predictable but was outside the 'language zone'. Given these findings, one wonders whether the classical conception of the language zone [as presented elsewhere in this work (cf pp. 168-171 and Fig. 8-5)] should not be critically reconsidered.

5 THE LANGUAGE ZONE

It has long been known that certain abnormal behaviours observed in clinical neurology are specifically related to the onset of precisely localized cerebral lesions.* Bouillaud[142] taught, as early as 1825, that the site of a lesion could be deduced from knowledge of the signs and symptoms which it caused (see Chapter 1). It is thus also known that the abnormal behaviours related to particular sites of lesion are not observed in the presence of lesions located elsewhere in the brain. Finally, it is known that certain predictable behaviours can be elicited through the application of electrical stimulation to certain precise points of the brain (see Chapter 7). These behaviours may, or may not, correspond to phenomena observed in normal individuals in natural situations and they may, or may not, correspond to disturbances observed following lesions of these same regions. It was on the basis of these facts that neurologists of the past century and the beginning of the present one developed the concept that different anatomical *centres* constituted the specific *sites* of different psychological *functions*. Within this conceptual framework, it was maintained that a psychological *function* is *localized* or *represented* in a specific zone of the central nervous system. Explicitly rejected by Freud in 1891[143], this notion of a *centre as a site of function* is almost obsolete today (Insertion 8.6). It must nevertheless be recognized that certain parts of the brain are essential, in a specific way, for certain functions such as visual perception, auditory perception, recognition of the body[145], language, etc. In other words, it must be recognized that the notions of *cerebral localization* and *functional specialization* are based on solid anatomoclinical foundations. This is true even if the effects of the lesion of a given area may vary, to a certain extent, according to the patient's age and the aetiology of the lesion (see Chapter 9), if they may also vary according to the time of evolution of the pathological process and even if the effects of the lesion may differ from those of surgical excision or from those of electrical stimulation.

There is no doubt that man's acquisition, comprehension, and production of articulated language (see Sections 8-1 and 8-3) are, in the final analysis, dependent upon the activity of his central nervous system. Neither is there any doubt that a very large number of neural structures somehow participate in the elaboration of linguistic behaviours. For example, since a state of alertness is necessary for most linguistic exchanges, it can be asserted that the reticular formation is not extraneous to language behaviour. To give another example, the blind naming of an object palpated with the left hand depends on information initially addressed, at the cortical level, to a right parietal area, so that it may be

* For example, physicians of ancient Egypt knew that a hemispheric lesion causing hemiplegia is contralateral to the side of hemiplegia (Edwin Smith's papyrus).

Insertion 8.6

Here is what one of us (F.L.) said in this regard in the context of his inaugural lesson[144]: 'What are then the relationships which exist between the lesion of the brain and the functional disorganizations which are the consequence?

The facts are well known: circumscribed lesions situated in different regions of the brain disorganize, in a varied manner, visual and auditory perception, recognition of the body, orientation in space, constructional activities, abstract thought.

It was not long ago, but this time is now past, when, confounding the lesion with the disturbances it caused, neurologists drew a map of the brain, a mosaic of functions and of fragments of consciousness. Such interpretations are no longer conceivable. The impairment of any one activity does not mean that the function is located in the lesioned part of the central nervous system, but only that this [part of the central nervous system] is essential to its accomplishment. The complex activities which we have in mind are integrated in a series of cerebral mechanisms so complicated that we are unable to identify with precision structure and function. The whole brain participates in them, but, depending on the activity considered, the different regions have roles of unequal importance, dominant for some, unobtrusive—at least apparently unobtrusive—for others.'

asserted that this area is required for completely normal linguistic behaviour. Although the number of such examples can be easily multiplied, they in no way constitute a denial of the predominant role played by certain hemispheric structures (left hemisphere in the vast majority of cases) in regard to language. It is these structures, generally identified through the application of the anatomoclinical method (see Chapter 8-4, pp. 195-196) which are collectively designated by the name *speech area*, *language area*, *language territory* or *language zone*.

We have already discussed elsewhere in this work the most generally taught conception (the so-called *classical* conception) of the language zone (see Chapter 8-1). With only very rare exceptions, the 'language zone' has remained resolutely bidimensional since the work of Gall[146]. It has nevertheless shown, depending on the observations and hypotheses of different individuals, a peculiar tendency to move about, to occupy a more extensive territory at certain times and a more restricted one at other times.

Gall and Spurzheim, whose principal arguments were not those which we have enumerated here (see Chapter 1), recognized the existence of various *organs* (parts of the cortical mantle) which constituted the seats of an equal number of 'moral and intellectual faculties'. They thus localized loyalty, patriotism, magnanimity, dependence, attraction to wine, parental love, domestic instincts, courage, reticence, modesty, sexual drive and *memory*. The seat of memory, which was soon destined to become *verbal memory*,* was situated in the anterior lobules of the brain at the level of the orbital surfaces[146]. The first in the list of the language zones was thus bilateral and situated on the inferior surface of the frontal lobes (Fig. 8-30).

Although they engaged in passionate polemics about Gall's teaching, XIXth century physicians scarcely sought empirical verification of the phrenological postulates. There was, however, one important exception which should be mentioned. In regard to *verbal memory*, henceforth considered as a *faculty* or as a *function*, the validity of the *centre* (anatomical site of a psychological function) was, in fact, soon questioned. The language zone then underwent the first of a series of metamorphoses.

In 1825, 18 years after Gall settled in Paris and three years before his death, Bouillaud[142] maintained, on the basis of his anatomoclinical studies, that 'the loss of speech corresponds to a lesion of the anterior lobules of the brain'. This original work merits several comments: it inaugurated the era of major anatomoclinical studies of aphasia; although Bouillaud was clearly con-

* This change was no doubt fostered by the fact that Gall's arguments concerning what he called *memory* were largely based on the observation of linguistic behaviours.

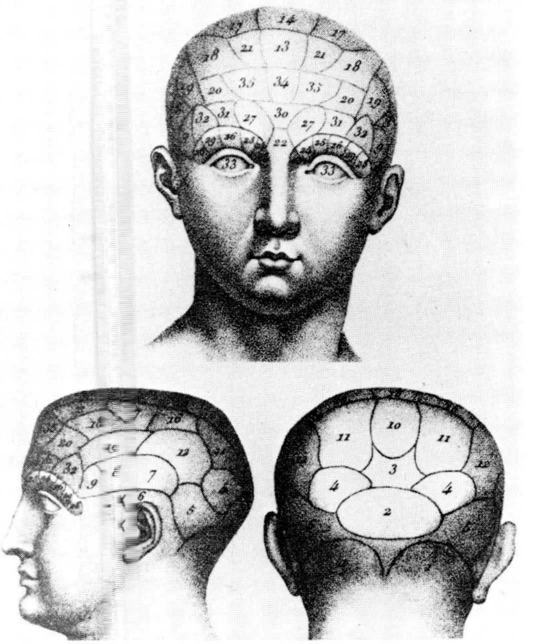

Fig. 8-30 *Phrenological localizations according to François Joseph Gall. The seat of verbal 'memory' is at 33, which corresponds to the orbital surfaces of the frontal lobes.*

vinced that his observations confirmed Gall's teachings, he spoke of the seat of *articulated language* (see Chapter 1) rather than of the seat of *verbal memory*; Bouillaud was concerned only with negative expressive symptomatology, that is, with a loss of speech (his patients would now be called Broca's aphasics or else global aphasics); like Gall, Bouillaud considered the seat of language to be bilateral but, unlike Gall, he did not specify a precise localization at the level of the orbital surfaces. The language zone, consisting of the whole of the frontal lobes, thus gained considerable territory with Bouillaud (Fig. 8-31).

In 1836 Dax[15, 147, 148] argued, also on the basis of anatomoclinical evidence, that aphasia was caused by cerebral diseases of the left hemisphere and not by those of the right. The wording of Dax's discussion suggests that he did not restrict the localization of 'verbal memory' to the left frontal lobe and that, unlike Bouillaud, he took different clinical forms of aphasia into consideration. With Dax, the language zone thus lost prerolandic territory on the right but gained approximately equal retrorolandic territory on the left.

Broca's modifications were made at two different times. Like Bouillaud, Broca was only concerned with the aphasic disorder which was eventually to bear his name. In 1861[149–151], and again in 1863[152], he emphasized that aphemia was caused by lesions located on the lateral surface of the frontal lobe (without precision regarding laterality) and not on the orbital surfaces which, he specified, were intact. In 1865, Broca[16, 153] attributed a lateralized, and very precisely circumscribed territory to the language zone (or the *seat of the faculty of articulated language*). He considered lesions of the pars opercularis and pars triangularis of the left, third frontal convolution to be the cause of aphemia (in right-handers).

From Gall to Broca, the language zone was viewed in terms of a *centre*. Wernicke[60] thereafter developed an *associationist model*. The hypothesis which he presented in 1874 can be summarized as follows: there is a *centre of motor word images* (*Bewegungsvorstellungen*) (Insertion 8.7) composed of the caudalmost part of the left, third frontal convolution; a lesion of this area results in the onset of a *motor aphasia* [i.e., of Broca's *aphemia* (see Chapters 1-1 and 10)]. There is also a centre of *auditory word images*, localized in the posterior half of the left, first temporal convolution; a lesion of this area results in a sensory aphasia [i.e., in Baillarger's[154] terms, in *aphasia with perversion of the faculty of language* (see Chapter 10)]. These two centres are connected by long axons; an isolated lesion of these axons would result in a third type of language disturbance, namely, conduction aphasia (*Leitungsaphasie*). Thus, with Wernicke, the language zone remained on the left but became a discontinuous territory including two centres linked to each other by long association fibres.

In 1881, Exner[155] suggested that the caudalmost part of the left, second frontal convolution constituted a graphic motor centre which had the same importance for written language as did the caudalmost part of the left, third frontal convolution for oral language.

The associationist model became more complex with the work of Bastian[156–159], Charcot[160, 161], Lichteim[162, 163], etc. According to Bastian, language is governed by four centres and their interconnections. The centre of *glossokinaesthetic* word images corresponds to the caudalmost part of the left, third frontal convolution and that of their *cheirokinaesthetic* images to the caudalmost part of the left, second frontal convolution; the centre of auditory word images

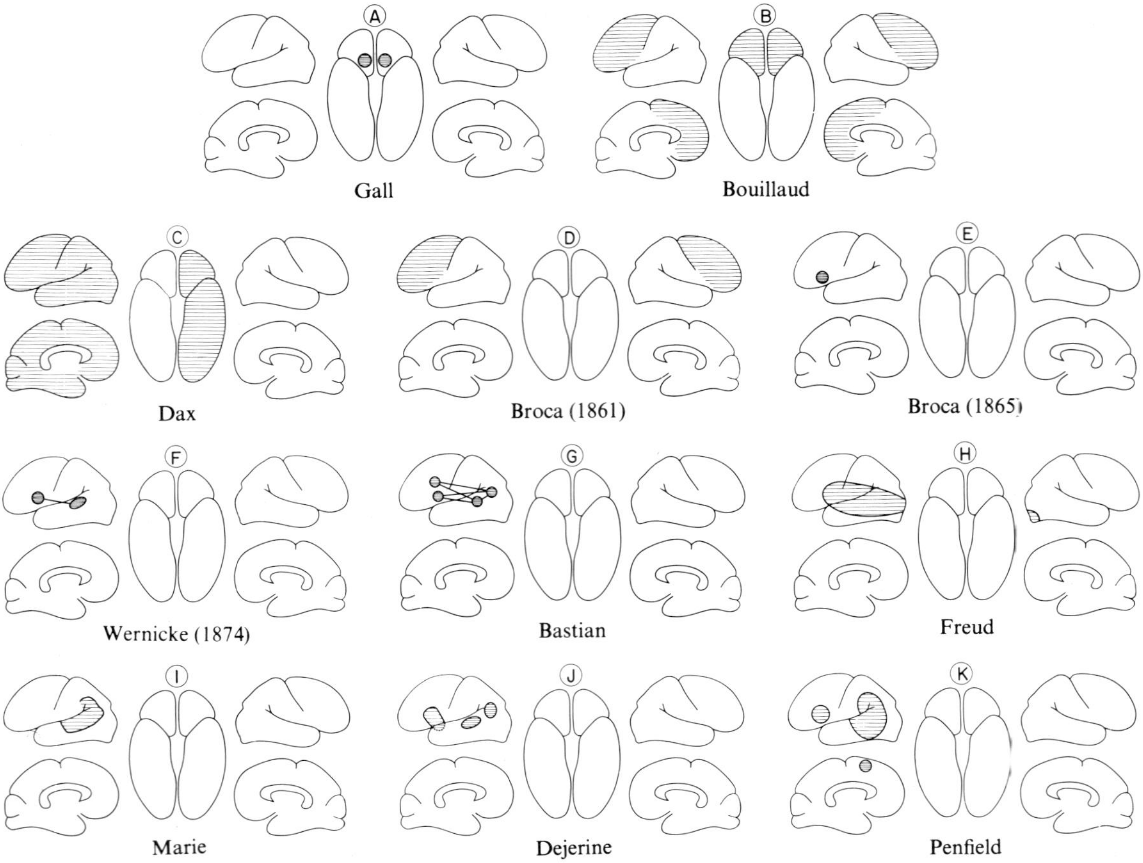

Fig. 8–31 *Metamorphoses of the language zone from François Joseph Gall to Wilder Penfield. Commentary in the text.*

Insertion 8.7

'for reasons to be later discussed, it must be assumed that movements of the body and changes in the state of the musculature generate sensations, memory images of which are also stored in the cerebral cortex. For the sake of brevity, we shall call these memory images of movement sensations either movement representations or movement images.' [Translated from Wernicke[17].]

corresponds to the caudal half of the left, first temporal convolution and that of their visual images is located in the left, inferior parietal lobule. While remaining discontinuous and lateralized, the language zone thus reacquired a part of the territory lost through the works of Dax to those of Wernicke.

At the end of the last century, Pierre Marie[83, 164, 165], who also followed the anatomoclinical method, concluded that it did not validate the associationists' assertions. Although he considered that the notions of *centres* and *images* had no empirical bases, he nevertheless maintained that aphasia was caused by lesions of a continuous retrorolandic area, namely, Wernicke's territory. According to Marie, this territory includes the caudal half of the left, first temporal convolution as well as the adjacent portion of the second temporal convolution, and the supramarginal and angular gyri on the same side.

Lesions at any point within this territory disturb all aspects of linguistic behaviour (with the severity of the aphasia being proportional to the size of the lesion), so that there is no reason to subdivide Wernicke's territory into several centres. As for anarthria, Marie considered it to be a different disorder from aphasia and the result of a subcortical lesion involving the lenticular zone [Pierre Marie's quadrilateral (see Fig. 8-20)]. If the doctrinal implications of Marie's terminological choices are ignored, his teachings could be said to involve another modification of the language zone (Fig. 8-31): it lost its frontal component;* enlarged its temporal component and acquired a parietal component; and for the first time acquired an explicit subcortical component (the quadrilateral), that is, a third dimension. It even regained some territory on the right since, according to Pierre Marie, lesions of the region which cause anarthria may be situated in either the left or the right hemisphere[166].

During the same period, the language zone was also defined by Dejerine[89, 90, 101, 108, 167], whose conclusions were also based on anatomoclinical studies and reflected his characteristic precision. Dejerine's *Broca's area* was enlarged and became *Broca's territory*, combining the pars opercularis and the pars triangularis of the left, third frontal convolution, including the corresponding frontal operculum, the adjacent caudalmost part of the left, second frontal convolution and ('possibly') the anterior part of the insula; Dejerine explicitly excluded the rolandic operculum and all of the precentral gyrus. Besides Broca's region, the language zone included Wernicke's region (the caudal half of the left, first and second temporal convolutions) and a posterior portion corresponding to the left angular gyrus.† Dejerine considered this last component to be the centre of *visual word images*. Like the Germans and the English, Dejerine recognized that the language zone included an association network[1]: he described it very precisely and emphasized the importance of the 'association fibres and, in particular, [of the] fibres of the superior longitudinal or arcuate fasciculus which connect Broca's region to the angular gyrus and to Wernicke's region' (see Fig. 8-6).

In 1891, Freud[143] resolutely rejected current fashions in thinking about the language zone. According to Freud, the language zone is composed of 'a continuous cortical region occupying the space between the terminations of the optic and acoustic nerves and of the areas of the cranial and certain peripheral motor nerves in the left hemisphere.'‡ Although Freud did not agree with the postulates of anatomic associationism, his writings, like those of Dejerine, were very explicit about the connections linking the different parts of the language zone to each other and to the rest of the brain, callosal connections included. With Freud, the language zone thus underwent a considerable superficial extension (Fig. 8-32): it included the insula and, significantly, acquired primary cortical components.

Curiously enough, it was a combination of Wernicke's and Pierre Marie's views which finally prevailed and thus became the classical conception of the language zone (see Section 8-5 and Fig. 8-5). Restrictive in terms of its frontal component (limited to the caudalmost part of F3), it was more inclusive in its retrorolandic components (posterior part of T1, supramarginal gyrus, angular gyrus). For some time now, certain aphasiologists have also considered the language zone to include another component, namely the caudal-internal part of the first frontal convolution, namely *Penfield's supplementary motor area*[14] (see Chapter 7) (Fig. 6-1).

The classical conception of the language zone has certain advantages: first, it is reassuring because it is consistent with tradition and is almost universally accepted and taught; furthermore, lesions of its various components are, in

---

* During a meeting of the *Societé de Neurologie de Paris* (9 July 1908), Madame Dejerine (Augusta Klumpke)[139] presented sections horizontally crossing the quadrilateral above the level selected by Pierre Marie and demonstrated that there were close anatomical connections between the third frontal convolution and the superior, anterior and external sectors of the quadrilateral. Contrary to Pierre Marie's assertions, the quadrilateral is not entirely caudal to the third frontal convolution: at least a third of it is situated directly beneath the third frontal convolution.

† It is difficult to determine whether or not Dejerine considered the supramarginal gyrus to be an integral part of the language zone (see Chapter 10).

‡ In modern terms, this would correspond to a continuous cortical area of the left hemisphere, extending from the termination of the acoustic and optic pathways to the region of the motor pathways governing the buccophonatory and dominant-hand musculature.

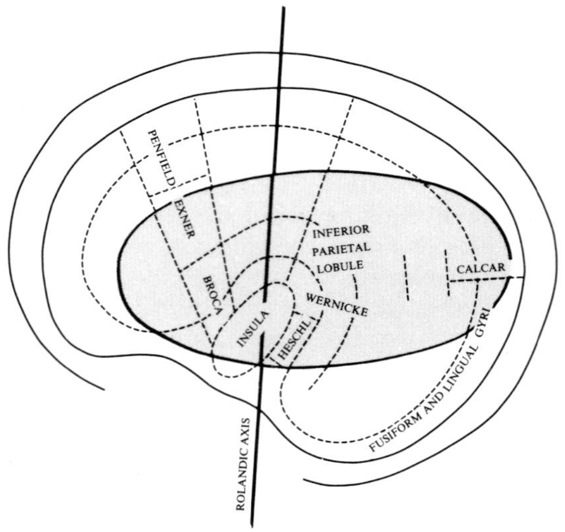

Fig. 8–32 *The language zone according to the anatomoclinical definition suggested by Sigmund Freud*[85]. *It is represented here in a Mercator projection (see Fig. 7–3). Commentary in the text.*

fact, among the most aphasiogenic. In our opinion, the major disadvantage is that this conception is not sufficiently operational, that is, its empirical utility is limited. Consider, for example, the implications of the classical conception in regard to the phonetic disintegration syndrome: if it occurs as an isolated or nearly isolated disturbance, it is called pure anarthria and it is not considered a form of aphasia but rather as a type of apraxia resulting from a lesion outside the language zone; on the other hand, when the same disturbance occurs within a more complex symptomatological context, one speaks of Broca's aphasia, that is, of the effect of a lesion of the language zone, and the phonetic disintegration is considered to be an essential characteristic of this form of aphasia. A similar line of reasoning can be followed in regard to word deafness: if it occurs in an isolated or nearly isolated state, revealing the presence of a lesion outside the language zone, it is asserted that it is not a form of aphasia but rather a type of agnosia; on the other hand, if it occurs within the more complex symptomatological context of a Type I Wernicke's aphasia, following a lesion of the caudal portion of the left, first temporal gyrus, it is considered to be one of the essential characteristics of this form of aphasia. Resulting, at least partially, from the fact that the lesions causing anarthria and word deafness may be situated outside the classical language zone, this manner of subdividing clinical reality does not facilitate reflection in physiopathological terms: it sometimes leads to the view that aphasia and apraxia, and aphasia and agnosia, are mutually exclusive and it sometimes implies that one is simply an aspect of the other.

There are many reasons to wish for the formulation and widespread acceptance of a less restrictive definition of the language zone, among them the following:

(a) Such a definition would emphasize that disturbances, which in any case are studied together, are actually members of the same physiopathological family. (Is it conceivable that pure word blindness would be omitted from an aphasiological treatise on the pretext that it is a type of agnosia?)
(b) It would also (partially) reduce the terminological imbroglios which are more misleading to students than pleasing to the experts. (Is it not curious that the aphasias which are called 'pure' are, in fact, those which result from a lesion situated outside the 'language zone'? Or again, that the notion of 'pure' aphasia is contrasted with that of 'true' aphasia?)
(c) A less restrictive definition of the language zone would reduce the hiatus between anatomophysiological and linguistic conceptions of aphasia. (If an acquired disturbance of the third linguistic phase is not an aphasia, why should that of the second phase be so considered: in other words, if anarthria is not an aphasia, why should conduction aphasia be considered an aphasia?)

Among the conceptions of the language zone discussed in the previous pages, there is one, namely that of Freud[143] (Fig. 8–32) which, in our opinion, proves more useful in clinical aphasiology than does the classical formulation. Thus Freud's conception will be one of the bases for an aphasia classification which will be presented in a later chapter of this work (see Chapter 10): we shall there discuss three groups of disturbances related to the malfunctioning of the various cortical components of the language zone and/or of their afferents or efferents (Insertion 8.8).

Although the Freudian conception of the language zone provides a more complete and more coherent frame of reference than does the classical conception, it clearly does not solve all the

Insertion 8.8

The cortical surface of the Freudian language zone can be subdivided into three compartments:

(a) A primary compartment including, on the motor side, the lower half of the precentral gyrus and, on the sensory side, the lower half of the postcentral gyrus, Heschl's gyri and the calcarine cortex. Obviously, the notion of functional specialization and localization does not apply to this primary compartment as it does to the other two.

(b) A specific association compartment including, on the motor side, Broca's area (caudalmost part of F3 on the left) and Exner's area (caudalmost part of F2 on the left) and, on the sensory side, a somaesthetic association zone (located in the middle parietal region and no doubt overlapping the lower part of the postcentral gyrus and the supramarginal gyrus), Wernicke's area (caudal half of T1 and T2 on the left) and at least a part of the visual association cortex (including the lingual and fusiform gyri on the left).

(c) A non-specific association compartment including, on the motor side, the prefrontal components of F3 and F2 on the left and, on the sensory side, the major part of the left inferior parietal lobule.

In the ontogenesis of the brain, maturation of the primary compartment begins and ends before that of the specific association compartment and maturation of this compartment begins and ends before that of the non-specific association compartment[11, 57, 61] (see Chapter 8–2).

problems of a clinician who, on the basis of his observations of abnormal linguistic behaviours, attempts the blind prediction of the site of eventual cerebral lesions. Several predictions remain guarded and a fair number prove to be inaccurate. This is partially due to presently limited knowledge of variables related to individual variations in the degree of functional lateralization for speech and language (see Chapter 11) and to even more limited knowledge of individual variations related to age and, especially for written language, to teaching methods and the intensity of the learning experience. Hesitant or inaccurate predictions are also due to the general persistence of a bidimensional view of the language zone, regardless of which particular conception is taken as a reference,. It is known, however, that deep lesions may play a role in the onset of several clinical forms of aphasia. This was mentioned long ago by Pierre Marie[166] in regard to the region of the lenticular nucleus and by Dejerine[167] in regard to the long axons connecting the visual cortices to the angular region (see Fig. 8–20 and 8–21). Similarly, several more recent works on lesions and stimulation of the thalamus have emphasized the possible role of deep lesions in the origin of certain disturbances which fall within the general domain of aphasia (see Chapter 7–2 and Fig. 7–5). In other words, it will probably be appropriate, at some time in the near future, to develop and, above all, to teach, a tridimensional conception of the neuronal networks which underlie man's acquisition, comprehension and production of speech and language. This tridimensional view would no doubt involve consideration of the following facts: lesions of the components of the classical language zone (see Fig. 8–5) remain the most specifically aphasiogenic; the problems of functional localization and of lateralized hemispheric specialization are not the same for all structures which participate in the control of speech and language behaviours [left dominance is clearer and functional localization is less diffuse for the (association) components of the classical language zone than for the primary cortical components of the Freudian zone or for certain subcortical structures (see Chapter 11)]; hemispheric dominance becomes increasingly clear as the behaviours considered become more complex and more highly integrated; it becomes less and less obvious as behaviours become increasingly automatized (see Chapter 8–4 and Insertion 11.2); certain thalamic relay nuclei no doubt play, as part of the anatomical foundations of speech and language[168] (see Chapter 7), a role which is clearly less important and less specific than those of their corresponding primary cortices; among the thalamic association nuclei, it appears that the ventral lateral and the pulvinar (and probably also the lateral posterior), particularly on the left, should immediately be included in a tridimensional model of the language zone (see Chapter 7): this may also be the case for other subcortical structures such as the caudate and pallidum.

REFERENCES

1. Dejerine, J. (1901) *Anatomie des centres nerveux*. Paris: Rueff.
2. Crosby, E.C., Humphrey, T. & Laver, E.W. (1962) *Correlative Anatomy of the Nervous System*. New York: Macmillan.
3. Peele, T.L. (1961) *The Neuroanatomic Basis for Clinical Neurology*. New York: McGraw-Hill.
4. Haymaker, W. (Ed.) (1969) *Bing's Local Diagnosis in Neurological Diseases*. St Louis, MO: Mosby.
5. Haymaker, W. (Ed.) (1972) *Diagnostic des localisations en neurologie*. Paris: Maloine.
6. Truex, R. & Carpenter, M.B. (1969) *Human Neuroanatomy*. Baltimore, MD: Williams and Wilkins.
7. Carpenter, M.B. (1973) *Core Text of Neuroanatomy*. Baltimore, MD: Williams and Wilkins.
8. Brodal, A. (1948) The cranial nerves. In *Neurological Anatomy in Relation to Clinical Medicine*. p. 188. Oxford: Clarendon.
9. Chatelain, E. (1883) *Lexique latin-français*. Paris: Hachette.
10. Penfield, W. & Rasmussen, Th. (1950) *The Cerebral Cortex of Man; a Clinical Study of Localization of Function*. New York: Macmillan.
11. Flechsig, P. (1920) *Anatomie des menschlichen Gehirns und Rückenmarks*. Leipzig: Thieme.
12. Pandya, D.N., Karol, E.A. & Heilbronn, D. (1971) The topographical distribution of interhemispheric projections in the corpus callosum of the rhesus monkey. *Brain Research*, **32,** 31.
13. Pandya, D.N. & Sanides, F. (1973) Architectonic parcellation of the temporal operculum in rhesus monkey and its projection pattern *Zeitschrift für Anatomie und Entwicklungsgeschichte*, **139,** 127.
14. Penfield, W. & Roberts, L. (1963) *Langage et mécanismes cérébraux*. Paris: Presses Universitaires de France. (Translated by J.-C. Gautier.)
15. Dax, M. (1865) Lésions de la moitié gauche de l'encéphale coïncidant avec l'oubli des signes de la pensée. *Gazette hebdomadaire de Médecine et de Chirurgie*, **33,** 259.
16. Broca, P. (1865) Du siège de la faculté du langage articulé. *Bulletin de la Société d'Anthropologie*, **7,** 377.
17. Wernicke, C. (1874) *Der aphasische Symptomenkomplex*. Breslau: Cohn and Weigert.
18. Eberstaller, O. (1884) Zur Oberflächenanatomie der Grosshirnhemisphären. *Wiener Medizine Blaetter*, **7,** 479, 542 and 644,
19. Economo, C. (von) & Horn, L. (1930) Uber Windungsrelief, Masse und Ridenarchitektonik der Supratemporalfläche, ihre individuellen und ihre seiten Unterschiede. *Zentralblatt für die gesamte Neurologie und Psychiatrie*, **130,** 678.
20. Pfeiffer, R.A. (1936) Pathologie der Horstrahlung und der corticalen Horsphäre. In *Handbuch der Neurologie* (Ed.) Bumke, O. & Foerster, O. p. 533, Vol. 6. Berlin: Springer.
21. Kakeshita, T. (1925) Zur Anatomies der operkularen temporal Region (vergleichende Untersuchungen der rechten und linken Seite). *Arbeiten aus dem neurologischen institulander weiner Universität*, **27,** 292.
22. Geschwind, N. & Levitsky, W. (1968) Human brain: left–right asymmetries in temporal speech region. *Science*, **161,** 186.
23. Teszner, D. (1972) *Etude anatomique de l'asymétrie droite-gauche du planum temporale*. Medical thesis, Paris.
24. Teszner, D., Tzavaras, A., Gruner, J. & Hécaen, H. (1972) L'asymétrie droite-gauche du planum temporale; à propos de l'étude anatomique de 100 cerveaux. *Revue neurologique*, **126,** 444.
25. Wada, J. (1974) Morphologic asymmetry of human cerebral hemispheres: temporal and frontal speech zones in 100 adult and 100 infant brains. *Neurology*, **24,** 349.
26. Wada, J., Clark, R. & Hamm, A. (1975) Cerebral hemispheric asymmetry in humans. *Archives of Neurology* (Chicago), **32,** 239.
27. Bonin, G. (von) (1967) Anatomical asymmetries of the cerebral hemispheres. In *Interhemispheric Relations and Cerebral Dominance* (Ed.) Mountcastle, V.B. p. 1. Baltimore, MD: Johns Hopkins.
28. Geschwind, N. (1974) *Selected Papers on Language and the Brain*. Dordrecht and Boston, MA: Reidel.
29. Hécaen, H. & Ajuriaguerra, J. (de) (1963) *Les gauchers*. Paris: Presses Universitaires de France.
30. Subirana, A. (1952) La droiterie. *Archives suises de Neurologie et de Pychiatrie*, **69,** 321.
31. Subirana, A. (1964) The relationship between handedness and language function. *International Journal of Neurology*, **4,** 215.
32. Subirana, A. (1969) Handedness and cerebral dominance. In *Handbook of Clinical Neurology* (Ed.) Vinken, P.J. & Bruyn, G.W. Vol. 4, p. 248. Amsterdam: North-Holland.
33. Lhermitte, F., Lecours, A.R., Ducarne, B. & Escourolle, R. (1974) Unexpected anatomical findings in a case of fluent jargon aphasia. *Cortex*, **10,** 83.
34. Yakovlev, P.I. (1962) Morphological criteria of growth

and maturation of the nervous system in man. *Research Publications, Association for Research in Nervous and Mental Diseases*, **39,** 3.

35. Kaes, T. (1907) *Die Grosshirnrinde des Meschen in ihrem Massen und in ihrem Fasengehalt*. Iéna: Fischer.
36. Kemper, T.L., Lecours, A.R., Gates, M.J. & Yakovlev, P.I. (1973) Retardation of the myelo- and cytoarchitectonic maturation of the brain in the congenital rubella syndrome. *Early Development, Research Publication of the Association for Research in Nervous and Mental Disease*, **51,** 23.
37. Altman, P. & Dittmar, D. (1962) *Growth*. Washington: Federation of American Societies of Experimental Biology.
38. Larroche, J.C. (1967) Maturation morphologique du système nerveux central: ses rapports avec le développement pondéral du fœtus et son âge gestationnel. In *Regional Development of the Brain in Early Life*. (Ed.) Minkowski, A. p. 247. Oxford: Blackwell.
39. Torgersen, J.M. (1954) The occiput, the posterior cranial fossa and the cerebellum. In *Aspects of Cerebellar Anatomy*. (Ed.) Jansen, J. & Brodal, A. p. 396. Olso: Grundt Tanum.
40. Dullemeijer, P. (1971) Comparative ontogeny and cranio-facial growth. In *Cranio-facial Growth* (Ed.) Meyers, R.E. & Krogman, W.M. p. 45. New York: Pergamon.
41. Epstein, H.T. (1974) Phrenoblysis: special brain and mind growth periods. I. Human brain and skull development. *Developmental Psychobiology*, **7,** 207.
42. Epstein, H.T. (1974) Phrenoblysis: special brain and mind growth periods. II. Human mental development. *Developmental Psychobiology*, **7,** 217.
43. Yakovlev, P.I. (1948) Motility, behavior and the brain. Stereodynamic organization and neural co-ordinates of behavior. *Journal of Nervous and Mental Diseases*, **107,** 313.
44. Yakovlev, P.I. (1963) Telokinesis and handedness (an empirical generalization). In *Recent Advances in Biological Psychiatry* (Ed.) Wortis, J. Vol. 6, p. 21. New York: Plenum Press.
45. Yakovlev, P.I. (1968) Telencephalon 'impar', 'semipar' and 'totopar' (morphogenetic, tectogenetic and architectonic definitions). *International Journal of Neurology*, **6,** 245.
46. Yakovlev, P.I. (1970) The structural and functional 'trinity' of the body, brain and behavior. *Topical Problems in Psychiatrical Neurology*, **10,** 197.
47. Yakovlev, P.I. (1972) A proposed definition of the limbic system. In *Limbic System Mechanisms and Autonomic Function* (Ed.) Hockman, C.H. p. 241. Springfield, IL: Thomas.
48. Gratiolet, L.P. (1854) *Mémoire sur les plis cérébraux de l'homme et des primates*. Paris: Bertrand.
49. Lilly, J.C. (1963) Critical brain size and language. *Perspectives in Biology and Medicine*, **6,** 246.
50. Rakič, P. & Yakovlev, P.I. (1968) Development of the corpus callosum and cavum septi in man *Journal of Comparative Neurology*, **132,** 45.
51. Lecours, A.R. (1982) Correlates of developmental behavior in brain maturation. In T. Bever (Ed.), *Regression in Development* (Ed.) Bever, T. Hills Dale: LEA Press.
52. Flechsig, P. (1901) Developmental (myelogenetic) localization of the cerebral cortex in the human subject. *Lancet*, **2,** 1027.
53. Flechsig, P. (1927) *Meine myelogenetische Hirnlehre*. Berlin: Springer.
54. Vogt, C. (1900) *Etude sur la myélinisation des hémisphères cérébraux*. Medical thesis, Paris.
55. Vogt, C. & Vogt, O. (1904) Die Markreifung des Kindergehirns während der ersten vier Lebensmonate und ihre methodogische Bedeutung. In *Neurobiologische Arbeiten* (Erster Serie, Erster Band) (Ed.) Vogt, O. Jèna: Fischer.
56. Langworthy, O. (1933) Development of behavior patterns and myelination of the nervous system in the human foetus and infant. *Contributions to Embryology*, **139,** 1.
57. Yakovlev, P.I. & Lecours, A.R. (1967) The myelogenetic cycles of regional maturation of the brain. In *Regional Development of the Brain in Early Life* (Ed.) Minkowski, A. p. 3. Oxford: Blackwell.
58. Bertrand, I. (1930) *Techniques histologiques de neuropathologie*. Paris: Masson.
59. Bailey, P. & Bonin, G. (von) (1951) *The Isocortex of Man*. Urbana, IL: University of Illinois Press.
60. Wernicke, C. (1966) The symptom complex of aphasia. In *Boston Studies in the Philosophy of Science*, (Ed.) Cohen, R.S. & Watofsky, M.W. Vol. 4. Boston, MD: O. Riedel.
61. Lecours, A.R. (1975) Myelinogenetic correlates of the development of speech and language. In *Foundations of Language Development: a Multidisciplinary Approach* (Ed.) Lenneberg, E. & Lenneberg, E. Vol. I, p. 121. New York: Academic Press.
62. Ey, H., Bernard, P. & Brisset, C. (1963) *Manuel de psychiatrie*. Paris: Masson.
63. Berry, M.F. (1968) *Language Disorders of Children: the Bases and Diagnosis*. New York: Appleton.
64. Gesell, A. (1940) *The First Five Years of Life*. New York: Harper.
65. Gesell, A. & Amatruda, C.S. (1947) *Developmental Diagnosis*. New York: Hoeber.
66. Gruber, J.S. (1967) Topicalization in child language. *Foundations of Language*, **3,** 37.
67. Osterrieth, P. (1966) *Introduction à la psychologie de l'enfant*. Paris: Presses Universitaires de France.
68. Lenneberg, E.H. (1967) *Biological Foundations of Language*. New York: Wiley.
69. Lecours, A.R. & Vanier-Clément, M. (1976) Schizophasia and jargonaphasia. A comparative description with comments on Chaika's and Fromkin's respective looks at 'schizophrenic' language. *Brain and Language*, **3,** 516.
70. Brain, R. & Walton, J.N. (1969) *Brain's Diseases of the Nervous System*. London and New York: Oxford University Press.

71. Piaget, J. (1949) *La psychologie de l'intelligence*. Paris: A. Colin.
72. Piaget, J. (1954) Le langage et la pensée du point de vue génétique. *Acta Psychologica*, **10,** 51.
73. Piaget, J. (1959) *La formation du symbole chez l'enfant*. Paris: Delachaux et Niestlé.
74. Piaget, J. (1965) Langage et pensée. *Revue pratique* (Paris), **15,** 2253.
75. Piaget, J. (1967) *Biologie et connaissance*. Paris: Gallimard.
76. Brodmann, K. (1925) *Vergleichende Lokalisationslehre der Grosshirnrinde*. Leipzig: Barth.
77. Bailey, P. & Bonin, G. (von) (1957) Evolution of the cerebral cortex, organ of the mind. *What's new*, **198,** 13.
78. Conel, J.L. (1941–1967) *The Postnatal Development of the Human Cerebral Cortex*. Cambridge, MA: Harvard University Press, 1941 to 1967, and London: Oxford University Press, 1964.
79. Purpura, D.P., Shofer, R.J., Housepian, E.M. & Noback, C.R. (1964) Comparative ontogenesis of structure–function relations in cerebral and cerebellar cortex. *Progress in Brain Research*, **4,** 187.
80. Purpura, D.P. (1967) Discussion de Gruner, J.E. and Zahnd, J.-P:, Sur la maturation synaptique dans le cortex visuel du lapin. In *Regional Development of the Brain in Early Life* (Ed.) Minkowski, A. p. 125. Oxford and Edinburgh: Blackwell.
81. Jacobson, M. (1970) *Developmental Neurobiology*. New York: Holt, Rinehart and Winston.
82. Woerdeman, M.W. (1950) *Atlas of Human Anatomy*. Vol. II, Philadelphia and Toronto: Blakiston.
83. Marie, P. (1926) *Travaux et mémoires*. Vol. I. Paris: Masson.
84. Marie, P. & Foix, C. (1917) Les aphasies de guerre. *Revue neurologique*, **1,** 53.
85. Freud, S. (1891) *Zur Auffasung der Aphasien* Vienna: Deuticke.
86. Broca, P. (1888) *Mémoires sur le cerveau de l'homme*. Paris: Reinwald.
87. Lhermitte, F., Lecours, A.R., Ducarne, B. & Escourolle, R. (1973) Unexpected anatomical findings in a case of fluent jargon aphasia. *Cortex*, **9,** 433.
88. Lecours, A.R. & Lhermitte, F. (1976) The 'pure forme' of the phonetic disintegration syndrome ('pure anarthria'); anatomo-clinical report of a historical case. *Brain and Language*, **3,** 88.
89. Dejerine, J. (1906) A propos de la localisation de l'aphasie motrice. *Presse médicale*, **56,** 742.
90. Dejerine J. (1906) L'aphasie motrice; sa localisation et sa physiologie pathologique. *Presse médicale*, **57,** 453.
91. Ladame, P.L. (1906) Aphasie et anarthrie (avec réponse de M.J. Dejerine). *Presse médicale*, **102,** 826.
92. Marie, P. (1906) Révision de la question de l'aphasie: la troisième circonvolution frontale ne joue aucun rôle spécial dans la fonction du langage. *Semaine médicale* (Paris), **26,** 241.
93. Luria, A.R. (1964) Factors and forms of aphasia. In *Disorders of Language* (Ed.) de Reuck, A.V.S. & O'Connor, M. p. 143. London: Churchill.
94. Geschwind, N. (1965) Disconnexion syndromes in animals and man. *Brain*, **88,** 237 and 585.
95. Benson, D.F. & Geschwind, N. (1977) The aphasias and related disturbances. In *Clinical Neurology* (Ed.) Baker, A. & Baker, L. Vol. 1, p. 1. Hagerstown: Harper and Row.
96. Benson, D.F., Sheremata, W.A., Bouchard. R. Segarra, J.M., Price, D & Geschwind, N. (1973) Conduction aphasia. A clinicopathological study. *Archives of Neurology* (Chicago), **28,** 339.
97. Lecours, A.R. (1975) Aphasie. *Encyclopédie médico-chirurigale, 17019 A^{10}*, 7, Paris.
98 Alajouanine, Th. & Lhermitte, F. (1964) The phonemic and semantic components of jargon aphasia. *Journal of Neurology*, **4,** 277-286.
99. Goldstein, K. (1948) *Language and Language Disturbance*. New York: Grune and Stratton.
100. Whitaker, H.A. (1976) Disorders of speech production mechanisms. In *Handbook of Perception* (Ed.) Carterette, E. & Friedman, M. Vol. 7, p. 429. New York: Academic Press.
101. Dejerine, J. (1906) L'aphasie sensorielle; sa localisation et sa physiologie pathologique. *Presse médicale*, **55,** 437.
102. Lecours, A.R. & Lhermitte, F. (1973) Phonemic paraphasias; linguistic structures and tentative hypotheses. In *Psycholinguistics and Aphasia* (Ed.) Goodglass, H. & Blumstein, S. p. 69. Baltimore, MD: Johns Hopkins University Press.
103. Jakobson, R. (1956) Two aspects of language and two types of aphasic disturbances. In *Fundamentals of Language* (Ed.) Jakobson, R. & Halle, M. p. 55. The Hague: Mouton.
104. Lecours, A.R., Deloche, G. & Lhermitte, F. (1973) Paraphasies phonémiques; description et simulation sur ordinateur. In *Colloques IRIA—Informatique médicale*, p. 311. Institut de recherche d'informatique et d'automatique, Rocquencourt.
105. Lecours, A.R. & Rouillon, F. (1976) Neurolinguistic analysis of jargonaphasia and jargonagraphia. In *Studies in Neurolinguistics* (Ed.) Avakian-Whitaker, H. & Whitaker, H. Vol. 2, p. 95. New York: Academic Press.
106. Geschwind, N., Quadfasel, F.A. & Segarra, J. (1968) Isolation of the speech area. *Neuropsychologia*, **6,** 327.
107. Dejerine, J. (1891) Sur un cas de cécité verbale avec agraphie, suivi d'autopsie. *Mémoires de la Société de Biologie*, **3,** 197.
108. Dejerine, J. (1892) Des différentes variétés de cécité verbale. *Mémoires de la Société de Biologie*, **4,** 1.
109. Dejerine, J. (1892) Contribution à l'étude anatomopathologique et clinique des différentes variétés de cécité verbale. *Mémoires de la Société de Biologie*, **4,** 61.
110. Pitres, A. (1898) L'aphasie amnésique et ses variétés cliniques. *Progrès médicale* (Paris), **7,** 321, 337, 369 and 401.
111. Pitres, A. (1898) L'aphasie amnésique et ses variétés cliniques. *Progrès médicale* (Paris), **8,** 17 and 65.
112. Pitres, A. (1898) *L'aphasie amnésique et ses variétés cliniques*. Paris: Alcan.

113. Lhermitte, F. (1965) Séméiologie de l'aphasie. *Revue pratique*, (Paris), **15,** 1.
114. Botez, M. . (1974) Frontal lobe tumours. In *Handbook of Clinical Neurology* (Ed.) Vinken, P.J. & Bruyn, G.W. Vol. 17, p. 234. Amsterdam: North-Holland, and New York: American Elsevier.
115. Lhermitte, F. & Derouesné, J. (1976) L'aphasie amnésique: étude de 25 cas. *Revue neurologique*, **132,** 669.
116. Geschwind, N. (1971) Aphasia. *New England Journal of Medicine*, **284,** 654.
117. Lhermitte, F., Chain, F., Escourolle, R., Ducarne, B., Pillon, B. & Chedru, F. (1971) Etude des troubles perceptifs auditifs dans les lésions temporales bilatérales. A propos de trois observations dont deux anatomo-cliniques. *Revue neurologique*, **124,** 329.
118. Peronnet, F. & Michel, F. (1977) The asymmetry of the auditory evoked potentials in normal man and in patients with brain lesions. *Progress in Clinical Neurophysiology*, **2,** 130.
119. Bouche, P. (1975) *Les lésions cérébrales de l'agnosie visuelle*. Medical thesis, Paris.
120. Geschwind, N. & Fusillo, M. (1966) Color-naming defects in association with alexia. *Archives of Neurology* (Chicago), **15,** 137.
121. Lhermitte, F., Chain, F., Aron, D., Leblanc, M. & Souty, C. (1969) Les troubles de la vision des couleurs dans les lésions postérieures du cerveau, à propos de 42 observations. *Revue neurologique*, **121,** 5.
122. Gerstmann, J. (1940) Syndrome of finger agnosia, disorientation for right and left, agraphia and acalculia. *Archives of Neurology and Psychiatry* (Chicago), **44,** 398.
123. Benton, A.L. (1977) Reflections on the Gerstmann syndrome. *Brain and Language*, **4,** 45.
124. Dejerine, J. (1908) Address to the meeting of the Société Neurologique de Paris, 9 July 1908. *Revue neurologique*, **16,** 977–990.
125. Dejerine, J. (1926) *Séméiologie des affectations du système nerveux*. p. 109. Paris: Masson.
126. Alajouanine, Th., Lhermitte, F., Ledoux, Renaud, D. & Vignolo, L.A. (1964) Les composantes phonémiques et sémantiques de la jargonaphasie. *Revue neurologique*, **110,** 5.
127. Lhermitte, F., Chain, F., Escourolle, R., Ducarne, B. & Pillon, B. (1972) Etude anatomoclinique d'un cas de prosopagnosie. *Revue neurologique*, **126,** 329.
128. Alajouanine, Th., Ombredane, A. & Durand, M. (1939) *Le syndrome de désintégration phonétique dans l'aphasie*. Paris: Masson.
129. Ombredane, A. (1926) Sur le mécanisme de l'anarthrie. *Journal de Psychologie normale et pathologique*, **61,** 940.
130. Penfield, W. & Roberts, L. (1959) *Speech and Brain Mechanisms*. Princeton, NJ: Princeton University Press.
131. Signoret, J.L. (1966) *Etude d'un apprentissage associatif chez 26 sujets présentant une aphasie par lésion cérébrale localisée*. Medical thesis, Paris.
132. Alajouanine, Th., Pichot, P. & Durand, M. (1949) Dissociation des altérations phonétiques avec conservation relative de la langue la plus ancienne dans un cas d'anarthrie pure chez un sujet français bilingue. *Encéphale*, **28,** 245.
133. Alajouanine, Th. & Lhermitte, F. (1960) Les troubles des activités expressives du langage dans l'aphasie; leurs relations avec les apraxies. *Revue neurologique*, **102,** 66.
134. Denny-Brown, D. (1963) The physiological basis of perception and speech. In *Problems of Dynamic Neurology* (Ed.) Halpern, L. p. 1. Jerusalem: Jerusalem Post Press.
135. Denny-Brown, D. (1965) Physiological aspects of disturbances of speech. *Australian Journal of Experimental Biology and Medical Science*, **43,** 455.
136. Weisenburg, T.H. (1934) A study of aphasia. *Archives of Neurology and Psychiatry* (Chicago), **31,** 1.
137. Weisenburg, T.H. & McBride, K.E. (1935) *Aphasia*. New York: Commonwealth Fund.
138. Weisenburg, T.H. & McBride, K.E. (1964) *Aphasia: a Clinical and Psychological Study*. New York: Hafner.
139. Klippel, M.M. (Ed.) (1908) Compte rendu de la réunion de la société neurologique de Paris du 9 juillet 1908: discussion sur l'aphasie (suite). *Revue neurologique*. **16,** 974. (Voir l'intervention de Mme Dejerine sur les limites supérieure et inférieure du quadrilatère de Pierre Marie.)
140. Bay, E. (1964) Principles of classification and their influence on our concepts of aphasia. In *Disorders of Language* (Ed.) de Reuck, A.V.S. & O'Connor, M. p. 122 London: Churchill.
141. Ombredane, A. (1951) *L'aphasie et l'élaboration de la pensée explicite*. pp. 398–399. Paris: PUF.
142. Bouillaud, J.B. (1825) Recherches cliniques propres à démontrer que la perte de la parole correspond à la lésion des lobules antérieurs du cerveau et à confirmer l'opinion de M. Gall, sur le siège de l'organe du langage articulé. *Archives générales de Médecine*, **8,** 25.
143. Freud, S. (1953) *On Aphasia; a Critical Study*. New York: International Universities Press.
144. Lhermitte, F. (1964) *Leçon inaugurale. Chaire de Neurologie et Neuropsychologie*. Paris: Masson.
145. Lhermitte, J. (1939) *L'image de notre corps*. Paris: Editions de la Nouvelle Revue Critique.
146. Gall, F.J. (1825) *Sur les fonctions du cerveau et sur de chacune de ses parties*. Paris: Baillière.
147. Joynt, R.L. & Benton, A.L. (1964) The memoir of Marc Dax on aphasia. *Neurology*, **14,** 851.
148. Benton, A.L. (1964) Contributions to aphasia before Broca. *Cortex*, **1,** 314.
149. Broca, P. (1861) Perte de la parole. Ramollissement chronique et destruction partielle du lobe antérieur gauche du cerveau. *Bulletin de la Société d'Anthropologie*, **2,** 235.
150. Broca, P. (1861) Remarques sur le siège de la faculté du langage articulé, suivies d'une observation d'aphémie. *Bulletin de la Société d'Anthropologie*, **6,** 330.
151. Broca, P. (1861) Nouvelle observation d'aphémie produite par une lésion de la troisième circonvolution frontale. *Bulletin de la Société d'Anthropologie*, **6,** 398.
152. Broca, P. (1863) Remarques sur le siège, le diagnostic et

la nature de l'aphémie. *Bulletin de la Société d'Anthropologie*, **38,** 379 and 393.

153. Hécaen, H. & Dubois, J. (1969) *La naissance de la neuropsychologie du langage*. Paris: Flammarion.

154. Baillarger, J. (1890) De l'aphasie au point de vue psychologique. Aphasie simple. Aphasie avec perversion de la faculté du langage. In *Recherches sur les maladies mentales* (Ed.) Baillarger, J. p. 584. Paris: Masson (première édition en 1865).

155. Exner, S. (1881) *Untersuchungen über die Lokalisation der Funktionen in der Grosshirnrinde des Menschen*. Vienna: Wilhelm Braumuller.

156. Bastian, H.C. (1869) On the various forms of loss of speech in cerebral disease. *British and Foreign Medico-chirurgical Revue*, **43,** 209 and 470.

157. Bastian, H.C. (1896) *The Brain as an Organ of the Mind*. New York: Appleton.

158. Bastian, H.C. (1887) On different kinds of aphasia, with special reference to their classification and ultimate pathology. *British Medical Journal*, **2,** 931.

159. Bastian, H.C. (1897) Some problems in connexion with aphasia and other speech defects. *Lancet*, **1,** 933, 1005, 1131 and 1187.

160. Charcot, J.M. (1883) Des différentes formes de l'aphasie. I. De la cécité verbale; II. Aphasie motrice. *Le progrès médical, 11e année*, 441, 469, 487, 521 and 859.

161. Charcot, J.M. (1884) *Differente formi d'afazia; lezioni fatte nella Salpêtrière nel semestre d'estate dell'anno 1883*. Milan: Antica casa editrice Dr Francesco Vallardi.

162. Lichtheim, L. (1885) Uber Aphasie. *Deutsches Archiv für klinische Medizin*, **36,** 204.

163. Lichtheim, L. (1885) On aphasia. *Brain*, **7,** 433.

164. Marie, P. (1906) Révision de la question de l'aphasie: l'aphasie de 1861 à 1866: essai de critique historique sur la genèse de la doctrine de Broca. *Semaine médicale* (Paris), **26,** 565.

165. Marie, P. (1922) Existe-t-il chez l'homme des centres préformés ou innés du langage? In *Questions neurologiques d'actualité* (Ed.) Wilson, S.A.K. & Chatelin, C. p. 527. Paris: Masson.

166. Marie, P. (1926) La troisième circonvolution frontale gauche ne joue aucun rôle spécial dans la fonction du langage. In *Travaux et mémoires* (Ed.) Marie, P. Vol. 1. Paris: Masson.

167. Dejerine, J. (1914) *Séméiologie des affections du système nerveux*. Paris: Masson.

168. Elghozi, D. (1977) *Discussion sur le rôle du thalamus dans l'activité du langage*. Medical thesis, Paris.

BIBLIOGRAPHY

Abbott, K.H. (1939) Total aphasia from a parietal lesion. *Bulletin of the Los Angeles Neurological Society*, **4,** 84.

Adams, A.E. (1972) Neurologie der Sprache. *Deutsche Medizin Wochenschrift*, **97,** 1065.

Adams, A.E. (1973) Uber Sprache und Gedächtnis bei Aphasikern. *Archiv für Psychiatrie und Nervenkrankheiten*, **217,** 25.

Adams, R.D. (1959) Concerning certain psychological principles which have been derived from clinico-pathologic study. *Transactions and Studies of the College of Physicians of Philadelphia*, **27,** 1.

Ahrens, R. (1958) Zum Problem der impressiven Sprachstorugen. *Nervenartz*, **29,** 488.

Ajuriaguerra, J. (de) & Hécaen, H. (1956) Examen anatomique d'un cas d'aphasie de conduction. *Revue neurologique*, **94,** 434.

Ajuriaguerra, J. (de), Inhelder, B. & Sinclair, H. (1965) L'ontogenèse du langage. *Revue pratique* (Paris), **15,** 2241.

Alajouanine, Th. (1955) Essai d'une approche neurophysiologique du langage pathologique. In *Les grandes activités du lobe temporal* (Ed.) Alajouanine, Th. p. 179. Paris: Masson.

Alajouanine, Th. (1955) Essai d'une approche neurophysiologique du langage pathologique. *Acta Neurologica Belgica*, **5,** 373.

Alajouanine, Th. & Lhermitte, F. (1964) Aphasia and physiology of speech. *Disorders of Communication*, **42,** 204.

Alford, L.B. (1948) Cerebral localization. *Journal of Nervous and Mental Diseases*, **77** (*monographie*).

Allison, R.S. (1962) *The Senile Brain*. London: Arnold.

Altman, J. (1967) Postnatal growth and differentiation of the mammalian brain with implications for a morphological theory. In *The Neurosciences* (Ed.) Quarton, G.S., Melnechuk, T. & Schmitt, F. p. 723. New York: Rockefeller University.

Avramov, S. & Raichev, R. (1970) Recherche clinique électro-encéphalographique chez les malades atteints d'aphasie d'origine vasculaire. *Nauchni Trudove*. **17,** 309. (In Russian.)

Azcoaga, J. (1972) Actualidad de la afasia. *Acta Audiologica y Foniatrica Hispana-americana*, **9,** 153.

Bailey, P.A. (1924) Contributions to the study of aphasia and apraxia. *Archives of Neurology and Psychiatry* (Chicago), **11,** 501.

Ballet, G. (1903) Un cas de surdité verbale par lésion sous-nucléaire (sous-corticale) avec atrophie secondaire de l'écorce de la première temporale. *Revue neurologique*, **11,** 685.

Barrett, A.M. (1910) A case of pure word-deafness with autopsy. *Journal of Nervous and Mental Diseases*, **37,** 73.

Bay, E. (1975) Ontogeny of stable speech areas in the human brain. In *Foundations of Language Development: a Multidisciplinary Approach* (Ed.) Lenneberg, E. & Lenneberg, E. Vol. II, p. 21. New York: Academic Press.

Bazier, M.A.B. (Ed.) (1960) *The Central Nervous System and Behavior*. New York: Josiah Macy Jr Foundation and The National Science Foundation.

Bell, A.G. (1916) *The Mechanisms of Speech*. New York: Funk and Wagnalls.

Benson, D.F. (1967) Fluency in aphasia: correlation with radioactive scan localization. *Cortex*, **3,** 373.

Benson, D.F. & Patten, D.H. (1967) The use of radioactive isotopes in the localization of aphasia-producing lesions. *Cortex*, **3,** 258.

Berendes, J. (1954) Elektrophysiologie des inneren internal Sprechens. *Archiv für Ohren-, Nasen- und Kehlkopfheilkunde*, **165** 635.

Birch, H.G. & Lee, J. (1955) Cortical inhibition in expressive aphasia. *Archives of Neurology* (Chicago), **54,** 514.

Blakemore, C.B. & Falconer, M.A. (1967) Long-term effects of anterior temporal lobectomy on certain cognitive functions. *Journal of Neurology, Neurosurgery and Psychiatry*, **30** 364.

Blinkov, S.M. & Arutyunova, A.S. (1966) Reaction time and conducting pathways of the brain. *Neuropsychologia*, **4,** 177.

Bocca, E. & Calearo, C. (1963) Central hearing processes. In *Modern Developments in Audiology* (Ed.) Jerger, J. p. 337. New York: Academic Press.

Bollinger, M. (1976) Meaning and memory, *Forum Linguisticum*, **1,** 1

Bonhoeffer, K. (1914) Klinischer und anatomischer Befund zur Lehre von der Apraxie under der 'motorischen Sprachbahn'. *Monatschrift für Psychiatrie und Neurologie*, **35,** 11 .

Bonhoeffer, K, (1923) Zurklinik und Lokalisation der Agrammatismus und der Rechts-Links-Desorientierung. *Monatschrift für Psychiatrie und Neurologie*, **54,** 11.

Bonin, G. (von) (1950) *Essay on the Cerebral Cortex*. Springfield Thomas.

Bonin, G. (von) (1960) *Some Papers on the Cerebral Cortex*. Springfield, IL: Thomas.

Borrell, A. & Despoulos, J.L. (1973) Vers l'acquisition de la syntaxe par l'enfant. *Annales*, **9,** 69.

Bosma, J., Grossman, R. & Kavanagh, J. (1967) Impairment of somesthetic perception and motor function in the oral and pharyngeal area. *Neurology*, **17,** 649.

Brage, D. (1950) Psicopatologia del languajen. *Semana Médica*, (B. Aires), **14,** 521.

Brain, R. (1961) *Speech Disorders*. Washington: Butterworth.

Branco-Lefevre, A.F. (1950) Contribuçiào para o estudo da psicopatologia da afasia em crianças. *Archivos de Neuro-psiquiatria*, **8,** 345.

Brodal, A. (1973) Self-observations and neuro-anatomical considerations after a stroke. *Brain*, **96,** 675.

Brown, D. (1956–1957) What is the basic language skill? Evidence from aphasia studies on importance of auditory language. *ETC, a Review of General Semantics*, **14,** 103.

Brown, J.R. & Simonson, J. (1957) A clinical study of 100 aphasic patients: 1. Observations on lateralization and localization of lesions. *Neurology*, **7,** 777.

Brown, J.W. (1974) The neural organization of language; aphasia and neuropsychiatry. In *American Handbook of Psychiatry* (Ed.) Arieti, S. Vol. 4, p. 244. New York: Basic Books.

Bruner, J.S. (1968) The course of cognitive growth. In *Contemporary Issues in Development Psychology* (Ed.) Endler, N.S., Boulter, L.S. & Osser, H. p. 476. New York: Holt, Rinehart and Winston.

Campain, R. & Minckler, J. (1976) A note on the gross configurations of the human auditory cortex. *Brain and Language*, **3,** 318.

Canter, G.J. (1967) Neuromotor pathologies of speech. *American Journal of Physical Medicine*, **46,** 659.

Carmon, A. & Nachshon, I. (1971) Effect of unilateral brain damage on perception of temporal order, *Cortex*, **7,** 410.

Carrow, M.A. (1968) The development of auditory comprehension of language structure in children. *Journal of Speech Disorders*, **33,** 99.

Castaigne, P. & Lecasble, R. (1960) L'électroencéphalogramme. Sa valeur localisatrice dans les lésions des hémisphères cérébraux. *Revue pratique* (Paris), **10,** 1275.

Cermak, L.S. & Moreines, J. (1976) Verbal retention deficits in aphasic and amnesic patients. *Brain and Language*, **3,** 16.

Chafe, J. (1973) Language and memory. *Language*, **49,** 261.

Charlton, M.H. (1963) Aphasia: a review. *American Journal of Psychiatry*, **119,** 872.

Chmidt, E.V. (1962) Essai d'une interprétation physiologique de certaines manifestations de l'aphasie. *World Neurology*, **3,** 602.

CIBA symposium (1964) *Disorders of Language*. London: Churchill.

Cohn, R. (1959) Dyscalculia: a clinical study with some neuropathologic correlations. *Transactions of the American Neurological Association*, **84,** 118.

Cohn, R. (1962) A study in aphasia. *Transactions of the American Neurological Association*, **87,** 187.

Cohn, R. (1971) Differential cerebral processing of noise and verbal stimuli. *Science*, **172,** 599.

Contamin, F. (1972) Quelques aspects sémiologiques et physiopathologiques des aphasies. *Le Langage et l'Homme*, **18,** 7.

Critchley, M. (1939) *The Language of Gesture*. London: Arnold.

Critchley, M. (1953) *The Parietal Lobes*. London: Arnold.

Critchley, M. (1962) Speech and speech loss in relation to the quality of the brain. In *Interhemispheric Relations and Cerebral Dominance* (Ed.) Mountcastle, V.B. p. 208. Baltimore, MD: Johns Hopkins.

Critchley, M., Russell, W.R. & Zangwill, O.L. (1951) Discussion on parietal lobe syndromes. *Proceedings of the Royal Society of Medicine*, **44,** 337.

Cutting, J.E. (1974) Two left hemisphere mechanisms in speech perception. *Perception and psychophysics*, **16,** 601.

Daujat, C., Gainotti, G. & Tissot, R. (1959) Sur quelques aspects des troubles de la compréhension dans l'aphasie. *Cortex*, **10,** 347.

Davis, D.O. & Pressman, B.D. (1974) Computerized tomography of the brain. *Radiologic Clinics of North America*, **12,** 297.

Debray-Ritzen, P., Hirsch, J.-F., Pierre-Kahn, A., Bursztejn, C. & Labbé, J.-P. (1977) Atteinte transitoire du langage écrit en rapport avec un hématome du lobe temporal gauche chez une adolescente de quatorze ans. *Revue neurologique*, **133,** 207.

Denny-Brown, D. (1950) Disintegration of motor function resulting from cerebral lesions. *Journal of Nervous and Mental Diseases*, **112,** 1.

Denny-Brown, D. & Chambers, R.A. (1958) The parietal lobe and behavior. *Research Publications, Association for Research in Nervous and Mental Diseases*, **36,** 35.

Efron, R. (1963) Temporal perception aphasia and 'déjà vu'. *Brain*, **86,** 403.

Eimas, P., Siqueland, E., Jusczyr, P. & Vigorito, J. (1971) Speech perception in infants. *Science*, **171,** 303.

Eisenson, J. (1964) Aphasia: a point of view as to the nature of the disorder and factors that determine prognosis for recovery. *International Journal of Neurology*, **4,** 287.

Ertl, J. & Schafer, E.W.P. (1967) Cortical activity preceding speech. *Life Sciences*, **6,** 473.

Ettlinger, G. (Ed.) (1965) *Functions of the Corpus Callosum*. Boston, MA: Little Brown.

Ettlinger, G., Jackson, C.V. & Zangwill, O.C. (1955) Dysphasia following right temporal lobectomy in a right-handed man. *Journal of Neurology, Neurosurgery and Psychiatry*, **18,** 214.

Fant, C.G.M. (1960) *Acoustic Theory of Speech Production*. The Hague: Mouton.

Fedio, P. & Weinberg, L.K. (1971) Dysnomia and impairment of verbal memory following intracarotid injection of sodium amytal. *Brain Research*, **31,** 159.

Fiorio, V. & Agostine, L. (1950) Amnesic aphasia due to lesions of second parietal gyrus. *Revue neurologique*, **83,** 145.

Foix, Ch. (1928) Aphasies. In *Nouveau Traité de Médecine* (Ed.) Roger, G., Widal, F. & Teissier, P.J. p. 135. Masson: Paris.

Foulis, D.A. (1897) A case in which there was destruction of the third left frontal convolution without aphasia. *British Medical Journal*, **1,** 383.

Fox, W.C. & German, W.J. (1935) Observations following left (dominant) temporal lobectomy. Report of case. *Archives of Neurology and Psychiatry*, **33,** 791.

Freidman, D.G. & Fisher, C.M. (1964) Case records of the Massachusetts general hospital; multiple occlusions in a forty-four years old woman. *New England Journal of Medicine*, **271,** 837.

Gaillard, L. (1881) Aphasie avec lésion classique. *Progrès médicale* (Paris), **9,** 422.

Galaburda, A. (1980) La région de Broca: observations anatomiques fait un siècle après la mort de son découvrer. *Revue neurologique*, **136,** 609.

Galaburda, A. & Sanides, F. (1980) Cytoarchitectonic organization of the human auditory cortex. *Journal of Comparative Neurology*, **190,** 597.

Galaburda, A.M., Le May, M., Kemper, T.L. & Geschwind, N. (1978) Right-left asymmetries in the brain. *Reprint Series*, **199,** 852.

Galaburda, A., Sanides, F. & Geschwind, N. (1978) Human brain: cytoarchitectonic left-right asymmetries in the temporal speech region. *Archives of Neurology*, **35,** 812.

Geschwind, N. (1962) The anatomy of acquired disorders of reading. In *Reading Disability* (Ed.) Money, J. p. 115. Baltimore, MD: Johns Hopkins.

Geschwind, N. (1964) The development of the brain and the evolution of language. In *Monograph Series on Language and Linguistics 17* (Ed.) Stuart, C.I.J.M. p. 155. Washington: Georgetown University Press.

Geschwind, N. (1969) Problems in the anatomical understanding of the aphasias. In *Contributions to Clinical Neuropsychology* (Ed.) Benton, A.L. p. 107. Chicago: Aldine.

Geschwind, N. (1970) The organization of language and the brain. *Science*, **170,** 940.

Geschwind, N. (1972) Language and the brain. *Scientific American*, **226,** 76.

Gilbert, J.H. (Ed.) (1972) *Speech and Cortical Functioning*. New York: Academic Press.

Godfrey, C.M. & Douglass, E. (1959) The recovery process in aphasia. *Canadian Medical Association Journal*, **8,** 618.

Goldberg, H.K., Marshall, C. & Sims, E. (1960) The role of brain damage in congenital dyslexia. *American Journal of Ophthalmology*, **50,** 586.

Goldstein, K. (1932) Restitution in injuries of the brain cortex. *Archives of Neurology and Psychiatry* (Chicago), **27,** 736.

Goldstein, K. Modifications of behavior consequent to cerebral lesions. *Psychiatry Quarterly*, **10,** 586.

Goldstein, K. (1942) *After-effects of Brain Injuries in War; Their Evaluation and Treatment*. New York: Grune and Stratton.

Gordinier, H.C. (1899) A case of brain tumor at the base of the second left frontal convolution. *American Journal of the Medical Sciences*, **117,** 526.

Gordinier, H.C. (1903) Arguments in favor of the existence of a separate center for writing. *Transactions of the Medical Society*, **126,** 231.

Green, E. & Boller, F. (1974) Features of auditory comprehension in severely impaired aphasics. *Cortex*, **10,** 2.

Grégoire, A. (1933) L'apprentissage de la parole pendant les deux premières années de l'enfance. *Journal of Psychology*, **30,** 375.

Gross, M.M. (1972) Hemispheric specialization for processing of visually presented verbal and spatial stimuli. *Perception and Psychophysics*, **12,** 357.

Gubbay, S.S., Ellis, E., Walton, J.N. & Court, S.D. (1965) Clumsy children; a study of apraxic and agnosic defects in 21 children. *Brain*, **88,** 295.

Guillaume, P. (1927) Les débuts de la phrase dans le langage de l'enfant. *Journal of Psychology*, **24,** 26.

Guillaume, P. (1927) Le développement des éléments formels dans le langage de l'enfant. *Journal of Psychology*, **24,** 203.

Hadziselimovic, H. & Cus, M. (1966) The appearance of internal structures of the brain in relation to configuration of the human skull. *Acta Anatomica*, **63,** 289.

Hadziselimovic. H. & Ruzdic, N. (1968) Appearance of the

base of the brain in relation to the configuration of the human skull. *Acta Anatomica* (Basel), **65,** 146.

Hahn, E. (1895) Pathologisch-anatomische Untersuchung des Lissauerschen Falles von Seelenblindheit. *Arbeiten aus der psychiatrischem Klinica*, **21,** 107.

Hansen, S., Perry, T.L. & Wada, J. (1972) Amino acid analysis of speech areas in human brains; absence of left-right asymmetry. *Brain Research*, **45,** 318.

Hardy, J.C. (1967) Suggestions for physiological research in dysarthria. *Cortex*, **3,** 128.

Hayes, J. (Ed.) (1970) *Cognition and the Development of Language*. New York: Wiley.

Head, H. (1925) Speech and cerebral localization. *West London Medical Journal*, **28,** 99.

Hécaen, H. (1967) Brain mechanisms suggested by studies of parietal lobes. In *Brain Mechanisms Underlying Speech and Language* (Ed.) Millikan, C. & Darley, F. p. 146. New York: Grune and Stratton.

Hécaen, H. (1969) Clinico-anatomical and neurolinguistic aspects of aphasia. In *The Pathology of Memory* (Ed.) Talland, A. & Waugh, N.C. p. 9. New York: Academic Press

Hécaen, H. & Ajuriaguerra, J. (de) (1955) Le syndrome praxique et gnosique au cours des lésions de l'hémisphère droit; rôle respectif des lésions des hémisphères droit et gauche dans les troubles des fonctions symboliques. *Presse médicale*, **63,** 401.

Hécaen, H. & Angelergues, R. (1961) Etude anatomo-clinique de 280 cas de lésions rétrorolandiques unilatérales des hémisphères cérébraux. *Encéphale*, **6,** 533.

Hécaen, H. & Angelergues, R. (1965) *Pathologie du langage*. Paris: Larousse.

Hécaen, H., Dell, M.B. & Roger, A. (1955) L'asphasie de conduction. *Encéphale*, **44,** 170.

Hécaen, H., Dubois, J. & Marcie, P. (1967) Aspects linguistiques des troubles de la vigilance au cours des lésions temporales antéro-internes droite et gauche. *Neuropsychologia*, **5,** 311.

Hécaen, H., Gastaut, H., Bancaud, J. & Rebufat-Deschamps, M. (1964) Clinical and EEG aspects of the problem of cortical localization. In *Cerebral Localization and Organization* (Ed.) Schaltenbrand, G. & Woolsey, C.N. p. 67. Madison, WI: University of Wisconsin Press.

Heilman, K.M., Wilder, B.J. & Malzone, W.F. (1972) Anomic aphasia following anterior temporal lobectomy. *Transactions of the American Neurological Association*, **97,** 291.

Heilman, K.M., Pandya, D.W., Karol, E.A. & Geschwind, N. (1971) Auditory inattention. *Archives of Neurology* (Chicago), **24,** 323.

Held, R. & Freedman, S.F. (1963) Plasticity in human sensorimotor control. *Sciences*, **142,** 455.

Hillier, W. (1954) Total left cerebral hemispherectomy for malignant glioma. *Neurology*, **4,** 718.

Hirsh, I.J. (1959) Auditory perception of temporal order, *Journal of the Acoustical Society of America*, **31,** 759.

Hirsh, I.J. & Sherrick, C.E. (1961) Perceived order in different sense modalities. *Journal of Experimental Psychology*, **62,** 423.

Hoeft, H.J. (1957) Klinisch-anatomischer Beitrag zur Kenntnis der Nachsprechaphasie (Leitungsaphasie). *Deutsche Zeitschrift für Nervenheilkunde*, **175,** 560.

Hoff, H. (1961) Die Lokalisation der Aphasie. *Proceedings of the VIIth International Congress of Neurology, Rome*, 55.

Hoffman, M.L. (Ed.) (1964) *Review of Child Development Research*. New York: Russell Sage Foundation.

Hohl, G.F. & Tschabitscher, H. (1953) Uber einen Fall von Amusia. *Wiener Zeitschrift für Nervenheilkunde*, **10,** 219.

Holmes, H.L. (1965) *Disordered Perception of Auditory Sequences in Aphasia*. Unpublished thesis, Harvard University.

Howes, D. (1967) Hypotheses concerning the functions of the language mechanisms. In *Research in Verbal Behavior and Some Neurophysiological Implications* (Ed.) Salzinger, K. & Salzinger, S. p. 429. New York: Academic Press.

Huber, M. (1946) Paragnosia and paraphasia. *Journal of Speech Disorders*, **11,** 321.

Hudson, A.J. (1968) Perseveration. *Brain*, **91,** 571.

Illingworth, R.S. (1963) *The Development of the Infant and Young Child, Normal and Abnormal*. Edinburgh: Livingstone.

Ingham, S.D. & Nielsen, J.M. (1937) Interpretation dissociated from recognition of visual, verbal (varied) symbols; illustrated by case of complete major (left) temporal lobectomy. *Bulletin of the Los Angeles Neurological Society*, **2,** 1.

Ingram, D. (1975) Cerebral speech lateralization in young children. *Neuropsychologia*, **13,** 103.

Jackson, J.H. (1874) On the nature of the duality of the brain. *Medical Press and Circular*, **1,** 19.

Jackson, J.H. (1915) Hughlings Jackson on aphasia and kindred affections of speech, together with a complete bibliography of his publications on speech and a reprint of some of the more important papers. *Brain*, **38,** 1.

Jacobsen, C.F. (1935) Functions of the frontal association in primates. *Archives of Neurology and Psychiatry* (Chicago), **33,** 558.

Jacobson, M. (1975) Brain development in relation to language. In *Foundations of Language Development: a Multidisciplinary Approach* (Ed.) Lenneberg, E. & Lenneberg, E. Vol. I, p. 105. New York: Academic Press.

Jarvis, P.E. (1968) Verbal control of sensory-motor performance: a test of Luria's hypothesis. *Human Development*, **11,** 172.

Jeffress, L.A. (Ed.) (1951) *Cerebral Mechanisms in Behavior*. New York: John Wiley.

Jerger, J., Weikers, N., Sharbrough, F. & Jerger, S. (1969) Bilateral lesions of the temporal lobe. *Acta oto-laryngologia* (*suppl. 258*).

John, E.R. (1967) *Mechanisms of Memory*. New York: Academic Press.

Karasseva, T.A. (1972) The role of the temporal lobe in human auditory perception. *Neuropsychologia*, **10,** 227.

Karis, R. & Horenstein, S. (1976) Localization of speech parameters by brain scan. *Neurology*, **26,** 226.

Keenan, J. (1968) The nature of receptive and expressive impairments in aphasia. *Journal of Speech Disorders*, **33,** 20.

Kerschensteiner, M., Poeck, K., Huber, W. & Stachowiak, F.J. (1975) Die Untersuchung auf Aphasie. *Aktuelle Neurologie*, **2,** 151.

Kertesz, A. & Benson, F. (1970) Neologistic jargon: a clinicopathological study. *Cortex*, **6,** 362.

Kim, Y.C. (1976) Deficits in temporal sequencing of verbal material: the effect of laterality of lesion. *Brain and Language*, **3,** 507.

Kimble, D.P. (Ed.) (1963) *The Anatomy of Memory*. Palo Alto, CA: Science and Behavior Books.

Kimura, D. (1961) Some effects of temporal lobe damage on auditory perception. *Canadian Journal of Psychology*, **15,** 156.

Kinsbourne, M. (1971) The minor cerebral hemisphere as a source of aphasic speech. *Archives of Neurology* (Chicago), **25,** 302.

Kinsbourne, M. (1972) Behavioral analysis of the repetition deficit in conduction aphasia. *Neurology*, **22,** 1126.

Kinsbourne, M. (1972) Contrasting patterns of memory span decrement in ageing and aphasia. *Journal of Neurology, Neurosurgery and Psychiatry*, **35,** 192.

Kinsbourne, M. (1975) Minor hemisphere language and cerebral maturation. In *Foundations of Language Development: a Multidisciplinary Approach* (Ed.) Lenneberg, E. & Lenneberg, E. Vol. II, p. 107. New York: Academic Press.

Kinsbourne, M. & Rosenfield, D. (1974) Agraphia selective for written spelling: an experimental case study. *Brain and Language*, **1,** 215.

Kinsbourne, M. & Warrington, E.K. (1962) A variety of reading disabilities associated with right hemisphere lesions. *Journal of Neurology, Neurosurgery and Psychiatry*, **25,** 339.

Klosovskii, B.N. (1963) *The Development of the Brain and Its Disturbance by Harmful Factors*. Oxford: Pergamon Press.

Korzybski, A. (1966) The role of language in perceptual processes. In *Perception: An Approach to Personality* (Ed.) Blake, R. & Ramasy, G. p. 1. New York: International non-Aristotelian Library.

Krechesvsky, I. (1937) Brain mechanism and variability: III. Limitations of the effect of cortical injury upon variability. *Journal of Comparative Psychology*, **23,** 351.

Kreindler, A. & Fradis, A. (1961) The Bucharest symposium on aphasia. *World Neurology*, **2,** 986.

Kreindler, A. & Fradis, A. (1964) A study on changes in the latency period of verbal and nonverbal performances in aphasics. *International Journal of Neurology*, **4,** 265.

Krieg, W.J.S. (1953) *Functional Neuroanatomy*. New York: Blakiston.

Kubik, C.S. & Adams, R.D. (1946) Occlusion of the basilar artery—a clinical and pathological study. *Brain*, **69,** 73.

Laguna, G. (de) (1927) *Speech—Its Function and Development*. New Haven, CT: Yale University Press.

Lane, H. (1965) The motor theory of speech perception: a critical review. *Psychological Review*, **4,** 275.

Lashley, K.S. (1937) Functional determinants of cerebral localization. *Archives of Neurology and Psychiatry* (Chicago), **38,** 371.

Lashley, K.S. (1951) The problem of serial order in behavior. In *Cerebral Mechanisms in Behavior* (Ed). Jeffress, L.A. p. 112. New York: Wiley.

Lenneberg, E.H. (1967) *Biological Foundations of Language*. New York: Wiley.

Lenneberg, E.H. (1969) On explaining language. *Science*, **164,** 635.

Lenneberg, E.H. (1973) The neurology of language. *Daedalus*, **102,** 115.

Lenneberg, E.H. (Ed.) (1975) Language and brain: developmental aspects. *Neurosciences Research Program Bulletin*, **12,** 513.

Lenneberg, E.H. & Lenneberg, E. (Ed.) (1975) *Foundations of Language Development: a Multidisciplinary Approach*. Vol. I and II. New York: Academic Press.

Leonhard, K. (1965) Uber parietale Aphasia. *Psychiatrie, Neurologie und medizinische Psychologie* (Leipzig), **17,** 162.

Lhermitte, F. (1968) Bases physiologiques de la mémoire. *Evolution psychiatrique*, **33,** 579.

Lhermitte, F. & Gautier, J.C. (1965) Corrélations anatomocliniques de l'aphasie. *Revue pratique* (Paris), **15,** 2309.

Lhermitte, F., Lecours, A.R. & Bertaux, D. (1969) Activation and seriation of linguistic units in aphasic transformations. In *Biocybernetics of the Central Nervous System* (Ed.) Proctor, L.D. p. 389. Boston, MA: Little and Brown.

Lhermitte, F. & Signoret, J.L. (1972) Analyse neuropsychologique et différenciation des syndromes amnésiques. *Revue neurologique*, **126,** 161.

Lhermitte, J. (1925) *Les fondements biologiques de la psychologie*. Paris: Gauthier-Villars.

Liberman, A.A., Cooper, F.S., Shankweiler, D.P. & Studdert-Kennedy, M. (1967) Perception of the speech code. *Psychological Review*, **74,** 431.

Liepmann, H. (1900) *Das Krankheitsbild der Apraxie*. Berlin: Karger.

Liepmann, H. (1900) Das Krankheitsbild des Apraxie ('motorischen Asymbolie') auf Grund eines Failes von einseitiger Apraxie. *Monatschrift für Psychiatrie und Neurologie*, **8,** 15, 102 and 182.

Liepmann, H. (1908) *Drei Aufsätze aus dem Apraxiegebiet*. Berlin: Karger.

Liepmann, H. (1912) Anatomische Befunde bei Aphasischen und Apraktischen. *Neurologisches Zentralblatt*, **31,** 1524.

Lipsitt, L.P. & Spiker, C.C. (1963) *Advances in Child Development and Behavior*. New York: Academic Press.

Lissauer, H. (1889) Ein Fall von Seelenblindheit nebst einem Beitrage zur Theorie derselben. *Archiv für Psychiatrie und Nervenkrankheiten*, **21,** 222.

Lotmar, F. (1936) Neuere Kämpfe um die Auffasung Aphasischer Störungen. *Schweizer Archiv für Neurologie und Psychiatrie*, **38,** 97.

Luria, A.R. (1961) *The Role of Speech in the Regulation of Normal and Abnormal Behaviour*. Oxford: Tizard.

Luria, A.R. (1965) Aspects of aphasia. *Journal of the Neurological Sciences*, **2**, 278.

Luria, A.R. (1965) L.S. Vygotsky and the problem of localization of functions. *Neuropsychologia*, **3**, 387.

Luria, A.R. (1966) *The Human Brain and Psychological Processes*. New York: Harper and Row.

Luria, A.R. (1973) *The Working Brain. An Introduction to Neuropsychology*. London: Penguin Press.

Luria, A.R. (1973) Towards the mechanisms of naming disturbance. *Neuropsychologia*, **11**, 417.

Luria, A.R. & Karasseva, T.A. (1968) Disturbances of auditory-speech memory in focal lesions of the deep regions of the left temporal lobe. *Neuropsychologia*, **6**, 97.

Luria, A.R. & Yudovich, F. (1959) *Speech and the Development of Mental Processes in the Child*. London: Staples Press.

Luria, A.R., Sokolov, E.N. & Klimkowski, M. (1967) Towards a neurodynamic analysis of memory disturbances with lesions of the left temporal lobe. *Neuropsychologia*, **5**, 1.

McNeilage, P.F. (1970) Motor control of serial ordering of speech. *Psychological Review*, **77**, 182.

McNeilage, P.F. (1972) Speech physiology. In *Speech and Cortical Functioning* (Ed.) Gilbert, J.H. p. 1. New York: Academic Press.

McNeilage, P.F., Rootes, T.P. & Chase, R.A. (1967) Speech production and perception in a patient with severe impairment of somesthetic perception and motor control. *Journal of Speech Research*, **10**, 449.

Mamo, H. (1972) Bases physiologiques du système nerveux. In *Système nerveux et muscles* (Ed.) Vallery-Radot, P., Hamburger, J. & Lhermitte, F. Collection La nouvelle pathologie médicale, fascicule 6, p. 4. Paris: Flammarion.

Mann, M.B. & Chubrich, R.C. (1970) Binaural stimulation of aphasic patients. Effects on oral reading. *New York State Journal of Medicine*, **70**, 2815.

Martin, .E. (1951) Cortical neurology: disturbance of speech and of the body image. *Medical Journal of Australia*, **2**, 363.

Masland, R.L. (1967) Brain mechanisms underlying the language function. *Bulletin of the Orton Society*, **17**, 1.

Masland, R.L. (1968) Some neurological processes underlying language. *Annals of Otolaryngology* (St Louis), **77**, 787.

Mattingly, I.G. & Liberman, A.M. (1969) The speech code and the physiology of language. In *Information Processing in the Nervous System* (Ed.) Leibovic, K.N. p. 97. New York: Springer-Verlag.

McFie, J. (1969) The diagnostic significance of disorders of higher nervous activity—syndromes related to frontal, temporal, parietal and occipital lesions. In *Handbook of Clinical Neurology* (Ed.) Vinken, P.J. & Bruyn, G.W. Vol. 4 p. 1. Amsterdam: North-Holland.

McNeill, D. (1970) *The Acquisition of Language: the Study of Developmental Linguistics*. New York: Harper and Row.

Meir, G. & Muller-Hermann, D. (1955) Etudes aphasiologiques: la signification, en recherche aphasiologique, des théories pavloviennes de l'activité nerveuse supérieure. *Psychiatrie, Neurologie und medizinische Psychologie (Leipzig)*, **7**, 347. (In German.)

Mempel, E., Zarski, S., Subczynska, J. & Srebrznska, J. (1963) Compensation of speech disorders by the non-dominant cerebral hemisphere in adults. *Journal of Neurology, Neurosurgery and Psychiatry*, **26**, 96.

Menyuk, P. (1972) *The Development of Speech*, Indianapolis: Bobbs-Merill.

Millikan, C.H. & Darley, F. (1967) *Brain Mechanisms Underlying Speech and Language*. New York: Grune and Stratton.

Mills, C. & McConnell, K. (1895) The naming center. *Journal of Mental and Nervous Diseases*, **21**, 1016.

Mills, C. (1904) Aphasia and the cerebral zone of speech. *American Journal of the Medical Sciences*, **128**, 375.

Milner, B. (1954) Intellectual function of the temporal lobes. *Psychological Bulletin*, **51**, 42.

Milner, B. (1958) Psychological defects produced by temporal-lobe excision. *Research Publications, Association for Research in Nervous and Mental Diseases*, **36**, 244.

Milner, B. (1967) Brain mechanisms suggested by studies of temporal lobes. In *Brain Mechanisms Underlying Speech and Language* (Ed.) Millikan, C. & Darley, F. p. 122. New York: Grune and Stratton.

Minkowski, A. (Ed.) (1967) *Regional Development of the Brain in Early Life*. Oxford: Blackwell.

Mohr, J.P. (1976) Broca's area and Broca's aphasia. In *Studies in Neurolinguistics* (Ed.) Whitaker, H & Whitaker, H. Vol. 2, p. 201. New York: Academic Press.

Monakow, C. (von) (1910) *Uber Lokalisation der Hirnfunktionen*. Wiesbaden: Verlag von Bergmann.

Morel, F. (1935) L'audition dans l'aphasie sensorielle. *Encéphale*, **2**, 533.

Mourgue, R. (1921) Disorders of symbolic thinking due to local lesions of brain. *British Journal of Psychology*, **1**, 97.

Moutier, F. (1908) *L'aphasie de Broca*. Paris: Steinheil.

New, P.F.J., Scott, W.R., Schnur, J.A., Davis, K.R. & Taveras, J.M. (1974) Computerized axial tomography with the Emi scanner. *Radiology*, **110**, 109.

Newmann, J. (von) (1958) *The Computer and the Brain*. New Haven: Yale University Press.

Nielsen, J.M. (1940) Unsolved problems in aphasia. *Bulletin of the Los Angeles Neurological Society*, **5**, 78.

Nielsen, J.M. (1944) Functions of the minor cerebral hemisphere in language. *Bulletin of the Los Angeles Neurological Society*, **9**, 67.

Nielsen, J.M. (1944) The unsolved problems in aphasia: I. Alexia in motor aphasia. *Bulletin of the Los Angeles Neurological Society*, **9**, 114.

Nielsen, J.M. (1950) Cerebral-localization in aphasia and agnosia. *Archives of Neurology and Psychiatry* (Chicago), **5**, 748.

Nielsen, J.M. (1953) Spontaneous recovery from aphasia: autopsy. *Bulletin of the Los Angeles Neurological Society*, **18**, 147.

Nielsen, J.M. (1957) Motor aphasia with recovery: report of

a case with autopsy verification. *Bulletin of the Los Angeles Neurological Society*, **22,** 148.

Nielsen, J.M. (1965) *Agnosia, Apraxia, Aphasia. Their Value in Cerebral Localization*. New York: Hafner.

Nielsen, J.M. & Raney, R.B. (1938) Symptoms following surgical removal of major (left) angular gyrus. *Bulletin of the Los Angeles Neurological Society*, **3,** 42.

Nielsen, J.M. & Raney, R.B. (1939) Recovery from aphasia studied in cases of lobectomy. *Archives of Neurology and Psychiatry* (Chicago), **42,** 189.

Niessi, V. & Mayendorf, E. (1911) *Die aphasischen Symptome und ihre kortikale Lokalisation*. Leipzig: Barth.

Odom, G.L. & Lyman, R.S. (1946) Speech disorder following excision of post central gyrus. *Transactions of the American Neurological Association*, **71,** 67.

Offret, G. (1946) De quelques travaux modernes concernant la physiologie et la psychophysiologie des lobes pariéto-occipitaux du cerveau. *Archives d'Ophthalmologie* (Paris), **6,** 145.

Ogle, W. (1867) A case of softening of the brain with aphasia. *Lancet*, **11,** 736.

Oller-Daurella, L. & Dini, J. (1970) L'E.E.G. des syndromes aphasiques. *Revista Clinica Española*, **117,** 63. (In Spanish.)

Ombredane, A. (1935) Etude sur le langage, sur les premières manifestations du langage enfantin et sur la prétendue loi de Fritz Schultze. *Hygiène mentale*, **30,** 69.

Osborne, J. (1833) On the loss of the faculty of speech depending on forgetfulness of the art of using the vocal organs. *Dublin Journal of Medical and Chemical Sciences*, **4,** 157.

Palmer, M.F. (1940) The speech development of normal children. *Journal of Speech Disorders*, **5,** 185.

Panse, F. (1950) Sprache als Bewegung. *Archiv für Psychiatrie und Nervenkrankheiten*, **185,** 423.

Park, G.E., Bimmerle, J.F., Schmieding, A., Lorimer, F., Grams, A., Tarsitano, R. & Krause, V. (1955) Biological changes associated with dyslexia. *Archives of Pediatrics*, **72,** 71.

Peiper, A. (1964) *Cerebral Function in Infancy and Childhood*. New York: International Behavioral Sciences Series.

Pena-Casanova, J. (1976) La apraxia constructiva y problemas de desarrollo y aprendizaje en neurologia. *Revue neurologique*, **4,** 267.

Penfield, W. (1954) Mechanisms of voluntary movements. *Brain*, **77,** 1.

Penfield, W. (1965) Conditioning of uncommitted cortex for language learning. *Brain*, **88,** 787.

Perkell, J.S. (1969) *Physiology of Speech Production*. Cambridge, MA: MIT Press.

Pershing, H.T. (1900) A case of Wernicke's conduction aphasia with autopsy. *Journal of Nervous and Mental Diseases*, **27,** 369.

Pichon, E. (1936) *Le développement psychique de l'enfant et de l'adolescent*. Paris: Masson.

Poeck, K. (1969) Pathophysiology of emotional disorders associated with brain damage. In *Handbook of Clinical Neurology* (Ed.) Vinken, P.J. & Bruyn, G.W. Vol. 3, p. 343. Amsterdam: North-Holland.

Poeck, K. (1972) Stimmung und Krankheitseinsicht bei Aphasien. *Archiv für Psychiatrie und Nervenkrankheiten*, **216,** 246.

Poeck, K., Hartje, W., Kerschensteiner, M. & Orgass, B. (1973) Sprachverständnisstörungen bei aphasischen und nicht aphasischen Hirnkranken. *Deutsch Medizin Wochenschrift*, **98,** 139.

Poeck, K., Kerschensteiner, M., Stachowiak, F.J. & Huber, W. (1975) Die Aphasien. *Aktuelle Neurologie*, **2,** 159.

Preacher, W.G. (1945) Speech disorders in World war II. *Journal of Speech Disorders*, **10,** 155.

Preacher, W.G. (1949) Neurological factors in the etiology of delayed speech. *Journal of Speech Disorders*, **14,** 147.

Pribram, K.H. (1958) Neocortical function in behavior. In *Biological and Biochemical Bases of Behavior* (Ed.) Harloing, H.F. & Woolsey, C.N. p. 151. Madison: University of Wisconsin Press.

Pribram, K.H. (1958) *Comparative Neurology and Evolution of Behavior*. New Haven, CT: Yale University Press.

Pribram, K.H. (1960) A review of theory in physiological psychology. *Annual Review of Psychology*, **11,** 1.

Pribram, K.H. (1971) *Languages of the Brain: Experimental Paradoxes and Principles in Neuropsychology*. Englewood Cliffs, NJ: Prentice Hall.

Pribram, K.H. & Broadbent, D.E. (Ed.) (1970) *Biology of Memory*. New York: Academic Press.

Proctor, L.D. (Ed.) (1969) *Biocybernetics of the Central Nervous System*. Boston: Little and Brown.

Raines, G.N. & Cohn, R. (1951) Intravenous sodium amytal in generalized language dysfunction. *Neurology*, **1,** 299.

Riese, W. (1960) Dynamics in brain lesions. *Journal of Nervous and Mental Disorders*, **131,** 291.

Rioch, D. & Weinstein, E. (Ed.) (1964) *Disorders of Communication*. New York: Research Publications of the Association for Research in Nervous and Mental Disease.

Robb, J.P. (1946) *A Study of the Effects of Cortical Excision on Speech in Patients with Previous Cerebral Injuries*. Medical Thesis, McGill University, Montreal.

Robb, J.P. (1948) Effect of cortical excision and stimulation of the frontal lobe on speech with a review of aphasia and cerebral physiology related to speech. *Research Publications, Association for Research in Nervous and Mental Diseases*, **27,** 587.

Roberts, L. (1951) Localization of speech in the cerebral cortex. *Transactions of the American Neurological Association*, **76,** 43.

Roberts, L. (1958) Functional plasticity in cortical speech areas and the integration of speech. *Archives of Neurology and Psychiatry* (Chicago), **79,** 275.

Rouvière, H. (1974) *Anatomie humaine, descriptive et topographique*. 3 tomes; 11e édition, Paris: Masson.

Russell, J. (1866) Loss of the faculty of expression in connection with injury to the portion of the skull corresponding with the left anterior lobe of the brain. *British Medical Journal*, **1,** 567.

Russell, W.R. (1951) Disability caused by brain wounds; a review of 1166 cases. *Journal of Neurology, Neurosurgery and Psychiatry*, **14,** 35.

Russell, W.R. (1961) Anatomical aspects of aphasia. *Scottish Medical Journal*, **6**, 237.

Russell, W.R. (1963) Some anatomical aspects of aphasia. *Lancet*, **1**, 1173.

Russell, W.R. & Espir, M.L.E. (1961) *Traumatic Aphasia*. London: Oxford University Press.

Sanders, W.E. (1866) Aphasia with right hemiplegia. Lesion in the island of Reil extending into the external frontal convolution. *Lancet*, **1**, 656.

Sanides, F. (1975) Comparative neurology of the temporal lobe in primates including man with reference to speech. *Brain and Language*, **2**, 396.

Santha, K. (1947) Fasttotale obtragung der linken dritten Stirnwindung ohne motorische Aphasie. Zur Frase der amnestischen Aphasie frontalen choprunges. *Monatschrift für Psychiatrie und Neurology*, **114**, 179.

Scheinker, I.M. & Kuhr, B.M. (1948) Motor aphasia and agraphia caused by a small vascular lesion confined to third and second convolutions of left frontal lobe. *Research Publications, Association for Research in Nervous and Mental Diseases*, **27**, 582.

Schiller, F. (1947) Aphasia studied in patients with missile wounds. *Journal of Neurology, Neurosurgery and Psychiatry* **10**, 183.

Schlanger, B. (1959) A longitudinal study of speech and language development of brain damaged retarded children. *Journal of Speech Disorders*, **24**, 354.

Schott, B., Trillet, M. & Bourrat, C. (1975) Syndrome temporal, *Encyclopédie médico-chirurgicale, 17036 E*[10], **1**.

Schubert, K. & Panse, F. (1953) Audiologische Befunde bei sensorischer Aphasie. *Archiv für Ohren-, Nasen- und Kehlkopfheilkunde* **164**, 23.

Schuell, H. & Jenkins, J.J. (1959) The nature of language deficit in aphasia. *Psychological Review*, **66**, 45.

Schulman, C.L. (1965) *Brain Damage and Behavior*. Springfield, IL: Thomas.

Scott, C. & Ringel, R.L. (1971) Articulation without oral sensory control. *Journal of Speech Research*, **14**, 804.

Scott, C.M. & Ringel, R.L. (1971) The effects of motor and sensory disruptions on speech: a description and articulation. *Journal of Speech Research*, **14**, 819.

Segalowitz, S.J. & Gruber, F.A. (1977) *Language Development and Neurological Theory*. New York: Academic Press.

Selnes, O.A. (1974) The corpus callosum: some anatomical and functional considerations with special reference to language. *Brain and Language*, **1**, 111.

Shimrat, N. (1973) The impact of laterality and cultural background on the development of writing skills. *Neuropsychologia*, **11**, 239.

Singer, H.D. & Low, A.A. (1933) Brain in a case of motor aphasia in which improvement occurred with training. *Archives of Neurology and Psychiatry* (Chicago), **29**, 162.

Singh, S. & Schlanger, B.B. (1969) The effects of delayed sidetone on the speech of aphasic, dysarthric, and mentally retarded subjects. *Language and Speech*, **12**, 167.

Sipos, J. & Hagert, J. (1972) Kurrzverfahren zur Erfassung von aphasischen Störungen. *Nervenarzt*, **43**, 207.

Sklar, M. (1963) Relation of psychological and language test scores and autopsy findings in aphasia. *Journal of Speech Research*, **6**, 84.

Smith, F. & Miller, G.A. (1966) *The Genesis of Language: a Psycho-linguistic Approach*, Cambridge, MA: MIT Press.

Smith, K.U. (1951) Learning and associative pathways of the human cerebral cortex. *Science*, **114**, 117.

Sokolov, A.N. (1967) Speech-motor afferentation and the problem of brain. *Soviet Psychology*, **1**, 3.

Sperry, R.W. (1961) Cerebral organization and behavior. *Science*, **133**, 1749.

Sperry, R.W. (1964) The great cerebral commissure. *Scientific American*, **210**, 42.

Sperry, R.W., Gazzaniga, M.S. & Bogen, J.E. (1969) Interhemispheric relationships: the neocortical commissures; syndromes of hemisphere disconnection. In *Handbook of Clinical Neurology* (Ed.) Vinken, P.J. & Bruyn, G.W. Vol. 4, p. 273. Amsterdam: North Holland.

Spiller, W.G. (1906) Lesions of the left first temporal convolution in relation to sensory aphasia. *Review of Neurology and Psychiatry*, **4**, 329.

Starr, M.A. (1889) The pathology of sensory aphasia with an analysis of 50 cases in which Broca's centre was not destroyed. *Brain*, **12**, 82.

Stengel, E. (1950) Borderlands of neurology and psychiatry. *Recent Progress in Psychiatry*, **2**, 416.

Stengel, E. (1964) Psychopathology of dementia. *Proceedings of the Royal Society of Medicine*, **57**, 911.

Stevens, K.N. & House, A.S. (1972) Speech perception. In *Foundations of Modern Auditory Theory* (Ed.) Tobias, J. Vol. 2, p. 1. New York: Academic Press.

Street, B.S. (1957) Hearing loss in aphasia. *Journal of Speech Disorders*, **22**, 60.

Strub, R.L. & Gardner, H. (1974) The repetition defect in conduction aphasia: mnestic or linguistic? *Brain and Language*, **1**, 241.

Stutte, H. (1968) Wann soltten wir von Rindlicher Aphasie sprechen? *Acta Paedopsychiatrica*, **35**, 1.

Subirana, A. (1953) *Sur les bienfaits éventuels de certaines maladies neurologiques*. Livre jubilaire du professeur Roger. Marseille: Faculté de médecine.

Teitelbaum, H.A. (1943) An analysis of the disturbances of the higher cortical functions: agnosia, apraxia and aphasia. *Journal of Nervous and Mental Diseases*, **97**, 44.

Teuber, H.L. (1951) Book review: Wepman, Joseph M., 'Recovery from aphasia'. *J. abnorm. Soc. Psychol.*, **46**, 610.

Teuber, H.L. (1955) Physiological psychology. *Annual Review of Psychology*, **6**, 267.

Teuber, H.L. (1960) The premorbid personality and reaction to brain damage. *American Journal of Orthopsychiatry*, **30**, 322.

Teuber, H.L. (1964) Discussion. In *Disorders of Language* (Ed.) de Reuck, A.V.S. & O'Connor, M. p. 177. London: Churchill.

Teuber, H.L. (1965) Some needed revisions of the classical views of agnosia. *Neuropsychologia*, **3**, 371.

Tikofsky, R.S., Kooi, K.A. & Thomas, M.H. (1960) Electroencephalographic findings and recovery from aphasia. *Neurology*, **10**, 154.

Tissot, R. (1966) *Neuropsychopathologie de l'aphasie*. Paris: Masson.

Trevarthen, C. (1974) The psychobiology of speech development. *Neurosciences Research Program Bulletin*, **12**, 570.

Turkewitz, G., Gordon, E.W. & Birch, H.G. (1965) Head turning in the human neonate: spontaneous patterns. *Journal of Genetic Psychology*, **107**, 143.

Twitchell, T.E., Lecours, A.R., Rudel, R.G. & Teuber, H.L. (1966) Minimal cerebral dysfunctions in children: motor deficits. *Transactions of the American Medical Association*, p. 353.

Tzortzis, C. & Albert, M.L. (1974) Impairment of memory for sequences in conduction aphasia. *Neuropsychologia*, **12**, 355.

Ungar, J. (1972) Le code moléculaire de la mémoire. *La Recherche*, **3**, 19.

Vrtunski, P.B., Mack, J.L., Boller, F. & Kim, Y. (1976) Response to delayed auditory feedback in patients with hemispheric lesions. *Cortex*, **12**, 395.

Vygotsky, L.S. (1965) Psychology and the localization of functions. *Neuropsychologia*, **3**, 381.

Warren, L.R., Peltz, L. & Haueter, E.S. (1976) Patterns of EEG alpha during word processing and relations to recall. *Brain and Language*, **3**, 283.

Warrington, E.K. & Shallice, T. (1969) The selective impairment of auditory verbal short-term memory. *Brain*, **92**, 885.

Warrington, E.K., Logue, V. & Pratt, R.T.C. (1971) The anatomical localization of selective impairment of auditory verbal short-term memory. *Neuropsychologia*, **9**, 377.

Wechsler, L. (1937) Excision of the speech area without resultant aphasia. *Archives of Neurology and Psychiatry* (Chicago), **38**, 430.

Weiss, D.A. (1948) Organic lesions leading to speech disorders. *Nervous Child*, **7**, 29.

Wen, I.C. (1933) A study of the occipital region of the Chinese fetal brain. *Journal of Comparative Neurology*, **57**, 477.

Wepman, J.M., Jones, L.V., Bock, R.D. & Pelt, D. (van) (1960) Studies in aphasia: background and theoretical formulations. *Journal of Speech Disorders*, **25**, 323.

Werner, H. & Kaplan, E. (1952) *An Acquisition of Word Meanings: a Developmental Study*. Evanston, IL: Child Development Publications.

West, S. (1885) A case of aphasia in which the chief lesion was seated in the supramarginal gyri. Broca's convolution being unaffected. *British Medical Journal*, **1**, 1242.

Whitaker, H.A. & Selnes, O.A. (1975) Broca's area: a problem in language-brain relationships. *Linguistics*, **154**, 91.

Whitty, C.W.M. & Newcombe, F. (1965) Disabilities associated with lesions in the posterior parietal region of the non-dominant hemisphere. *Neuropsychologia*, **3**, 175.

Wilks, S. (1872) A case of aphasia with remarks on the faculty of language and the duality of the brain. *Guy's Hospital Reports*, **17**, 145,

Williams, D. (1968) Man's temporal lobe. *Brain*, **91**, 639.

Winchester, R.A. & Hartman, B.T. (1955) Auditory differentiation in the dysphasic. *Journal of Speech Disorders*, **20**, 178.

Witelson, S. (1977) Developmental dyslexia: two right hemispheres and none left. *Science*, **195**, 309.

Witelson, S. & Pallie, W. (1973) Left hemisphere specialization for language in the newborn. Neuroanatomical evidence of asymmetry. *Brain*, **96**, 641.

Woerkom, W. (van) (1921) La signification de certains éléments de l'intelligence dans la genése des troubles aphasiques. *Journal of Psychology*, **18**, 730.

Yakovlev, P.I. & Rakič, P. (1966) Patterns of decussation of bulbar pyramids and distribution of pyramidal tracts on two sides of the spinal cord. *Transactions of the American Neurological Association*, **91**, 366.

Zangwill, O.L. (1951) Discussion on parietal lobe syndromes. *Proceedings of the Royal Society of Medicine*, **44**, 343.

Zavala, C. (1972) Genética y problemas de la communicación linguística. *Acta Audiologica y Foniatrica Hispano-Americana*, **9**, 173.

Zucker, K. (1934) An analysis of disturbed function in aphasia. *Brain*, **57**, 109.

9. Aetiology of the Aphasias

'There: that makes three days. Here, there: that was cut. I was given a shot. Then he opened that. He opened the other one, underneath. Those above were scraped. He scraped them because that, that exploded. I had a pressure: nearly thirty. Then, everything burst. He scraped them well. He sewed them up again. It's only the first, there [speech]: it's that one which breaks down. That one is not working. He will be responsible for looking after it. He says to me: "But Sir, move this hand." And: "Jump to the left." And: "Jump to the right." You can do anything. You can with your feet in the air. One can walk on one's hands. Everything is absolutely impeccable. There is only this one, poor thing, which is mistaken inside.'

(*Conversation with Mr Les.; May 1969*)

Aphasiology is primarily based on the study of language disturbances observed, in adults, following certain lesions of the left cerebral hemisphere. Such lesions may be caused by various diseases. The aetiological analysis of the aphasias is concerned with the relationships between particular causal diseases and the origin, nature, site and extent of lesions of the language zone and of associated structures (see Chapter 8-1 and 8-5). Such analysis is intended to further understanding of the clinical manifestations and the evolution of these lesions.

CEREBRAL VASCULAR DISEASES

Cerebral vascular accidents are the most frequent cause of aphasia in adults. These diseases are, in fact, frequently accompanied by circumscribed and permanent cerebral lesions. The neuropathological study of such lesions, in association with the study of the abnormal linguistic behaviours which they may cause, has contributed in a very large measure to the anatomical description of the aphasias and, consequently, to the identification of the role of several parts of the brain in linguistic functioning (see Chapters 3 to 8). As a matter of fact, the systematic analysis of the linguistic anomalies attributable to localized cerebrovascular lesions remains the starting point—or the stumbling block—of all theories which attempt to relate the most specific of all human behaviours to its particular substratum.

The term 'cerebral vascular disease' refers to a large number of pathological conditions characterized by modifications of the structure of the vessels which irrigate the brain and/or of the blood supply which nourishes it. Whether there is occlusion of an artery by a thrombus or an embolus, an anomaly in the wall of a vessel which reduces its diameter and flow, modifies its permeability or causes its rupture, or circulatory insufficiency from a drop in systemic arterial pressure, a critical reduction of the blood supply has immediate effects on the cerebral parenchyma. A brief interruption, of less than three minutes' duration, produces transient ischaemia with a reversible functional deficit, whereas prolonged circulatory arrest is accompanied by irreversible necrosis of cerebral tissue (cerebral softening) and a long-standing deficit. In the case of vascular rupture subsequent to a congenital or acquired anomaly, the harmful effects of the intraparenchymatous haemorrhage may add to those of the ischaemia or constitute a genuine expansive cerebral lesion which is itself the cause of a major neurological disorder.

The typical example of a cerebral vascular accident (*stroke*) is that of apoplexy, resulting from a massive cerebral haemorrhage, in which the patient falls, suddenly paralysed, rapidly becomes comatose and dies within a few hours. In other cases, hemiplegia appears within a few minutes or hours and the victim remains conscious, without other apparent deficits. It is then evident that s/he will survive the stroke, with or without functional recovery. Most often, the cerebral vascular accident is accompanied by a constellation of neurological symptoms and signs, for example, deficits of muscular strength, of sensation, of vision, etc. (see Chapters 4 and 16) and, possibly, aphasia. In other cases—and this is rare and depends on the site of lesion (see Chapter 8-3 and 8-4)—aphasia may be the sole manifestation of a cerebral vascular accident, particularly in certain forms of Wernicke's aphasia.

The aetiology of aphasia-producing cerebral vascular disease naturally influences the mode of onset and the clinical form of the resulting aphasia, as well as the evolution of the language disturbance. Nevertheless, once the presence of a vascular disease has been recognized, aetiological factors seldom determine the distinctive features of an aphasia. On the other hand, the study of the symptomatology of the aphasia, like the study of all other neurological signs, can contribute to the identification of the underlying pathological process.

CEREBRAL THROMBOSIS

Cerebral thrombosis may be defined as the occlusion of one or more cerebral arteries by the formation of a thrombus at the level of an anomaly* of the vascular wall[1–8]. By extension, this term is also commonly used to designate the resulting cerebral lesion, that is, cerebral softening.

Cerebral softening is most often caused by atherosclerosis of the cervical arteries. Atheromatous deposits form at points of bifurcation or curvature in arteries of large or medium calibre, selectively affecting the carotid and vertebrobasilar arteries and the extracerebral portion of their terminal branches, the anterior, middle and posterior cerebral arteries (Fig. 9-1). Thrombosis generally occurs at the site of maximal narrowing within the vessel. Consequently, those which cause aphasia are very often located at the origin of the internal carotid in the neck (carotid sinus) and in the carotid siphon; less frequently (4 to 5 per cent of the cases), they are located in the first third of the middle cerebral artery (Fig. 9-1). Arterial hypertension and diabetes contribute to the extension of the atherosclerotic process to the small arteries and, in these diseases, there are often small areas of softening secondary to the occlusion of the intraparenchymatous branches of the cerebral arteries. These small lesions are called lacunae[3, 9–12].

The effect of an atherosclerotic thrombosis on the cerebral parenchyma varies considerably among different individuals. The topography and the extent of the softening depend, in fact, upon the availability of collateral circulation. Substitutions may occur through the anastomotic circle of Willis at the base of the brain, through anastomoses (the joining together of two vessels) between the superficial (cortical) branches of the cerebral arteries and through a reversal in the direction of blood flow in the ophthalmic artery, allowing the external carotid to compensate for the obstruction of the corresponding internal carotid[13–15] (Fig. 9-1). In some cases, the collateral circulation is well enough developed that complete occlusion of an artery, the internal carotid for instance, remains completely unnoticed[16]. In contrast, in other cases, thrombosis of a vessel is accompanied by softening of the entire territory which it supplies. Between these two extremes, all intermediates are possible, thus explaining the variation in the localization as well as the extent of superficial and/or deep cerebral softenings and, consequently, the variation in the clinical pictures observed. When the lesion involves the whole territory vascularized by the left middle cerebral artery, one sees global aphasia associated with sensorimotor impairment of the right side of the body[1]. On the other hand, if damage is limited to the territory of the more anterior branches of this artery, it is Broca's aphasia which occurs, often with an associated hemiplegia[1]. Finally, if the lesioned region is that vascularized by the most posterior branches of the sylvian artery, one of the forms of Wernicke's† aphasia is observed, often accompanied by a right hemianopsia (or a quadranopsia)[1]. The presence of partial softenings affecting several components of the same

* Almost always an atheromatous patch.

† Charles Foix thus distinguished between the effects of softenings of the respective territories of the posterior temporal branch of the left sylvian artery, its posterior parietal branch and its so-called angular gyrus branch (see Chapter 10).

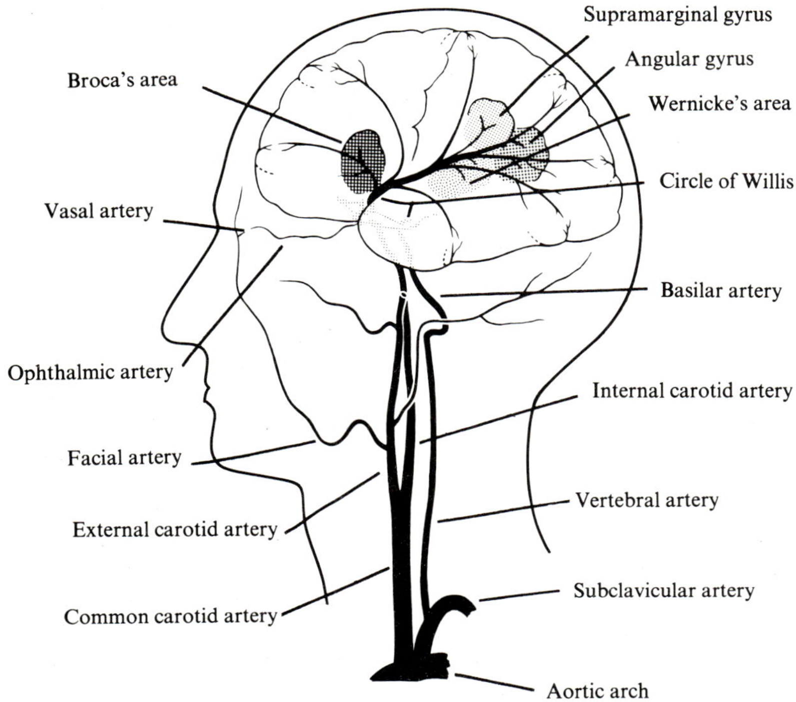

Fig. 9–1 *Arterial vascularization of the left cerebral hemisphere and, particularly, of the language zone. Adapted from G. Lazorthes*[51].

arterial territory frequently complicates the symptomopathological analysis of cerebral thrombosis.

Atherosclerotic cerebral thrombosis is more frequent in males than in females. Its incidence increases with age. In younger individuals, it is usually associated with predisposing pathological conditions such as familial or acquired hypercholesterolaemia and diabetes. At older ages, it most often occurs in the context of generalized atherosclerosis, with coronary insufficiency and/or circulatory insufficiency of the lower limbs[3].

The clinical picture of cerebral thrombosis differs from those of embolism or cerebral haemorrhage (cf. below), and also shows much greater individual variation than either of the latter. In many cases, the onset of a permanent deficit is preceded by premonitory signs of varying severity which may last a few seconds, minutes or hours, and appear one or more times before the installation of a permanent disturbance. These are transient ischaemic attacks, manifesting a temporary circulatory failure in a restricted vascular territory (Insertion 9.1).

Whether or not preceded by prodromes (premonitory symptoms), aphasia resulting from cerebral thrombosis most often develops in the course of a single episode which lasts a few mintues or hours and occurs indifferently during sleep or wakefulness. Less frequently, the language disturbance develops in an intermittent fashion over a period of hours or days and, during this time, moments of increased severity or transient remission can be observed. This pattern of evolution, observed especially in Wernicke's aphasias, is so characteristic that it permits an immediate aetiological diagnosis.

Besides atherosclerosis, there are many other diseases which may cause cerebral thrombosis manifested, in some cases, by aphasia. These pathologies are relatively rare in Western Europe and North America. They include, for example, meningovascular syphilis, purulent or tuberculous meningitis, cerebral thrombophlebitis secondary to ear infections or post-partum, migraine accompanied by a permanent neurological deficit, complications arising from arteriography[17].

CEREBRAL EMBOLISM

A cerebral embolism is the sudden obliteration, by a foreign body (embolus) mobilized in the

Insertion 9.1

Transient ischaemic attacks may sometimes be manifested by aphasia. The type of aphasia varies in different cases and may or may not be associated with a sensorimotor or visual disturbance. In most cases, these attacks last only a few minutes. A small number may occur on an occasional basis or several may occur daily. Their occurrence can often be recognized to be related to changes of position, to violent emotions, to exercise, fatigue, defecation or coughing. Between each episode, the neurological examination is normal. On the other hand, vascular examination will often demonstrate the presence of stenosis (atherosclerotic narrowing) of the internal carotid[4, 5]. Eventual complication of the disease by cerebral thrombosis is not uncommon, but there are also cases in which the attacks disappear spontaneously and without sequelae.

circulatory system, of an artery which nourishes the brain. Most cerebral embolisms are due to the fragmentation of an intracardiac thrombus or of a thrombus of the aortic arch or of the carotid bifurcation[3, 5–8, 17].

An embolus may be voluminous enough to block the internal carotid in the neck. However, most of the fragments cast into the carotid or vertebral circulation are smaller and will lodge in the cerebral arteries. When an embolus stops at the site of a bifurcation or an atherosclerotic narrowing, it blocks the circulation and causes softening downstream to the obstacle, as in the case of thrombosis. If the fragment disintegrates, the return of circulation to an ischaemic territory may be accompanied by extravasation of blood (haemorrhagic softening[3, 5–8, 17, 18]). Because embolic occlusion occurs very suddenly, collateral circulation is generally not sufficient to prevent necrosis of the nervous tissue; the territory distal to the obstruction is therefore less frequently spared than in thrombosis. Embolisms sometimes affect only the small branches of the cerebral arteries. They may then result in very circumscribed cortical or cortical-subcortical lesions whose clinical manifestations, in certain cases of damage of the left cerebral hemisphere, involve only a particular aspect of linguistic functioning. This type of aetiology is associated with many of the cases of 'pure disorders'—pure anarthria, conduction aphasia, agnosic alexia (see Chapters 3 to 5)—observed in clinical neurology.

For reasons related to circulatory dynamics, the territory most frequently affected by cerebral embolisms is that of the sylvian artery[6]. Consequently, aphasia is one of the common clinical manifestations of this disease. The language disorder always appears suddenly, without premonitory signs, and seldom progresses thereafter. On the other hand, a global impairment, caused for example by an embolus which stops at the bifurcation of the carotid, may rapidly give way to an aphasia of more limited symptomatology: it can then be concluded that the extent of the threatened zone has been reduced through the fragmentation of the embolus and its dispersal in one or more distal branches of the vessel. The disorders associated with a cerebral embolus may be transient or permanent; as in the case of thrombosis, their severity and the nature of their evolution depend on the site and extent of parenchymatous destruction subsequent to vascular obstruction and ischaemia.

Certain diseases involve repeated embolisms. They often damage different regions of the brain and thus give rise to disparate neurological disorders which may include aphasia. In such cases of multifaceted symptomatology, diagnosis and localization may be particularly difficult and uncertain.

The most frequent causes of cerebral embolism include auricular fibrillation, myocardial infarction with mural thrombus[19], and valvular, aortic or carotid atherosclerosis.[17].

INTRACRANIAL HAEMORRHAGE

Haemorrhage from arterial hypertension

Cerebral haemorrhages associated with arterial hypertension are the most frequent of the intracranial haemorrhages[3, 17]. They result from the rupture of an intraparenchymatous branch of a cerebral artery. The extravasation* of blood caused by the lesion may be violent enough to destroy a portion of the cerebral parenchyma; it may also impair the local vascularization of the tissue and, through compression, damage neighbouring regions (see Fig. 5–1 and 9–2).

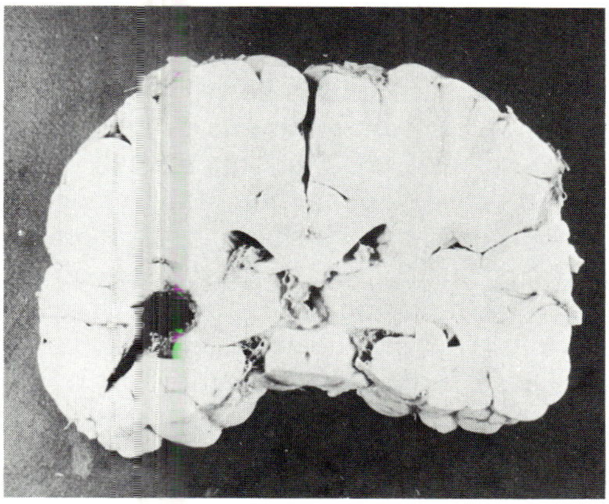

Fig. 9-2 *Simulation of a recent intracerebral haemorrhage located beneath Wernicke's area and extending into the axis of the left, second temporal convolution. Courtesy of Dr Luis Oliva, Department of Neuropathology, Queen Elizabeth Hospital, Montreal.*

If the intraparenchymatous mass of blood is voluminous, it may enter the ventricular cavity. As may be verified through a lumbar puncture, the cerebrospinal fluid is then tinged with blood. The form and size of the haematoma are variable. If the patient survives, reabsorption of the clot, which may take from two to six months, leaves a scar consisting of only a thin yellowish slash. This is particularly characteristic in the case of haemorrhages occurring at the cortical–subcortical junction or in the axis of a convolution (Fig. 9–3).

In cerebral haemorrhages associated with hypertension, the neurological deficit appears suddenly, with no premonitory signs (other than those of the hypertension) and rarely during sleep. The patient's status deteriorates within a few hours or days and death follows in more than two-thirds of the cases. When the intracerebral extravasation of blood is massive, ventricular inundation, herniation of the temporal lobe and/or compression of the mesencephalon (upper part of the brainstem) lead to death (see Chapter 8–1 and Fig. 8–1). When the extravasation is small in volume, survival is the rule. Haemorrhage rarely recurs during evolution and functional recovery is often considerable. Unlike softening, a cerebral haemorrhage causes greater displacement than destruction of the cerebral parenchyma.

Intracerebral haemorrhages are less frequent than thromboembolic softenings. However, when the former result in aphasia, its clinical form is usually more characteristic than in thromboembolic accidents. Through its repercussions on the whole of the language zone, the classical capsulolenticular haemorrhage of hypertension often causes global aphasia when

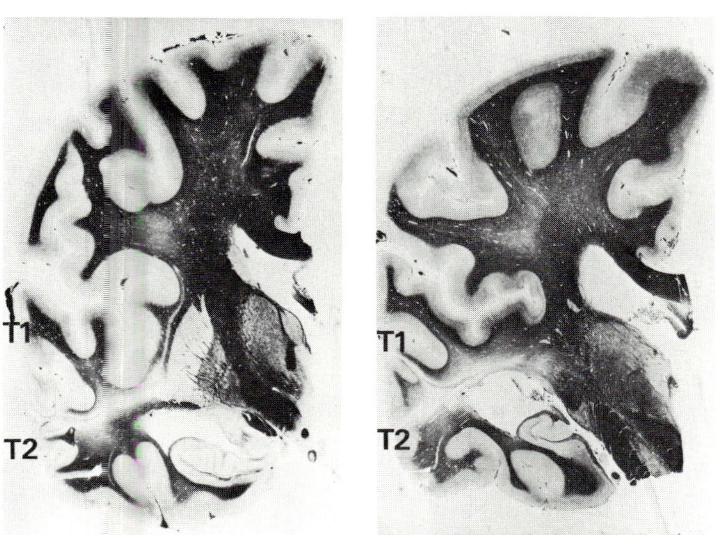

Fig. 9-3 *An old intracerebral haemorrhage (coronal sections of the left cerebral hemisphere; Loyez staining). The cicatricial slash is located in the axis of the left, second temporal convolution (T2) and extends beneath to the putamen; the lesion thus isolates a large part of Wernicke's area proper (T1: left, first temporal convolution). In its prototypic phase, the clinical picture was that of Wernicke's aphasia proper with logorrhoeic jargon. Case C-91, Laboratoire Théophile Alajouanine, Centre de Recherche du Centre Hospitalier Côte-de-Neiges, Montreal.*

* The escape of fluids (in this case, blood) into the surrounding tissue.

it is in the left hemisphere; in this case, a right hemiplegia is also present. Moreover, a haemorrhage of the left, temporo-parieto-occipital junction causes one form or another of Wernicke's aphasia (Fig. 9-2). The limited knowledge presently available on language disorders related to natural thalamic lesions has been almost entirely acquired through the study of cases of hypertensive haemorrhages of the left thalamus (see Chapter 7-3)[20-24].

Haemorrhage by the rupture of an arterial aneurysm

Aneurysmal haemorrhage is the fourth cause of cerebral vascular accidents[3, 17], following, in order of frequency, atherosclerotic thrombosis, embolism and hypertensive haemorrhage. It is usually caused by the rupture of a sacculated aneurysm. Such aneurysms, either single or multiple, are situated at the origin and/or bifurcations of the cerebral arteries. They involve a genuine hernia of the arterial wall which appears with age as a result of localized anomalies in the development of the muscular and elastic layers of the arteries (Fig. 9-4).

Before it ruptures, an aneurysm is generally asymptomatic.* The moment of rupture is usually marked by a brutal, violent headache which is sometimes soon followed by a loss of consciousness. There are also cases in which a loss of consciousness occurs immediately without any prodrome. The rupture of the aneurysm causes a haemorrhage which is at first subarachnoid, that is, meningeal; the extravasation may be limited to the meningeal space but, in many cases, it damages the subjacent cerebral parenchyma. Depending on the site and extent of the damage, the rupture of an aneurysm may cause

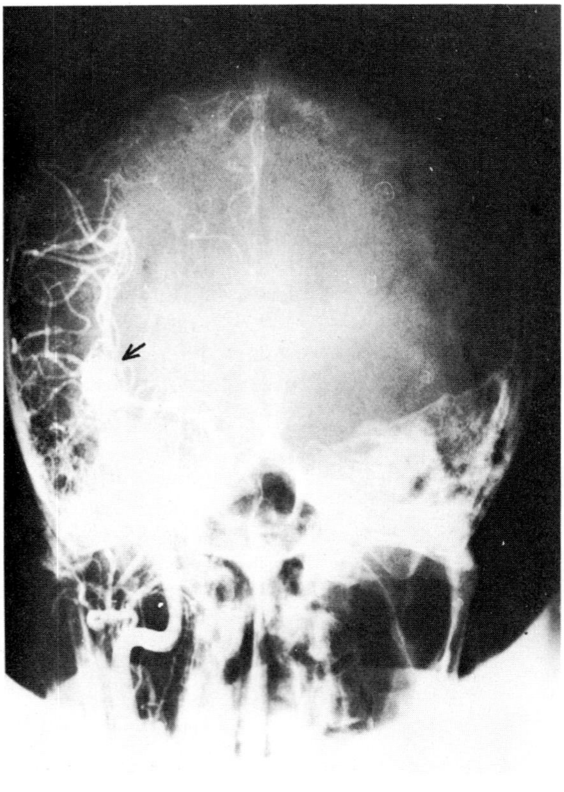

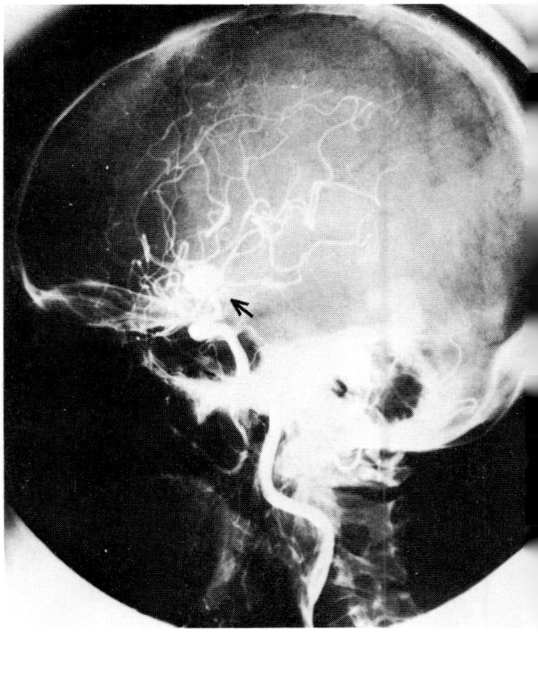

Fig. 9-4 *Subarachnoid haemorrhage in the left sylvian territory by the rupture of a sacculated aneurysm; the only localizing clinical signs observed in this case were those of a mild Wernicke's aphasia (C-398, Laboratoire Théophile Alajouanine, Centre de Recherche du Centre Hospitalier Côte-de-Neiges, Montreal). The aneurysm is visible on the above arteriographic plates (face on the left and profile on the right); it is situated at the level of the sylvian trifurcation (arrows). Courtesy of Dr Marc Aubé, Département de Radiologie, Hôtel-Dieu, Montreal.*

* In cases where death is not attributable to neurological disease, it is not uncommon that autopsy reveals the presence of one or several non-ruptured aneurysms.

different neurological disorders including aphasia. These disorders may correspond to one or both of two different mechanisms: we have already mentioned the possibility of parenchymatous destruction through adjacency to the meningeal extravasation of blood; in these cases, an arterial spasm frequently occurs and, in turn, causes ischaemic necrosis in the territory of the abnormal vessel. Since the carotid siphon and the middle cerebral artery (see Fig 9-1) are the site of 60 per cent of all sacculated aneurysms, the sylvian territory—which, on the left, includes the language zone (see Chapter 8-1)—is often damaged.

Transient aphasia may be present for some minutes after the rupture of an aneurysm and then disappear leaving no sequelae; this type of evolution indicates, of course, that there was no significant parenchymatous destruction within the language zone. A more serious and persistent disorder may nevertheless occur, caused by either or both of the two mechanisms discussed above, particularly when the ruptured aneurysm is situated at the bifurcation of the left, middle cerebral artery (Fig. 9-4) or at its origin in the anastomotic circle of Willis (see Fig. 9-1). In these cases, the aphasia is, as a general rule, either a global aphasia or Wernicke's type of aphasia (see Chapter 4). The abrupt onset of such an aphasia, in a young right-handed adult, immediately suggests the diagnosis of the rupture of a sacculated aneurysm of the left, middle cerebral artery.

A ruptured aneurysm has an unfavourable prognosis. When the patient survives, a second bleeding, which occurs in more than half of the cases, may be fatal or again cause severe and permanent neurological disorders. The difficulties of surgical treatment, and its complications, add to the seriousness of the disease. However, in certain cases, this treatment permits a most favourable evolution.

Haemorrhages by the rupture of an arteriovenous aneurysm

The arteriovenous aneurysm[3, 17, 25] of interest in the present context is a congenital malformation, consisting of an abnormal vascular network allowing communication between arteries and veins. It is more frequent in women than in men. Its volume may increase over time. Given the clinical manifestations of an arteriovenous aneurysm (atypical headaches and/or attacks of epilepsy), it is not uncommon that it is discovered in the absence of a rupture. In many respects, the signs of a rupture of a cerebral angioma* resemble those of a rupture of a sacculated aneurysm. Depending on whether or not the malformation is superficial, its rupture will result in a subarachnoid haemorrhage or intraparenchymatous haemorrhage. It may possibly cause both at once. The neurological disturbances which mark the rupture of a cerebral angioma vary with its location. In cases of involvement of the language zone, the disturbances include aphasia; the clinical features of the language disorder will then vary according to the localization and the extent of the lesions within the language zone. In addition to the rupture of a sacculated aneurysm (cf. p. 234), the abrupt onset of aphasia in a young subject also suggests the diagnosis of rupture of an arteriovenous aneurysm.

MIGRAINE

Migraine is a very particular type of headache. Pulsatile and hemicranially located, it occurs in intermittent attacks. Migraine often begins during childhood or adolescence and, as a general rule, the attacks become less frequent with age. Migraine often occurs in several members of the same family.

In certain individuals, an impending attack of migraine is signalled by the onset of transient neurological disorders and one then speaks of accompanied migraine[3, 17, 26]. These disorders often affect visual functions (scotoma, hemianopsia); sensory disturbances (paraesthesias) may also occur.† In certain cases, aphasia is a prodrome of migraine. The language disorder immediately precedes the headache and rarely lasts more than 20 to 30 minutes. The aphasia is sometimes global. In other cases, dissociated disturbances of verbal expression or comprehension may be observed or, more rarely, alexia or agraphia. These transient aphasic disorders are thought to reflect a circulatory disturbance with reversible ischaemia in the territory of the left sylvian artery.

* In the present context, a synonym for cerebral arteriovenous aneurysm.

† An episode of migraine is sometimes followed by persistent hemiplegia. It is then not an accompanying phenomenon but a post-migraine disturbance having different physiopathology.

CRANIAL TRAUMA

In present times, the frequency of cranial trauma is progressively increasing due to a growing number of automobile and occupational accidents. Cranial trauma represents an important cause of aphasia[27–29], particularly in young adults. The aetiological diagnosis raises no difficulty but it is more difficult to determine the nature and importance of the cerebral lesions and, as a consequence, to anticipate the occurrence of complications and the severity of sequelae.

Cranial trauma, either with or without cranial fracture, is often accompanied by a cerebral contusion, that is, a macroscopic lesion consisting of an area of dilaceration and haemorrhagic necrosis, to which cerebral oedema is temporarily added. It follows that this type of parenchymatous lesion may give rise to neurological and neuropsychological localizing signs, including aphasia. These signs generally become clear secondarily, that is, after the regression of impaired consciousness resulting from the initial concussion.

Depending on the localization and the extent of the contused region, any of the clinical forms of aphasia may be observed (see Chapters 3 to 8). The rather high frequency of contusions of limited extent (classically situated on the top of a cerebral convolution and having the form of an inverted cone with its base on the cortical surface and its apex in the subcortical white matter) explains the occurrence of disturbances more or less specifically affecting a particular aspect of linguistic functioning. The fact that these contusions often affect the temporal lobe explains the rather high incidence of a Wernicke's type of aphasia (sometimes including an element of severe jargonaphasia). When the evolution is favourable, word-finding difficulty (see Chapter 4) is often the last disturbance to disappear; either at onset or after evolution, amnesic aphasia (or an analogous picture) is not uncommon following cranial trauma.

Whether or not aphasia is present, the post-traumatic syndrome often includes a loss of academic knowledge which may, in certain cases, be very pronounced. When associated with aphasia, this loss may contribute to the anomalies of linguistic behaviour. It may then be difficult to identify which aspects of the impairment are specifically aphasic.

CEREBRAL TUMOURS

Cerebral tumours (Fig.9–5) are also a frequent cause of aphasia[30–37] during the first half of life, a period during which cerebral vascular accidents are relatively rare. Whether the tumours are primary or metastatic, there is progressive formation of an intracranial mass which displaces or invades the cerebral parenchyma. Primary tumours develop in situ from the constituents of nervous tissue itself or from adjacent extra-encephalic structures (bones, meninges, hypophysis, cranial nerves): one commonly speaks of *benign tumours*, namely ones which are well localized, do not invade the cerebral tissue, develop slowly and are surgically accessible, and of *malignant tumours*, namely ones which are infiltrating, rapidly growing and rarely susceptible to definitive surgical treatment. Metastatic tumours are neoformations distant from their point of origin. For example, a pulmonary neoplasm may migrate towards the brain and give rise to one, or, even more characteristically, to several cerebral metastases.

The compression or destructive invasion of the cerebral parenchyma by a tumour results in several neurological manifestations. Some are said to be focal because they depend on the site of the tumour. The others reflect the effects of the neoformation on the entire encaphalic mass (cerebral oedema, intracranial hypertension) and have no localizing value. Aphasia is usually a focal manifestation.

One of the particular aspects of the aphasic symptomatology of cerebral tumours is paroxysmal aphasia, which corresponds to a focal epileptic attack (see Chapter 6)[38–43]. Focal or generalized epilepsy may, in fact, constitute the first sign of a cerebral tumour; it sometimes precedes other manifestations by several years. This mode of appearance is especially observed in slowly developing tumours (meningiomas, astrocytomas, oligodendrogliomas). The first attack typically occurs during adult life (tardy epilepsy). The onset of paroxysmal aphasia strongly suggests the presence of a lesion in the

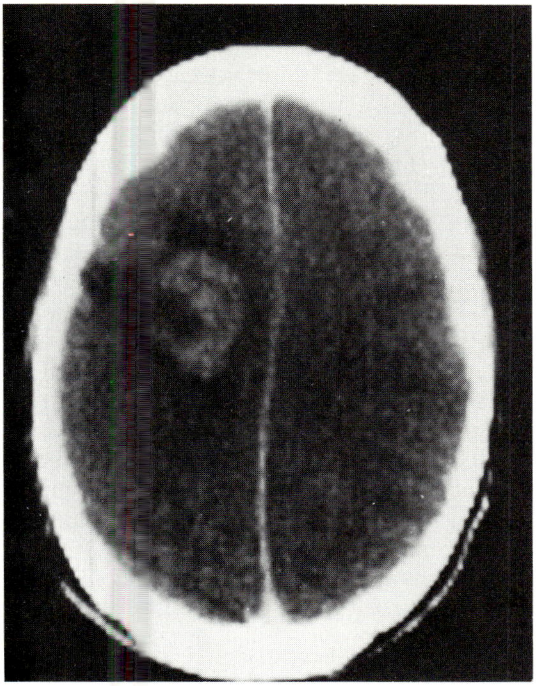

Fig. 9-5 *CT scan: haemorrhage within a left frontal glioblastoma in a 17-year-old patient. The clinical picture included a Broca's type aphasia manifested primarily by severe reduction without an obvious comprehension disturbance. Courtesy of Dr Marc Aubé,* Service de Neuroradiologie, Hôtel-Dieu, Montreal.

language zone or in neighbouring regions (see Chapter 8-1 and 8-5).

Linguistic aspontaneity, which is sometimes observed in lesions of the prefrontal convexity (see Chapter 6), often results from tumours of this region[37] (see Insertion 6.3). In contrast, the classical picture of Broca's aphasia (see Chapter 4), as caused by cerebrovascular accidents, almost never occurs in the case of cerebral tumours* although they may nevertheless be the source of predominantly expressive aphasic disorders. Tumoral and vascular symptomatology is more similar in regard to left temporal and temporoparietal lesions. The different clinical forms of Wernicke's aphasia may indeed occur with tumours of these regions; on the other hand, the clinical picture of conduction aphasia is very seldom observed with tumours. In aphasias resulting from tumours, the clinical signs appear gradually rather than brutally, as in the case of vascular accidents and trauma (for example, while paraphasic productions may be included in the clinical picture of various cerebral tumours, unequivocal jargon is never observed unless there is an intratumoral haemorrhage). Botez's work[34, 37] showed that word-finding difficulty may be a very early sign of a cerebral tumour: as a general rule, its presence as an isolated disturbance is then more prolonged in prerolandic than in retrorolandic tumours (see Chapter 6).

Despite certain similarities between aphasias subsequent to cerebral vascular accidents and those resulting from tumoral aetiology, the latter have, like some other signs of a cerebral tumour, certain distinctive characteristics. One of the most obvious is certainly the insidious and regular evolution towards increased severity with the growth of the tumoral mass. Certain intercurrent phenomena may nevertheless modify this slowly progressive evolution: thus necrosis and an intratumoral haemorrhage are sometimes accompanied by a sudden aggravation;† similarly, the severity of the aphasia varies significantly in certain cases as a result of fluctuations in the peritumoral oedema, fluctuations which may themselves be linked to the action of various therapeutic agents. In the long term, deterioration is inevitable and the aphasia becomes of secondary importance in the picture of extensive left hemisphere involvement; the symptomatological analysis of the language disorder—or even its identification—is then compromised. If this progressive course is modified through surgery, the postoperative symptomatology may differ in certain respects from the preoperative symptomatology; the residual disorder, which is often very severe, should then be considered as the result of the combined effects of the tumour and of the surgical intervention.

* With the exception of cases in which a haemorrhage is formed from neovessels of the tumoral tissue, thus abruptly changing the nature of the clinical picture and its mode of evolution, one never sees agrammatism, for example, in aphasias resulting from cerebral tumours.

† For example the transition from conversational behaviour including occasional phonemic paraphasic deviations to clearly jargoned discourse marks, in an almost pathognomonic way, the occurrence of a haemorrhage within a tumoral lesion of the left temporal or temporoparietal region.

DEGENERATIVE DISEASES

This heading refers to a heterogeneous group of diseases attributable to a progressive loss of nerve cells in more or less definite regions of the neural axis. When such pathology affects the cerebral covering to a major or predominant extent, the result is an organic dementia, that is, a gradual deterioration of intellectual functions (attention, memory, judgement, reasoning ability, etc.). Unlike the transient impairments of higher mental functions which accompany toxi-infectious or metabolic confusional states (see below), this deterioration is slowly progressive and irreversible.*

At present, several types of organic dementia are recognized in adults. While probably of varied aetiology,† their symptomatology and the nature of their evolution justify, within the present context, the grouping of the following conditions: senile dementia, Alzheimer's disease, Pick's disease, Creutzfeldt-Jakob disease, Huntington's chorea. Most of the patients suffering from these diseases sooner or later present a language disorder[44–46]. The onset is insidious and the disorder initially appears attributable to impairments of thought, of inner language, of the ability to abstract or to generalize. The patient's attention and his memory of linguistic messages are implicated. The degree of semantic and syntactic complexity of heard or produced discourse, as well as its more or less concrete or abstract nature, also enter into account. Word-finding difficulty, which is sometimes very clear and primarily manifested in conversation, constitutes an early sign in some cases. On the other hand, the flow of speech, as well as transposition activities (see Chapter 15) may remain normal during a certain period. However, this does not last and, in most cases, disturbances soon appear whose nature is more clearly aphasic: naming gives rise to numerous verbal paraphasias, paragraphic transformations abound in written expression, etc. On the other hand, repetition may remain intact for a long time in certain patients and echolalic phenomena are frequent; the picture then observed (in the linguistic sphere) is that of a Type II Wernicke's aphasia (see Chapter 4).

Although aphasia may sometimes be seen among the first signs of a degenerative disease, or may even constitute the earliest sign,‡ the language disorder soon occurs within the context of a multitude of neuropsychological disorders which also includes agnosic, apraxic and amnesic elements. Perseverative phenomena may then appear in almost all of the patient's behaviours, including those related to language. At this time, the aphasia is only one facet of a progressively generalized cortical disease. It is then often impossible to carry out a rigorous symptomatological analysis of the aphasia itself.

METABOLIC OR DEFICIENCY DISEASES AND POISONING

Metabolic diseases, deficiency diseases and exogenous poisoning rarely result in a typical aphasia. Rather, these conditions tend to be accompanied by confusional states with impaired vigilance; they may also take the form of pseudodemential syndromes. Certain of these conditions should nevertheless be mentioned since the encephalopathies which they induce may lead to the formation of localized cerebral lesions. Such lesions may cause aphasia when they affect the left hemisphere. For example, it was on the basis of a case of carbon-monoxide poisoning, with lesions surrounding the language zone, that Geschwind et al[47] recently specified the symptomatology of one of the clinical forms of Wernicke's aphasia (*isolated speech area*) (see Chapters 4 and 8–3).

Anoxic and hypoglycaemic encephalopathies

* From a clinical and therapeutic point of view it is therefore important to utilize all possible means in order to distinguish between dementias related to degenerative diseases and other—curable—organic pathological states which may resemble degenerative diseases in certain respects (chronic subdural haematoma, frontal meningioma, normotensive hydrocephalus in certain cases, neurosyphilis, myxoedema, bromide poisoning, and other disorders of infectious, toxic or metabolic origin).

† Work by Gajdusek and his collaborators has recently shown that Creutzfeldt-Jakob disease, one of the classical 'degenerative diseases', is related to the invasion of the organism by a slow virus.

‡ The clinical picture is then that of amnesic aphasia (see Chapter 4), a picture comparable with that also observed in certain cases of an abscess, haematoma or tumour of the left, temporoparietal region.

may be complicated by a localized cerebral softening, especially in the presence of arterial circulation already compromised by pre-existing vascular disease. The occurrence of a language disorder has also been reported in certain cases of encephalopathies of hepatic or renal origin.

INFECTIOUS DISEASES

Infections of the central nervous system are seldom the cause of aphasia. A temporal lobe abscess, of bacterial, mycotic or parasitical origin is, however, an important exception[48–50]. This lesion is a purulent collection, more or less completely encapsulated, depending on the duration of it evolution, which is often accompanied by cerebraloedema and intracranial hypertension. With the exception of the phenomena related to the infection itself, its manifestations are similar to those of a cerebral tumour in the same location. However, surgical treatment, combined with eradication of the causal agent by antibiotics or chemotherapy, is effective in a large number of patients. An aphasia, either with or without hemiplegia, remains as a sequel in 30 per cent of the patients who survive.

Certain cases of meningitis may be accompanied by inflammatory vascular lesions which may cause cerebral softenings. They may affect the language areas. The use of antibiotics has considerably reduced the frequency of such complications.

Viral encephalitis may also cause significant necrosis of temporoparietal regions. Nevertheless, in cases where an aphasia can be identified, it represents, in these patients (for example, those with herpetic encephalitis), only one of the many manifestations or sequelae attesting to a massive destruction of the cerebral parenchyma.

REFERENCES

1. Foix, C. & Lévy, M. (1927) Les ramollissements sylviens—syndromes des lésions en foyer du territoire de l'artère sylvienne et de ses branches. *Revue neurologique*, **35**, 1.
2. Fisher, C.M. (1961) Clinical syndromes in cerebral arterial occlusion. In *Pathogenesis and Treatment of Cerebrovascular Disease* (Ed.) Fields, W. p. 1. Springfield, IL: Thomas.
3. Fisher, C.M., Praful, M.D. & Adams, R.D. (1962) Cerebrovascular disease and the stroke syndrome. In *Principles of Internal Medicine* (Ed.) Harrison, T.R. et al. p. 1748. New York: McGraw-Hill.
4. Lhermitte, F., Gautier, J.C. & Derouesné, C. (1966) Anatomopathologie et physiopathologie des sténoses carotidiennes. *Revue neurologique*, **115**, 641.
5. Gautier, J.C. (1967) Sténoses et occlusions de l'artère carotide interne. *Gazette médical de France*, **1**, 3901.
6. Lhermitte, F., Gautier, J.C., Derouesné, C. & Guiraud, B. (1968) Ischemic accidents in the middle cerebral artery territory. *Archives of Neurology* (Chicago), **19**, 248.
7. Waddington, M.M. & Ring, B.A. (1968) Syndromes of occlusion of middle cerebral artery branches. *Brain*, **91**, 658.
8. Castaigne, P., Lhermitte, F., Gautier, J.C., Escourolle, R. & Derouesné, C. (1970) Internal carotid artery occlusion. A study of 61 instances in 50 patients with postmortem data. *Brain*, **93**, 231.
9. Alvarez, W.C. (1955) More about little strokes. *Geriatrics*, **10**, 555.
10. Fisher, C.M. & Curry, H.B. (1964) Pure motor hemiplegia. *Transactions of the American Neurological Association*, **89**, 94.
11. Fisher, C.M. & Curry, H.B. (1965) Pure motor hemiplegia of vascular origin. *Archives of Neurology* (Chicago), **13**, 30.
12. Fischer C.M. (1967) Lacunar stroke: the dysarthria-clumsy hand syndrome. *Neurology*, **17**, 614.
13. Lazorthes, G., Gouazé A. & Salamon, G. (1976) *Vascularisation et circulation de l'encéphale* (*vol. I*): *Anatomie descriptive et fonctionnelle*. Paris: Masson.
14. Lazorthes, G. & Gouazé A. (1968) Les voies anastomotiques de suppléance de la vascularisation artérielle cérébro-spinale. *Bulletin de l'Association des Anatomistes* (Nancy), *139 bis*, 1.
15. Bes, A. & Géraud, G. (1974) *Circulation cérébrale—Physiologie*. Rueil-Malmaison: Sandoz.
16. Lhermitte, F. (1960) Les thromboses bilatérales de la carotide interne. *Acquisitions médicales récentes*, **15**, 37.
17. Fisher, C.M., Mohr, J.P. & Adams, R.D. (1972) Maladies cérébro-vasculaires. In *Principes de médecine interne*. (Ed.) Harrison, T.R. p. 1752. Paris: Flammarion.
18. Down, L. (1871) Right hemiplegia with loss of speech due to red softening of the brain. *Lancet*, **1**, 852.
19. Boudin, G. & Sabouraud, O. (1950) Hémiplégie droite avec aphasie révélatrice d'une endocardite infectieuse chez une mitrale. Guérison. *Bulletin et Mémoires de la Societé médicale des Hôpitaux de Paris*, **66**, 160.
20. Fisher, C.M. (1959) The pathologic and clinical aspects of thalamic hemorrhage. *Transactions of the American Neurological Association*, **84**, 56.

21. Bugiani, O., Conforto, C. & Sacco, G. (1969) Aphasia in thalamic haemorrhage. *Lancet*, **24,** 1052.
22. Ciemins V.A. (1970) Localized thalamic hemorrhage: a case of aphasia. *Neurology*, **20,** 776.
23. Fazio, C., Sacco, G. & Bugiani, O. (1973) The thalamic haemorrhage. An anatomo-clinical study. *European Neurology*, **9,** 30.
24. Mohr, J.P., Watters, W.C. & Duncan, G.W. (1975) Thalamic hemorrhage and aphasia. *Brain and Language*, **2,** 3.
25. Pluvinage, R. (1960) Les angiomes cérébraux. *Revue pratique* (Paris), **10,** 3395.
26. Masson, M. (1973) Migraines et algies faciales. In *Collection Nouvelle pathologie médicale (fascicule 6): Système nerveux et muscles* (Ed.) Lhermitte, F. p. 294. Paris: Flammarion.
27. Alajouanine, Th., Castaigne, P., Lhermitte, F., Escourolle, R. & Ribaucourt, B. (de) (1957) Etude de 43 cas d'aphasie post-traumatique. Confrontation anatomoclinique et aspects évolutifs. *Encéphale*, **46,** 1.
28. Ritchie Russell, W. & Espir, M.L.E. (1961) *Traumatic Aphasia*. London: Oxford University Press.
29. Heilman, K.M., Safran, A. & Geschwind, N. (1971) Cranial trauma and aphasia. *Journal of Neurology, Neurosurgery and Psychiatry*, **34,** 265.
30. Smythe, G.E. & Stern, K. (1938) Tumors of the thalamus. *Brain*, **61,** 339.
31. Metzer, O. & Kammerer, T. (1951) Alexie et troubles aphasiques dans un cas de méningiome temporo-pariétal gauche. *Revue oto-neuro-ophtalmologie*, **23,** 239.
32. McKissock, W. & Paine, K.W.E. (1958) Primary tumors of the thalamus, *Brain*, **81,** 41.
33. Arseni, C. & Botez, M.I. (1961) Speech disturbances caused by tumors of the supplementary motor area. *Acta Psychiatrica Scandinavica*, **36,** 279.
34. Botez, M.I. (1962) *Aphasia and Correlated Syndromes in Intracranial Expanding Processes*. Bucharest: Academici R.S.R.
35. Peyton, W.T., French, L.A. & Baker, A.B. (1962) Intracranial neoplasms. In *Clinical Neurology* (Ed.) Baker, A.B. Vol. I, p. 460. New York: Hoeber-Harper.
36. Smith, A. (1966) Intellectual functions in patients with lateralized frontal tumors. *Journal of Neurology, Neurosurgery and Psychiatry*, **29,** 52.
37. Botez, M.I. (1974) Frontal lobe tumours. In *Handbook of Clinical Neurology* (Ed.) Vinken, P.J. & Bruyn, G.W. Vol. 17, p. 234. Amsterdam and New York: North Holland and American Elsevier.
38. Winkler, E.G., Freiman, G.V. & Lieberman, S.S. (1951) Astrocytoma of the left temporal lobe: contribution to the problem of psycho-pathology of epileptic personality disorders and to the problem of semantic aphasia. *American Journal of Psychiatry*, **108,** 343.
39. Hécaen, H. & Piercy, M. (1956) Paroxysmal dysphasia and the problem of cerebral dominance. *Journal of Neurology, Neurosurgery and Psychiatry*, **19,** 194.
40. Hécaen, H. & Angelergues, R. (1960) Epilepsie et troubles du langage. *Encéphale*, **49,** 138.
41. Falconer, M.A. & Serafetinides, E.A. (1962) The incidence and significance of speech disturbances during temporal seizures. *Journal of Neurology, Neurosurgery and Psychiatry*, **25,** 394.
42. Serafetinides, E.A. & Falconer, M.A. (1963) Speech disturbances in temporal lobe seizures. *Brain*, **86,** 333.
43. Geets, W. (1975) Crises agnosiques avec troubles du langage et anomalies asymétriques de l'EEG. *Acta Neurologica Belgica*, **75,** 160.
44. Haag, M. & Brabant, P. (1963) Le langage de 15 déments séniles dans la perspective de leur perte de l'attitude catégorielle de K. Goldstein. In *Recherches sur les maladies mentales* (Ed.) Daumézon, G. p. 111. Paris: Imprimerie municipale.
45. Tissot, R., Richard, J., Duval, F. & Ajuriaguerra, J. (de) (1967) Quelques aspects du langage des démences dégénératives du grand âge. *Acta Neurologica Belgica*, **67,** 911.
46. Escourolle, R. (1973) Démences. In *Système nerveux et muscles* (Ed.) Lhermitte, F. & Mamo, H. p. 313, fascicule 6, Collection Nouvelle Pathologie médicale. Paris: Flammarion.
47. Geschwind, N., Quadfasel., F.A. & Segarra, J. (1968) Isolation of the speech area. *Neuropsychologia*, **6,** 327.
48. Gehuchten, A. (van). & Goris, C. (1901) Un cas de surdité verbale pure par abcès du lobe temporal gauche; trépanation, guérison. *Névraxe*, **3,** 65.
49. Harper, A.R. (1951) Aphasia as a symptom of otogenic brain abscess. *Journal of Laryngology*, **65,** 89.
50. Lechevalier, B. (1973) Abcès du cerveau. In *Système nerveux et muscles* (Ed.) Lhermitte, F. & Mamo, H. p. 344, fascicule 6, Collection Nouvelle Pathologie médicale. Paris: Flammarion.
51. Lazorthes, G. (1961) Vascularisation et circulation cérébrales. Paris: Masson.

BIBLIOGRAPHY

Alajouanine, Th. & Sabouraud, O. (1960) Les perturbations du langage dans l'épilepsie. *Encéphale*, **49,** 95.

Amyes, E.W. & Nielsen, J.M. (1955) Clinicopathologic study of vascular lesions of the anterior cingulate region. *Bulletin of the Los Angeles Neurological Society*, **20,** 112.

Angelergues, R., Hécaen, H. & Ajuriaguerra, J. (de) (1955) Les troubles mentaux au cours des tumeurs du lobe frontal. *Annales médico-psychologiques*, **2,** 577.

Baruk, H. (1926) *Les troubles mentaux dans les tumeurs cérébrales*. Paris: Doin.

Bes, A., & Géraud, G. (1974) *Circulation cérébrale-Physiologie*. Rueil-Malmaison: Sandoz.

Bingley, T. (1958) Mental symptoms in temporal lobe epilepsy and temporal lobe gliomas. *Acta Psychiatrica Scandinavica*, **33** (suppl. 120), 1.

Bocca, E., Calearo, C., Cassinari, V. & Migliavacca, F.

(1951) Testing 'cortical' hearing in temporal lobe tumours. *Acta Oto-laryngologica* (Stockholm), **45,** 289.

Botez, M.I. (1960) Clinical contributions to the study of the tumoral frontal syndrome. *Psychiatria et Neurologia,* **140,** 351.

Botez, M.I. (1968) The tumoral temporohinencephalic syndrome of the dominant hemisphere. *Confinia Neurologica* (Basel), **30,** 349.

Boudouresque, J., Roger, J. & Gastaut, H. (1962) Crises aphasiques subintrantes chez un épileptique temporal. Etude électro-clinique. *Revue neurologique,* **106,** 381.

Buge, A., Escourolle, R., Rancurel, G. & Poisson, M. (1975) 'Mutisme akinétique' et ramollissement bicingulaire. *Revue neurologique,* **131,** 121.

Castaigne, P., Lhermitte, F. & Gautier, J.C. (1960) Formes topographiques des ramollissements cérébraux. *Revue pratique* (Paris), **10,** 3709.

Castaigne, P., Lhermitte, F. & Gautier, J.C. (1960) Physiopathologie des accidents ischémiques cérébraux. *Revue pratique* (Paris), **10,** 3705.

Cambier, J. (1960) Physiologie de la circulation cérébrale. *Revue pratique* (Paris), **10,** 3699.

Chavany, J.-A., Lobel, G. & Hagenmuller, D. (1956) Etude clinique des troubles du langage d'essence épileptique. *Presse médicale,* **64,** 1449.

Cole, F. (1883–84) Amnesic aphasia resulting from railroad accident. *Georgia Medical Monthly,* **4,** 339.

Collier, J.S. (1899) A contribution to the study of aphasia. A case in which complete destruction of Broca's convolution by a neoplasm in a right handed person produced no aphasia. *Lancet,* **1,** 824.

Critchley, M. (1960) Troubles de la parole dans les cas d'épilepsie. *Encéphale,* **49,** 134.

Davidson, C., Goodhart, P. & Needles, W. (1934) Cerebral localization in cerebro-vascular disease. *Research Publications, Association for Research in Nervous and Mental Diseases,* **13,** 435.

Delay, J. & Brion, S. (1962) *Les démences tardives.* Paris: Masson.

Driver, M.V., Falconer, M.A. & Serafetinides, E.A. (1964) Ictal speech automatism reproduced by activation procedures. A case report with comments on pathogenesis. *Neurology,* **5,** 455.

Falconer, M.A. & Serafetinides, E.A. (1963) A follow-up study of surgery in temporal lobe epilepsy. *Journal of Neurology, Neurosurgery and Psychiatry,* **26,** 154.

Fiolle, J. (1950) Anévrysme traumatique de la carotide primitive compliqué d'hémiplégie et d'aphasie; résection; amélioration fonctionnelle. *Marseille chirurgical,* **5,** 690.

Fisher, C.M., Mohr, J.-P. & Adams, R.D. (1970) Cerebrovascular diseases. In *Harrison's Principles of Internal Medicine* (Ed.) Wintrobe, M.M. et al. p. 1227. New York: Blakiston.

Forest, R.E. (ed), (Ed.) (1966) *Proceedings of the National Stroke Congress.* Springfield, IL: Thomas.

Frazier, C.H. & Ingham, S.D. (1920) A review of the effects of gunshot wounds of the head based on the observation of two hundred cases at U.S. general hospital. *Archives of Neurology and Psychiatry* (Chicago), **3,** 17.

Freemon, F.R. (1971) Akinetic mutism and bilateral anterior cerebral artery occlusion. *Journal of Neurology, Neurosurgery and Psychiatry,* **34,** 693.

Gautier, J.C. (1960) Le dispositif artériel cérébral. *Revue pratique* (Paris), **10,** 3691.

Gautier, J.C., Rosa, A. & Lhermitte, F. (1974) Accidents vasculaires cérébraux et contraceptifs oraux. *Revue neurologique,* **130,** 217.

Geschwind, N. & Sherwin, I. (1967) Language-induced epilepsy: case history. *Archives of Neurology* (Chicago), **16,** 25.

Hécaen, H. & Angelergues, R. (1960) Epilepsie et troubles du langage. *L'encéphale,* **49,** 138.

Hécaen, H. & Ajuriaguerra, J. (de) (1956) *Troubles mentaux au cours des tumeurs intracrâniennes.* Paris: Masson.

Heilman, K.M. (1974) Neuropsychologic changes in the stroke patient. *Geriatrics,* **29,** 153.

Jakab, I. (1950) L'aphasie dans la dêmence infantile de Heller. *Encéphale,* **39,** 220.

Lazorthes, G. (1961) *Vascularisation et circulation cérébrales.* Paris: Masson.

Lazorthes, G., Gouazé, A. & Salamon, G. (1976) *Vascularisation et circulation de l'encéphale.* Vol. I. Paris: Masson.

Lhermitte, F. & Mammo, H. (Ed.) (1973). Collection Nouvelle Pathologie médicale, fascicule 6: *Système nerveux et muscles.* Paris: Flammarion.

Miles, A. & Shennan, T. (1899) On a case of cerebral abscess illustrating certain forms of aphasia. *Lancet,* **1,** 1143.

Mugler, A. (1950) Aphasie chez un goutteux, guérie par la colchicine. *Strasbourg médicale,* **8–9,** 485.

Oettinger, L., Nikonishe, H. & Gill, I.G. (1967) Cerebral dysrythmia induced by reading (subclinical reading epilepsy). *Developmental Medicine and Child Neurology,* **9,** 191.

Page, I.H. (1963) *Strokes: How They Occur and What Can Be Done About Them.* New York: Macmillan.

Perevoschikova, G.F. & Tonkonoghy, I.M. (1967) Aphasie paroxystique avec localisation bilatérale à la partie caudale de la troisième circonvolution frontale. *Zhurnal Nevropatologii i Psikhiatrii,* **12,** 1772. (In Russian.)

Petit-Dutaillis, D., Guiot, G., Messimy, R. & Bourdillon, C. (1954) A propos d'une aphémie par atteinte de la zone motrice supplémentaire de Penfield, au cours de l'évolution d'un anévrysme artério-veineux; guérison de l'aphémie par ablation de la lésion, *Revue neurologique,* **90,** 95.

Pluvinage, R. (1960) Les angiomes cérébraux. *Revue pratique* (Paris), **10,** 3395.

Riese, W. (1949) Aphasia in brain tumors, its appearance in relation to the natural history of the lesion. *Confinia Neurologica* (Basel), **9,** 64.

Ritchie, D. (1961) *Stroke, a Study of Recovery.* New York: Garden City.

Ritchie-Russell, W. & Espir, M.L.F. (1961) *Traumatic Aphasia.* London: Oxford University Press.

Robillard, R. (1962) L'athéromatose cérébrale, *Union médical du Canada,* **91,** 415.

Scheenberg, P.A. (1958) A critical review of circulatory physiology as it applies to cerebral vascular disease. *Annals of Internal Medicine*, **48,** 1001.

Segarra, J.M. (1970) Cerebral vascular disease and behavior. *Archives of Neurology* (Chicago), **22,** 408.

Serafetinides, E.A. & Falconer, M.A. (1963) Speech disturbances in temporal lobe seizures: a study in 100 epileptics submitted to anterior temporal lobectomy. *Brain*, **86,** 333.

Solomon, A. (1957) An unusual receptive aphasia as a manifestation of temporal lobe epilepsy. Report of a case treated by surgery. *New England Journal of Medicine*, **257,** 313.

Wechsler, A.F. (1977) Presenile dementia presenting as aphasia. *Journal of Neurology, Neurosurgery and Psychiatry*, **40,** 303.

Williams, D. (1966) Temporal lobe epilepsy. *British Medical Journal*, **1,** 1439.

Winkler, E.G., Freiman, G.V. & Lieberman, S.S. (1951) Astrocytoma of the left temporal lobe: contribution to the problem of psycho-pathology of epileptic personality disorders and to the problem of semantic aphasia. *American Journal of Psychiatry*, **108,** 343.

Zangwill, O.L. (1954) Agraphia due to a left parietal glioma in left-handed man. *Brain*, **77,** 510.

10. Classifications of the Aphasias

> 'The essential of all work to be completed is a classification of work corresponding to ... to the human physique. That's to say that the human physique, uh, animal and vegetal is first classified, naturally, by the heavenly body. And the human classifies the heavenly body as well. They are continual classifications. An itinerant bureau, a living corpse—itinerant bureau for some—where some clay earth formed, from above, to the classifying bases from below ... Uh, continuously, a classification. It's a continual classification. Continual. What one sees, everywhere, what one does, a kind of photography: the eyes are cameras which classify the visual. Good! Properly to call. Properly to speak.'
>
> (*Conversation with Mr Gn.; April 1966*)

Aphasiology—should one be surprised?—became precociously addicted to the game of linguistic ambiguities [recall, for example, the debate between Broca and Trousseau over the meaning of the terms *aphemia* and *aphasia*[1] (see Chapter 1)]. More than any other medical discipline, with the possible exception of psychiatry, aphasiology generated and tolerated (apparent) terminological confusions in its own vocabulary and, particularly, in its classifications. These confusions appear to be related to several factors.

The first involves the almost indifferent usage of various terms to refer to the same phenomenon. For example, with only a few subtle differences, the terms *Broca's aphasia*, *motor aphasia*, *central motor aphasia* (for certain authors only), *cortical motor aphasia*, *kinetic efferent motor aphasia*, *expressive aphasia*, *verbal aphasia*, *aphasia of phonematic realization*, etc., all refer to the same clinical picture. Many of these terms serve to point out, rightly or wrongly, that their authors made—in this case with regard to Broca's aphasia—an anatomopathological, physiopathological or neurolinguistic discovery which was sufficiently important, universal and definitive to justify a change of label.

Conversely, the same term may be employed, according to different usages, to refer to different clinical phenomena. For example, for many associationists, a *central aphasia* attests to a lesion or dysfunction of a *centre*; that is, of the anatomical site of a psychological function. On the other hand, for many globalists, who object to the notion of a centre, a central aphasia* is one resulting from the lesion of the middle of the language zone [*the centre of the speech area* (Goldstein)].

Often deliberate for reasons of convenience, the semantic ambivalence of certain terms also enters into account. There are, for example, several classifications in which the notion of *aphasia* excludes those of *agnosia* and *apraxia* with regard to certain headings but includes one or the other with regard to other headings. Thus Foix considered *pure word deafness* to be an *agnosia* and not an *aphasia*, and then taught that (Wernicke's *aphasia* includes an *agnosic element* (cf. p. 253). To take another example, in discussions of *pure agraphia* it is generally not specified whether it should be compared with *Broca's aphasia* (which is suggested by the localization of the lesion attributed to it) or to *pure anarthria* [which corresponds more closely to the observed features of this clinical picture which, furthermore, is quite rare (see Chapters 3 and 6)].

Although this appears paradoxical, great semantic precision in terminology (i.e., a lack of ambiguity), especially in taxonomies which include particularly homogeneous terms, may constitute an even more formidable snare. For

* A conduction aphasia in the terminology of this text (pp. 90–93).

example, in the classification proposed by Wernicke after Lichteim's work (cf. pp. 248–249), the symmetry which is established between *subcortical, cortical* and *transcortical motor aphasias* and *subcortical, cortical* and *transcortical sensory aphasias* is very clear and appealing. It nevertheless suggests that *sensory aphasia* cannot include primary expressive symptoms, that *subcortical aphasia* necessarily results from a subcortical lesion, etc., all of which assertions follow from belief in a theoretical scheme rather than from clinical and anatomoclinical observation. To take another example, Head's classification (cf. pp. 254–255), with its four linguistic headings, may appear very pertinent and reassuring since the issue at hand is precisely the classification of language disorders. It would, nevertheless, be wrong to suppose that *syntactic aphasia* specifically disorganizes syntax or that *verbal aphasia* does not disorganize it at all. It would also be wrong to suppose that semantic inadequacy is present only in *semantic aphasia* or that difficulty in evoking names is a feature of *nominal aphasia* only.

This lack of etymological rigour is not exceptional. The terms *anarthria* and *dysarthria* are contrasted (at least in French), not to indicate different degrees of the same articulatory disturbance, as would appear logical, but rather to indicate different sites of lesion. The name *dynamic aphasia* is used to refer to a mode of discourse whose essential characteristic is its adynamism and the name *semantic jargon* is used to refer to a mode of discourse whose essential characteristic is its asemantism. One speaks of *dyssyntaxia*[2–5] to refer to behaviour in which the disturbance of syntax is no doubt a secondary phenomenon, occurring mainly when the selection of grammatical monemes is defective [see examples (2.45) to (2.47), (2.66), (2.78) to (2.80)], as is that of lexical monemes[6] (paradigmatic disorganization[7–9]), and one speaks of *agrammatism*[5, 10, 11] to designate behaviour in which the syntactical disturbance is probably more specific (syntagmatic disorganization[7–9]). Although these examples could be easily multiplied, it must be admitted that traditional usage has finally endowed many of these terms with such force that the change to an etymologically more appropriate name, while desirable a priori, is in fact scarcely possible.

The preceding reservations were purely ones of form and were in no way concerned with the appropriateness of a taxonomic approach. Indeed, such an approach largely provides the basis for possible discussions of aphasia (of its clinical manifestations, linguistic characteristics, physiopathology and pathological anatomy). Although an aphasia classification was suggested by previous discussion in several other sections of this text (see Chapters 3 to 8), this classification has not yet been presented systematically. We shall present it now and then try to indicate the main points of correspondence between this classification and those which the reader will encounter in other works on aphasia.

CLASSIFICATION OF THE APHASIAS IN THE CONTEXT OF THE PRESENT TEXT

The main characteristics of our classification are as follows: its three major divisions are based on functional anatomy (cf. pp. 165–167 and Insertion 8.8); its foremost aims are, however, clinical (to the extent that it is intended to permit easy labelling of as large a number of cases as possible); terminological homogeneity has been sacrificed, as has etymological rigour on some occasions, in order to retain the commonest terms in the lexicon of the French school (particularly the eponymous terms which have the advantage of being unbiased with regard to the physiopathology and the anatomopathology of aphasia); the notion of *aphasia* in no way excludes those of *apraxia*, *agnosia* or *amnesia*. We have thus discussed, in previous pages of this text, 11 symptom constellations (in addition to *global aphasia* and *mixed aphasias*).

(a) Clinical pictures generally attributed to lesions which impair the functioning of either a primary cortex,* the part of a specific association cortex most closely linked to its corresponding primary cortex,† the axons

* This may be the case in certain patients presenting 'pure anarthria'[12, 13] (cf. pp. 190–191).

† This may be the case in certain patients presenting 'pure word deafness'[14] (cf. p. 194).

entering or leaving these cortical zones* (cf. p. 249; *subcortical aphasias* in Wernicke's nomenclature) or of several of these structures at once. Certain authors (cf. pp. 252 and 264) group these disturbances under the name of *pure aphasias*.

(i) *Pure word deafness* is manifested by a disturbance in oral language comprehension, in repetition, and in writing to dictation (see Chapters 5 and 8–3).

(ii) *Pure word blindness* is manifested by a disturbance in written language comprehension, in oral reading, and in copying (see Chapters 5 and 8–3).

(iii) *Pure anarthria* is manifested by an isolated articulatory disturbance; that is, by a specific disorganization of the third phase of oral language[19] (see Chapters 2, 3 and 8–3).

(iv) *Pure agraphia* is manifested, according to the conception which we have presented, by the presence of an isolated graphic disturbance (see Chapters 2, 3, 6 and 8–3).

(b) Clinical pictures attributed to lesions which impair the functioning of a specific association cortex and/or of the associative axons immediately entering or leaving it. This group includes the classical *Broca's* and *Wernicke's aphasias*.

(i) *Wernicke's aphasia proper or Type I Wernicke's aphasia*. Articulatory production is normal and discourse is jargoned; comprehension and repetition are impaired; a component of *word deafness* may dominate the clinical picture (see Chapters 4 and 8–3).

(ii) *Type III Wernicke's aphasia*. All aspects of language are impaired with the exception of articulation; the disturbance of written expression and the alexia are nevertheless very clearly predominant (see Chapter 4). For Dejerine[15], the alexic element can be likened to a component of *word blindness*. Since the localization of the causal lesions is not precisely known (see Chapter 8–3), it is the parallel which can easily be drawn between *Type I* and *Type III Wernicke's aphasia* which led us to classify them under the same general heading.

(iii) *Broca's aphasia*. In the absence of an immediately apparent comprehension disturbance, it is *anarthria* (an articulatory disturbance) and *reduction* which constitute the principal clinical features of Broca's aphasia (see Chapters 4 and 8–3); whether it be a case of *Broca's aphasia almost limited to an articulatory disturbance* or of the *common form of Broca's aphasia*, both of these clinical features partially mask the production of paraphasic and paragraphic transformations. Such productions are nevertheless undeniable when a certain capacity for oral and written expression is retained.

If only because they sometimes correspond to (favourably) evolving forms of *Wernicke's aphasia proper*, we shall include the following two clinical pictures under the same general heading.

(iv) *Conduction aphasia*. Comprehension is comparable with that in Broca's aphasia and articulatory production is comparable with that in Wernicke's aphasia; discourse and repetition include numerous phonemic transformations (this may also be true of oral reading) (see Chapters 4 and 8–3). In certain cases, the phonemic transformations may be so predominant that they readily suggest, in regard to oral expressive symptomatology, a specific disorganization of the second linguistic phase[6, 19] (see Chapter 2).

(v) *(Pitres') Amnesic aphasia*. The clinical picture is essentially composed of word-finding difficulty manifested, chiefly by more or less adequate periphrastic productions, in discourse and in attempts at naming; performance is often impaired on comprehension tests requiring fine semantic discrimination (see Chapters 4, 8–3 and 12).

(c) Clinical pictures attributed to lesions which impair the functioning of a non-specific association cortex and/or of the associative axons immediately entering or leaving it. These are the *transcortical aphasias* in Wernicke's terminology (cf. p. 249).

(i) *Type II Wernicke's aphasia*. Articulatory

---

* Although not the general rule, this may be the case in certain patients presenting 'pure word blindness'[15–18] (cf. pp. 194–195).

production is normal; discourse is more or less abundant but is characterized by numerous verbal transformations and evident word-finding difficulty; language comprehension is impaired but repetition is not; a tendency towards echolalia (see Chapters 4 and 8–3) may be observed. In certain cases, the verbal transformations may be so predominant that they readily suggest, in regard to oral expressive symptomatology, a specific disorganization of the first phase of language (see Chapter 2).

(ii) *Aspontaneity* (in linguistic behaviour). The essential clinical feature is a *lack of verbal incentive* manifested, in discourse, by a major quantitative reduction; the same is true of spontaneous written expression. Articulatory production is normal; both naming and transposition activities remain possible (see Chapters 6 and 8–3).

APHASIA CLASSIFICATIONS

Written with the goal of facilitating understanding of different aphasia classifications, the following pages contain a schematic presentation of several classifications, each one representing the thoughts of a particular investigator. The reader will quickly realize that the aims of certain (empirical) classifications, like the one just discussed, are essentially clinical (Alajouanine, Goodglass) or anatomoclinical (Dejerine, Foix), whereas the primary aim of others is to place the problem of aphasia within a conceptual framework. In the latter case, the author's main concern may be related to the functional anatomy (Lichteim, Wernicke) and physiology (Luria) of language, to its psychopathology (Goldstein) or to the neurolinguistic (Hécaen) or properly linguistic (Jakobson) aspects of aphasia.

BAILLARGER (1865)

Considering two anomalies of discourse, that is, two features of oral expressive symptomatology (see Chapter 4), Baillarger[20] developed his dichotomous classification of aphasic syndromes (see Chapter 1) almost ten years before the publication of Wernicke's[21] monograph. The first of these anomalies concerns the flow of speech (which may or may not be quantitatively reduced, perhaps even non-existent) and the second concerns certain linguistic characteristics of discourse (which, beyond properly articulatory production, may or may not be qualitatively transformed).

(a) *Simple aphasia*. The disorder is characterized by a more or less complete loss of speech. Baillarger distinguished two subgroups:

(i) In certain patients presenting *simple aphasia*, the disorder impairs both speech and writing. According to Baillarger, this form of aphasia 'is explained in the most simple way by amnesia.' This clinical picture corresponds, in our classification, to the *common form of Broca's aphasia* and to certain forms of *global* or *mixed aphasia* (see Chapter 4).

(ii) In other patients, *simple aphasia* impairs speech but spares writing. Baillarger noted that in such patients 'the involuntary verbal incentive persists whereas the voluntary verbal incentive is abolished': he considered this fact to be of prime importance in regard to the psychopathology of the disorder. This second picture of *simple aphasia* probably corresponds to *pure anarthria* in our classification (see Chapter 3).

(b) *Aphasia with perversion of the faculty of language*. The clinical pictures discussed under this heading have jargonaphasic production as their common feature. They correspond, in our classification, to *Types I* and *II Wernicke's aphasia* and probably also to *conduction aphasia* (see Chapter 4). Baillarger considered that the notion of automatic–voluntary dissociation was also relevant in the case of aphasia with perversion of the faculty of language. He wrote, on this matter, that 'the dysfunction again consists in the substitution of automatic speech for the voluntary verbal incentive'.

JACKSON (1868)

During a scientific meeting also attended by Broca (Norwich, 1868), Jackson[22–24] presented a classification which was very similar to that of Baillarger. He first distinguished between patients with *paralytic articulation disorders* and those with *true aphasic disorders* ('true affections of speech', in Head's words[24]), and then identified two classes of patients among the latter:

(a) In the case of a *paralytic articulation disorder*, the patient can write normally. This disorder corresponds to the second picture of *simple aphasia* in Baillarger's classification[20] and to that of *pure anarthria* in ours (see Chapter 3).
(b) When *true aphasia* is present, *intellectual language* is more impaired than *emotional language*. It is in these cases that the effects of the automatic–voluntary dissociation are observed (quoting Head[24]: 'Jackson then passes on to show that the general law underlying these disturbances of speech is that voluntary power is diminished with retention of the power to carry out the same movement in a more automatic manner'). Jackson identified two clinical groups of true aphasia:
    (i) *Class 1.* In Head's words[24], Jackson defined his *Class 1* in the following way: 'Severe cases in which the patient is speechless or nearly so, or in which speech is very much damaged. In the worse of these cases the patient can only utter some one unvarying word or two words of some jargon.' The reduction affects written language as well as oral language. Thus the disorder corresponds completely to the first picture of *simple aphasia* in Baillarger's classification[20] and, in ours, to the *common form of Broca's aphasia* and to certain forms of *global* or *mixed aphasia* (see Chapter 4).
    (ii) *Class 2.* In Head's words[24], Jackson defined his *Class 2* in the following way: 'Cases in which there are plentiful movements, but wrong movements, or plenty of words, but mistakes in words.' Here again, written language is impaired. The clinical picture corresponds, in Baillarger's classification[20], to *aphasia with perversion of the faculty of language* and, in ours, to the forms of jargonaphasia (*Types I* and *II Wernicke's aphasia, conduction aphasia*) (see Chapter 4).

Although the clinical pictures discussed by Baillarger and Jackson are clearly the same, Jackson's grouping differs from that proposed by Baillarger. This change is not insignificant for it suggests the terms of the dichotomy which would later be established by Marie[25] (cf. pp. 250–251). Furthermore, while Baillarger claimed to have observed the effects of the automatic–voluntary dissociation in some patients presenting simple aphasia with preserved writing, Jackson observed these phenomena in patients whose written language was not spared (i.e., in patients whom he considered to have true aphasia).

WERNICKE (1874)

According to Wernicke[21], the biological substratum of thought is anatomically distinct from that of language. In right-handers, linguistic behaviour is specifically subtended by two left hemisphere regions. One region, namely the first temporal convolution, constitutes an *auditivo-verbal centre* which contains stored memory images of auditory sensations corresponding to the audition of spoken language. The other region, namely the caudalmost part of the third frontal convolution, identified by Broca in 1865[26], constitutes a *verbo-motor centre* which contains stored memory images of the sensations of movement (*Bewegungsvorstellungen*) corresponding to the production of articulated language (see Insertions 8.6, 10.1 and 10.4). These two centres are linked by an association pathway [which Wernicke considered to be subinsular (see Chapter 1)]. On the basis of this model, Wernicke recognized, in 1874, two forms of aphasia and postulated the existence of a third clinical picture.

(a) *Motor aphasia.* The clinical manifestations correspond to those which we have grouped, elsewhere in this text, under the heading of *Broca's aphasias* (see Chapter 4). Wernicke considered this clinical picture to be the effect of a lesion of the *verbo-motor centre*. This lesion causes a more or less total loss of *motor word images*, a loss which is manifested by a severe reduction in the capacity for oral expression and by a distortion of residual productions.
(b) *Sensory aphasia.* The clinical manifestations correspond to the picture which we have described under the name of *Wernicke's aphasia proper* or *Type I* (see Chapter 4). For Wernicke, this clinical picture is the effect of a lesion of the *auditivo-verbal centre*. This

Insertion 10.1

In his 1891 monograph, Freud[27] maintained that Wernicke believed each one of his memory images to be localized in a particular cell. While not going this far, Wernicke did indeed write that 'the cerebral cortex ... with its 600 million cells according to Meynert's estimate, provides a sufficient number of storage areas in which the countless sense impressions delivered by the outside world can be stored in succession'. [Translated from Wernicke[21].]

lesion causes a more or less total loss of *auditory word images*, a loss which is manifested by disturbed comprehension and repetition and, to the extent that the patient no longer has auditory control over his own production, by paraphasic expression.

(c) *Conduction aphasia*. Wernicke predicted that a lesion of the pathways associating the auditivo-verbal centre to the verbo-motor centre would cause the onset of aphasia combining paraphasic discourse with normal comprehension. He gave this clinical picture the name of *conduction aphasia* (*Leitungsaphasie*). In our opinion, the validity of the physiopathological implication of this term has not been conclusively demonstrated (see Chapter 8–3). Since its usage is nevertheless very widespread, we have retained it in our classification (see Chapter 4).

Finally, Wernicke recognized that certain lesions of the visual cortical region could affect written language (reading and writing), perhaps even in a specific way, while spoken language would remain normal. He considered that this clinical picture—which is sometimes referred to today by the name of *Dejerine's alexia-agraphia*[15, 16]—should be placed among the *asymbolias* rather than among the *aphasias* ('that disturbance would, however, not properly have anything to do with aphasia'[28]).

LICHTEIM (1844) AND WERNICKE (1885–1886)

Starting from the associationist model formulated ten years earlier by Wernicke, Lichteim gave it, in 1884,* a much more elaborate form. In doing so, he actually carried Wernicke's postulates to their logical conclusion. To the latter's original scheme (essentially composed of an *auditivo-verbal centre*, a *verbo-motor centre* and an axonal link between them), Lichteim[29, 30] added the *immediate afferents of the auditivo-verbal centre*, the *immediate efferents of the verbo-motor centre* and the *immediate associative links* of each of these two centres with the various association areas which form a large part of the remainder of the cerebral cortex (see Chapters 8–1 and 8–5). In Lichteim's sketch (Fig. 10–1):

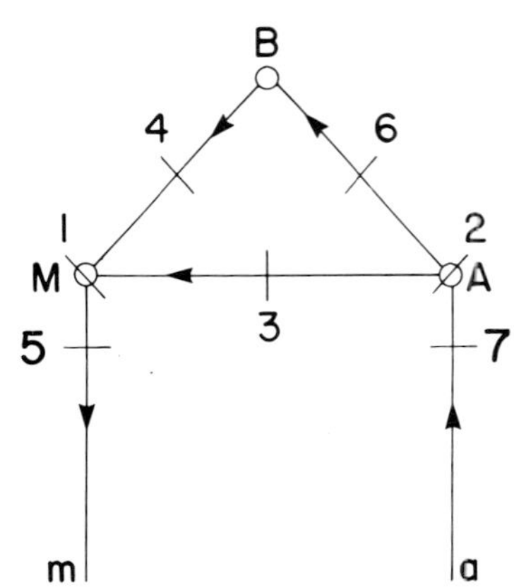

Fig. 10–1 *Anatomical associationism. Ludwig Lichteim's scheme. Commentary in the text. From Lichteim*[30].

A corresponds to the auditivo-verbal centre, that is, to a precisely localized cortical area (the posterior half of the left, first temporal convolution); M corresponds to the verbo-motor centre, that is, to another precisely localized cortical area (the caudalmost half of the left, third frontal convolution); B corresponds to all of the association cortices directly linked to the auditivo-verbal centre or to the verbo-motor centre (thus it does not represent a precisely localized cortical area); the arrow $a \rightarrow A$ corresponds to the imme-

* Cited by Freud in 1891[27].

diate afferents of the auditivo-verbal centre; the arrow $m \leftarrow A$ corresponds to the immediate efferents of the verbo-motor centre; the arrow M←A corresponds to the axonal link connecting the auditivo-verbal centre to the verbo-motor centre, that is, presumably, to the arcuate fasciculus; the arrow M←B corresponds to the link connecting the verbo-motor centre to the rest of the associative cortex; finally, the arrow A→B corresponds to the link connecting the auditivo-motor centre to the rest of the association cortex.

On the basis of this theoretical sketch, Lichteim hypothesized the existence of seven forms of aphasia. Two of them are *central aphasias* (*centre aphasias*), one *motor* and the other *sensory* (Fig. 10–1; lesions in *1* and *2*). The five others are *commissural aphasias*. Two of this group are *peripheral commissural aphasias*, one *motor* and the other *sensory* (Fig. 10–1; lesions in *5* and *7*); the other three are *central commissural aphasias* (Fig. 10–1; lesions in *4*, *3* and *6*).

Wernicke, who by Freud's account[27], 'closely followed Lichteim's work', was soon to reconsider this scheme and to modify its terms (but not its contents). This led to the following classification of the aphasias:

(a) *Motor aphasias*
  - (i) *Subcortical motor aphasia* (Fig. 10–1; lesion in *5*). The clinical picture is that which we have designated, following Marie's terminology[25], as *pure anarthria* (see Chapters 1 and 3).
  - (ii) *Cortical motor aphasia* (Fig. 10–1; lesion in *1*). This is the motor aphasia of Wernicke's first classification (cf. p. 247). It corresponds, in our terminology, to the *common form of Broca's aphasia* (see Chapter 4).
  - (iii) *Transcortical motor aphasia* (Fig. 10–1; lesion in *4*). The clinical picture approximates the one which we have discussed under the name of *aspontaneity* in linguistic behaviour (see Chapter 6).

(b) *Conduction aphasia* (Fig. 10–1; lesion in *3*). This term, proposed by Wernicke[21], is one which we have retained here (see Chapter 4). The presence of the characteristic repetition disturbance was subsequently recognized by Lichteim[29,30] (see Chapter 1).

(c) *Sensory aphasias*
  - (i) *Subcortical sensory aphasia* (Fig. 10–1; lesion in *7*). The clinical picture is that which we have identified, following Bastian* and Dejerine[16], by the name of *pure word deafness* (see Chapter 5).
  - (ii) *Cortical sensory aphasia* (Fig. 10–1; lesion in *2*). This is the *sensory aphasia* of Wernicke's first classification (cf. p. 247). It corresponds to *Wernicke's aphasia proper* in our classification (see Chapter 4).
  - (iii) *Transcortical sensory aphasia* (Fig. 10–1; lesion in *6*). The clinical picture is similar to that which was discussed here under the name of *Type II Wernicke's aphasia* (see Chapter 4).

In 1886, Wernicke† considered the disorders which would theoretically follow from an analogous model applied, this time, to written language: *subcortical*, *cortical* and *transcortical agraphias*; *conduction agraphia*; and *subcortical*; *cortical* and *transcortical alexias*. Comparison of this hypothetical model and clinical reality led Wernicke to accept the notion of a visuo-verbal centre but to reject that of a graphic motor centre; it also led him to accept only the clinical existence of *subcortical alexia* and *cortical alexia*. The first of these clinical pictures corresponds to *pure word blindness* in our classification (see Chapter 5) and the second is probably related to that which we have described under the name of *Type III Wernicke's aphasia* (see Chapter 4).

FREUD (1891)

Freud[27], who employed the term *association* only in accordance with its accepted psychological meaning, opposed the *idea of a word* or *word concept*[31] to the *idea of an object* or *object concept*[31] (Fig. 10–2). A word concept corresponds to a closed, complex network of associations between bits of information of auditory, visual and kinaesthetic origin. An object concept also corresponds to a complex network but this time it is an open network of associations between very diverse bits of information, that is, visual, auditory, tactile, kinaesthetic and other. The bond between the idea of a word and the idea of an object would be mainly established through an association between the auditory component

* According to Head[illegible].

† Cited by Freud, in 1891[27].

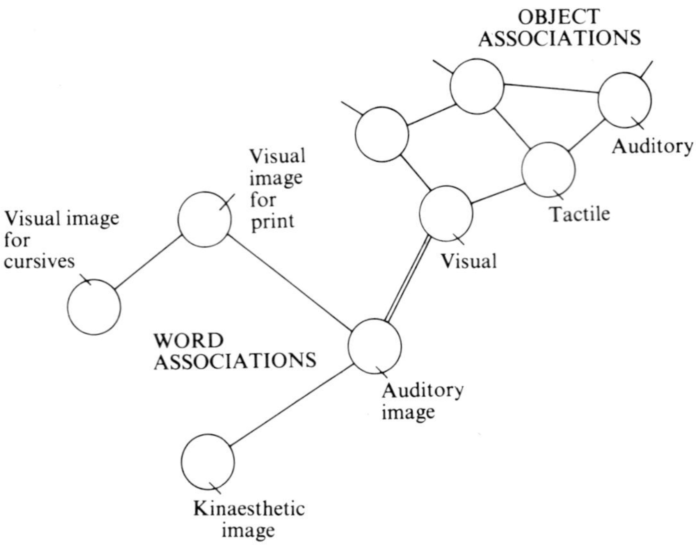

Fig. 10-2 *Psychological associationism. Sigmund Freud's scheme. Commentary in the text. From Freud*[27].

of the word concept and the visual component of the object concept. After having specified that this scheme would be strictly applicable only in the case of substantives (nouns[31]), Freud deduced from it the principle of an aphasia classification having three headings.

(a) *Verbal aphasia.* The disturbance selectively affects associations between the constituent elements of word concepts.
(b) *Asymbolic aphasia.* The disturbance affects associations between word concepts and the corresponding object concepts.
(c) *Agnosic aphasia.* This condition would be observed only in the presence of extensive bilateral cortical lesions. Such lesions would cause a language disturbance because all stimuli leading to spontaneous discourse come from the constituent associations of object concepts.

It appears to us that Freud (who emphasized the high frequency of mixed forms of aphasia which were both verbal and asymbolic) viewed his classification less as a clinical tool than as the result of a psychophysiological conception of language. However this may be, we did not find it possible to identify correspondences between this classification and the others considered in this chapter.

PIERRE MARIE (1906)

Marie's[25] original doctrine on language and aphasia can be easily summarized (see Chapter 1): thought and language are biologically indissociable; the notion of a centre and that of a memory image, as well as the associationists' hypotheses derived from them, have no anatomoclinical basis; there is only one clinical form of aphasia,* namely *Wernicke's aphasia*, and it represents a particular variety of intellectual deterioration; there is another condition, namely *anarthia*, which is completely separate from aphasia and represents a disorganization of speech rather than of language; Broca's aphasia corresponds to the co-occurrence of (Wernicke's) aphasia and anarthria. This last assertion has long been known by the name of *Pierre Marie's law*. It implies the following classification:

(a) *Anarthria.* This corresponds to *pure anarthria* in our classification (see Chapter 3). It can be assumed that Marie would also have placed, among his files on anarthria, those of

* 'Aphasia is one,' said Marie
But others contend that can't be.
They claim three forms, or four,
Sometimes five, even more.
There's no number on which all agree. [B.B.]

patients presenting the picture which we have identified by the name of *Broca's aphasia almost limited to an articulatory disturbance* (see Chapter 4).

(b) *Wernicke's aphasia.* Marie wrote, in 1906[32], that 'Wernicke's aphasia is a syndrome which appears with all of its components, as soon as there is a lesion, even limited, of Wernicke's zone [posterior half of the first two temporal convolutions, inferior parietal lobule] in no matter which of its points'. His *Wernicke's aphasia*, in reference to our classification, corresponds to all the clinical pictures which we have grouped under the headings of *Wernicke's aphasia* (*conduction aphasia, Type I, II and III Wernicke's aphasia*) and *amnesia aphasia** (see Chapter 4).

(c) *Broca's aphasia.* The clinical picture corresponds, in our classification, to the common form of Broca's aphasia and to global aphasia (see Chapter 4).

DEJERINE (1914)

In his teaching on aphasiology, Dejerine[16] placed particular emphasis on the need to resort to the anatomoclinical method and he himself carried out exemplary work in this sense. His aphasia classification is largely based on a distinction between the clinical effects of lesions which directly affect the *language zone* and the effects of lesions which spare it, but isolate it from *its physiological connections*. Although this dichotomy seems, a priori, to be as valid as any other, we must admit that we were unable to grasp certain points. On one hand, Dejerine clearly maintained that the language zone includes, in the left hemisphere of a right-hander (or in the right hemisphere of a left-hander): (1) an anterior part or Broca's region composed of the pars opercularis and pars triangularis of the third frontal convolution, the caudalmost part of the second frontal convolution, the frontal operculum (with the exception of the rolandic operculum) and, perhaps, the rostral part of the insula; this is the *centre of motor images of articulation*; (2) an inferior part or Wernicke's region, composed of the posterior part of the first two temporal convolutions; this is the *centre of auditory word images*; (3) a posterior part ('which I played a part in localizing', Dejerine specifies) composed of the angular gyrus (*pli courbe*); this is the *centre of visual word images*. On the other hand, and in the same publication[16], Dejerine wrote as follows about the anatomoclinical correlates of aphasias from lesions of the language zone: 'the destruction of Broca's region produces a Broca-type motor aphasia; a lesion of the supramarginal gyrus produces sensory aphasia; word blindness is attributable to the destruction of the angular gyrus; word deafness is due to a lesion of the posterior part of the first temporal [convolution]'.† The ambiguity concerns sensory aphasia which, according to Dejerine, partakes of both word deafness and word blindness: it is classified among the aphasias from a lesion of the language zone and is given a supramarginal localization (which is in itself quite surprising) even though the supramarginal gyrus is not mentioned in the list of components of the language zone. Since Dejerine (and his wife Augusta Klumpke) were the outstanding neuroanatomists of their time, the problem—if it is in fact one—undoubtedly involves terminology more than the facts themselves. Whatever the case, we consider the following reconstitution of Dejerine's classification to be an accurate representation of his teachings.

(a) *True aphasias or aphasias resulting from lesions of the language zone* (aphasias with impaired inner language)

   (i) *Expressive aphasia* or *cortical motor aphasia* or *Broca's aphasia.* The clinical picture described by Dejerine corresponds to that which we have defined, elsewhere in this text, under the name of the *common form of Broca's aphasia* (see Chapter 4).

   (ii) *Comprehension aphasia* or *sensory aphasia* or *Wernicke's aphasia.* In reference to our classification, the clinical picture described by Dejerine first corresponds to *Wernicke's aphasia proper* or *Type I Wernicke's aphasia.* Modification of the clinical picture during evolution may lead to a clear predominance of symptomatology associated

---

* Marie denied the existence of pure word deafness and classified pure word blindness among the visual agnosias.

† Dejerine was speaking here about word deafness and word blindness and not about pure word deafness and pure word blindness.

with word deafness (in our terminology, *Type I Wernicke's aphasia* with an *auditory aspect*) or that reflecting word blindness (in our terminology, *Type III Wernicke's aphasia*, i.e., one with a *visual aspect*). In referring to these evolving forms, Dejerine spoke of *Wernicke's word deafness* and *Wernicke's word blindness*, probably in order to distinguish them from *pure word deafness* and *pure word blindness*. He maintained, moreover, that certain lesions of the angular gyrus may result, generally after a certain period of evolution, in a disorder limited strictly to reading and writing; he then spoke of *word blindness with agraphia*. These various clinical aspects of Wernicke's aphasias have already been presented in detail (see Chapter 4).

(iii) *Total aphasia* (*global aphasia*). Both the label and the clinical picture correspond to the account previously presented (see Chapter 4). The symptom constellation associates the expressive disturbance of cortical motor aphasia with the receptive disturbance of sensory aphasia.

(b) *Pure aphasias or aphasias resulting from lesions outside the language zone* (aphasias without impaired inner language)

(i) *Pure motor aphasia* or *subcortical aphasia* or *aphemia*. With the word *aphemia* (which was later adopted by Goodglass[33] as well), Dejerine returned to the term which Broca[1] had vainly tried to defend against Trousseau's attacks[34] (see Chapter 1). However, Dejerine used the term 'aphemia' in a much more restricted sense and the clinical picture corresponds to that which we have identified by the name of *pure anarthria* (Chapter 3). According to Dejerine, the lesion is subcortical; it damages fibres coming from Broca's area so that it is no longer able to control the muscles of the phonoarticulatory apparatus in a normal manner.

(ii) *Pure word deafness*. Like Bastien,* Dejerine used this name, which we have also retained (see Chapter 5), to refer to Wernicke's *subcortical sensory aphasia* (cf. p. 249). According to Dejerine, the clinical picture may result from a (left temporal) subcortical lesion damaging the pathways which associate the 'common and bilateral centre of the audition to the centre of auditory word images; in other cases, the disorder is related to a weakening of the functions of the common auditory centre by a bilateral temporal lesion'.

(iii) *Pure word blindness*. The term and the clinical description correspond to the account previously presented in this text (see Chapter 5). According to Dejerine, the clinical picture corresponds to a (left occipital) subcortical lesion damaging the pathways which associate 'the common and bilateral centre of vision to the centre of visual word images' (see Fig. 8-21).

(c) *Other types of aphasia* (without localizing value)

(i) *Verbal amnesia or amnesic aphasia*. The clinical picture is similar to that which we defined under the name of *amnesic aphasia* (see Chapter 4). Dejerine[16] taught that verbal amnesia is very seldom observed in an isolated state; on the other hand one may 'also see verbal amnesia in certain cases of motor aphasia, sensory aphasia and in global aphasia' (Dejerine added that 'it is to this last category of facts which belong the cases published by Pitres (1908) under the name of amnesic aphasia'[35].

(ii) *Transcortical aphasias*. Under this heading, Dejerine discussed the *transcortical motor aphasia* and *transcortical sensory aphasia* which Wernicke had accepted as existing forms (cf. p. 249). These clinical pictures correspond, in our classification, to those defined under the name of *aspontaneity* (in linguistic behaviour) (see Chapter 4) and *Type II Wernicke's aphasia* (see Chapter 4). Dejerine[16] wrote that 'They are interesting facts from the clinical point of view but [ones] whose interpretation is highly debatable and nothing yet proves that there exists a transcortical aphasia, [which is] localizable anatomically speaking'.

---

* Cited by Head[26].

FOIX (1917)

Like Marie, who was his mentor, Foix[36] excluded *anarthria* from the specific domain of aphasia. He taught that there is only one true aphasia, that is, *Wernicke's aphasia* and, second, that *Broca's aphasia* represents the co-occurrence of *Wernicke's* aphasia and *anarthria*. Nevertheless, Foix also maintained that the effects of a triple dysfunction can be recognized in the symptomatology of Wernicke's aphasia, that is, the effects of an amnesic element (according to Foix, the clinical picture of Pitres' amnesic aphasia is produced when this amnesic element selectively impairs the evocation of substantives), an agnosic element and a dysphasic element. According to Ombredane[37] 'the amnesic element groups the symptoms of an intellectual type, the agnosic element the symptoms of a sensory type, the dysphasic element (which is not an articulatory disturbance) the symptoms of an expressive if not motor type.' These notions were, however, much less important than anatomoclinical studies in leading Foix to differentiate four forms of Wernicke's aphasia to the point that each was given a different name. According to Foix, each of these forms results from a particular lesion of Wernicke's zone (as understood by Marie[25]: the caudal half of the first two temporal convolutions on the left and the left inferior parietal lobule); although all aspects of language are impaired in all cases, the site of lesion determines the predominant symptomatological characteristics. On the basis of this information, Foix's classification of acquired disorders of speech and language can be reconstituted as follows:

(a) *Non-aphasic disorders*

(i) *Anarthria* corresponds to *pure anarthria* in our classification (see Chapter 3).

(ii) *Pure agraphia*. The label is the same as that used elsewhere in this text (see Chapters 3 and 4). For Foix, it was a question of apraxia with the isolated nature of the writing impairment attesting to the particular fragility of this skill. This is related to both its relatively late acquisition and to the high degree of gestural differentiation.

(iii) *Pure word deafness*. The label and the description are the same as in the account presented elsewhere (see Chapter 5). For Foix, this clinical picture corresponds to a form of auditory agnosia.

(iv) *Pure alexia* corresponds to *pure word blindness* in our classification (see Chapter 5). Foix considered it to be a form of visual agnosia.

(b) *Aphasia* (*Wernicke's aphasia*)

(i) *Full Wernicke's aphasia* (*grande aphasie de Wernicke*). The lesion affects the entire posterior sylvian territory (see Chapter 9) which includes all the constituent structures of Wernicke's zone. The comprehension disturbance is severe and affects written language as much as oral language; the jargon may be spectacular and transposition activities are all impaired. In our classification, this clinical picture has been placed under the heading *Wernicke's aphasia proper* or *Type I Wernicke's aphasia* (see Chapter 4). Foix emphasized that full Wernicke's aphasia is often accompanied by neurological and neuropsychological disturbances, for example, a right homonymous hemianopsia and ideomotor or ideational apraxia.

(ii) *Temporal aphasia*. The lesion affects the territory vascularized by the posterior temporal branch of the sylvian artery, namely the territory which includes the temporal components of Wernicke's zone. The symptomatology approximates that of full Wernicke's aphasia but the disturbance of written expression and, especially, of written language comprehension may be less obvious. In our classification, this clinical picture was also placed under the heading of *Type I Wernicke's aphasia* (it probably corresponds, at least in certain cases, to a Type I Wernicke's aphasia with a predominant *auditory aspect*) (see Chapter 4).

(iii) *Aphasia from a lesion of the supramarginal gyrus*. The lesion affects the territory vascularized by the posterior parietal branch of the sylvian artery, that is the territory which includes the supramarginal component of Wernicke's zone. The clinical picture discussed by Foix, observed in a case of cerebral damage from gunshot injury, is similar in certain features (relative sparing of comprehension, production of phonemic transformations, word-finding difficulty) to that which we have identified by the name of *conduction aphasia* (see Chapter 4). However, because the patient presented an articulatory disturbance,* his disorder would correspond to a form of *mixed aphasia* in our classification.

(iv) *Aphasia from a lesion in the region of the angular gyrus (pli courbe).* The lesion affects the territory vascularized by the so-called angular gyrus artery, a branch of the sylvian artery. This territory includes the angular component of Wernicke's zone. Since written language, and particularly reading, is predominantly affected, it can be assumed that the clinical picture corresponds approximately to that which we have identified by the name of *Type III Wernicke's aphasia* (see Chapter 4).

(c) *Aphasia (Wernicke's) with concomitant anarthria*
Broca's aphasia. The clinical picture corresponds, in our classification to the common form of Broca's aphasia and to global aphasia (see Chapter 4).

HEAD (1926)

Head[24] taught, and this apparently constitutes the theoretical basis of his doctrine, that aphasia corresponds to *defects of symbolic formulation and expression.* Disturbances which are limited to the expressive and receptive poles (see Chapters 3 and 5) would therefore be excluded from the specific domain of aphasia. Head recognized four types of aphasia to which he assigned names with clearly linguistic connotations. While his terminology thus has the advantage of homogeneity, the reasons for the selection of particular terms are not equally clear in all cases. Head's classification has the following four headings:

(a) *Verbal aphasia.* The symptom constellations grouped under this heading mainly correspond to those which we have described as *Broca's aphasia* and, for cases of Head's *verbal aphasia* with an obvious comprehension disturbance ('comprehension is relatively intact, except in the most severe cases'), to certain of those which we have labelled as *mixed* or *global aphasias* (see Chapter 4). According to Head, verbal aphasia attests to 'a defective power of forming words, whether for external or internal use'[24].

(b) *Syntactic aphasia.* The clinical picture corresponds, in our classification, to *Wernicke's aphasia proper* or *Type I Wernicke's aphasia* (see Chapter 4). According to Head, it reflects 'a disturbance in the rhythmic aspects of symbolic formulation and expression'[24].

(c) *Nominal aphasia.* The main symptomatological features of Head's nominal aphasia are as follows: word-finding difficulty is present and is manifested by the production of circumlocutions (and sometimes of semantic paraphasias) as well as by disturbed comprehension of word meanings. On the other hand, repetition is normal or nearly so. Spontaneous writing is very reduced, dictated writing is dysorthographic and copying is servile. Comprehension of written language is impaired but may be facilitated if the stimuli are read aloud. Contrary to common belief, it is thus clear that Head's nominal aphasia does not correspond to the clinical picture described elsewhere in this text under the name 'amnesic aphasia' (see Chapter 4). In reference to our classification, *nominal aphasia* is quite similar to *Type II Wernicke's aphasia* (see Chapter 4). According to Head, this clinical picture attests to the 'loss of power to employ names together with want of comprehension of the nominal value of words and other symbols'[24].

(d) *Semantic aphasia.* The clinical picture is characterized, on the receptive side, by a disturbance in the comprehension of wholes (the comprehension of general propositions, composed of several elements, remains defective although shorter and more concrete

---

* Foix's description of the articulatory disturbance does not convey a very precise impression: 'Words are spontaneously pronounced with difficulty. [The patient] will say *craron* for *crayon*, *boutetelle* for *bouteille*, all with effortful and spastic articulation. Repeated speech is also affected and correct pronunciation of the tests is difficult: *artilleur* from *artillerie*, *tarte*, *tartare*, *tartelette* are impossible.' If the articulatory disturbance had been typical, Foix would probably have spoken—especially because his published report on this case was also signed by Pierre Marie[38]—of signs of anarthria in association with those of aphasia and would probably have pointed out the similarity between the aphasia resulting from a lesion of the supramarginal gyrus and Broca's aphasia. Given the clinical picture observed in Foix's patient, one may also wonder if it is not somehow related to that identified by Luria[39] under the name of afferent motor aphasia (cf. p. 259).

segments are normally understood) and, on the expressive side, by an inability to arrange the components of elaborated discourse in an appropriate order (in narration, for example). It appears that, for Head, semantic aphasia represents a disturbance which specifically affects the ability to perform logical operations (i.e., a 'loss of power to appreciate or to formulate the logical conclusion of a train of thought or action . . . of power to coordinate details into a general formula for internal or external statement'[24]. None of the clinical pictures previously discussed in this text correspond to Head's *semantic aphasia*. In our opinion this symptom complex, which also includes word-finding difficulty (and thus resembles *Pitres' amnesic aphasia*) should be considered within the context of evolution. It is, in fact, observed at the start of evolution in certain Wernicke's aphasias related to insidiously progressive disease (for example, tumours or degenerative diseases) and, on the other hand, after a more or less prolonged period, in certain cases of Wernicke's aphasia related to pathology characterized by a sudden onset and favourable evolution (for example, in certain cases of trauma or a cerebral vascular accident) (see Chapter 9).

Head's classification appears of limited use from a clinical point of view: first, because it does not include several pictures observed in clinical aphasiology and, second, because certain terminological implications do not correspond to observed facts (for example, as we have already pointed out, Head's syntactic aphasia does not involve a specific or even predominant disturbance of syntax). As for the theoretical value of this classification, we shall leave this for the reader to judge on the basis of Head's interpretations: each of the four preceding quotations was taken from an explanatory summary which Head provided, in his celebrated treatise[24], at the end of each of four sections devoted to his specific forms of aphasia.

GOLDSTEIN (1948)

As we have already mentioned, Goldstein[40] was one of the most vigorous supporters of the globalist theory of aphasia (see Chapter 1). It is nevertheless clear that this champion of the globalists' views did not consider this theoretical position to be incompatible with the division of aphasic behaviours into numerous symptom constellations. Indeed, Goldstein's nomenclature includes no less than 30 headings, a number which may appear astonishing when compared, for example, with the three headings in the original classification by Wernicke, an associationist (cf. pp. 247–248). Goldstein's terminological choices sometimes reflect clinical and anatomical observations and at other times are influenced by a psychophysiopathological scheme of interpretation linked to Gestalt theory ('our nomenclature cannot be very homogeneous')[40]. When considered with regard to the clinical pictures defined in other sections of this text (see Chapters 3 to 6), the principal terms of Goldstein's nomenclature permit the reconstitution* of the following classification of *aphasic symptom complexes*:

(a) *Aphasias from predominant or exclusive impairment of the instrumentalities of language*

(i) *Peripheral motor aphasia*. The essential disturbance is a *dedifferentiation of the Gestalten of speech*, that is, of a class of specific motor patterns acquired through learning; an inability to acquire new patterns of this type is usually present as well (and, adds Goldstein, there are some cases in which this latter element predominates). From a neurolinguistic point of view, this pathognomonic dedifferentiation of Goldstein's *peripheral motor aphasia* is no doubt equivalent to the *phonetic disintegration syndrome* of Alajouanine, Ombredane and Durand[41] (see Chapter 3). In reference to our classification, the observations cited by Goldstein[40] to illustrate the notion of *peripheral motor aphasia* correspond, depending on the case, to *pure anarthria*, to *Broca's aphasia almost limited to an articulatory disturbance*, to the *common form of Broca's aphasia* (the possible evolution towards agrammatism is pointed out) and even to a recovering form of *global aphasia* (with recovery of an elementary level of comprehension) (see Chapters 3 and 4).

---

* This classification was not presented as such by Goldstein. In our opinion, it is nevertheless implicit in his writings.

(ii) *Motor agraphia or pure agraphia.* The second of the terms used by Goldstein, namely *pure agraphia*, is the same as in our classification. It is a specific disturbance in which 'the patient can innervate the muscles by which writing is performed for other purposes but not for the production of letters'[40]. Goldstein's teachings on the clinical manifestations of pure agraphia and the localization of the cerebral lesions causing the disorder (caudalmost part of the left, second frontal convolution) reflect those of Exner[42] (see Chapter 6).

(iii) *Peripheral sensory aphasia.* This heading corresponds in all respects to *pure word deafness* in our classification (see Chapter 5).

(iv) *Primary alexia or visual agnosic alexia.* This heading corresponds to *pure word blindness* in our classification (see Chapter 5).

(b) *Aphasias linked to a dedifferentiation of inner language*

Central aphasia. The clinical picture defined by Goldstein corresponds very closely to *conduction aphasia* in our classification (see Chapter 4). According to Goldstein, the principal features of this clinical picture can be explained by a *dedifferentiation of inner language*. Contrary to Wernicke's belief[21], the causal lesion is cortical (probably left insular, at least in certain cases): 'If we want to bring the disturbance of repetition into relation with some anatomic defect, we cannot assume a defect of a simple fibre connection but dysfunction of a cortical apparatus. This is still more valid concerning the other symptoms which occur in these cases'[40] (see Chapter 8-3).

(c) *Aphasias linked to a disturbance of abstract attitude*

Amnesic aphasia. Except in a few small details, the clinical picture corresponds to that which we have designated by the name of *Pitres' amnesic aphasia* (see Chapter 4). Isolated or nearly isolated behaviours of word-finding difficulty constitute its primordial clinical feature. Goldstein attributes the word-finding difficulty of amnesic aphasia to a particular psychopathological mechanism: 'Only those cases with word-finding difficulties where this defect is related to impairment of abstract attitude should be called amnesic aphasia'[40] (Insertion 10.2).

(d) *Aphasias from concomitant impairment of the instrumentalities of language and of abstract attitude and which may include a dedifferentiation of inner language*

(i) *Central motor aphasia.* The main clinical characteristics of Goldstein's central motor aphasia are as follows: there is a massive (qualitative and quantitative) reduction; resulting from a loss of abstract attitude, it is reflected by a decrease in all the patient's activities. The articulatory disturbance (impairment of the instrumentalities) is generally much less apparent than in peripheral motor aphasia; it may completely disappear during recitation of overlearned sequences—where performance is usually successful—and be especially evident during repetition tasks (see Chapter 15); comprehension of spoken language is only possible at an elementary level and written language comprehension is even more impaired. Our own classification proves somewhat inadequate in regard to this symptom constellation whose clinical existence we cannot contest (see Insertion 17.3). Depending on the severity of the disturbances, we would no doubt speak of *mixed aphasia* or of *global aphasia* (see Chapter 4); in cases where the articulatory disturbance is particularly mild, we might refer to the idea of '*reduced Wernicke's aphasia*' (see Insertion 4.1).

(ii) *Central sensory aphasia.* The clinical picture defined by Goldstein corresponds to that which we have described under the name of *Wernicke's aphasia proper or Type I Wernicke's aphasia* (see Chapter 4). Goldstein considered that the comprehension disturbance results from the same mechanism as in peripheral sensory aphasia (impairment of *instrumentalities*), that the paraphasic transformations can be explained in the same way as in central aphasia (*dedifferentiation of inner language*) and that the word-finding difficulty is of the same type as in *amnesic aphasia* [a disorder of *abstract attitude* (Insertion 10.2)].

Insertion 10.2

Goldstein wrote as follows about the abstract attitude: 'Our actions are determined not so much by the objects before us as by the way we think about them; the individual thing becomes a mere accidental example or representative of a "category". Therefore, we also call this attitude the categorical or conceptual attitude. The abstract attitude is basic for the following potentialities:

1. Assuming a mental set voluntarily, taking initiative, even beginning a performance on demand.
2. Shifting voluntarily from one aspect of a situation to another, making a choice.
3. Keeping in mind simultaneously various aspects of a situation; reacting to two stimuli which do not belong intrinsically together.
4. Grasping the essential of a given whole, breaking up a given whole into parts, isolating them voluntarily, and combining them to wholes.
5. Abstracting common properties, planning ahead ideationally, assuming an attitude toward the "merely possible", and thinking or performing symbolically.
6. Detaching the ego from the outer world.

In all these potentialities, the patients are more or less impaired'.
[From Goldstein[40].]

(e) *Aphasias from anomalies of non-linguistic mental processes**
   (i) *Transcortical motor aphasia.* The clinical picture corresponds to that which we have defined under the name of *aspontaneity* (in linguistic behaviour) (see Chapter 6). Goldstein considers it the effect of a 'lack of the impulse to speak at all'[40].
   (ii) *Transcortical sensory aphasia.* As in the preceding case this term was borrowed from Wernicke's terminology (cf. p. 249). The clinical picture corresponds approximately to that which we have defined under the name of *Type II Wernicke's aphasia* (see Chapter 4). Goldstein's discussion of the psychopathology of this form of aphasia is particularly involved. Among other interpretations, he suggests that transcortical sensory aphasia could result from 'a defect of the relation between perception and understanding (the non-language mental processes'[40]). One inevitably wonders about the possible biological substratum of this relation.
   (iii) *Mixed transcortical aphasia.* Under this heading, Goldstein describes a clinical picture in which there is a severe reduction of spontaneous expression and disturbed comprehension while repetition remains nearly normal. Echolalic phenomena may also be observed. This clinical picture is also related to that which we have defined under the name of *Type II Wernicke's aphasia* (this time, in cases where spontaneous expression is reduced or becomes so during evolution).

BAY (1964)

Like Marie[25], Bay[13] recognized only one true form of aphasia (*die genuin Aphasie*). Although Bay did not propose an aphasia classification, his writings nevertheless permit a reconstitution of the following classification of the main clinical pictures which include an acquired disorder of speech and/or language (as a result of a hemispheric lesion):

(a) *Cortical dysarthria*
When it occurs in a pure state, Bay's *cortical*

* Pictures of speech disturbances due to disturbances of non-language mental processes'[40].

dysarthria corresponds to *pure anarthria* in our classification (see Chapters 3 and 8–4).

(b) *True aphasia*

(i) In a pure state, Bay's *true aphasia* corresponds approximately to the clinical picture described in this text under the name of *Pitres' amnesic aphasia* (see Chapter 4). Bay, however, emphasizes that this clinical picture includes a comprehension disturbance which is manifested, albeit mildly, on tests of word identification (see Chapter 12 and 15).

(ii) In the spirit of Pierre Marie's law, Bay maintains that the association of *true aphasia* and *cortical dysarthria* results in clinical pictures generally designated by the name of Broca's aphasia [or, in our classification, *Broca's aphasia almost limited to an articulatory disturbance* and the *common form of Broca's aphasia* (see Chapter 4)].

(iii) According to Bay, the clinical picture which we have here discussed under the name of *Wernicke's aphasia proper or Type I* (see Chapter 4) would represent the association of *true aphasia* and a *general mental disorder*. A *cortical acoustical disorder* would often be present as well. This last element probably corresponds to what other authors call *word deafness*.

(iv) Finally, there would be a symptom constellation in which *true aphasia* is associated with a *lack of ideas* (*Einfallsleere*). Despite the latter element, the patients 'display a marked echolalia which must be looked upon not as a particular aphasic feature but rather as a detour performance allowing speech activity in spite of the lack of ideas'[13]. This clinical picture is perhaps related, in certain respects, to *Type II Wernicke's aphasia* in our classification (see Chapter 4); Bay's discussion also calls to mind certain aspects of the disturbance which we have termed *aspontaneity* (in linguistic behaviour) (see Chapter 6).

LURIA (1964)

The Soviet psychologist, Luria, does not appear to have given much credit to aphasiological theories which preceded his own. In discussing *sensory aphasia*, Luria reviewed the associationist notion of auditory word images and the holistic notion of intellectual impairment and then rejected both ('time has revealed the fallacies of both points of view'[39]). In discussing *motor aphasia*, he noted that it has generally been attributed to a lesion of Broca's area (caudalmost half of the left, third frontal convolution) and that some aphasiologists have interpreted it in terms of a disturbance of motor word images, and then concluded that 'both views have turned out to be inexact'[39]. Having reached these conclusions, Luria[39] then carried out an analysis intended to be both anatomophysiological and linguistic. He maintained—and few would contest the soundness of this postulate—that language depends on the activity of several interdependent functional systems. Subtended by a precisely localized cortical zone and processing a particular aspect of the linguistic codes, each of these systems makes a specific contribution to the control of language. Thus Luria interprets aphasic behaviours in psychophysiopathological terms and it is this approach which accounts for the originality of his classification. In our opinion, however, its terms cannot be regarded as exhaustive for clinical and anatomoclinical purposes. Luria recognized the occurrence of six clinical forms of aphasia:

(a) *Sensory aphasia*. According to Luria, this clinical picture corresponds to a 'disintegration of phonemic hearing', that is, to 'a type of disturbance of the analysis and synthesis of speech sounds which arises when the cortical elements of the auditory analyser are impaired'[39]. The causal lesion generally destroys the posterior third of the left, first temporal convolution. According to Luria, the disintegration of phonemic hearing (which we presume would correspond to the word deafness of classical writers) is the source of all the anomalies which have been discussed elsewhere in this text under the heading of *Wernicke's aphasia proper or Type I Wernicke's aphasia* (see Chapter 4), including word-finding difficulty, jargon (Insertion 10.3) and certain intellectual disturbances [the last would be evident only during tasks involving a significant linguistic factor (see Chapter 16)]. Luria nevertheless specified that in some very rare cases, the disintegration of phonemic hearing may produce only the clinical picture described here under the name of *pure word deafness* (see Chapter 5). He is not very explicit about why the same dysfunction may be the source of clinical manifestations which differ widely in certain aspects 'Only in very rare cases of so-called pure verbal deafness can such a defect remain an isolated symptom. Usually, it leads to a whole system of secondary disorders which constitute the picture of sensory aphasia'[39].

(b) *Acoustic-amnestic aphasia.* Here again, the lesion affects the left temporal lobe of a right-hander. However, in the present case, it does not destroy the specific auditory association cortex ('the secondary areas of the auditory cortex') but does alter its functioning. Although 'phonemic hearing may remain relatively normal', this functional disturbance results in 'impaired retention of stable audiospeech traces'[39] (Insertion 10.4). From a purely clinical point of view, the symptomatology of Luria's *acoustic-amnestic aphasia* appears to resemble an attenuated form of *sensory aphasia*. For example, in order to demonstrate the repetition disturbance, the examiner must usually rely on multisyllabic stimuli or on series of words which are related in form (Insertion 10.3) (see Chapters 2 and 15). Luria's *acoustic-amnestic aphasia* has no exact equivalent in our classification but rather corresponds to a mild form of *Wernicke's aphasia proper*, that is, *Type I Wernicke's aphasia* (see Chapter 4). In regard to sensory and acoustic-amnestic aphasia, the use of Luria's terminology may have the advantage—or the disadvantage—of including an aetiological suggestion (particularly for clinical pictures considered soon after onset) in addition to the physiopathological implications outlined above. Trauma and cerebral vascular accidents would generally result in sensory aphasia and tumours and abscesses in acoustic-amnestic aphasia (see Chapter 9).

(c) *Afferent motor aphasia or kinaesthetic motor aphasia.* According to Luria, the lesion affects the opercular third of the postcentral gyrus. Like Freud[27, 31] then Dejerine[16], Luria[39] was thus willing to venture beyond the traditional limits of the language zone (see Chapter 8-1 and 8-5). In Luria's terms, the 'primary defect' is a 'disturbance of the articuleme' (Insertion 10.4). It results from a disruption of the 'continual afferent correction' which is normally ensured through proprioceptive feedback generated by the activity of the phonoarticulatory musculature. This disturbance may sometimes be severe enough to cause a total suppression (see Chapter 4). In other cases, oral production remains possible but is slow, awkward and transformed; these features are observable in spontaneous discourse, oral reading, and repetition (Insertion 10.3). Orthographic deviations are frequent (Insertion 10.3) and were considered by Luria to be secondary to the disturbance of the articulemes (he spoke of a loss of general articulatory schemata). The theoretical validity of the concept of afferent motor aphasia can scarcely be contested [although certain proprioceptive inputs are probably addressed to the precentral gyrus (see Chapter 7), it can be logically assumed that a lesion affecting the opercular third of the postcentral gyrus could cause a more or less significant loss of proprioceptive information coming from the phonoarticulatory apparatus: it could also be logically assumed that a loss of this type could impair articulatory production, at least temporarily]. We must nevertheless report our difficulty in clinically identifying *afferent motor aphasia* or even in distinguishing, among the characteristic transformations of *phonetic disintegration* in Broca's aphasics (see Chapters 3 and 4), which ones might be related to pathology of afferents rather than of efferents. This is why none of the clinical pictures which we have previously discussed corresponds to Luria's afferent motor aphasia. Faced with this type of expressive symptomatology, we would no doubt speak of *Broca's aphasia* if the disturbance observed in oral expression appeared to be especially of the phonetic type and we would speak of *conduction aphasia* if the disturbance appeared to be almost exclusively of a phonemic type (see Chapters 2, 3, and 4).

(d) *Efferent motor aphasia or kinetic motor aphasia.* According to Luria, this clinical picture results from the destruction of Broca's area and reflects a 'disturbance of serial organization of a spoken word'[39]. This disturbance would be the origin of most of the expressive anomalies (oral and written) which we have mentioned in regard to the *common form of Broca's aphasia* (see Chapter 4) including the evolution towards

Insertion 10.3

Luria appeared to consider certain paraphasic and paragraphic transformations as quasi-pathognomonic in relation to each of his first three clinical forms of aphasia (sensory, acoustic–amnestic, afferent motor). The following examples are cited in the report on a symposium held in London[43].

For sensory aphasia
(a) Repetition: /bapa/→/baba/ or /papa/;
(b) Writing to dictation: (bapa)→(baba) or (papa).

In these cases, Luria spoke of sound substitutions and cited, as a very characteristic example, the confusion between a voiced consonant and its unvoiced cognate [/d/↔/t/, /b/↔/p/].

For acoustic–amnestic aphasia
(a) Repetition: the patient makes mistakes when asked to repeat /bapaba/ or /pabapa/ or to repeat three or four words presented as a single stimulus.
(b) Writing to dictation: the patient makes mistakes when asked to write *zabor-sabor-zapor* (enclosure – church – bolt).

Luria emphasized the fact that patients with acoustic–amnestic aphasia can repeat pairs of similar phonemes, or even isolated words, but that mistakes occur as the information content of the stimuli is increased ('they lose their clear differentiation only when the amount of information impinging upon them is increased'[39]).

For afferent motor aphasia
(a) Repetition: the patient repeats /n/ or /d/ instead of /l/ ('a confusion of sounds made by the front part of the tongue') or else /m/ or /p/ instead of /b/ ('confusion of lip sounds')
(b) Writing: *khalat* (dress)→(khanat) or (khadat);
stol (table)→(snot) or (snol).

In this case, the confusions are not acoustic but rather articulatory and related to a disturbance of the articulemes.

We do not find these examples to be entirely convincing in regard to the differential diagnoses of aphasia. Consider the transformation /b/↔/p/ from a diagnostic point of view. It is cited first in relation to a disintegration of phonemic hearing, then as a reflection of the instability of an acoustic memory trace and, finally, as evidence of a disturbance of the articulemes. It is our opinion that the above transformations (oral and written) are probable in most of the clinical forms of Wernicke's aphasia (including, of course, conduction aphasia); they are also probable, if the articulatory and graphic disturbances are not taken into account, in the majority of Broca's aphasics who retain or recover a certain level of oral and written expression (see Chapters 2 and 4).

agrammatism (if this corresponds to what Luria[39] named a 'telegram style'). One of the primary impairments would originate from an inability to modify the articulatory production of a phonemic segment in accordance with its relations to other parts of the context in which it occurs ('Any disturbance of the ability to modify articulation depending on the place of the sound in the word unavoidably leads to a disturbance of the speech act... Patients with such impairment, unlike those with afferent motor aphasia, exhibit movements which are necessary for the articulation of separate sounds; however, they prove not to be in condition to change an articulation relative to its place in the word, to de-innervate a previous articulation, or to change smoothly from one articulation to another ... speech becomes de-automatized'[39] [see example (8.39)].

(e) *Semantic aphasia.* When speaking of semantic aphasia, Luria[39] claimed to be referring to the same clinical picture which Head[24] had designated by the same name: the similarity appears to us to be more evident in these authors' theoretical commentaries than in their clinical descriptions. According to Luria, the disorder affects the comprehension and repetition of segments having a complex grammatical structure and also results in word-finding difficulty ('amnestic aphasia ... is a typical component of this syndrome'[39]), which is usually facilitated by phonemic cues. The disorder reflects a 'primary disturbance of simultaneous synthesis', which is manifested by a 'disturbance of the semantic and logicogrammatical structure of speech'. In reference to our own classification, Luria's *semantic aphasia*, like that of Head, appears to represent an *initial stage, or a residual, of a Wernicke's aphasia* (cf. p. 255).

(f) *Dynamic aphasia.* The clinical picture is that which Lichteim and Wernicke, and later Goldstein, identified by the name of *transcortical motor aphasia* (cf. pp. 249 and 257); it corresponds, in our classification, to the clinical picture described under the name of *aspontaneity* (in linguistic behaviour). Luria[39] suggests that there may be a disturbance of *inner speech* which impairs its *predicative function.*

Insertion 10.4

According to Wernicke[21], sensory information from the extracerebral world leaves impressions in the cerebral cortex which have longer durations than those of the corresponding stimuli. These impressions, particularly when they have been reinforced through information of a repetitive type, can be evoked in the absence of external stimulation: Wernicke speaks of memory images (*Erinnerungsbilder*). Two classes of memory images are particularly important for linguistic functions: those corresponding to the sounds of spoken language (sound images) and those corresponding to its production (images of movements, representations of movements). This concept of images is apparently so naive that Luria[39], like others before him[24, 25], rejected it peremptorily. This raises two questions:

What is the essential difference between Luria's audiospeech traces, apparently registered in the cortex of the posterior half of the left, first temporal convolution, and the memory images of sounds which Wernicke stored in an auditivo-verbal centre in the same location?

What is the difference—if it is not only in their assigned cerebral localization—between Luria's articulemes and the memory images of movement as they were conceived by Wernicke? Indeed it will be remembered that, just as Luria was to do so 90 years later, Wernicke stressed the importance of afferents in the formation of images of movements: He taught that 'movements and changes in the state of the musculature give rise to sensations, memory images of which also remain in the cerebral cortex'[21].

JAKOBSON (1956 and 1964)

Emphasizing that language production presupposes a process of selection on the one hand and a process of combination on the other, the linguist Jakobson[7] recognized, in 1956, two classes of aphasic disorders (see Chapters 1 and 12).

(a) *Similarity disorder*. The disorder is related to a disturbance of the selection process, that is, to a disturbance of the paradigmatic function (see Chapter 2). Jakobson referred to the symptomatology of *Wernicke's aphasias* (see Chapter 4) when discussing *similarity disorders*.

(b) *Contiguity disorder*. The disorder is related to a disturbance of the combination process, that is, to a disturbance of the syntagmatic function (see Chapter 2). Jakobson referred to the symptomatology of *Broca's aphasias* (see Chapter 4) when discussing *contiguity disorders*.

In 1964, Jakobson[8] reviewed and refined his classification to incorporate his thoughts on the hypotheses of his compatriot, Luria[39].

Following an intellectual approach apparent in all his works, he characterized Luria's six aphasias on the basis of three dichotomies (Insertion 10.5): *a disorder of encoding versus one of decoding, a disorder of sequencing versus one of concurrence and a disorder of disintegration versus one of limitation*. These dichotomies permitted, so to speak, the identification of the *distinctive features* of each of Luria's aphasias.

(a) The *encoding–decoding* dichotomy
The *encoding disorder* corresponds to the *contiguity disorder* of the 1956 classification; it affects the process of combination, that is, the syntagmatic function. The three forms of aphasia which Luria attributed to central or precentral lesions—*afferent motor aphasia, efferent motor aphasia, dynamic aphasia*—are related, according to Jakobson, to an encoding disorder.
The *decoding disorder* corresponds to the *similarity disorder* of the 1956 classification; it affects the process of selection, that is, the paradigmatic function. The three forms of aphasia which Luria attributed to postcentral lesions—*semantic aphasia, sensory aphasia, acoustic–amnestic aphasia*—are related to a decoding disorder.

(b) The *sequence–concurrence* dichotomy
A disturbance of either encoding or decoding may affect units which are produced or perceived in *succession:* there is then a *disorder of sequencing*. Among the encoding disorders, sequencing is impaired in *dynamic aphasia* and in *efferent motor aphasia*: among the decoding disorders, it is impaired in *acoustic–amnestic aphasia*.
A disturbance of either encoding or decoding may affect units which are produced or perceived *simultaneously*: there is then a *disorder of concurrence* (co-occurrence). Among the encoding disorders, concurrence is impaired in *afferent motor aphasia* [a disturbance in the combination of features into phonemes, i.e., a disorganization of the third phase of oral language (see Chapters 2 and 3)]: among the decoding disorders, it is impaired in *semantic aphasia* and in *sensory aphasia*.

(c) The *disintegration–limitation* dichotomy
In either a disorder of encoding and sequencing or a disorder of decoding and concurrence, language production or reception may be impaired at the level of phonemic and/or grammatical sequences: Jakobson then spoke of a *disorder by disintegration* (*disruption*). Such would be the case in *efferent motor aphasia* on the one hand, and in *sensory aphasia* on the other.
In either a disorder of encoding and sequencing or a disorder of decoding and concurrence, language production or reception may be impaired only at the level of highly complex units (sentences↔utterances↔discourse): Jakobson then spoke of a *disorder by limitation*. Such would be the case in *dynamic aphasia* on the one hand and in *semantic aphasia* on the other.

The three dichotomies defined by Jakobson[8] permit the following reconstitution of his 1964 classification (having already discussed the terminological relationships between our classification and that of Luria[39], only the correspondences between Luria's and Jakobson's lexicon will be systematically indicated):

(a) *Aphasia from a disorder in the encoding of simultaneously produced units*. There is, in other words, a disorder in the combination of features into phonemes. In our opinion, this definition would at least partially correspond to the *phonetic disintegration syndrome* of Alajouanine et al[41]. However, Jakobson specifically relates it to Luria's *afferent motor aphasia*.

(b) *Aphasic disintegration from a disorder in the encoding of successively produced units*. According to Jakobson, this characterization specifically corresponds to Luria's *efferent motor aphasia*. In our opinion, it would be equally applicable to the phonemic and verbal transformations observed in most of the clinical forms of aphasia (of a Wernicke's type as well as of a Broca's type) (see Chapters 2 and 4).

(c) *Aphasic limitation from a disorder in the encoding of successively produced units*. This heading corresponds to Luria's *dynamic aphasia*, that is, to Lichteim's and to Wernicke's *transcortical motor aphasia*.

(d) *Aphasia from a disorder in the decoding of serially presented units* ('only items named serially are affected'). According to Jakobson this corresponds to Luria's *acoustic–amnestic aphasia*. In our opinion, it does not correspond, in a pure state, to any observed clinical picture.

(e) *Aphasic disintegration resulting from a disorder of decoding and concurrence*. This char-

Insertion 10.5

Jakobson's 1964 characterization of Luria's six forms of aphasia can be summarized as follows:

	Afferent motor aphasia	*Efferent motor aphasia*	*Dynamic aphasia*	*Semantic aphasia*	*Sensory aphasia*	*Acoustic-amnestic aphasia*
Disorder of:						
Encoding (or contiguity)	+	+	+			
Decoding (or similarity)				+	+	+
Sequencing (or succession)		+	+			+
Concurrence (or simultaneity)	+			+	+	
Disintegration		+			+	
Limitation			+	+		

acterization would correspond to Luria's *sensory aphasia*.

(f) *Aphasic limitation resulting from a disorder of decoding and concurrence*. This characterization would correspond to Luria's *semantic aphasia*.

ALAJOUANINE (1968)

Although it includes a few terms referring to the anatomy of the brain, Alajouanine's classification[44] is essentially clinical. Like the one used in this book (in which borrowings can be easily identified) and unlike those of Luria[39] and Jakobson[8] for example, Alajouanine's classification is empirically aimed at the unequivocal labelling of as many cases as possible. Alajouanine's affiliation with Marie is obvious in his initial division of the aphasias according to the presence or absence of an articulatory disturbance (impairment of verbal articulation). With the exception of isolated disturbances of the receptive and expressive poles, which are treated separately, Alajouanine thus classifies aphasic disorders under two major headings:

(a) Among the *aphasias without impaired verbal articulation* or *Wernicke's aphasias*, Alajouanine recognized five related clinical pictures:

(i) *Complete temporal aphasia*. The comprehension disturbance is severe and affects both spoken and written language. Oral expression is jargoned and logorrhoeic and written expression is generally very reduced. All transposition activities are impaired. The patient is excited, anosognosic and inattentive. The picture thus corresponds to the main symptomatological constellations which we have discussed under the heading of *Wernicke's aphasia proper* or *Type I Wernicke's aphasia* (see Chapter 4).

(ii) *Jargonaphasia*. For reasons which are not self-evident, Alajouanine reserved the label 'jargonaphasia' for Wernicke's aphasias in which nearly normal oral and written comprehension is associated with jargoned oral expression. This clinical picture can be seen to include the essential symptoms of *conduction aphasia* as originally conceived by Wernicke[21] (see Chapter 4).

(iii) *Temporal aphasia with sensory predominance*. Spoken language comprehension is severely disturbed, reflecting a major component of word deafness. On the other hand, written language comprehension is relatively spared or even quasi-normal. The production of paraphasias and, especially, of paragraphias (except in writing to dictation) may be relatively limited. We have discussed this clinical picture under the heading of *Wernicke's aphasia proper* or *Type I Wernicke's aphasia*, specifying that it is characterized by an *auditory aspect* (*versant auditif*) (see Chapters 4 and 5).

(iv) *Pitres' amnesic aphasia.* Both this label and the clinical picture identified by Alajouanine are consistent with our own description of this form of aphasia (see Chapter 4). Like Foix[36], Alajouanine[44] recognized that amnesic aphasia may emerge during recovery from a temporal aphasia; he also added that it may 'appear as the beginning of an aphasia which will become more complete ... especially in temporal tumours or in certain cerebral atrophies'.

(v) *The parieto-angular gyrus syndrome.* Alajouanine[44] referred to Foix's[45] anatomoclinical research in discussing this clinical picture (which we mention here even though Alajouanine treated it separately). He taught that 'partial softening of the posterior sylvian territory by isolated involvement of the last branches of the artery [may cause] a parieto-angular gyrus syndrome where the aphasia includes a marked predominance in written language [alexia, agraphia]'. This clinical picture corresponds to that which we have designated by the name of *Type III Wernicke's aphasia* (see Chapter 4).

(b) Two other symptom constellations are grouped under the heading *Aphasias with impaired verbal articulation* or *Broca's aphasias*.

(i) *Full Broca's aphasia or Dejerine's total aphasia.* The clinical picture corresponds to that of *global aphasia* as it was previously described (see Chapter 4). Alajouanine specified that patients with this form of aphasia include those whose oral expression is suppressed or reduced to a verbal stereotype (a type of linguistic production usually uttered without articulatory distortion). Given the wording of the second general heading in Alajouanine's classification, it must be concluded that the terms 'articulatory disturbance' or 'impairment of verbal articulation' refer to an absence of production as much as to the appearance of the *phonetic disintegration syndrome* (see Chapters 3 and 4).

(ii) *Broca's aphasia.* Alajouanine discussed *Broca's aphasia* in terms of *the common form*, cases where '*the syndrome is especially of an anarthric type*' and cases where '*it is the properly aphasic remainder which is in the foreground*'. With only a few exceptions, our description of *Broca's aphasias* (see Chapter 4) is thus consistent with that of Alajouanine[44].

(c) Under a final heading, Alajouanine[44] discussed each of the *isolated impairments of the receptive and expressive poles of language* (*pure aphasias, dissociated aphasias*).

(i) *Pure anarthria.* The terminology and discussion previously presented correspond to that of Alajouanine (see Chapter 3).

(ii) *Pure agraphia.* We have discussed this clinical picture under the same name, as well as under that of *frontal agraphia* (see Chapters 3 and 6).

(iii) *Pure word deafness.* The terminology and the discussion previously presented correspond to that of Alajouanine (see Chapter 5).

(iv) *Pure alexia.* We have discussed this clinical picture under the name of *pure word blindness* (see Chapter 5).

HÉCAEN (1972)

Hécaen[46] provided what he rightly described as a neurolinguistic description and classification of the aphasias. It was indeed based both on anatomoclinical findings and on certain properly linguistic characteristics which he and Dubois[47] identified in the various forms of aphasic discourse. Hécaen thus classified the aphasias under three major headings:

(a) *Expressive aphasias*

(i) *Aphasia of phonematic realization.* The clinical picture which Hécaen discusses under this heading corresponds very closely to that which we have identified by the names of *Broca's aphasia almost limited to an articulatory disturbance* and the *common form of Broca's aphasia* (see Chapter 4); it might also include the picture which we have labelled *pure anarthria* (see Chapter 3). In speaking of *phonematic realization*, Hécaen undoubtedly wished to emphasize the *phonetic disintegration* component; in the terminology of our own discussion, this would correspond to a disorganization of the third phase of oral language and to phonetic transformations (see Chapters 2 and 3).

(ii) *Agrammatic aphasia* or *disorder of syntactic realization.* We have already stated that agrammatism almost always represents a stage in the evolution of a Broca's aphasia (see Chapters 2 and 4). Hécaen[46], for his part, places more emphasis on its individual identity, probably because this clinical picture is of great interest from a linguistic point of view. He nevertheless recognizes that agrammatic aphasia is *more of a variant* (of aphasia of phonematic realization) *than a distinct form.*

(iii) *Conduction aphasia* or *disorder of sentence programming.* We have retained only the first of these terms as the heading for the description of this clinical picture (see Chapter 4). Hécaen[46] maintains that the discourse of conduction aphasics is very characteristic because 'sentences are limited to outlines or to simple unlinked propositions, with pauses and the insertion of adverbs such as "then", "after", at each change of utterance, which removes all fluency from discourse' [see example (4.5)]. In many classifications, conduction aphasia is grouped with the Wernicke's aphasias, that is, with the disorders related to the presence of a retrorolandic lesion. In Hécaen's classification, it appears under the same major heading as aphasia of phonematic realization (Broca's aphasia): the soundness of this grouping can scarcely be contested when one considers that Hécaen chose to classify the aphasias under the headings of expressive aphasias and sensory aphasias rather than under the headings of Broca's aphasias and Wernicke's aphasias.

(b) *Amnesic aphasias or disorders of morpheme selection.* The pluralization of the word 'aphasia' in the above heading can probably be explained by the fact that nearly isolated word-finding difficulty may appear in different ways. Although it is sometimes present at onset and persists in a pure state, it may also represent the initial stage of an aphasia which will worsen or be the sequel of an aphasia (expressive or sensory) which has evolved favourably. However this may be, the heading *amnesic aphasias* in Hécaen's classification closely corresponds to the clinical picture which we have defined under the name of *amnesic aphasia* (see Chapter 4).

(c) *Sensory aphasias*

(i) *Pure word deafness.* The heading and the description correspond to the account presented earlier in this text (see Chapter 5).

(ii) *Sensory aphasias.* Hécaen here distinguishes three main symptom constellations:

—*A form with predominant word deafness.* We have spoken, in reference to this clinical picture, of the *auditory aspect* sometimes observed in Wernicke's aphasia proper or Type I Wernicke's aphasia (see Chapter 4). Oral expression is jargoned, repetition is very disturbed, comprehension of spoken language is much more impaired than that of written language and the disorganization of written expression especially affects writing to dictation.

—*A form with a predominant disturbance of verbal comprehension.* Comprehension is severely disturbed and there is no dissociation between spoken and written language (see Insertion 8.2). This is the main symptom constellation described, elsewhere in this book, under the heading of *Wernicke's aphasia proper* or *Type I Wernicke's aphasia* (see Chapter 4).

—*Attentional disorganization.* The clinical picture which Hécaen terms 'attentional disorganization' is in many ways similar to that which Bay[13] described under the name of *Einfallsleere* and which we discussed under the name of *Type II Wernicke's aphasia* (fluent discourse attesting to word-finding difficulty and especially including verbal transformations, preserved repetition, presence of echolalic phenomena). It nevertheless differs because, in Hécaen's attentional disorganization, there is not usually a major disturbance of comprehension.

Like Wernicke* in his classification of 1885–1886, Hécaen[46] considered separately the (nearly) isolated disorders of written language. He accepts the existence of *pure agraphia*, a clinical picture which we have discussed under the same label and under that of *frontal agraphia* (see Chapters 3 and 6). He also recognizes, among

* Cited by Freud in 1891[27].

the agraphias, an *agraphia from an encoding disturbance* or *apraxic and alexic agraphia* as well as the existence, this time among the alexias, of an *alexia-agraphia*. These two headings appear to us to cover a single clinical picture which is analogous to that which we have discussed under the name of *Type III Wernicke's aphasia* (see Chapter 4). Finally, Hécaen described the *pure word blindness* of our classification (see Chapter 5).

GOODGLASS (1972)

An empirical approach, reminiscent of that which characterized Alajouanine's work (see Chapter 12), can readily be perceived (and appreciated) in Goodglass' research and publications. In an excellent monograph published in collaboration with Kaplan, Goodglass[48] presented a classification and description of the aphasias based on an exceptionally rigorous method of clinical observation. The clinical pictures described as existing forms of aphasia are, in general, very consistent with those previously discussed in this text (see Chapter 4). Thus we shall simply note the headings used by Goodglass and Kaplan and point out the corresponding terms in our own classification.

(a) *Broca's aphasia*
Discussed here under the headings of *Broca's aphasia almost limited to an articulatory disturbance* and *the common form of Broca's aphasia* (see Chapter 4).

(b) *Wernicke's aphasia*
Discussed here under the heading of *Wernicke's aphasia proper* or *Type I Wernicke's aphasia* (see Chapter 4).

(c) *Anomic aphasia*
Discussed here under the heading *Pitres' amnesic aphasia* (see Chapter 4).

(d) *Conduction aphasia*
Discussed here under the same heading (see Chapter 4).

(e) *Transcortical sensory aphasia*
Discussed here under the name of *Type II Wernicke's aphasia* (see Chapter 4).

(f) *Transcortical motor aphasia*
Discussed here under the name of *aspontaneity* (in linguistic behaviour) (see Chapter 4).

(g) *Alexia with agraphia*
Discussed here under the heading *Type III Wernicke's aphasia* (see Chapter 4).

(h) *Pure aphasias*
- (i) *Pure alexia* or *pure word blindness*. Discussed here under the second of these labels (see Chapter 5).
- (ii) *Pure word deafness*. Discussed here under the same heading (see Chapter 5).
- (iii) *Pure agraphia*. Discussed here under the same heading (see Chapter 3).
- (iv) *Aphemia*. Discussed here under the heading *pure anarthria* (see Chapter 3): Goodglass thus gives the term 'aphemia' a much more specific and restricted meaning than that which was originally attributed to it by Broca[1] (see Chapter 1).

REFERENCES

1. Broca, P. (1969) Sur les mots aphémie, aphasie et aphrasie. Lettre à M. le professeur Trousseau. In *La naissance de la neuropsychologie du langage* (Ed.) Hécaen, H. & Dubois, J. p. 267. Paris Flammarion.
2. Cyr-Stafford, C. & Boisclair-Papillon, R. (1974) *La dyssyntaxie: éssai de définition*. Medical thesis, Montreal.
3. Ducarne, B. & Préneron, C. (1976) La dyssyntaxie. *La linguistique*, **12,** 33.
4. Lecours, A.R. & Rouillon, F. (1976) Neurolinguistic analysis of jargonaphasia and jargonagraphia. In *Studies in Neurolinguistics* (Ed.) Avakian-Whitaker, H. & Whitaker, H. Vol. 2, p. 95. New York: Academic Press.
5. Rouillon, F. (1971) *A propos de quelques observations d'agrammatiques et de dyssyntaxiques; essai d'analyse comparative de certaines de leurs performances grammaticales*. Mémoire, Faculté de Médecine, Paris.
6. Martinet, A. (1967) *Eléments de linguistique générale*. Paris: A. Colin.
7. Jakobson, R. (1956) Two aspects of language and two types of aphasic disturbances. In *Fundamentals of Language* (Ed.) Jakobson, R. & Halle, M. p. 55. The Hague: Mouton.
8. Jakobson, R. (1964) Towards a linguistic typology of aphasic impairments. In *Disorders of Language* (Ed.) de Reuck, A.V.S. & O'Connor, M. p. 21. London: Churchill.
9. Sabouraud, O., Gagnepain, J. & Sabouraud, A. (1963) Vers une approche linguistique des problèmes de l'aphasie. *Revue de Neuropsychiatrie de l'Ouest*, **1; 2; 3; 4;** 6; 3; 3; 3.
10. Dordain, G. (1968) *Contribution à l'étude neurolinguistique de l'aphasie. Analyse comparative des performances grammaticales de 28 aphasiques dont 14 agrammatiques*. Medical thesis, Paris.
11. Tissot, R., Mounin, G. & Lhermitte, F. (1973) *L'agrammatisme. Etude neuropsycholinguistique*. Brussels: Dessart.

12. Lecours, A.R. & Lhermitte, F. (1976) The 'pure form' of the phonetic disintegration syndrome (pure anarthria); anatomo-clinical report of a historical case. *Brain and Language*, 3, 88.
13. Bay, E. (1964) Principles of classification and their influence on our concepts of aphasia. In *Disorders of Language* (Ed.) de Reuck, A.V.S. & O'Connor, M. p. 122. London: Churchill.
14. Lhermitte, F., Chain, F., Escourolle, R., Ducarne, B., Pillon, B. & Chedru, F. (1971) Etude des troubles perceptifs auditifs dans les lésions temporales bilatérales. A propos de trois observations dont deux anatomo-cliniques. *Revue neurologique*, **124**, 329.
15. Déjerine, J. (1892) Contribution à l'étude anatomopathologique et clinique des différentes variétés de cécité verbale. *Mémoires de al Société de Biologie*, **4,** 61.
16. Déjerine, J. (1914) *Séméiologie des affections du système nerveux*. Paris: Masson.
17. Geschwind, N. & Fusillo, M. (1966) Color-naming defects in association with alexia. *Archives of Neurology* (Chicago), **15,** 137.
18. Geschwind, N. (1965) Disconnexion syndromes in animals and man. *Brain*, **88,** 237 and 585.
19. Buyssens, E. (1967) *La communication et l'articulation linguistique*. Paris: Presses universitaires de France.
20. Baillarger, J. (1890) De l'aphasie au point de vue psychologique. Aphasie simple. Aphasie avec perversion de la faculté du langage. In J. Baillarger, *Recherches sur les maladies mentales*. p. 584. Paris: Masson. (First edition, 1865.)
21. Wernicke, C. (1874) *Der aphasische Symptomenkomplex*. Breslau: Cohn and Weigert.
22. Jackson, J.H. (1958) *Selected Writings of John Hughlings Jackson*. New York: Basic Books.
23. Head, H. (1915) Hughlings Jackson on aphasia and kindred affections of speech. *Brain*, **38,** 190.
24. Head, H. (1926) *Aphasia and Kindred Disorders of Speech* London: Cambridge University Press.
25. Marie, P. (1926) *Travaux et mémoires*. Vol. I. Paris: Masson.
26. Broca, P. (1865) Du siège de la faculté du langage articulé. *Bulletin de la Société d'Anthropologie*, **7,** 377.
27. Freud, S. (1891) *Zur Auffasung der Aphasien*. Vienna: Deuticke.
28. Wernicke, C. (1966) The symptom complex of aphasia. In *Boston Studies in the Philosophy of Science* (Ed.) Cohen, R.S. & Watofsky, M.W. Vol. 4. Boston, MA: O. Reidel.
29. Lichteim, L. (1885) Uber Aphasie. *Deutsches Archiv für Klinische Medizin*, **36,** 204.
30. Lichteim, L. (1885) On aphasia. *Brain*, **7,** 433.
31. Freud, S. (1953) *On Aphasia; a Critical Study*. New York: International Universities Press.
32. Marie, P. (1906) Révision de la question de l'aphasie: que faut-il penser des aphasies souscorticales (aphasies pures)? *Semaine médicale* (Paris), **26,** 493.
33. Goodglass, H. & Kaplan, E. (1972) *The Assessment of Aphasia and Related Disorders*. Philadelphia, PA: Lea & Febiger.
34. Trousseau, A. (1877) De l'aphasie. In A. Trousseau, *Clinique médicale de l'Hôtel-Dieu de Paris*. Vol. 2, p. 669. Paris: Baillière.
35. Pitres, A. (1898) L'aphasie amnésique et ses variétés cliniques. *Progrès médicale*, **7,** 321, 337, 369 and 401; **8,** 17, 65.
36. Foix, C. (1928) Aphasies. In *Nouveau traité de médecine* (Ed.) Roger, G. et al. p. 135. Paris: Masson.
37. Ombredane, A. (1950) *L'aphasie et l'élaboration de la pensée explicite*. Paris: Presses Universitaires de France.
38. Marie, P. & Foix, C. (1917) Les aphasies de guerre. *Revue neurologique*, **1,** 53.
39. Luria, A.R. (1964) Factors and forms of aphasia. In *Disorders of Language* (Ed.) de Reuck, A.V.S. & O'Connor, M. p. 143. London: Churchill.
40. Goldstein, K. (1948) *Language and Language Disturbances*. New York: Grune and Stratton.
41. Alajouanine, Th., Ombredane, A. & Durand, M. (1939) *Le syndrome de désintégration phonétique dans l'aphasie*. Paris: Masson
42. Exner, S. (1881) *Untersuchungen über die Lokalisation der Funktionen in der Grosshirnrinde des Menschen*. Vienna: Wilhelm Braumuller.
43. Reuck, A.V.S. (de) & O'Connor, M. (Ed.) (1964) *Ciba Foundation Symposium on Disorders of Language*. London: Churchill.
44. Alajouanine, Th. (1968) *L'aphasie et le langage pathologique*. Paris: Baillière.
45. Foix, C. & Levy, M. (1927) Les ramollissements sylviens—syndromes des lésions en foyer du territoire de l'artère sylvienne et de ses branches. *Revue neurologique*, **35,** 1.
46. Hécaen, H. (1972) *Introduction à la neuropsychologie*. Paris: Larousse.
47. Dubois, J. & Hécaen, H. (1967) Pathologie du langage. *Revue de l'enseignement* (suppl. 1-2), 31.
48. Goodglass, H. & Kaplan, E. (1972) *The Assessment of Aphasia and Related Disorders*. Philadelphia, PA: Lea and Febiger.

BIBLIOGRAPHY

Bay, E. (1967) The classification of disorders of speech. *Cortex*, **3,** 26.

Hécaen, H. & Dubois, J. (1967) Critères neurolinguistiques d'une classification des aphasies. *Acta Neurologica Belgica*, **67,** 959.

Ingram, T.T.S. (1962) A description and classification of the common disorders of speech in childhood. *Archives of Diseases in Childhood*, **34,** 444.

Ingram, T.T.S. (1969) Developmental disorders of speech. In *Handbook of Clinical Neurology* (Ed.) Vinken, P.J. & Bruyn, G.W. p. 407. Amsterdam: North-Holland.

Jakobson, R. (1963) Linguistic types of aphasia. In *Brain*

Function (Ed.) Carterette, E. Vol. 3, p. 67. California: University of California Press.

Jakobson, R. (1973) Un enfoque linguistico de la afasia. *Acta audiologica y foniatrica hispano-americana*, **10,** 101.

Kerschensteiner, M., Poeck, K. & Brunner, E. (1972) The fluency-nonfluency hypothesis in the classification of aphasic speech. *Cortex*, **8,** 233.

Kertesz, A. & Phipps, J.B. (1977) Numerical taxonomy of aphasia. *Brain and Language*, **4,** 1.

Wepman, J.M. & Jones, L.V. (1964) Five aphasias: a commentary on aphasia as a regressive linguistic phenomenon. In *Disorders of Communication* (Ed.) Rioch, D. & Weinstein, E. p. 190. Baltimore, MD: Williams and Wilkins.

Wepman, J. & Jones, L. (1964) The brain and disorders of communication in five aphasics: a commentary of aphasia as a regressive linguistic phenomenon. *Research Publications, Association for Research in Nervous and Mental Diseases*, **42,** 190.

11. Cerebral Dominance and Language

'Ah yes! The things themselves . . . secondary, I can do them with my left hand; but the pre . . . precise things, it was my right hand. There, at present, it's good . . . a bit: I don't have control over it; I'm not able to . . . to lead it where I want. I tried to cut my meat with my right hand but that . . . that tires me. I succeed but that is tiring then, when I get angry, I say to it: 'My damned one, you are going to work!' . . . Yes, if I . . . if I made comparisons between the two: I'm . . . I'm right-handed; I would be expected to play the piano faster with that hand; but there, it's the opposite, I go faster . . . faster with the other, eh.'

(*Conversation with Mr Bl.; November 1971*)

Cerebral dominance for linguistic behaviour, that is, the functional specialization of one half of the brain as the biological substratum of language, was recognized on the basis of anatomoclinical work carried out during the last century. The knowledge then accumulated* included the contralaterality of hemispheric lesions causing aphasia and, from the outset, a parallel was drawn between manual dominance and dominance for language. A general rule was first formulated about pathology of the left half of the brain in right-handers: in 1836, Dax[2,3] stated that left hemisphere diseases, but not those of the right impaired verbal memory; in 1865, Broca[4] maintained that damage to the caudalmost portion of the left, third frontal convolution caused aphemia; in 1874, Wernicke[5] taught that a lesion of the caudal half of the left first temporal convolution causes sensory aphasia and that consistent with Broca's views, a lesion in the caudalmost half of the left, third frontal convolution causes motor aphasia (see Chapter 1 and 10). As a complement, attempts were made to determine the significance of exceptions to this rule: in 1865, Bouillard[6] and Broca[4] expressed the opinion that a right hemisphere lesion could impair the faculty of articulated language in left-handers. A definite conclusion based, according to Broca, on knowledge of nervous system embryology[7] (see Chapter 1) as well as on anatomoclinical observations, then appeared obvious, namely, that the same hemisphere usually had an exclusive and permanent monopoly over manual dominance and dominance for language: this would be the left hemisphere in right-handers and the right hemisphere in certain exceptional individuals, namely left-handers[4]. By relating most of the apraxias (see Chapter 4) to left hemispheric lesions, Liepmann[8-12] was to give still greater weight to this view which limited the concept of cerebral dominance solely to the realms of language and manual ability and attributed dominance to a single hemisphere, the major hemisphere.

A nearly absolute doctrine on cerebral dominance had thus been formulated by the second half of the last century. It was later to undergo certain modifications. The main factors which guided the development of thinking on this matter were as follows:

(a) Detailed studies of different aspects of manual behaviour indicated that the phenomenon of manual dominance must be defined in relative terms in a large number of people.
(b) Similarly, clinical and anatomoclinical studies of aphasia led to the suggestions that cerebral dominance for language is another

* Earlier than 1320 BC, the Edwin Smith papyrus mentions that right or left cranial lesions can cause hemiplegia on the side opposite to the lesion[1].

phenomenon which should generally be considered in relative, rather than absolute, terms and that there are important individual variations in this regard. The pertinence of the first suggestion was recently confirmed through observations of certain aspects of linguistic behaviour after surgical section of the large interhemispheric commissures[13].

(c) Techniques were developed to permit the study, in normal speakers, of the respective participation of the left and the right hemisphere in speech and language. These techniques permitted experimental verification of the nineteenth-century neurologists' assertion regarding the ipsilaterality of cerebral dominance for manual ability and for language.

(d) Longitudinal observations of the effects of cerebral lesions sustained during childhood indicated that the ontogenesis of cerebral dominance is largely postnatal and reaches completion only after several years. It was thus possible to speak, depending on an individual's age, of the functional plasticity of the brain[14].

(e) On the basis of neuroanatomical studies, a possible link was suggested between cerebral dominance for language and the presence of morphological asymmetries observed on the surface of the cerebral hemispheres.

(f) Neuropsychological research demonstrated that the concept of cerebral dominance is equally valid for behaviours other than those related to language or to manual preference and, especially, that each of an individual's two cerebral hemispheres may assume relative functional dominances[15].

We shall now discuss in turn each of the factors listed above and then attempt to specify the essential features of a contemporary definition of cerebral dominance.

LEFT-HANDERS AND RIGHT-HANDERS

Motor pre-eminence (and possibly sensory as well) of one limb over its contralateral homologue is only present, or at least immediately obvious, in the human species. In man, movements requiring the greatest precision are generally executed with the right hand. This habitual dextrality has been noted since prehistoric times but has not yet been satisfactorily explained.

Infants do not show manual preference at birth. According to Gesell[16], the first, and very precarious, signs appear at about the age of one year. There is much variation but as a general rule, the preferred use of one of the hands is gradually established and becomes stabilized between the ages of six and eight years.

Manual dominance in normals

In a normal individual, the laterality of the dominant hand is related to two major factors, one being genetic and the other sociocultural. There are undeniable cases in which the latter (in the form of tools and objects designed only for use by right-handers, educational practices emphasizing use of the right hand, sometimes through coercion, the view of sinistrality as a pathological state, etc.) has effectively countered a spontaneous biological tendency. At present, there are no physical attributes or even electroencephalographic characteristics which are known to be valid predictors of the eventual side of manual dominance in a normal individual.

Possible effects of pathology

Pathology which impairs the cerebral hemisphere destined to control the dominant hand may be followed by functional reorganization of the healthy hemisphere and results, even if the process of lateralization has already begun, in a change of laterality of the dominant hand. In contrast, it has not been demonstrated that an acquired disability (present or future) of the preferred hand can have a significant effect on the functional organization of the cerebral hemispheres.

'Left-handers'

The proportion of left-handers is probably not the same from one population to another. The figures given in different reports are nevertheless so diverse (from 1 to 25 per cent) that they more obviously reflect varying definitions of dextrality and sinistrality than actual differences between the populations studied. There are, for example, three obvious consequences of defining a left-hander as an individual who writes with the left hand: (a) the proportion of left-handers is relatively small; (b) the proportion of left-handers decreases as the stigma associated with sinistrality increases in the populations studied (left-handers who have shifted are counted among the right-handers); (c) illiterates are neither left-handed nor right-handed. Such a definition is clearly too incomplete and thus inadequate: through the use of insufficiently detailed questionnaires, some clinicians nevertheless accept it in their routine clinical work.

It may prove interesting, even from a purely biological point of view, to know the percentage of individuals in a given population who write with their left hand only (it has been suggested that the learning of written expressive language may play a significant role in determining the extent of lateralization for language). It would nevertheless be wrong to suppose that the problem of dextrality and sinistrality can be adequately treated solely on the basis of observations of writing behaviour.

Subirana's work

Many discussions of manual dominance erroneously suggest that right-handers and left-handers constitute homogeneous groups. It is now known that, within a normal population, manual dominance may vary over the entire range from the extreme of absolute dextrality to that of relative sinistrality.* Investigations by the Spanish neurologist, Subirana[18–22], largely contributed to the acquisition of this knowledge and appear particularly valuable because they were based on the systematic observation of several well-defined behaviours (writing, eating, combing one's hair, throwing a ball, dealing cards, threading a needle etc.). Subirana's conclusions can be summarized as follows:

(a) Approximately 25 per cent of the human population are absolute right-handers. These individuals show preferred use of the right hand in all one-handed tasks and, in bimanual tasks, execute the more precise movements with the right hand.

(b) Approximately 40 per cent are preferred right-handers. The preferred use of the right hand is very clear in most tasks but certain acts are preferentially executed with the left hand or indifferently performed with either hand.

(c) Approximately 25 per cent are ambidexterous. Preferred use of the right hand varies across tasks or in particular tasks and is approximately equal to the preferred use of the left hand.

(d) Approximately 10 per cent are preferred left-handers.† The preferred use of the left hand is very clear in most tasks but certain acts are preferentially executed with the right hand or indifferently performed with either hand.

(e) An absolute left-hander, or someone who always prefers to use the left hand, is an exceptional individual.

In summary, if Subirana's findings are accepted, cerebral dominance for handedness has its biological foundations exclusively in the left hemisphere in only one-quarter of the population; the foundations are bilateral but with a net gradient in favour of the left hemisphere in two-fifths of the population; they are bilateral and without a clear predominance of one hemisphere over the other in a quarter of the population; they are bilateral with a gradient in favour of the right hemisphere in one-tenth of the population; finally, within a normal population, their exclusive lateralization to the right hemisphere is exceptional.

Shared dominance, either with or without a gradient favouring one hemisphere (usually the left) is thus frequent in regard to manual behaviour. We shall now examine reasons to believe that dominance may also be shared, to a certain degree, in regard to cerebral activities linked to the comprehension and production of articulated (i.e., multiphased) language.

* A monograph by Hécaen and Ajuriaguerra[17] on handedness and cerebral dominance includes a review of the most significant publications on this topic before 1963. The reader is advised to consult this excellent work for further information.

† Studying only gestures whose execution is not usually codified by social convention, such as those involving the manipulation of an object like a hammer or a face-cloth, one of us (F.L.) found that left-handers presently comprise 5 per cent of the contemporary French population. In a study of Anglo-Saxons, Annett[23–25] observed the manual behaviour of more than 2000 subjects on 12 different tasks: of the 30 per cent who were not right-handed, 3 per cent showed a left-hand preference on all tasks (i.e., were exclusively left-handed).

FINDINGS FROM APHASIOLOGY

As previously mentioned, it was observations of aphasia which led nineteenth-century neurologists to formulate a doctrine of cerebral dominance for language (cf. p. 12). It was also clinical and anatomoclinical studies of aphasia which, to a very large extent, permitted the subsequent refinement of this doctrine.

LEFT HEMISPHERE LESIONS IN RIGHT-HANDERS

Aphasia belongs to the clinical picture associated with the onset of a lesion in the left sylvian region in more than 95 per cent of right-handers who sustain such a lesion. The severity, duration and evolution of the different clinical manifestations of the aphasia then vary according to the localization and the extent of the lesions and the aetiology of the disease causing these lesions (see Chapters 3 to 9). They also vary depending on whether the affected individual is an absolute right-hander or a preferred right-hander and on whether or not there is a familial history of sinistrality and/or ambidexterity. A study by Luria and another by Subirana appear of particular interest in this regard:

(a) Luria[26] studied 120 right-handers who became aphasic after a left hemisphere lesion. He considered 64 patients within this group to be absolute right-handers* and 56 to be preferred right-handers. Considerable language recovery occurred in only two of the absolute right-handers (3 per cent) but was observed in 29 of the preferred right-handers (52 per cent).
(b) Subirana[22] studied 113 right-handers who became aphasic and hemiplegic after a cerebral vascular accident affecting the left sylvian region. The right hemiplegia persisted in all cases. The aphasia also persisted in 76 patients: only 20 per cent of this group were preferred right-handers with a familial history of sinistrality or ambidexterity. Recovery from aphasia occurred in the 37 other patients: 80 per cent of this group were preferred right-handers with a familial history of sinistrality or ambidexterity.

These two investigations strongly suggest that dominance for language, like that for manual ability, is often shared between the two hemispheres and that, in right-handers at least, dominance for language is often shared in those same individuals who show shared dominance for manual ability (with a pre-eminence of the left hemisphere in both cases) (Insertions 11.1 and 11.2). These considerations should be borne in mind by therapists considering a possible programme of aphasia therapy (see Chapter 17).

RIGHT HEMISPHERE LESIONS IN RIGHT-HANDERS

A right-hander rarely becomes aphasic following a right hemisphere lesion. If an aphasia is observed, it should be asked whether the patient has not been a victim of a left hemisphere lesion at some time in the past and particularly during childhood (cf. p. 280). Proof of such a lesion cannot usually be established so that it may then be asked if this is not a case in which the aphasia represents the consequence, in a normal right-hander, of a lesion limited strictly to the right hemisphere; such cases are extremely rare.† Two comments should be made:

(a) On one hand, the fact that right hemisphere lesions do not cause aphasia in right-handers does not necessarily imply that the right hemisphere plays no role in the normal linguistic behaviour of right-handers[28] (Insertion 11.2). The only definite conclusion which can be drawn is that a right-hander's left hemisphere can ensure, in the presence of a right hemisphere lesion, linguistic behaviour which does not differ from the norm (or at least does not differ in an immediately obvious way).
(b) On the other hand, to state that a right hemisphere lesion in a right-hander is not accom-

* These figures suggest that Luria and Subirana did not define absolute right-handedness in the same way; Subirana's definition was probably more restrictive.

† It occurs in right-handers whose family also includes left-handers; one then speaks of crossed aphasia, a clinical picture whose onset suggests that there may be a dissociation between the genetic factors linked to manual preference and those linked to language. See Boller's discussion on this topic[27].

Insertion 11.1

> With the aim of identifying the eventual role of the right cerebral hemisphere in the residual linguistic behaviour of right-handed aphasics having a left hemisphere lesion, Kinsbourne[29] subjected three patients [one case with Broca's aphasia, one with conduction aphasia and one with a mixed aphasia (see Chapter 4)] to the Wada test (cf. p. 277). The injection of sodium Amytal into the left internal carotid (see Chapter 9) did not alter the patients' linguistic behaviour; in contrast, injection on the right resulted in a transient suppression in all three cases. This study thus confirmed a fact established long ago through the application of the anatomoclinical method (see Chapter 8–4).

panied by aphasia is to say only that the signs and symptoms classically recognized as those of aphasia do not occur in right-handers after a right hemisphere lesion. This does not rule out, a priori, the possibility that particularly detailed and refined tests of certain aspects of linguistic functioning might permit a demonstration, in a right-hander with a right hemispheric lesion, of minor (and perhaps transient) anomalies which are not usually classified among the manifestations of aphasia[28].

LEFT HEMISPHERE LESIONS IN AMBIDEXTRALS AND IN LEFT-HANDERS

Although in a less predictable way than in right-handers, a left hemisphere lesion may, and often does, cause aphasia in an ambidextral or left-hander. This is illustrated by findings from different investigations carried out during the last 2[illegible] years:

(a) Goodglass and Quadfasel[30] studied 123 cases of left-handers with a unilateral hemispheric lesion; of the 65 who had a left hemisphere lesion, 53 (81 per cent) presented aphasia.
(b) Botez and Calcainu[33] studied 17 cases of left-handers with a unilateral cerebral lesion; of the nine who had a left hemisphere lesion, six (67 per cent) presented aphasia.
(c) Hécaen[17, 34, 35] studied 59 cases of left-handers with aphasia; 37 of the patients (63 per cent) had a unilateral left hemisphere lesion.
(d) Subirana[22] studied six cases of left-handers with aphasia; four of these patients (67 per cent) had a unilateral left hemisphere lesion; recovery from aphasia occurred in all four cases.
(e) Luria[26] studied 19 cases of left-handers who became aphasic after a lesion of the left sylvian region; the aphasia was transient in 11 cases and permanent in the eight other cases.

On the basis of these and other studies, the following points can be noted: aphasia from a unilateral left hemisphere lesion is frequent in left-handers and in ambidextrals and is probably even more frequent than aphasia from a unilateral right hemisphere lesion (unlike right-handers, left-handers do not show systematic ipsilaterality of dominance for language and for manual ability); recovery from aphasia resulting from a left hemisphere lesion is more frequent and more rapid in left-handers and ambidextrals than in right-handers (shared dominance for language is more frequent and more marked in left-handers and ambidextrals than in right-handers); following a left hemisphere lesion, comprehension disturbances are less frequent, less severe and of shorter duration in left-handers and ambidextrals than in right-handers (the bilaterality of representation in left-handers and ambidextrals is perhaps particularly marked and effective in regard to language comprehension).

RIGHT HEMISPHERE LESIONS IN AMBIDEXTRALS AND IN LEFT-HANDERS

While a right hemisphere lesion almost never causes aphasia in right-handers, it frequently does so in ambidextrals and in left-handers. Here again, the probability of an aphasia is nevertheless lower than in the case of a lesion of the left sylvian region in a right-hander. We shall

Insertion 11.2

Sperry and his collaborators[31] studied the behaviour of right-handers who had undergone a complete section of the large interhemispheric commissures (anterior commissure and corpus callosum), the effect of this intervention presumably being to isolate each of the two cerebral hemispheres completely from the other. The results suggest that, in the absence of any aphasiogenic lesion of the left hemisphere, the linguistic capacity of the right hemisphere in right-handers is limited but undeniable. This capacity is particularly related to language comprehension (both spoken and written language); through blind palpation with the left hand, the patient could find, among an array of objects, the one which was named or described by the examiner; when a written word was tachistoscopically projected to the left visual half field, the patient could not 'read' it and verbally denied its presentation but could nevertheless find the matching object through blind palpation with the left hand. Generally speaking, these performances were only possible with familiar objects. In addition to this linguistic capacity, it was also shown that the right hemisphere of a right-hander can itself ensure the 'conceptualization' of the features of familiar objects: thus, after a picture of a small flat key (car key) had been briefly projected to the left visual half field, the patient—who could not name the picture and denied its presentation—was able to match this stimulus with a large round key (from an old lock). On the other hand, the expressive capacities of the right hemisphere were found to be almost non-existent in the patients studied by Sperry et al; only a few very short and familiar words could be composed (through blind palpation of large plastic letters with the left hand).

It is interesting to consider these observations in relation to two findings from aphasiology[32]: (a) depending on the aetiology of the causal disease, partial recovery from an aphasic comprehension disturbance may often be observed, particularly in regard to the comprehension of concrete messages (see Chapters 4 and 9); (b) in a right-hander who becomes aphasic after a left hemisphere lesion, the later onset of a right hemisphere lesion may abolish all reacquired language regardless of the extent of linguistic recovery.

reconsider, in this regard, certain investigations already cited:

(a) Goodglass and Quadfasel[30] studied 123 cases of left-handers with a unilateral hemispheric lesion; of the 58 with a right hemisphere lesion, 50 (85 per cent) presented aphasia.
(b) Botez and Calcainu[33] studied 17 cases of left-handers with a unilateral hemispheric lesion; of the eight with a right hemisphere lesion, seven (87 per cent) presented aphasia.
(c) Hécaen[17, 34, 35] studied 59 cases of left-handers with aphasia; 22 of them (37 per cent) had a unilateral right hemisphere lesion.
(d) Subirana[22] studied six cases of left-handers with aphasia; two of them (33 per cent) had a unilateral right hemisphere lesion; recovery from aphasia occurred in both cases.

On the basis of these and other studies, the following points can be made: although quite frequent in left-handers, aphasia from a unilateral right lesion is perhaps rarer than aphasia from a unilateral left lesion and is much less frequent than aphasia from a unilateral left lesion in right-handers (more often than otherwise and contrary to assertions by Bouillard[6] and Broca[4], a 'left-hander' is not necessarily an individual endowed with dominance which is both strong and generally ipsilateral for manual ability and for language); recovery from aphasia in left-handers, whether the aphasia resulted from a right or a left hemisphere lesion, is more frequent and more rapid than recovery from aphasia in right-handers (shared dominance for language—bilateral representation—is more frequent and more marked in left-handers than in right-handers); for a given clinical picture of aphasia there is a greater chance of error in attempting to predict the localization of a right hemisphere lesion than in attempting to predict the localization of a left hemisphere lesion (if there is significant right hemisphere representation of language, it is possibly more diffuse anatomically—perhaps even functionally less specific—than is left hemisphere representation).

THALAMIC STIMULATION AND THALAMIC LESIONS

We have previously discussed the effects of electrical stimulation of the pulvinar and the ventral lateral nucleus of the thalamus as well as the effects of surgical and natural lesions of this structure (see Chapter 7). We then maintained that the thalamus probably participates in linguistic functioning and that such participation is more evident, in right-handers, for the left thalamus than for the right thalamus; we added that the functional lateralization of the thalamus, in this regard, appears to be less pronounced and weaker than that of the cortex.

APHASIA AND CEREBRAL DOMINANCE FOR LANGUAGE

Although the ipsilaterality of strong cerebral dominance for language and strong cerebral dominance for handedness is less universal than was believed by investigators of the past century, the biological organization subtending cerebral dominance for language is probably very similar to that subtending dominance for manual ability. This is in any case what is suggested, first by the fact that strong dominance for manual abilities is usually accompanied by strong dominance for language and, second, by the fact that shared dominance for manual ability is often accompanied by shared dominance for language. This being so, it is not surprising that aphasiological data concerning cerebral dominance for language have been and continue to be reported in conjunction with information on manual preference in the patients studied. The following statements summarize the position of contemporary aphasiology on the topic of cerebral dominance for language:

(a) Strong unilateral representation is more frequent than bilateral representation.

(b) The notion of strong unilateral representation does not exclude the possibility that the non-dominant hemisphere may play a certain role in linguistic functioning, particularly in regard to language comprehension (cf. above and Insertion 11.2); neither does it exclude the possibility that activities of the non-dominant hemisphere may be the source of certain residual behaviours of aphasics or even play a role in recovery from aphasia (whether the recovery be significant or so partial that it has little effect on communication with others).

(c) It can generally be assumed that strong unilateral representation is increasingly absolute as manual dominance is more absolute.

(d) Strong unilateral language representation is a characteristic of nearly all right-handers and of a fairly large number of ambidextrals and left-handers. It involves left hemispheric lateralization in nearly all right-handers and in a significant proportion of non right-handers.

(e) Bilateral representation, in which the extent of shared dominance is sufficient to have a significant influence on the onset and evolution of aphasic disturbances, is more frequent in non-right-handers than in right-handers. It may also enter into account in certain preferred right-handers, particularly in those with a familial history of ambidexterity or sinistrality.

(f) The degree of anatomical definition and of functional specialization of the nervous structures ensuring language production and comprehension possibly varies, to a certain extent, among different individuals. If so, an absolute right-hander is perhaps an individual whose neurobiological support for language is anatomically the least diffuse and functionally the most specialized.

(g) With respect to aphasia, bilaterality of language representation has both a disadvantage and an advantage: as recognized by Conrad[36], Brain[37], Subirana[22], Hécaen[17], Brown[38], and others, it explains the presence of aphasia in a large number of non-right-handers after a unilateral lesion of either hemisphere; it also explains, with due regard to the aetiology of the causal lesions, why the prognosis for recovery from aphasia is far better—and the results of therapy far superior (see Chapter 17)—in a large number of non-right-handers than in most right-handers.*

*It would nevertheless be wrong to assume that bilaterality of language representation is the only factor which can explain the favourable evolution of an aphasia and the efficacy of aphasia therapy. Besides the quality of the therapy programme, other important factors include the aetiology of the causal lesions as well as their site and extent (see Chapters 8–1, 8–3, 9 and 17). Similarly, the possibility of ipsilateral substitution (within the limits of certain functional territories), rather than contralateral substitution, cannot be ruled out in a large number of cases.

Insertion 11.3

Consider, for example, the following case.

A 25-year-old school teacher was admitted to the *Salpêtrière* with complete occlusion of the left sylvian artery (verified by arteriography).

The patient was ambidexterous (although she usually wrote with her right hand she knew, from having experimented on several occasions, that she could write very normally with her left hand). Several members of her family were left-handed or ambidexterous.

No neurological antecedents were reported in this patient's case; her early development and educational progress were such that they completely ruled out the possibility of a disorder of spoken or written language acquisition (i.e., there was no developmental dysphasia or dyslexia-dysgraphia).

The neurological examination indicated involvement of the entire territory irrigated by the left sylvian artery (see Chapter 9). Observations included severe right hemiplegia, maximal in the face and upper limb; apraxia of the left upper limb which, while mild and variable, was undeniable (observed on imitation as well as in response to oral and written verbal commands); exceptionally severe buccofacial apraxia (on imitation as well as in response to spoken and written commands); a primary sensory deficit affecting the entire right side of the body, finger agnosia; a right homonymous hemianopsia; marked dyscalculia; and aphasia.

The aphasia included both disturbed expression and comprehension:

(a) Oral expression was reduced to 'Yes' and 'No', which were always used propositionally. No audible production occurred during attempts at repetition and oral reading.

(b) Written expression was only possible with the left hand. Production was rapid and regular with letters normally formed (there was no disturbance of graphism proper). Copying was completely normal. Mild word-finding difficulty and the production of a few literal paragraphias were observed during written naming. Productions written to dictation showed a tendency towards agrammatism and contained literal and verbal paragraphias (see Chapter 2). The agrammatism was even more obvious in samples of spontaneous writing (essentially composed of juxtaposed substantives); word-finding difficulty was evident and there were numerous literal and verbal paragraphias.

(c) Spoken language was completely understood in certain situations but very partially apprehended in others. The patient was very attentive to her interlocutors' linguistic interventions. She responded affirmatively when asked if she 'understood everything' and appeared to do so from her consistently appropriate replies of 'yes' or 'no' and from her spontaneous facial expressions. Spoken words were rapidly and correctly identified by pointing to the appropriate picture when the series of matching pictures *crossed categories* (see Chapter 15), that is, were conceptually unrelated (e.g., book, horse, pipe, etc.). On the other hand, spoken word identification was grossly abnormal when the series of matching pictures represented *within category* items, that is, semantically related words (e.g., carnation, tulip, peony, daffodil, etc.). The same was true for the identification of the spoken names of body parts, parts of a car, coloured tokens, etc. (122 errors in identifying 300 stimuli). Identification of spoken stimuli by pointing to the appropriate written word was rapid and normal when the words were semantically unrelated but very abnormal for semantically related words. Failures occurred on the first part of the *Token Test* (see Chapter 16).

(d) Comprehension of written language was normal in all respects. Written words were correctly matched to pictures presented in both *crossed categories* or *within category* series. Written commands led to the correct identification of body parts, parts of a car, coloured tokens, etc. (no errors for 300 stimuli). Performance on a written version of the *Token Test* was correct until the fifth part of the test.

Given the (presumed) extension of the left hemisphere lesion and the very unusual nature of the symptomatological dissociations, especially concerning oral versus written language comprehension[39], it can be logically suggested that this patient's residual behaviours may constitute evidence of right hemisphere participation in the control of certain aspects of her linguistic functioning.

(h) With respect to linguistic behaviour, unilaterality and (relative) exclusivity of language representation may include an advantage: it is certainly possible that the harmonious acquisition of language and the degree of mastery in the use of language are favoured—among other factors and to a certain extent—by functional specialization which is biologically well-defined.

(i) In clinical aphasiology, unexpected symptom constellations, [i.e., unclassifiable clinical forms (see Chapter 10)] and intriguing dissociations (which are justifiably considered of great interest in regard to theories about the interrelationships of the brain and language) are more frequently observed in non-right-handers than in right-handers (Insertion 11.3).

(j) There is one form of aphasia, discussed elsewhere under the name of aspontaneity or under that of transcortical motor aphasia (see Chapters 6 and 10), in which left lateralization of the causal lesions is clearly not as well recognized as in the other clinical forms of aphasia.

The confidence which should be accorded to each of the above assertions is probably best estimated by considering each of them individually.

LANGUAGE DOMINANCE IN NORMAL ADULT SPEAKERS

Until about 30 years ago, investigators had no means of determining the respective participation of each cerebral hemisphere in the linguistic activities of a normal speaker. The anatomoclinical study of aphasia—which permitted the observation, in right-handers, of the common association between this condition and right hemiplegia—was the only basis on which it could be presumed, with a certain degree of confidence, that the chief cerebral structures linked to language production and comprehension (see Chapter 8-1 and 8-3) were lateralized to the left hemisphere. At present, a few techniques are available which permit the study (as yet still limited) of cerebral dominance for language in normal speakers.

THE WADA METHOD

Described in 1949, the *Wada technique*[40, 41], or *Amytal test*, consists of the rapid injection (over one to two seconds), into the common carotid artery, of 150 to 200 mg of a 10 per cent solution of sodium Amytal. This substance impregnates the hemispheric structures ipsilateral to the side of injection and results in transient neurological disturbances. Use of the Amytal test is generally considered justified when the dominant hemisphere for language must be identified in a particular individual in order to reach a decision on the advisability of neurosurgical intervention.

In all cases, the injection of sodium Amytal is followed by a hemianopsia, hemianaesthesia and hemiplegia of the side contralateral to the impregnated cerebral hemisphere. The hemiplegia is complete for two to three minutes with gradual recovery then occurring over two to six minutes. As a general rule, injection ipsilateral to the dominant hemisphere for language is accompanied by a brief state of confusion followed by a phase in which the subject can follow simple orders but presents linguistic suppression (see Chapter 4). It usually persists over the entire period of complete hemiplegia and then linguistic performance improves rapidly: the subject is first able to reply, by 'yes' or 'no', to (simple) questions; there then follows a brief period (one to three minutes) in which the production of characteristic aphasic transformations may be observed (paraphasias, perseverative phenomena, etc. demonstrated through the use of naming, oral reading and serial recitation tasks); linguistic behaviour returns to normal approximately eight minutes after the injection.

From the point of view of neurolinguistic research, the brevity of the observed disturbances is an obvious limitation of the Wada technique. Its use has nevertheless revealed several interesting facts concerning cerebral dominance for language. Thus Milner and her collaborators[42–44] in Montreal studied 212 normal adult speakers (95 right-handed and 117 left-handed or ambidexterous subjects including 74 without and 43 with clinical evidence of the onset of a left cerebral lesion during childhood). The results indicated that more than 99 per cent (94 of the 95) of the right-handers and 69 per cent of the left-handers and ambidextrals without an early left hemisphere lesion had left cerebral dominance for language. In contrast, dominance for language was firmly established in the right hemisphere in 54 per cent of the left-handers and ambidextrals with clinical evidence of the onset of left hemisphere lesion at a young age (cf. p. 280). Of the 74 left-handed or ambidexterous subjects without clinical evidence of an early left hemisphere lesion, 13 per cent showed bilateral language representation and 18 per cent showed dominant representation in the right hemisphere; of the 43 left-handed or ambidexterous subjects with clinical evidence of an early left hemisphere lesion, 16 per cent showed bilateral language representation and 30 per cent showed dominant representation in the left hemisphere. In certain respects, this study confirmed the hypotheses of Russel and Espir[45] who, in their conclusions about cerebral lesions from gunshot injury, emphasized the relative rarity of aphasia, in left-handers and ambidextrals, after limited lesions of the right hemisphere. This study, and others which followed, also permitted more precise documentation of the occurrence of shared dominance (bilaterality). Observed by Milner et al[43] in 18 individuals of whom only one was a right-hander, this phenomenon appeared of interest from several points of view with the most spectacular finding undoubtedly being that in half of these subjects, the transient aphasia, while obvious after the injection of sodium Amytal on the right as well as on the left, was manifested differently depending on the hemisphere impregnated. In seven of these nine cases, sodium Amytal injection on the left resulted in an almost isolated naming disturbance (after a period of suppression when this occurred) while injection on the right caused an almost isolated difficulty in the production of familiar verbal sequences (for example, the days of the week); the opposite dissociation was observed in the two other cases. To a certain extent, this observation can be related to Jakobson's contrast[46] between a similarity disorder and a contiguity disorder and might even provide it with experimental support (see Chapter 10).

ELECTRICAL STIMULATION

The effects of electrical stimulation applied to different points of the cortex were discussed elsewhere in this text (see Fig. 7-5). In general, the results of electrical stimulation have permitted confirmation of left hemispheric dominance for language.

DICHOTIC LISTENING

Developed by Broadbent in 1954[47], the technique known as dichotic auditory stimulation involves the simultaneous presentation, through earphones, of different acoustic stimuli to each ear. The subject is asked to report, either verbally or otherwise, what he heard. Depending on the nature of the stimuli (words, noises, melodies, etc.) and the particular aspects of the stimulus to which the subject must attend, one of the two ears may show significant superiority in terms of the number of stimuli adequately reported. Since the arrangement of the auditory pathways is such that the functional link between each ear and the contralateral hemisphere is more efficient than the functional link between each ear and the ipsilateral hemisphere (Fig. 11-1 and 8-14), the superiority of one ear on a dichotic listening task can be interpreted as an indication of the (relative) dominance of the contralateral hemisphere for a given class of stimuli.

Kimura, in 1961[48] presented dichotic verbal stimuli to 120 subjects whose cerebral dominance for language had been previously established by

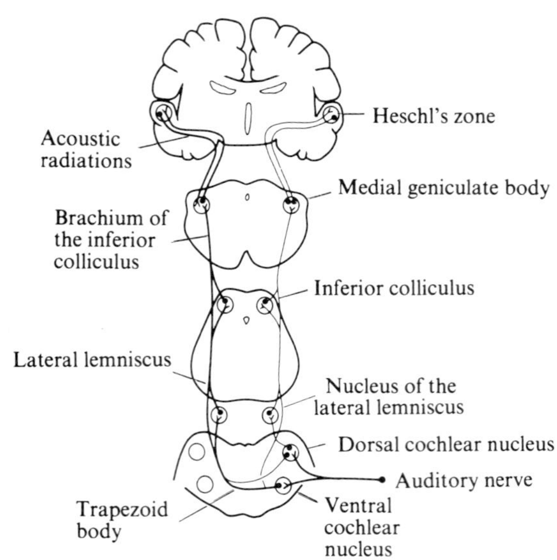

Fig. 11-1 *Anatomy of the acoustic pathways showing only the pathways for information coming from the left ear; because there is only partial decussation at the trapezoid level, this information reaches Heschl's region on both the left and the right side.*

the Amytal test. The left hemisphere was dominant in a group of 107 right-handers, left-handers and ambidextrals while the right hemisphere was dominant in 13 ambidextrals and left-handers. The results of the two procedures were in complete agreement: the 107 subjects found to have left hemisphere dominance on the Amytal test all showed right ear superiority during dichotic presentation of linguistic stimuli; the 13 subjects found to have right hemisphere dominance on the Amytal test all showed left ear superiority during dichotic presentation of linguistic stimuli. Seemingly valid, and certainly less dangerous than the sodium Amytal test, dichotic listening has proved to be a useful method of identifying hemispheric dominance for language in normal speakers.

In 1968, Milner et al[49] used Broadbent's method with split brain subjects, that is, subjects who had undergone sectioning of the large interhemispheric commissures (Insertion 11.2). Their results merit reflection: when asked to report verbally series of digits presented as stimuli, performance by right-handed commissurotomized subjects was equivalent, in monaural listening, to that of normals for the left ear as well as for the right. It can thus be concluded, with regard to the left ear, that the ipsilateral auditory representation is entirely sufficient to permit an adequate verbal report of stimuli presented in this condition. During dichotic listening (right ear stimuli differ from left ear stimuli), the number of digits reported by normal right-handers is usually slightly larger for the right than for the left ear. This difference was greatly exaggerated in right-handed commissurotomized subjects: the number of digits reported was completely normal for the right ear but was far below normal for the left ear. In other words, in a dichotic listening condition and in the presence of a section of the commissures, ipsilateral auditory information coming from the left ear may be almost totally suppressed in the left hemisphere by concurrent contralateral information coming from the right ear.* On the other hand, by using tasks in which the required response is non-verbal (for example a blind, matching-to-object response by palpation with the left hand), it can be shown that in a dichotic listening situation, the linguistic message addressed contralaterally from the left ear to the right hemisphere (of a right-hander) may also suppress, to a large extent, the competing message coming ipsilaterally from the right ear[32]. If, after this type of matching between a left auditory stimulus and an object palpated and recognized with the left hand, subjects are asked to name the object which they are holding in their hands, they will often utter the word corresponding to the auditory stimulus which was just presented to his right ear. Like other observations of this type, this extinction of ipsilateral information in favour of contralateral information demonstrates the possible occurrence of isolated hemispheric functioning in commissurotomized subjects; it also provides, in the case of either the right or the left hemisphere, a supplementary demonstration of the physiological pre-eminence, in man, of the contralateral auditory projections (Fig. 11.1).

TACHISTOSCOPIC STIMULATION

Investigations have also been carried out[50, 51] on the identification of (simple) written linguistic stimuli in extramacular tachistoscopic vision (rapid projection in a single half field or, simultaneously, in both half fields). The results of these studies suggest the presence, at least in right-handers, of a usual relative superiority of the right visual half field for the recognition of written language symbols, that is, there is relatively better processing of written verbal information when it is initially addressed to the left cerebral hemisphere. The relative nature of this phenomenon is obvious in normal subjects, namely when the corpus callosum is intact. It is still perceptible, but of course to a lesser degree, after section of the large interhemispheric commissures (Insertion 11.2); for example, Gazzaniga[13, 52] maintains that commissurotomized right-handers can recognize—although they are unable to read them aloud—some short, simple, concrete and frequently used substantives when presented tachistoscopically in the left visual half field.

ELECTROENCEPHALOGRAPHY

Over the past years an increasing number of electroencephalographic studies have attempted

* François Michel and his collaborators in Lyon recently observed analogous phenomena of verbal extinction. They also used dichotic listening tasks but with subjects having left or right temporal lesions.

to identify relationships between the electrical activity of the brain and speech production and reception. Thus Low, Wada and Fox[53], from Vancouver, studied over 50 adults and children (the youngest being five years old) and demonstrated the presence of electrical asymmetry between left and right in the mean of the slow wave potentials immediately prior to articulatory production. The slow waves were found, on the average, to be more negative in the hemisphere contralateral to the dominant hand than in the ipsilateral hemisphere. Even more convincing was the finding that the electroencephalographic data permitted accurate prediction of the dominant hemisphere for language in 10 of the 11 cases where a preoperative sodium Amytal test was considered necessary (cf. p. 277); right cerebral dominance was predicted in two of these cases.

XENON-133 TECHNIQUE

The xenon-133 technique permits computerized detection of minimal changes in the regional cerebral blood flow. In 1974, the Swedish scientist Ingvar[54, 55] used this method in a study of the dominant hemisphere. He reported a circumscribed increase of the blood flow within the precentral regions, particularly in their parasylvian parts, during automatized verbal production (e.g., when naming days of the week, months of the year) and during oral reading. Moreover, the last activity was accompanied by increased blood flow within the occipital regions.

MANUAL DOMINANCE AND DOMINANCE FOR LANGUAGE

Broca[4] maintained, in the nineteenth century, that the left hemisphere is dominant for language in right-handers and the right hemisphere is dominant in left-handers (cf. p. 12). The findings discussed in the previous pages agree with only the first part of this assertion. In other words, it appears that in a neurologically normal population of literate adults, left hemispheric dominance is even more widespread for language than for handedness (being characteristic of virtually all right-handers and of approximately 70 per cent of left-handers and ambidextrals). It appears that right hemisphere dominance for language, although indeed present in a certain proportion of left-handers and ambidextrals, is scarcely more frequent in these groups than is shared dominance between the two hemispheres.

HEMISPHERIC LESIONS IN CHILDHOOD

Research results published by Basser in 1962[56], on the linguistic development of 102 children who sustained a large hemispheric lesion during early childhood, have provided a better understanding of the ontogenesis of cerebral dominance for language. The characteristics of the population studied by Basser can be summarized as follows:

(a) The patients were very young. Hence, the idea of manual dominance cannot generally be considered.
(b) Basser considered that 72 of his subjects had sustained their lesion before the first phase of language acquisition while 30 sustained it later. Within the first group, 34 subjects had a left hemisphere lesion and 38 had a right hemisphere lesion; within the second group, 15 had a right lesion and 15 had a left lesion.
(c) Of the 72 children who sustained a lesion before language acquisition, 19 showed significant intellectual deterioration (8 left and 11 right lesions) while 53 did not (26 left and 27 right lesions). The former never acquired spoken language whereas the 53 children in the latter group acquired language at the same time, and by the same means, as normal children; 15 of them (eight left and seven right lesions) nevertheless presented dysarthria (see Chapter 3) or stuttering.
(d) Of the 30 children who sustained a lesion after language acquisition, 20 became aphasic (13 left and seven right lesions) while 10 did not (two left and 10 right lesions). None of the 20 aphasic children appeared to have presented an obvious comprehension disturbance; on the other hand, the aphasia was initially manifested by severe reduction in one child and by complete suppression (see Chapter 4) in the 19 others. The aphasia decreased in all cases, over a period of a few days to two years; with the exception of a

small number of cases in which the lesion had resulted in considerable intellectual deterioration, recovery from the oral expressive disturbance was eventually judged to be complete.

(e) Because of uncontrollable epileptic phenomena or severe behavioural disturbances, a hemispherectomy was eventually carried out on 72 of the 102 children in this series.

The following statements summarize the conclusions which can be drawn from Basser's research:

(a) An extensive hemispheric lesion, sustained during early childhood, does not necessarily result in significant intellectual deterioration. In the absence of such deterioration, the process of language acquisition is not hindered by either a left or a right hemispheric lesion if it is sustained before the first phases of language learning. At birth, each of the two hemispheres thus possesses, and retains for a certain period, sufficient potential to control the progressive appearance of articulated language. Functional lateralization related to language, which is characteristic of most adults although to different degrees, is therefore established only during subsequent phases of language acquisition.

(b) While it is known that strong functional lateralization for language is well established in the majority of normal speakers, at least in literate populations, it is not known at what age this process of functional lateralization is completed nor what may be the normal range of variation. However, Basser's research provides some information pertaining to these questions.

(i) Certain of Basser's observations suggest that strong lateralization may be established rather early, either on the left or on the right. Among the 10 cases having an extensive hemispheric lesion without aphasia, and for whom it can be presumed that the process of language lateralization was well advanced, there were two subjects, aged 18 and 21 months respectively, who presented right hemiplegia (right lateralization for language) and two subjects, aged 12 and 36 months, who presented left hemiplegia (left lateralization for language); in these four children, a subsequent hemispherectomy was not followed by any postoperative aphasic phenomena, even of a transient nature.

(ii) On the other hand, bilaterality of language representation is more frequent in young children than in adults. This fact has long been recognized in paediatric neurology where transient aphasias resulting from unilateral lesions, either left or right, are observed far more frequently than in adult neurology. One of Basser's patients was a six year old who presented severe aphasia after an extensive left hemisphere lesion; complete recovery occurred in four weeks. Another child, 30 months of age, became aphasic after a right hemisphere lesion; as in the preceding case, complete recovery occurred in four weeks. In both cases, the presence of aphasia following the cerebral lesion demonstrates the premorbid participation of the damaged hemisphere in linguistic functioning and the rapid recovery suggests that contralateral language representation also existed before onset of the disease.

(c) When an extensive lesion of the hemisphere already dominant for language is sustained at an early age and does not cause intellectual deterioration, it does not prevent the reacquisition of normal language functioning. In other words, the plasticity of the non-dominant hemisphere for language may remain sufficient, over a certain period, to permit its eventual control of linguistic functioning.

(i) Such functional transfer may be total: among Basser's subjects, an 18-month-old child became aphasic after a left hemisphere lesion and a five year old became aphasic after a right hemisphere lesion. In both cases, the aphasia persisted for about two years and then completely disappeared; a subsequent hemispherectomy was not followed by any aphasic disturbances, even of a transient nature.

(ii) The functional transfer may also be partial: one of Basser's patients became aphasic at the age of 20 months following an extensive left hemisphere lesion. The aphasia completely disappeared in 16 months and then recurred after a hemispherectomy. As in this child, whose second aphasic episode was very brief (one month), the potential of the

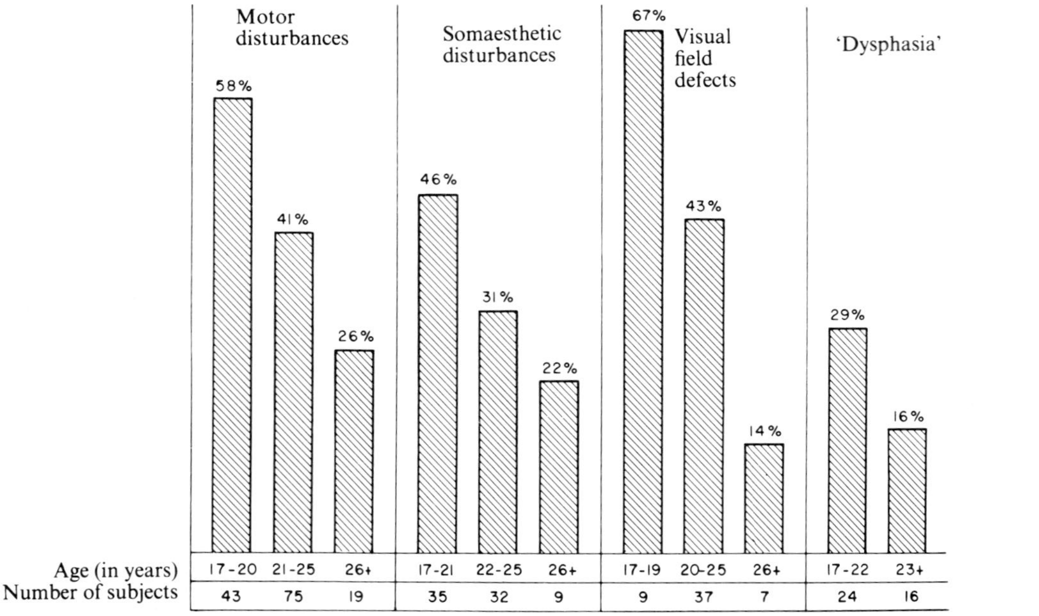

Fig. 11-2 *Functional recovery from different neuropsychological disturbances, as a function of age, in American veterans wounded in action (Second World War, Korea, Vietnam). The prognosis for recovery from aphasia is better in the 17- to 22-year age group than in those aged 24 and over. From Teuber*[14].

non-lesioned hemisphere is such, in this type of case, that a complete progressive transfer of language representation remains possible.

(iii) The remaining possibility is a complete, or almost complete, absence of functional transfer (this would correspond to a type of evolution whose frequency increases with the age of the patients in adult aphasiology). An absence of transfer could theoretically occur after destruction of the cerebral hemisphere in which strong functional lateralization had been precociously established (cf. p. 275). None of Basser's cases provided convincing evidence of this possibility unless it is assumed that strong precocious lateralization was the only factor accounting for two of his patients, described as severely mentally retarded (see Chapter 16), who never acquired or recovered language after an extensive unilateral hemispheric lesion.

Three additional remarks appear relevant in concluding this section of our discussion:

(d) In the series of children studied by Basser, the achievement of, or return to, linguistic normalcy was always judged in terms of spoken language; little is known concerning the development of written language in these children.

(e) It may be that detailed neurolinguistic investigations would demonstrate, in patient samples analogous to that of Basser's study, the presence of sequellae which escape notice during routine examinations: this might be expected considering, for example, Dennis' research[57, 58] on syntactical comprehension after hemidecortication.

(f) The functional plasticity of the child's brain in relation to linguistic functioning, which was clearly demonstrated by Basser's research, probably does not totally disappear after childhood. A certain ipsilateral or contralateral plasticity, which varies among individuals, may partially or completely explain cases of (relative) recovery observed in adult aphasiology, including those of right-handers. During a seminar in Montreal in 1974, Teuber reported findings on young adults who had become aphasic following cerebral damage from gunshot injury: the results showed that recovery from aphasia, in a group of adults of whom the great majority were less than 30 years of age, was generally more complete in the younger subjects[14] (Fig. 11-2).

LANGUAGE DOMINANCE AND MORPHOLOGICAL ASYMMETRY OF THE CEREBRAL HEMISPHERES

Considering cerebral dominance in terms of findings on language and manual dexterity, Broca[4] maintained that one manifestation of its biological foundations could be observed, during embryogenesis, in the usually more precocious development of primary fissures in the left hemisphere than in the right hemisphere (see Chapter 1). Indeed, there are periods during which asymmetries may be observed, in certain human fetuses, between the left and right cerebral hemispheres, particularly at the level of the rolandic regions (see Fig. 1-1). However, these phenomena have not been demonstrated to be as systematic as implied by Graliolet[7] and Broca[4]. Certain contemporary investigators, such as Geschwind[59] and Wada[60] are nevertheless convinced that there is a mutual relationship between certain anatomical asymmetries and cerebral dominance for language. Supporting arguments can be based on the following morphological observations:

(a) According to Eberstaller[61], the average length of the Fissure of Sylvius (see Fig. 8-2) is greater in the left hemisphere (58.2 mm) than in the right hemisphere (51.8 mm); it can be assumed this corresponds to a quantitatively greater importance of Wernicke's area than of its counterpart in the right hemisphere.

(b) According to Kodama[62], the length and height of the insula are greater in the left hemisphere (56.4 and 38.1 mm respectively) than in the right hemisphere (52.8 and 37.5 mm, respectively); depending on whether or not the insula is considered to be an integral part of the language zone (see Fig. 8-32), this fact may or may not be regarded as an indication of the quantitatively greater importance of the language zone than of its counterpart in the right hemisphere.

(c) According to Kakeshita[64], von Economo and Horn[65], Pfeiffer[66], Geschwind and Levitsky[67], Tezner[68, 69] and Wada, Clark and Hamm[60], the surface of the planum temporale (see Chapter 8-1 and Fig. 8-5) is, in general, noticeably larger in the left hemisphere than in the right hemisphere (in a study of 200 brains, Wada et al observed the opposite asymmetry in only 22 cases); this finding thus indicates that Wernicke's area is, in general, quantitatively more important than its counterpart in the right hemisphere (see Fig. 8-5). Wada et al claim that this asymmetry can be observed after the twenty-ninth week of gestation. They add that it is, in general, relatively more obvious in the adult female than in the adult male, an observation which we do not think should serve as a basis for hasty conclusions.

RIGHT HEMISPHERE SPECIALIZATION IN RIGHT-HANDERS

In right-handers, linguistic expression in all modalities appears to be under the nearly exclusive control of the left hemisphere; the same control appears to be generally true for manual ability. Regardless of the input modality, language comprehension is also under the dominant control of the left hemisphere in right-handers; there are, however, reasons to believe that this dominance is less absolute for comprehension than for expression (cf. p. 275). Linguistic and manual behaviours are probably the types which most often lead to the establishment of strongly lateralized functional specialization. Nevertheless, they are not the only ones for which it is appropriate to consider the idea of hemispheric specialization. Given the frequency and the nature of certain disorders observed in clinical neuropsychology following right hemisphere lesions in right-handers (for example, an inability to reproduce two or three dimensional models, difficulty in spatial orientation, etc.), it was assumed that there is a relative right hemisphere superiority for the integration of visuospatial information[70]. This fact was confirmed in normal right-handers through tachistoscopic investigations (cf. p. 279): certain ones by Kimura[51] demonstrated better localization of a point (presented in two- or three-dimensional space) when stimuli were presented in the left visual half-field than when presented in the right half-field. Concurrent studies of dichotic listening (cf. p. 278) revealed right hemisphere superiority in right-handers for the processing of different types of non-linguistic auditory information (melodies, noises such as coughing, crying, etc.). In summary, it is now taught that, in right-handers, it is the left hemisphere which ensures language production, controls the majority of the most highly refined gestural activities and is by far superior to the left hemisphere in regard to language comprehension; it is also taught that, in right-handers, the right hemisphere is superior to the left, at least for several types of sensory information, in perception of the non-linguistic environment.

In our opinion, a contemporary definition of cerebral dominance should include the following information:

(a) Dominance is a question of the relative functional specialization of one hemisphere in comparison to the other.
(b) This relative functional specialization is probably more pronounced for the cortical components of the dominant hemisphere than for its deep subcortical components (see Chapter 7).
(c) For a given function, the degree of functional lateralization varies among different individuals.
(d) For a given individual, either the left or right hemisphere may be dominant depending on the sensorimotor foundations of the behaviour considered (the notions of a major, or globally dominant hemisphere and that of a minor, or globally non dominant hemisphere are outdated).
(e) In the majority of normal speakers, dominance for language is among the most strongly lateralized and is, as a general rule, lateralized to the left hemisphere.
(f) Cerebral dominance is established gradually, as learning progresses with the biological maturation of the brain (see Chapter 8-2).
(g) It may be, at least in the case of language, that certain morphological asymmetries between the cerebral hemispheres are related to the phenomenon of functional lateralization and cerebral dominance.

REFERENCES

1. Margotta, R. (1968) *Histoire illustrée de la médecine*. Paris: Editions des Deux Coqs d'Or.
2. Dax, M. (1865) Lésions de la moitié gauche de l'encéphale coïncidant avec l'oubli des signes de la pensée. *Gazette hebdomadaire de Médecine et de Chirurgie*, **33,** 259.
3. Joynt, R.J. & Benton, A.L. (1964) The memoir of Marc Dax on aphasia. *Neurology*, **14,** 851.
4. Broca, P. (1865). Du siège de la faculté du langage articulé. *Bulletin de la Société d'Anthropologie*, **7,** 377.
5. Wernicke, C. (1874) *Der aphasische Symptomenkomplex*. Breslau: Cohn and Weigert.
6. Bouillaud, J.B. (1864–1865) Discussion du rapport de Lélut. *Bulletin de l'Académie de Médecine*, **30.**
7. Gratiolet, L.P. (1854) *Mémoire sur les plis cérébraux de l'homme et des primates*. Paris: Bertrand.
8. Liepmann, H. (1900) *Das Krankheitsbild der Apraxie*. Berlin: Karger.
9. Liepmann, H. (1900) Das Krankheitsbild der Apraxie ('motorischen Asymbolie') auf Grund einès Falles von einseitiger Apraxie. *Monatschrift für Psychiatrie und Neurologie*, **8,** 15, 102 and 182.
10. Liepmann, H. (1908) *Drei Aufsätze aus dem Apraxiegebiet*. Berlin: Karger.
11. Liepmann, H. (1912) Anatomische Befunde bei Aphasischen und Apraktischen, *Neurologisches Zentralblatt*, **31,** 1524.
12. Liepmann, H. & Maas, O. (1907) Fall von linksseitiger Agraphie und Apraxie bei rechtsseitiger Lähmung. *Journal für Psychologie und Neurologie* (Leipzig), **10,** 214.
13. Gazzaniga, M.S. (1970) *The Bisected Brain*. New York: Appleton-Century Crofts.
14. Teuber, H.L. (1975) Recovery of function after brain injury in man. In *Outcome of Severe Damage to the Central Nervous System* (Ed.) Ciba Foundation. p. 159 Amsterdam: North-Holland.
15. Harnad, S., Doty, R.W., Goldstein, L., Jaynes, J. & Krauthamer, G. (Ed.) (1977) *Lateralization in the Nervous System*. New York: Academic Press.
16. Gesell, A. (1940) *The First Five Years of Life*. New York: Harper.
17. Hécaen, H. & Ajuriaguerra, J. (de) (1963) *Les gauchers*. Paris: Presses Universitaires de France.
18. Subirana, A. (1952) La droiterie. *Schweizer Archiv für Neurologie und Psychiatrie*, **69,** 321.
19. Subirana, A. (1958) The prognosis in aphasia in relation to cerebral dominance and handedness. *Brain*, **81,** 415.
20. Subirana, A. (1964) The relationship between handedness and language function. *International Journal of Neurology*, **4,** 215.
21. Subirana, A. (1965) *La neuro-psicologia y el problema de la dualidad cerebral*. Madrid: Libro de Ponencias del VIII Congreso Nacional de Neuro-psiquiatria.
22. Subirana, A. (1969) Handedness and cerebral dominance. In *Handbook of Clinical Neurology* (Ed.) Vinken, P.J. & Bruyn, G.W. Vol. 4, p. 248. Amsterdam: North-Holland.
23. Annett, M. (1964) A model of the inheritance of handedness and cerebral dominance. *Nature*, **204,** 59.
24. Annett, M. (1970) A classification of hand preference by association analysis. *British Journal of Psychology*, **61,** 303.

25. Annett, M. (1973) Handedness in families. *Annals of Human Genetics*, **37**, 93.
26. Luria, A.R. (1970) *Traumatic Aphasia*. The Hague: Mouton.
27. Boller, F. (1973) Destruction of Wernicke's area without language disturbance. *Neuropsychologia*, **11**, 243.
28. Eisenson, J. (1959) Language dysfunctions associated with right brain damage. *Journal of the American Speech Association*, **1**, 107.
29. Kinsbourne, M. (1971) The minor cerebral hemisphere as a source of aphasic speech. *Archives of Neurology* (Chicago), **25**, 302.
30. Goodglass, H. & Quadfasel, F.A. (1954) Language laterality in left-handed aphasics. *Brain*, **77**, 521.
31. Sperry, R.W., Gazzaniga, M.S. & Bogen, J.E. (1969) Interhemispheric relationships: the neocortical commissures; syndromes of hemisphere disconnection. In *Handbook of Clinical Neurology* (Ed.) Vinken, P.J. & Bruyn, G.W. Vol. 4, p. 273. Amsterdam: North-Holland.
32. Lecours, A.R. & Poncet, M. (1975) Syndrome calleux. *Encyclopédie médico-chirurgie, 17036 C[10]*, **1**.
33. Botez, M.I. & Calcainu, G. (1961) Afaziia u Levsei. *Zhurnal Neuropatologii i Psikhiatrii*, **61**, 820.
34. Hécaen, H. (1959) Dominance hémisphérique et préférence manuelle. *Evolution psychiatrique*, **1**, 1.
35. Hécaen, H. (1962) Clinical symptomatology in right and left hemispheric lesions. In *Interhemispheric Relations and Cerebral Dominance* (Ed.) Mountcastle, V.B. p. 215. Baltimore, MD: Johns Hopkins.
36. Conrad, K. (1949) Uber aphasische Sprachstörungen bei hirnverletzten Linkshändern. *Nervenarzt*, **20**, 148.
37. Brain, R. (1945) Speech and handedness. *Lancet*, **2**, 837.
38. Brown, J.W. & Hécaen, H. (1976) Lateralization and language representation. *Neurology*, **26**, 183.
39. Al Chérif, A. (1972) *Considérations sur les troubles de l'expression orale et de la compréhension verbale présentés par deux malades aphasiques*. Medical thesis, Marseilles.
40. Wada, J. (1949) Une nouvelle méthode pour l'identification de l'hémisphère cérébral dominant pour le langage. Un rapport préliminaire sur l'injection intracarotidienne d'amytal sodique chez l'homme. *Igaku to Seibutsugaku*, **14**, 221. (In Japanese.)
41. Wada, J. & Rasmussen, Th. (1960) Intracarotid injection of sodium amytal for the lateralization of cerebral speech dominance. *Journal of Neurology*, **17**, 266.
42. Milner, B., Branch, C. & Rasmussen, Th. (1964) Observations on cerebral dominance, In *Disorders of Language* (Ed.) de Reuck, A.V.S. & O'Connor, M. p. 200. London: Churchill.
43. Milner, B., Branch, C. & Rasmussen, Th. (1966) Evidence for bilateral speech representation in some non-right-handers. *Transactions of the American Neurological Association*, **91**, 306.
44. Milner, B. (1973) Hemispheric specialization: scope and limits. In *The Neurosciences: Third Study Program* (Ed.). Schmitt, F.O. & Worden, F.G. Boston, MA: MIT Press.
45. Russell, W.R. & Espir, M.L.E. (1961) *Traumatic Aphasia*. London: Oxford University Press.
46. Jakobson, R. (1956) Two aspects of language and two types of aphasic disturbances. In *Fundamentals of Language* (Ed.) Jakobson, R. & Halle, M. p. 55. The Hague: Mouton.
47. Broadbent, D.E. (1954) The role of auditory localization in attention and memory span. *Journal of Experimental Psychology*, **47**, 191.
48. Kimura, D. (1961) Cerebral dominance and the perception of verbal stimuli. *Canadian Journal of Psychology*, **15**, 166.
49. Milner, B., Taylor, L. & Sperry, R.W. (1968) Lateralized suppression of dichotically-presented digits after commissural section in man. *Science*, **161**, 184.
50. Kimura, D. (1969) Spatial localization in left and right visual fields. *Canadian Journal of Psychology*, **23**, 445.
51. Kimura, D. (1973) The asymmetry of the human brain. *Scientific American*, **228**, 70.
52. Gazzaniga, M.S. & Hillyard, S.A. (1971) Language and speech capacity of the right hemisphere. *Neuropsychologia*, **9**, 415.
53. Low, M.D., Wada, J.A. & Fox, M. (1973) Electroencephalographic localization of connative aspects of language production in the human brain. *Transactions of the American Neurological Association*, **98**, 129.
54. Ingvar, D.H. (1973) Speech functions of the dominant hemisphere studied by regional cerebral blood flow measurements. *Excerpta Medica*, **296**, 158.
55. Ingvar, D.H. & Schwartz, M.S. (1974) Blood flow patterns induced in the dominant hemisphere by speech and reading. *Brain*, **97**, 273.
56. Basser, L.S. (1962) Hemiplegia of early onset and the faculty of speech with special reference to the effects of hemispherectomy. *Brain*, **85**, 427.
57. Dennis, M & Kohn, B. (1975) Comprehension of syntax in infantile hemiplegics after hemidecortication: left hemisphere superiority. *Brain and Language*, **2**, 472.
58. Dennis, M. & Whitaker, H.A. (1976) Language acquisition following hemidecortication: linguistic superiority of the left over the right hemisphere. *Brain and Language*, **3**, 404.
59. Geschwind, N. (1974) *Selected Papers on Language and the Brain*. Dordrecht: Reidel.
60. Wada, J., Clark, R. & Hamm, A. (1975) Cerebral hemispheric asymmetry in humans. *Archives of Neurology* (Chicago), **32**, 239.
61. Eberstaller, O. (1884) Zur Obeflächenanatomie der Grosshirnhemisphären. *Wiener Medizine Blaetter*, **7**, 479, 542 and 644.
62. Kodama, K. (1934) Beitrage zur Anatomie des Zentralnervensystems der Japaner: VIII. Insula Reilii. *Folia Anatomica Japonica*, **12**, 423.
63. Bonin, G. (von) (1962) Anatomical asymmetries of the cerebral hemispheres. In *Interhemispheric Relations and Cerebral Dominance* (Ed.) Mountcastle, V.B. p. 1. Baltimore, MA: Johns Hopkins.
64. Kakeshita, T. (1925) Zur Anatomies der operkularen temporal Region (vergleichende Untersuchungen der rechten und linken Seite). *Arbeiten aus dem Neurologischen Institut an der Wiener Universität*, **27**, 292.

65. Economo, C. (von) & Horn, L. (1930) Uber Windungsrelief, Masse und Rindenarchitektonik der Supratemporalfläche, ihre individuellen und ihre seiten Unterschiede. *Zentralblatt für die gesamte Neurologie und Psychiatrie*, **130,** 678.
66. Pfeiffer, R.A. (1936) Pathologie der Horstrahlung und der corticalen Horsphare In *Handbuch der Neurologie* (Ed.) Bumke, O. & Foerster, O. Vol. 6, p. 533. Berlin: Springer.
67. Geschwind, N. & Levitsky, W. (1968) Human brain: left–right asymmetries in temporal speech region. *Science*, **161,** 186.
68. Teszner, D. (1972) *Etude anatomique de l'asymétrie droite-gauche du planum temporal*. Medical thesis, Paris.
69. Teszner, D., Tzavaras, A., Gruner, J. & Hécaen, H. (1972) L'asymétrie droite-gauche du planum temporal à propos de l'etude anatomique de 100 cerveaux. *Revue neurologique*, **126,** 444.
70. Hécaen, H., Penfield, W., Bertrand, C. & Malmo, R. (1956) The syndrome of apractognosia due to lesions of the minor cerebral hemisphere. *Archives of Neurology and Psychiatry* (Chicago), **75,** 400.

BIBLIOGRAPHY

Akelaitis, A.J. (1943) Studies on the corpus callosum. VII. Study of language functions (tactile and visual lexia and graphia) unilaterally following section of the corpus callosum. *Journal of Neuropathology and Experimental Neurology*, **3,** 226.

Akelaitis, A.J. (1944) A study of gnosis, praxis and language following section of the corpus callosum and anterior commissure. *Journal of Neurosurgery*, **1,** 94.

Albert, M.L. (1972) Auditory sequencing and left cerebral dominance for language. *Neuropsychologia*, **10,** 245.

Albert, M.L., Goldblum, M.C., Benson, D.F. & Hécaen, H. (1971) Mechanisms of auditory comprehension. II. Cerebral dominance. *Transactions of the American Neurological Association*, **96,** 132.

Anastasopoulos, G.K. & Kokkini, D. (1960) De la dominance hémisphérique et de la localisation des centres de la parole. *Hellin. iatr.*, **29,** 785. (In Greek.)

Anastasopoulos, G.K. & Kokkini, D. (1962) Cerebral dominance and localization of the language functions. *Psychiatria et Neurologia* (Basel), **143,** 6.

Angelergues, R., Hécaen, H., Djindjian, R. & Jarrié-Hazan, N. (1962) Un cas d'aphasie croisée (thrombose de l'artère sylvienne droite chez une droitière). *Revue neurologique*, **107,** 543.

Annett, M. (1970) A classification of hand preference by association analysis. *British Journal of Psychology*, **61,** 303.

Archibald, Y.M. & Wepman, J.M. (1968) Language disturbances and nonverbal cognitive performance in eight patients following injury to the right hemisphere. *Brain*, **91,** 117.

Ardin-Delteil, Lévi-Valensi & Derrieu (1923) Deux cas d'aphasie. I. Aphasie de Broca par lésion de l'hemisphère droit chez une droitière. II. Aphasie avec hémiplégie-droite chez une gauchère. *Revue neurologique*, **30,** 14.

Bakan. P., Dibb, G. & Reed, P. (1973) Handedness and birth stress. *Neuropsychologia*, **11,** 363.

Bakker, D.J. (1969) Ear-asymmetry with monaural stimulation: task influences. *Cortex*, **5,** 36.

Bartholomeus, B. (1974) Effects of task requirements on ear superiority for sung speech. *Cortex*, **10,** 216.

Basser, L.S. (1962) Hemiplegia of early onset and the faculty of speech with special reference to the effects of hemispherectomy. *Brain*, **75,** 427.

Bauer, R.W. & Wepman, J.M. (1955) Lateralization of cerebral functions. *Journal of Speech Disorders*, **20,** 171.

Benton, A.L. (1964) Developmental aphasia and brain damage. *Cortex*, **1,** 40.

Benton, A.L. (1965) The problem of cerebral dominance. *The Canadian Psychologist*, **6a,** 332.

Benton, A.L., Meyers, R. & Polder, G.J. (1962) Some aspects of handedness. *Psychiatria et Neurologia* (Basel) **144,** 321.

Bergman, P.S. & Green, M. (1951) Aphasia: effect of intravenous sodium amytal. *Neurology*, **1,** 471.

Bever, T.G. (1971) The nature of cerebral dominance in speech behavior of the child and adult, In *Language Acquisition: Models and Methods* (Ed.) Huxley, R. & Ingram, D. p. 231. New York: Academic Press.

Bever, T.G. (1975) Cerebral asymmetries in humans are due to the differentiation of two incompatible processes: holistic and analytic. *Annals of the New York Academy of Sciences*, **263,** 251.

Bever, T.G. & Chiarallo, R.J. (1974) Cerebral dominance in musicians and nonmusicians. *Science*, **185,** 537.

Billow, B.W. Observation on the use of sodium Amytal in the treatment of aphasia. *Medical Record* (New York), **162,** 12.

Blau, A. (1946) The master hand; a study of the origin of right and left sidedness and its relation to personality and language. *Research Monograph of the American Orthopsychiatric Association*, **5.**

Blumstein, S., Goodglass, H. & Tartter, U. (1975) The reliability of ear advantage in dichotic listening. *Brain and Language*, **2,** 226.

Bogen, J.E. (1969) The other side of the brain: I. Dysgraphia and dyscopia following cerebral commissurotomy. *Bulletin of the Los Angeles Neurological Society*, **34,** 73.

Bogen, J.E., Fisher, E.D. & Vogel, P.J. (1965) Cerebral commissurotomy; a second case report. *Journal of the American Medical Association* **194,** 1328.

Bogen, J.E. & Gazzaniga, M.S. (1965) Cerebral commissurotomy in man: minor hemisphere dominance for certain visuo-spatial functions. *Journal of Neurosurgery*, **23,** 394.

Bogen, J.E. & Vogel, P.J. (1962) Cerebral commissurotomy in man; preliminary report. *Bulletin of the Los Angeles Neurological Society*, **27,** 169.

Bonkowski, R.J. (1967) Verbal and extraverbal components of language as related to lateralized brain damage. *Journal of Speech Research*, **10**, 558.

Botez, M.I. & Crighel, E. (1971) Partial disconnexion syndrome in an ambidextrous patient. *Brain*, **94**, 487.

Bramwell, E. (1899) On 'crossed' aphasia and the factors which go to determine whether the 'leading' or 'driving' speech-centres shall be located in the left or in the right hemisphere of the brain, with notes on a case of 'crossed' aphasia (aphasia with right-sided hemiplegia) in a left-handed man. *Lancet*, **1**, 1473.

Branch, C., Milner, B. & Rasmussen, T. (1964) Intracarotid sodium Amytal for lateralization of cerebral speech dominance. *Journal of Neurosurgery*, **21**, 399.

Brown, J.W. & Hécaen, H. (1976) Lateralization and language representation. *Neurology*, **26**, 183.

Brown, J.W. & Jaffe, J. (1975) Hypothesis on cerebral dominance. *Neuropsychologia*, **13**, 107.

Brown, J.W. & Wilson, F.R. (1973) Crossed aphasia in a dextral. A case report. *Neurology*, **23**, 907.

Bruce, W. (1868) Case of partial aphasia with left hemiplegia. *Medical Times*, **1**, 87.

Bryden, M.P. (1964) Tachistoscopic recognition, handedness and cerebral dominance. *Perceptual and Motor Skills*, **19**, 686.

Bryden, M.P. (1965) Tachistoscopic recognition, handedness, and cerebral dominance. *Neuropsychologia*, **3**, 1.

Bryden, M.P. (1975) Speech lateralization in families: a preliminary study using dichotic listening. *Brain and Language*, **2**, 201.

Buffery, A.W.H. (1971) Sex differences in the development of hemispheric asymmetry of function in the human brain. *Brain Research*, **31**, 364.

Burklund, C.W. (1972) Cerebral hemisphere function in the human: fact versus tradition. In *Drugs, Development and Cerebral Function* (Ed.) Smith, W.L. p. 8. Springfield, Ill.: Thomas.

Butler, S.R. & Norrsell, U. (1968) Vocalization possibility initiated by the minor hemisphere, *Nature*, **220**, 793.

Cameron, R., Currier, R. & Haerer, A. (1971) Aphasia and literacy. *British Journal of Communication*, **6**, 161.

Caplan, D., Holmes, J.M. & Marshall, J.C. (1974) Word classes and hemispheric specialization. *Neuropsychologia*, **12**, 331.

Carri, B.A. (1965) The occurrence of chronic aphasia in the left hemiplegia of adults. *Cerebral Palsy Review*, **4**, 16.

Carmon, A., Harishanu, Y., Lowinger, R. & Levy, S. (1972) Asymmetries in hemispheric blood volume and cerebral dominance. *Behavioral Biology*, **7**, 853.

Carmon, A., Nachson, I. & Starinsky, R. (1976) Developmental aspects of visual hemifield differences in perception of verbal material. *Brain and Language*, **3**, 463.

Catlin, J., Vanderveer, N.J. & Teicher, R.D. (1976) Monaural right-ear advantage in a target-identification task. *Brain and Language*, **3**, 470.

Chamberlain, H.D. (1928) The inheritance of left handedness. *Journal of Heredity*, **19**, 557.

Chesher, E.C. (1936) Some observations on the relation of handedness to language mechanism. *Bulletin of the Neurological Institute of New York*, **4**, 556.

Clark, B. & Zangwill, O. (1965) A case of 'crossed aphasia' in a dextral. *Neuropsychologia*, **3**, 81.

Claude, H. & Schaeffer, H. (1921) Un nouveau cas d'hémiplégie gauche avec aphasie chez un droitier. *Revue neurologique*, **28**, 170.

Crockett, H.G. & Estridge, N.M. (1951) Cerebral hemispherectomy: a clinical, surgical and pathological study of four cases. *Bulletin of the Los Angeles Neurological Society*, **16**, 71.

Crowell, D.H., Jones, R.H., Kapuniai, L.E. & Nakagawa, J.K. (1973) Unilateral cortical activity in newborn humans: an early index of cerebral dominance? *Science*, **180**, 205.

Cullen, J.K., Thompson, C.L., Hughes, L.F., Berlin, C.I. & Samson, D.S. (1974) The effects of varied acoustic parameters on performance in dichotic speech perception tasks. *Brain and Language*, **1**, 307.

Curry, F.K.W. (1967) A comparison of left-handed and right-handed subjects on verbal and non-verbal dichotic listening tasks. *Cortex*, **3**, 343.

Czopf, J. (1972) Uber die Rolle der nicht dominanten Hemisphären in der Restitution der Sprache der Aphasischen. *Archiv für Psychiatrie und Nervenkrankheiten*, **216**, 162.

Davis, J. & Wada, J. (1977) Lateralization of speech dominance by spectral analysis of evoked potentials. *Journal of Neurology, Neurosurgery and Psychiatry*, **40**, 1.

Déjerine, J. & Thomas, A. (1912) Contributions à l'étude de l'aphasie chez les gauchers et des dégénerations du corps calleux. *Revue neurologique*, **22**, 213.

Dennis. M, & Whitaker, H.A. (1976) Language acquisition following hemi-decortication. Linguistic superiority of the left or the right hemisphere. *Brain and Language*, **3**, 404.

Dirks, D. (1964) Perception of dichotic and monaural verbal material and cerebral dominance for speech. *Acta Otolaryngologica*, **58**, 73.

Doehring, D.G. (1972) Ear asymmetry in the discrimination of monaural tonal sequences. *Canadian Journal of Psychiatry*, **26**, 106.

Doehring, D.G. & Bartholomeus, B.N. (1971) Laterality effects in voice recognition. *Neuropsychologia*, **9**, 425.

Efron, R. (1963) The effects of handedness on the perception of simultaneity and temporal order. The effect of stimulus intensity on the perception of simultaneity in right and left-handed subjects. *Brain*, **86**, 261 and 285.

Eisenson, J. (1962) Language and intellectual modifications associated with right cerebral damage. *Language and Speech*, **5**, 47.

Ellis, H.D. & Shepherd, J.W. (1974) Recognition of abstract and concrete words presented in left and right visual fields. *Journal of Experimental Psychology*, **103**, 1035.

Ettlinger, G., Jackson, C.V. & Zangwill, O.C. (1956) Cerebral dominance in sinistrals. *Brain*, **79**, 569.

Gardner, W.J. (1941) Injection of procaine into the brain to locate speech area in left-handed persons. *Archives of Neurology and Psychiatry* (Chicago), **48**, 1035.

Gazzaniga, M.S. (1965) Psychological properties of the disconnected hemispheres in man. *Science*, **150,** 372.

Gazzaniga, M.S. (1970) *The Bisected Brain.* New York: Appleton-Century Crofts.

Gazzaniga, M.S. (1973) The split brain in man. *Scientific American*, **228,** 24.

Geffen, G. (1976) Development of hemispheric specialization for speech perception. *Cortex*, **12,** 337.

Geffen, G., Bradshaw, J.L. & Nettleton, N.C. (1972) Hemispheric asymmetry: verbal and spatial encoding of visual stimuli. *Journal of Experimental Psychology*, **93,** 25.

Geffen, G., Bradshaw, J.L. & Wallace, G. (1971) Interhemispheric effects on reaction time to verbal and nonverbal stimuli. *Journal of Experimental Psychology*, **85,** 415.

Giannitrapani, D. (1967) Developing concepts of lateralization of cerebral functions. *Cortex*, **3,** 353.

Gibson, A.R., Dimond, S.J. & Gazzaniga, M.S. (1972) Left field superiority for word matching. *Neuropsychologia*, **10,** 463.

Girard, P.F. (1952) A propos des troubles neurologiques et psychiatriques observés chez les gauchers; la notion de diphasie, dipraxie et diphrénie. *Semaine des Hôpitaux de Paris*, **28,** 750.

Gloning, I., Gloning, K., Haub, G. & Quatember, R. (1969) Comparison of verbal behavior in right-handed and non right-handed patients with anatomically verified lesion of one hemisphere. *Cortex*, **5,** 43.

Gloning, K. & Quatember, R. (1966) Statistical evidence of neuropsychological syndromes in left-handed and ambidextrous patients. *Cortex*, **2,** 484.

Gooddy, W. & Reinhold, M. (1961) Congenital dyslexia and asymmetry of cerebral function. *Brain*, **84,** 231.

Goodglass, H. & Calderon, M. (1977) Parallel processing of verbal and musical stimuli in right and left hemispheres. *Neuropsychologia*, **15,** 397.

Gordon, H.W. & Bogen, J.E. (1974) Hemispheric lateralization of singing after intracarotid sodium Amytal barbitone. *Journal of Neurology, Neurosurgery and Psychiatry*, **37,** 727.

Gott, P. (1973) Language following dominant hemispherectomy. *Journal of Neurology, Neurosurgery and Psychiatry*, **36,** 1082.

Gottlieb, G., Doran, C. & Whitley, S. (1964) Cerebral dominance and speech acquisition in deaf children. *Journal of Abnormal Social Psychology*, **69,** 182.

Gurd, F.B. (1920) Aphasia in a left-handed individual consequent upon a right cerebral lesion. *Canadian Medical Association Journal*, **10,** 270.

Halpern, Y., Nachshon, I. & Carmon, A. (1973) Shift in ear superiority in dichotic listening to temporal pattern nonverbal stimuli. *Journal of the Acoustical Society of America*, **53,** 46.

Harnad, S.R., Steklis, H.D. & Lancaster, J. (Ed). (1976) *Origins and Evolution of Language and Speech.* New York: The New York Academy of Sciences.

Hécaen, H. (1976) Acquired aphasia in children and the ontogenesis of hemispheric functional specialization. *Brain and Language*, **3,** 114.

Hécaen, H. & Ajuriaguerra, J. (de) (1956) Le problème de la dominance hémisphérique: les troubles du langage, des gnosies et des praxies chez les gauchers lors des lésions hémisphériques droites et gauches. *Journal of Psychology and Normal Pathology*, **53,** 473.

Hécaen, H. & Ajuriaguerra, J. (de) (1963) *Les gauchers.* Paris: Presses Universitaires de France.

Hécaen, H. & Assal, G. (1968) Les relations interhémisphériques et le problème de la dominance cérebrale. *L'année psychologique*, *68e* année, 491.

Hécaen, H. & Sauguet, J. (1971) Cerebral dominance in left-handed subjects. *Cortex*, **7,** 19.

Heilman, K. M., Coyle, J.M., Gonyea, E.F. & Geschwind, N. (1973) Apraxia and agraphia in a left-hander. *Brain*, **96,** 21.

Heilman, K.M., Gonyea, E.F. & Geschwind, N. (1974) Apraxia and agraphia in a right-hander. *Cortex*, **10,** 284.

Henschen, S.E. (1926) On the function of the right hemisphere of the brain in relation to the left in speech, music and calculation. *Brain*, **49,** 110.

Heuyer, G. & Feld M. (1954) Hémisphérectomie gauche pour atrophie cicatricielle chez un enfant droitier. *Revue neurologique*, **90,** 52.

Hochberg, F.H. & Lemay, M. (1975) Arteriographic correlates of handedness. *Neurology*, **25,** 218.

Holmes, J.A. & Sadoff, R.L. (1966) Aphasia due to a right hemisphere tumor in a right-handed man. *Neurology*, **16,** 392.

Humphrey, M.E. & Zangwill, O.I. (1952) Dysphasia in left-handed patients with unilateral brain lesions. *Journal of Neurology, Neurosurgery and Psychiatry*, **15,** 184.

Inglis, J. (1965) Dichotic listening and cerebral dominance. *Acta Oto-laryngologica*, **60,** 231.

Ingram, D. (1975) Cerebral speech specialization in young children. *Neuropsychologia*, **13,** 103.

Johnson, J.P., Sommers, R.K. & Weidner, W.E. (1977) Dichotic ear preference in aphasia. *Journal of Speech Research*, **20,** 116.

Kennedy, F. (1916) Stock-brainedness, the causative factors in the so-called 'crossed aphasias'. *Journal of Nervous and Mental Diseases*, **44,** 334.

Kertesz, A. & Geschwind, N. (1971) Patterns of pyramidal decussation and their relationship to handedness. *Archives of Neurology* (Chicago), **24,** 326.

Kimura, D. (1963) Speech lateralization in young children as determined by auditory test. *Journal of Comparative and Physiological Psychology*, **56,** 899.

Kimura, D. (1964) Left-right differences in the perception of melodies. *Quarterly Journal of Experimental Psychology*, **14,** 355.

Kimura, D. (1967) Functional asymmetry of the brain in dichotic listening. *Cortex*, **3,** 163.

Kimura, D. (1973) Manual activity during speaking: I. Right-handers. Manual activity during speaking: II. Left-handers. *Neuropsychologia*, **11,** 45 and 51.

Kimura, D. (1976) The neural basis of language qua gesture. In *Studies in Neurolinguistics* (Ed.) Whitaker, H. & Whitaker, H.A. Vol II, p. 145. New York: Academic Press.

Kimura, D. & Archibald, Y. (1974) Motor functions of the left hemisphere. *Brain*, **97**, 337

Kimura, D., Battison, R. & Lubert, B. (1976) Impairment of nonlinguistic hand movements in a deaf aphasic. *Brain and Language*, **3**, 566.

Kimura, D. & Folb, S. (1968) Neural processing of backwards-speech sounds. *Science*, **161**, 395.

King, F.L. & Kimura, D. (1972) Left-ear superiority in dichotic perception of vocal nonverbal sounds. *Canadian Journal of Psychology*, **26**, 111.

Kinsbourne, M. (1970) The cerebral basis of lateral asymmetries in attention. *Acta Psychologica*, **33**, 193.

Kinsbourne, M. (1970) The cerebral basis of lateral asymmetries in attention. In *Attention and Performance* (Ed.) Sanders, A.F. Vol. 3, p. 193. Amsterdam: North-Holland.

Kinsbourne, M. (1973) The control of attention by interaction between the cerebral hemispheres. In *Attention and Performance IV* (Ed.) Kornblum, S. p. 239. Amsterdam: North-Holland.

Kinsbourne, M. (1975) Cerebral dominance, learning, and cognition. In *Progress in Learning Disabilities* (Ed.) Helmer, R. & Myklebust, D. New York: Grune and Stratton.

Kinsbourne, M. (1975) The ontogeny of cerebral dominance. *Annals of the New York Academy of Sciences*, **263**, 244.

Kinsbourne, M. & Cook, J. (1971) Generalized and lateralized effects of concurrent verbalization in a unimanual skill. *Quarterly Journal of Experimental Psychology*, **23**, 34[illegible].

Klein, R. & Stack, J.J. (1953) Visual agnosia and alternating dominance, analysis of a case. *Journal of Mental Sciences*, **99**, 749.

Knox, C. & Kimura, D. (1970) Cerebral processing of nonverbal sounds in boys and girls. *Neuropsychologia*, **8**, [illegible]7.

Krashen, S. (1973) Lateralization, language learning and the critical period: some new evidence. *Language Learning*, **23**, 63.

Krashen, S. & Harshman, R. (1972) Lateralization and the critical period. *ULCA Working Papers in Phonetics*, **23**, 3.

Krynauw, R.A. (1916) Infantile hemiplegia treated by removing one cerebral hemisphere. *Journal of Nervous and Mental Diseases*, **44**, 334.

Lainé, E. & Gros, C. (1956) *L'hémisphérectomie*. Paris: Masson.

Lake, D.A. & Bryden, M.P. (1976) Handedness and sex differences in hemispheric asymmetry. *Brain and Language*, **3**, 266.

Lancker, D. (van) & Fromkin, V.A. (1973) Hemispheric specialization for pitch and 'tone': evidence from Thai. *Journal of Phonetics*, **1**, 101.

Lansdell, H. (1962) Laterality of verbal intelligence in the brain. *Science*, **135**, 922.

Lansdell, H. (1969) Verbal and nonverbal factors in right-hemisphere speech: relation to early neurological history. *Journal of Comparative and Physiological Psychology*, **69**, 734.

Le Fort, M. (1903) *Quelques considérations sur le rôle du cerveau droit dans les fonctions du langage*. Paris: Michalon.

Lemay, M. (1976) Morphological cerebral asymmetries of modern man, fossil man and nonhuman primate. *Annals of the New York Academy of Sciences*, **280**, 349.

Lemay, M. & Culebras, A. (1972) Morphologic differences in the hemispheres demonstrable by carotid arteriography. *New England Journal of Medicine*, **287**, 168.

Levy, J. (1969) Possible basis for the evolution of lateral specialization of the human brain. *Nature*, **224**, 614.

Levy, J., Nebes, R.D. & Sperry, R.W. (1971) Expressive language in the surgically separated minor hemisphere. *Cortex*, **7**, 49.

Levy, J. & Sperry, R.W. (1968) Differential perceptual capacities in major and minor hemispheres. *Proceedings of the National Academy of Sciences* (Washington), **61**, 1151.

Liberman, A.M. (1974) The specialization of the language hemisphere. In *Third Study Program* (Ed.) Schmitt, F.O. & Worden, F.G. p. 43. Cambridge, MA: MIT Press.

Lishman, W.A. & McMeekan, E.R.L. (1977) Handedness in relation to direction and degree of cerebral dominance for language. *Cortex*, **13**, 30.

Long, E. (1913) Aphasie par lésion de l'hémisphère gauche chez un gaucher. *Revue neurologique*, **21**, 339.

Long, E. (1913) Un cas d'aphasie par lésion de l'hémisphère gauche chez un gaucher (aphasie croisée et aphasie dissociée). *Encéphale*, **6**, 520.

Marcie, P., Hécaen, H., Dubois, J. & Angelergues, R. (1965) Les troubles de la réalisation de la parole au cours des lésions de l'hémisphère droit. *Neuropsychologia*, **3**, 217.

Morinesco, V., Grigoresco, D. & Axente S. (1938) Considérations sur l'aphasie croisée. *Encéphale*, **33**, 27.

Marshall, J.C. (1973) Some problems and paradoxes associated with recent accounts of hemispheric specialization. *Neuropsychologia*, **11**, 463.

Marshall, J.C., Caplan, D. & Holmes, J.M. (1975) The measure of laterality. *Neuropsychologia*, **13**, 315.

Matsumiya, Y., Tagliasco, V., Lombroso, C.T. & Goodglass, H. (1972) Auditory evoked response: meaningfulness of stimuli and interhemispheric asymmetry. *Science*, **175**, 790.

McFie, J. (1961) The effects of hemispherectomy on intellectual functioning in cases of infantile hemiplegia. *Journal of Neurology, Neurosurgery and Psychiatry*, **24**, 240.

McGlone, J. & Davidson, W. (1973) The relation between cerebral speech laterality and spatial ability with special reference to sex and hand preference. *Neuropsychologia*, **11**, 105.

McKeever, W.F. & Huling, M.D. (1971) Lateral dominance in tachistoscopic word recognition performances obtained with simultaneous bilateral input. *Neuropsychologia*, **9**, 15.

McKeever, W.F. & Huling, M.D. (1971) Bilateral tachistoscopic word recognition as a function of hemisphere stimulated and interhemispheric transfer time. *Neuropsychologia*, **9**, 281.

McRae, D.L., Branch, C.L. & Milner, B. (1968) The occipital horns and cerebral dominance. *Neurology*, **18**, 95.

Milner, B. (1962) Laterality effects in audition. In *Interhemispheric Relations and Cerebral Dominance* (Ed.) Mountcastle, V.B. p. 117. Baltimore, MD: Johns Hopkins.

Milner, B. (1971) Interhemispheric differences and psychological processes. *British Medical Bulletin*, **27**, 272.

Milner, B. (1973) Hemispheric specialization: scope and limits. In *The Neurosciences: Third Study Program* (Ed.) Schmitt, F.O. & Worden, F.G. p. 75. Boston, MA: MIT Press.

Molfese, D.L., Freeman, R.B. Jr & Palermo, D. (1975) The ontogeny of brain lateralization for speech and nonspeech stimuli. *Brain and Language*, **2**, 356.

Morrell, L.K. & Salamy, J.G. (1971) Hemispheric asymmetry of electrocortical responses to speech stimuli. *Science*, **174**, 164.

Moscovitch, M. (1972) A choice reaction time study assessing the verbal behavior of the minor hemisphere in normal, adult humans. *Journal of Comparative and Physiological Psychology*, **80**, 66.

Moscovitch, M. (1976) On the representation of language in the right hemisphere of right-handed people. *Brain and Language*, **3**, 47.

Mountcastle, V.B. (Ed.) (1962) *Interhemispheric Relations and Cerebral Dominance*. Baltimore, MD: Johns Hopkins.

Nagafuchi, M. (1970) Development of dichotic and monaural hearing abilities in young children. *Acta Otolaryngologica* (Stockholm), 69, 409.

Needles, W. (1942) Concerning transfer of cerebral dominance in function of speech. *Journal of Nervous and Mental Diseases*, **95**, 270.

Netley, C. (1972) Dichotic listening performance of hemispherectomized patients. *Neuropsychologia*, **10**, 233.

Newcombe, F. & Ratcliff, G. (1973) Handedness, speech lateralization and ability. *Neuropsychologia*, **11**, 399.

Nielsen, J.M. (1937) Unilateral cerebral dominance as related to mind blindness: minimal lesion capable of causing visual agnosia for objects. *Archives of Neurology and Psychiatry* (Chicago), **38**, 108.

Nottebohm, F. (1971) Neural lateralization of vocal control in a passerine bird. 1. Song. *Journal of Experimental Zoology*, **177**, 229.

Nottebohm, F. (1972) Neural lateralization of vocal control in a passerine bird. 2. Subsong, calls, and a theory of vocal learning. *Journal of Experimental Zoology*, **179**, 35.

Oldfield, R.C. (1971) The assessment and analysis of handedness: the Edinburgh inventory. *Neuropsychologia*, **9**, 97.

Orbach, J. (1967) Differential recognition of Hebrew and English words in right and left visual fields as a function of cerebral dominance and reading habits. *Neuropsychologia*, **5**, 127.

Oscar-Berman, M., Zurif, E.B. & Blumstein, S. (1975) Effects of unilateral brain damage on the processing of speech sounds. *Brain and Language*, **2**, 345.

Oxbury, J.M. & Oxbury, S.M. (1969) Effects of temporal lobectomy on the report of dichotically presented digits. *Cortex*, **5**, 3.

Piazza, D.M. (1977) Cerebral lateralization in young children as measured by dichotic listening and finger tapping tasks. *Neuropsychologia*, **15**, 417.

Piercy, M.F. & Smyth, V.O.G. (1962) Right hemisphere dominance for certain non-verbal intellectual skills. *Brain*, **85**, 775.

Pizzamiglio, L. & Cecchini, M. (1971) Development of the hemispheric dominances in children of 5 to 10 years of age and their relations with the development of cognitive processes. *Brain Research*, **31**, 363.

Ponzio, J. (1974) *L'écoute dichotique; étude théorique et application clinique*. Medical thesis, Marseilles.

Pratt, R., Warrington, E. & Halliday, A. (1971) Unilateral ECT as a test for cerebral dominance, *British Journal of Psychiatry*, **119**, 79.

Provins, K.A. & Cunlife, P. (1972) The reliability of some motor performance tests on handedness. *Neuropsychologia*, **10**, 199.

Renzi, E. (de) (1967) Nonverbal memory and hemispheric side of lesion. *Neuropsychologia*, **6**, 181.

Rife, D.C. (1940) Handedness with special reference to twins. *Genetics*, **25**, 178.

Roberts, L. (1955) Handedness and cerebral dominance. *Transactions of the American Neurological Association*, **80**, 143.

Roberts, L. (1966) Aphasia, apraxia and agnosia in abnormal states of cerebral dominance. In *Handbook of Clinical Neurology*. (Ed.) Vinken, P.J. & Bruyn, G.W. Vol. 4, p. 312. Amsterdam: North-Holland.

Robins, K.I. & Mac Adam, D.W. (1974) Interhemispheric alpha asymmetry and imagery mode. *Brain and Language*, **1**, 189.

Rosen, J., Curcio, F., Mackavey, W. & Herbert, J. (1975) Superior recall of letters in the right visual field with bilateral presentation and partial report. *Cortex*, **11**, 170.

Rossi, G.F. & Rosadini, G. (1967) Experimental analysis of cerebral dominance in man. In *Brain Mechanisms Underlying Speech and Language* (Ed.) Millikan, C.H. & Darley, F.L. p. 167. New York: Grune and Stratton.

Rubens, A.B., Mahowald, M.W. & Hutton, J.T. (1976) Asymmetry of the lateral (sylvian) fissures in man. *Neurology*, **26**, 620.

Rudel, R.G., & Denckla, M.B. (1974) Relations of forward and backward digit repetition to neurological impairment in children with learning disabilities. *Neuropsychologia*, **12**, 109.

Rudel, R.G., Denckla, M.B. & Hirsh, S. (1977) The development of left-hand superiority for discriminating Braille configurations. *Neurology*, **27**, 160.

Russell, J. (1874) Note on a case of left hemiplegia with loss of speech occurring in a left-handed patient. *Medical Times Gazette*, **2**, 36.

Satz, P. (1972) Pathological left-handedness: an explanatory model. *Cortex*, **8**, 121.

Satz, P. (1973) Left-handedness and early brain insult: an explanation. *Neuropsychologia*, **11**, 115.

Satz, P., Achenbach, I. & Fennell, E. (1967) Relations between assessed manual laterality and predicted speech laterality. *Neuropsychologia*, **5**, 295.

Saul, R.E. & Gott, P.S. (1973) Compensatory mechanisms in agenesis of the corpus callosum. *Neurology*, **23**, 443.

Saul, R.E. & Sperry, R.W. (1968) Absence of commissurotomy symptoms with agenesis of the corpus callosum. *Neurology*, **18**, 307.

Schulhoff, C & Goodglass, H. (1969) Dichotic listening, side of brain injury and cerebral dominance. *Neuropsychologia*, **7**, 149.

Seamon, J.C. & Gazzaniga, M.S. (1973) Coding strategies and cerebral laterality effects. *Cognitive Psychology*, **5**, 249.

Segalowitz, S. & Gruber, F.A. (Ed.) (1977) *Language Development and Neurological Theory*. New York: Academic Press.

Semmes J. (1968) Hemispheric specialization: a possible clue to mechanism. *Neurpsychologia*, **6**, 11.

Serafetinides, E.A., Hoare, R.D. & Driver, M.V. (1964) A modification of intracarotid amylobarbitone test: findings about speech and consciousness. *Lancet*, 249.

Serafetinides, E.A., Hoare, R.D. & Driver, M.V. (1965) Intracarotid sodium amylobarbitone and cerebral dominance for speech and consciousness. *Brain*, **88**, 107.

Shankweiler, D.P. (1967) Effects of temporal-lobe damage on perception of dichotically presented melodies. *Journal of Comparative and Physiological Psychology*, **62**, 115.

Shankweiler, D.P. & Studdert-Kennedy, M. (1975) A continuum of lateralization for speech perception? *Brain and Language*, **2**, 216.

Smith, A. (1971) Speech and other functions after left (dominant) hemispherectomy. *Journal of Neurology, Neurosurgery and Psychiatry*, **29**, 467.

Smith, A. (1972) Dominant and non-dominant hemispherectomy. In *Drugs, Development and Cerebral Function* (Ed.) Smith, W.L. p. 37. Springfield, IL: Thomas.

Smith, A. (1975) Development of above normal language and intelligence 21 years after left hemispherectomy. *Neurology*, **25**, 813.

Smith, A. & Burklund, C.W. (1966) Dominant hemispherectomy: preliminary report on neuropsychological sequelae. *Science*, **153**, 1280.

Souques, A. (1910) Aphasie avec hémiplégie gauche chez un droitier. *Revue neurologique*, **20**, 547.

Sousa-Poza, J.F., Rohrberg, R. & Shulman, E. (1973) Field dependence and self-disclosure. *Perceptual and Motor Skills*, **36**, 735.

Sparks, R. & Geschwind, N. (1968) Dichotic listening in man after section of neocortical commissures. *Cortex*, **4**, 3.

Springer, S.P. & Eisenson, J. (1977) Hemispheric specialization for speech in language-disordered children. *Neuropsychologia*, **15**, 287.

Studdert-Kennedy, M., Shankweiler, D. & Pisoni, D. (1972) Auditory and phonetic processes in speech perception evidence from a dichotic study. *Cognitive Psychology*, **3**, 455.

Sussman, H.M. & MacNeilage, P.F. (1975) Studies on hemispheric specialization for speech production. *Brain and Language*, **2**, 131.

Treisman, A. & Geffen, G. (1968) Selective attention and cerebral dominance in perceiving and responding to speech messages. *Quarterly Journal of Experimental Psychology*, **20**, 139.

Tsunoda, T. & Oka, M. (1971) Cerebral hemisphere dominance test and localization of speech. *Journal of Auditory Research*, **11**, 177.

Wechsler, A.F. (1976) Crossed aphasia in an illiterate dextral. *Brain and Language*, **3**, 164.

Weinstein, E.A. (1964) Affections of speech with lesions of the non-dominant hemisphere. *Research Publications, Association for Research in Nervous and Mental Diseases*, **42**, 220.

Weinstein, S. (1962) Differences in effects of brain wounds implicating right and left hemispheres: differential effects on certain intellectual and complex perceptual functions. In *Interhemispheric Relations and Cerebral Dominance* (Ed.) Mountcastle, V.B. p. 159. Baltimore, MD: Johns Hopkins Press.

Wertz, R.T., Messert, B., Collins, M., Rosenbeck, J.C. & Kao, C.C. (1977) Right-hemisphere language dominance in a case of left-hemisphere arteriovenous malformation. *Journal of Speech Disorders*, **42**, 106.

White, M.J. (1969) Laterality differences in perception: a review. *Psychological Bulletin*, **72**, 387.

Wilson, P.J.E. (1970) Cerebral hemispherectomy for infantile hemiplegia. A report of 50 cases. *Brain*, **93**, 147.

Witelson, S.F. (1974) Hemisphere specialization for linguistic and non-linguistic tactual perception using a dichotomous stimulation technique. *Cortex*, **10**, 3.

Zaidel, E. (1976) Auditory vocabulary of the right hemisphere following brain bisection of hemidecortication. *Cortex*, **12**, 191.

Zangwill, O.L. (1960) *Cerebral Dominance in Relation to Psychological Function*. Edinburgh: Oliver and Boyd.

Zangwill, O.L. (1964) The current status of cerebral dominance. *Research Publications, Association for Research in Nervous and Mental Diseases*, **42**, 103.

Zangwill, O.L. (1967) Speech and the minor hemisphere. *Acta Neurological Belgica*, **67**, 1013.

Zangwill, O.L. (1975) The ontogeny of cerebral dominance in man. In *Foundations of Language Development; a Multidisciplinary Approach* (Ed.) Lenneberg, E.H. & Lenneberg, E. Vol, I, p. 137. New York: Academic Press.

Zollinger, R. (1935) Removal of the left cerebral hemisphere: report of a case. *Archives of Neurology and Psychiatry* (Chicago), **34**, 1055.

Zurif, E.B. (1974) Auditory lateralization: prosodic and syntactic factors. *Brain and Language*, **1**, 391.

Zurif, E.B. & Bryden, M.P. (1969) Familial handedness and left-right differences in auditory and visual perception. *Neuropsychologia*, **7**, 179.

Zurif, E.B. & Mendelsohn, M. (1972) Hemispheric specialization for the perception of speech sounds: the influence of intonation and structure. *Perception and Psychophysics*, **11**, 329.

12. The Interaction between Linguistics and Aphasiology

> '[Are you reading ...] I read: no ... [the newspaper?] The newspaper: uh, that depends. The ... the words come back. But uh a ... It's ... it's ... it's ... it's funny. The words uh ... An easy text: I read. Difficult: I read also; uh the ... the medicine, particularly. It's funny, eh? And it has come back eh? A little, but ... but ... It's funny. But idiotic sentences, I can't. [What do you mean by "idiotic sentences"?] It's some little words. Uh some ... some "what", the "fors" some ... Uh ... And then, uh that makes me grumble, old chap! And then!'
>
> (*Conversation with Mr No.; October 1967*)

For most of its followers, modern linguistics has become a discipline which attempts to formulate and verify hypotheses about the structure and development of human language. This endeavour can be undertaken from one of two essentially different perspectives. Language can be considered in an ideal form (*la langue* of the Saussureians or the *competence* of the Chomskyans), that is, in an abstract form without regard to the many social, cultural, biological and other factors which influence the ways in which speakers actually use language; in taking this perspective, many investigators, from those in Port-Royal to those at the Massachusetts Institute of Technology, carried out work of major significance. Other than leading to the conclusion that aphasia is not a disorder of competence, this perspective is not, however, well suited to aphasiology since the main objective of this discipline is precisely the study of the influence of biopsychopathological factors on the language of a particular class of speakers (i.e., those with cerebral lesions). Language can also be considered in its actualized forms (*la parole* of the Saussureians or the *performance* of the Chomskyans), that is, in terms of empirical observations of the behaviours of individual speakers or groups of speakers: this is the perspective taken in psycholinguistic or neurolinguistic studies carried out on more or less well-defined groups (children in the language acquisition period, normal adult speakers, aphasic individuals, etc.).

The present chapter will therefore be mainly concerned with aphasic performance, usually studied with reference to a presumed or established norm. Whether applied by linguists or others, the methods of contemporary linguistics have contributed to a clearer definition of different aspects of aphasic language. Although the accumulated knowledge still remains very incomplete, it merits consideration because the interaction between linguistics and aphasiology during the past decades has proved to be mutually rewarding in several respects:

(a) The terminology of aphasiology has been refined and extended, thus permitting greater precision in the description of abnormal linguistic behaviours and in theoretical statements.
(b) Different linguistic theories provided the foundations for new categorizations—that is, for new classifications—of aphasic phenomena.
(c) The development of new techniques in linguistics, psychology and computer science permitted the study of the biology of language to be extended beyond the domain of aphasic pathology (we now speak of neurolinguistics: the study of the mutual relationships between the brain and language).
(d) Research on the linguistic behaviour of aphasics provided linguists with means of eventually confirming or refuting their

numerous hypotheses on the nature of normal language.

Certain aspects of the interaction between linguistics and aphasiology have already been discussed in previous sections of this text:

(a) With respect to historical background, we mentioned how, after precursory work, such as that of Lordat[1, 2] and Freud[3, 4] neurolinguistics was born when Alajouanine, a neurologist, Ombredane, a psychologist, and Durand, a linguist[5] described the phonetic disintegration syndrome (cf. p. 23; Chapters 1 and 3).

(b) The matter of linguistic vocabulary in aphasiology was subject of a detailed discussion (see Chapter 2). The works of Martinet[6] and Buyssens[7] had the greatest influence on our own choice of terminology[8, 9]: among the sources available, they appeared to provide the potentially most adequate means of organizing the undifferentiated mass of aphasic language by subdividing it in a systematic and hierarchical manner. Once selected and adapted as far as possible to our particular needs, this vocabulary was used as a descriptive tool in our discussion of linguistic behaviours in the different clinical forms of aphasia (see Chapters 3 to 7).

(c) Although the postulate that language is a multiphased activity was not based on an exhaustive classification of the aphasias, we have shown that it is relevant to aphasic disorganizations of language[10] (see Chapters 2 and 10) (phonetic disintegration and the third linguistic phase; conduction aphasia and the second linguistic phase; agrammatism, or certain jargons, and the first linguistic phase).

(d) The different linguistic classifications of aphasia were reviewed and the ways in which they correspond to our own were indicated (see Chapter 10). Head's classification[11] appears of little use from a neurolinguistic point of view because linguistics enters only into the headings, most of which are debatable (e.g., verbal aphasia because it involves a defective capacity to form words: could the same not be said of most of the clinical forms of aphasia?). Jakobson's classifications[12, 13], so fertile in terms of research hypotheses, are admirable for their theoretical coherence even if they cannot always be readily fitted to empirically observed facts. Finally, we discussed Hécaen's classification[14], which attempts to relate the linguistic and biological characteristics of the aphasias.

(e) The use of neurolinguistic techniques with normal speakers was discussed in regard to the phenomenon of cerebral dominance for language (see Chapter 11).

In order to complete this outline of the interaction between linguistics and aphasiology, the remainder of the present chapter will be devoted to a review of certain research findings which could be readily integrated into an introductory textbook on aphasia. We shall first discuss investigations of aphasic disorganizations of the phonetic and phonemic levels (disturbances of the third and second linguistic phases) and then studies of the syntactical, lexical, and semantic aspects of aphasia (disturbances of the first linguistic phase). We are aware that this division is somewhat artificial in certain regards. However it does permit emphasis of the possible relationships between properly linguistic concepts and the facts of cerebral pathology: it also ensures a certain coherence in the organization of the material to be discussed.

THIRD AND SECOND LINGUISTIC PHASES: PHONETIC AND PHONEMIC ASPECTS

In aphasiology, techniques and methods developed in linguistics were first applied to the study of disturbances of the simplest linguistic units, namely features and phonemes. Numerous studies have been carried out in this area over the past 30 years as indicated by the following examples.

In 1939, Alajouanine, Ombredane and Durand[5] published a phonetic description of the articulatory disturbances of Broca's aphasics which they named the 'phonetic disintegration syndrome' (see Chapters 3 and 4). In the most typical cases, the syndrome begins with a paretic phase manifested by weakness in the movements of the buccophonatory apparatus (lowering of high vowels, production of pseudo-diphthongs and pseudo-polyphthongs, nasalization of orals, inadequate occlusion and affrication of stops, voicing transformations, British pseudo-accent*). This phase is gradually followed by post-paralytic reorganization, that is, by a dystonic phase characterized by articulatory movements which are exaggerated in force and duration (raising of low vowels, pre-vocalic glottalization, production of pseudo-diphthongs and pseudo-polyphthongs, oralization of nasals, occlusion and affrication of fricatives, devoicing of voiced sounds, German pseudo-accent*). In addition to these phonetic transformations described in reference to phonemes considered individually, there are other anomalies related to the sequential structure of the phonemic chain (difficulty in the production of consonant clusters and production of initial vowels and final consonants, etc.); certain transformations are also observed, with varying frequency among different cases, which cannot be distinguished, on the basis of purely linguistic criteria, from the phonemic paraphasias observed in other forms of aphasia (see Chapters 3 and 4). It seems to be mainly transformations of this type which correspond to what Alajouanine et al referred to as the 'dyspraxic element of phonetic disintegration'.

Ten years later, Alajouanine and Durand, this time with Pichot's collaboration[15], reported a case study of pure anarthria† which completed their description of the dystonic phase of phonetic disintegration. In this phase, the rate of phonemic production is slowed, generally to less than half the normal rate; there is frequent partial or complete devoicing of voiced consonants [laryngeal vibration may be absent, intermittent or too brief (12.1) /ɔ̃noz/→ ≃/ɔ̃nozs/]; there is often partial or complete oralization of nasals [nasal resonance may be absent, intermittent or too brief; in the case of nasalized (French) vowels, this may result in the production of diphthongs or pseudo-polyphthongs (12.2) /lalɑ̃p/ → ≃/lalɑɑ̃p/]; the articulation of stop consonants is abnormally explosive; fricatives are frequently transformed through complete occlusion [(12.3) /mysik/→ ≃/mydik/] as well as by initial occlusion which results in the production of an affricate; laterals are often transformed into approximately corresponding stops [(12.4) /baʀtʀolɔ̃g/ → ≃/baʀtʀodɔ̃g/] and the articulation of /ʀ/ is usually exaggerated. Because of an instability in aperture and/or place of articulation, which is usually accompanied by some irregularity and lack of suppleness in palatal and laryngeal movements, vowels are often transformed into pseudo-diphthongs or pseudo-polyphthongs; pre-vocalic glottalization frequently occurs at the beginning of segments normally initiated with a vowel; epentheses, addition of a neutral vowel after a final consonant [(12.5) /œ̃naʀbʀ/ → ≃/œ̃naʀpœʀœ/] and other kindred phenomena are frequent; the occurrence of certain transformations which fit the definition of phonemic paraphasias is not uncommon.

In 1966, Marcie and his collaborators[16] carried out a spectrographic study of repetition by two patients who had undergone excision of a meningioma centred on the pars opercularis of the left, third frontal convolution. Both cases presented dysprosody with slowed speech and syllabification. Transformations were extremely rare in the first case [(12.6) /maʃinasjɔ̃/→ ≃/maʃinaʃjɔ̃/]. They were much more frequent in the second case and usually occurred in the form of phonetic approximations: typically, the initial phoneme was replaced by another which was similar in structure and the substitution was then corrected immediately. Marcie et al spoke of 'correction during programming: [the subject] succeeds in immediately changing the disposition of his articulatory organs in order to articulate the phoneme sought'. After having emphasized that all the phonemes in the language could be produced perfectly by both patients, even if this was not always done in the second case, Marcie et al suggested that both the phonetic transformations (the disturbance in the realization of the phonematic code) and the dysprosody (the disturbance in the realization of suprasegmental features) were evidence of a disorder in phonematic programming. The dysprosody, in the form of slowed syllabic speech, corresponds to an overcorrection 'of the difficulties of phonematic realization on the basis of auditory and/or kinaesthetic feedback'. As indi-

* In speakers of French or of other Latin languages. As far as we know, there are few published reports of a pseudo-accent in English-speaking aphasics. Should an identifiable accent be presented by an English-speaking patient, we would expect it to be that of the southern United States during the paretic phase and, depending on the severity, either French or German in the dystonic phase.

† An anatomoclinical discussion of this case has been previously presented in this text (cf. pp. 196–197).

cated by the name which he gave to Broca's aphasia [aphasia of phonematic realization (see Chapter 10)], Hécaen[14] believes that the characteristic transformations of phonetic disintegration (see Chapters 3 and 4) have their origin in a similar type of dysfunction.

Examining production during a repetition task, the linguist Fry (1959)[17] attempted to identify the relative difficulty of English phonemes in articulation disturbances associated with aphasia. The list of stimuli (single words) included all the phonemes of English presented in all positions in which they could appear. Like others, Fry noted the instability of the (voice) feature of consonants in phonetic disintegration and described the effects of this instability on phonemes in the immediate context; in contrast to the results obtained by other investigators, Fry did not observe a clear trend towards the replacement of voiced consonants by their unvoiced cognates. Neither did he observe a systematic relationship between his samples of pathological speech and speech produced by young children: he therefore challenged the validity of the hypothesis, put forward by Alajouanine et al[5] and Jakobson[18, 19], that the hierarchy of 'disintegration' observed in aphasia reflects, in inverse order, the hierarchical order of phoneme acquisition in children.

Shankweiler and Harris (1966)[20] also used a repetition task (200 monosyllabic English words) to examine the phonetic transformations of aphasics. Their patients, Broca's aphasics from a lesion of vascular origin, were examined after a rather long period of evolution and at a time when phonetic disintegration (see Chapters 3 and 4) was the only significant residual disturbance. Conclusions from this study were as follows: (a) the initial phonemes of the stimuli are the most frequently affected; (b) consonants are less stable than vowels; (c) consonant transformations most often affect fricatives and affricates (dystonic phase of phonetic disintegration); (d) certain consonant clusters are the source of particular difficulty. Shankweiler and Harris also noted that the 'phonetic simplifications' typically observed in the speech of young children were less frequent in phonetic disintegration than were other deviant forms which do not occur in children's speech; here again, the data contradicted the hypothesis of a parallel between phoneme acquisition and disintegration.

Alajouanine et al (1964)[21, 22] dissociated the phonemic and semantic components of jargonaphasia. They recognized that, in most cases, the jargon (of Wernicke's aphasics) includes both phonemic paraphasias and verbal transformations. They nevertheless emphasized that the transformations may be almost exclusively phonemic in certain cases and almost exclusively verbal in other cases. For these authors, the production of phonemic paraphasias reflects a 'disturbance of the patterns of auditory origin which subtend verbal expression'. They based their interpretation on the following arguments: in patients with phonemic paraphasias, oral reading was intact or, in any case, much better than repetition; unlike normal subjects, speech production in these patients was unaffected by delayed auditory feedback (DAF); spoken language comprehension was normal in these cases; finally, and especially, these patients were severely impaired on tests of non-linguistic audiophonatory transposition but not on analogous tests of visuophonatory transposition. In regard to the patients with semantic jargon, Alajouanine et al maintained that 'the same regression of semantic values' explains both the production of semantic paraphasias and the disturbance of oral language comprehension. The neurolinguistic findings observed in this study were integrated into the descriptions which were previously given of conduction aphasia (predominance of phonemic transformations), Type I Wernicke's aphasia (phonemic and verbal transformations) and Type II Wernicke's aphasia (predominance of verbal transformations) (see Chapter 4).

Hécaen et al (1964)[23] studied repetition in two cases of Wernicke's aphasia. Both patients produced phonemic paraphasias but they differed qualitatively: in the first case, the most characteristic transformations were substitutions between phonemes which differed in place of articulation [/t/↔/k/, /g/↔/d/]; in the second case, 'the disturbance of repetition is manifested especially on consonantal groups including a liquid [and] on the least frequent groups, that is, on the most difficult to pronounce'. On the basis of an exhaustive analysis of the residual linguistic abilities of their two patients, these authors claimed that the phonemic deviations reflected 'a disturbance of auditivo-verbal reception' in the first patient and a motor disorder (expressive, or 'emission', disorder) in the second. They suggested that the qualitative difference between the linguistic deviations of these two patients might be related to different sites of lesion within Wernicke's territory.*

de Renzi et al (1966)[24] compared the phonemic deviations of Broca's aphasics with those of Wernicke's aphasics and found them to be qualitatively similar. They thus maintained that the different clinical forms of aphasia could not be distinguished on the basis of linguistic criteria concerning the structure of phonemic transformations. This conclusion is consistent with our own[25, 26] and that of Poncet et al[27] and can be viewed as an instance of Marie's law (see Chapter 1): the production of Broca's aphasics includes phonetic and phonemic deviations whereas that of certain Wernicke's aphasics includes phonemic, but not phonetic, deviations.

In 1970, Johns and Darley[28] completed a study of speech in Broca's aphasia [which they named *apraxia of speech*]. Four of their findings distinguish phonetic disintegration from dysarthrias resulting from brain stem lesions (see Chapter 3): in the former case, the clinical picture included phonemic transformations as well as phonetic transformations; the disturbance was variable (discourse included both normal and abnormal segments with production of the same segment being more or less adequate at different times); spontaneous speech was less impaired than oral reading which, in turn, was less impaired than repetition; successive attempts usually resulted in improved production of the utterance. They confirmed, using English stimuli, that fricatives, affricates and consonant clusters are particularly difficult and that difficulty of production increases with word length.

In a series of articles published over the past years we have reported, in collaboration with Deloche[9, 10, 25-27, 29-32], on our studies of the linguistic structure of phonemic deviations in aphasia. We showed that phonemic paraphasias can be described in terms of elementary operations (phoneme omission, addition or displacement) or in terms of simple or multiple combinations of these elementary operations [see examples (2.73) to (2.77)]; we also discussed the structural relationships between phonemic paraphasias and literal paragraphias[33, 34] [see examples (2.54) to (2.59)]. Our descriptions of interphonemic substitutions included a study of replaced and replacing phonemes in terms of their constituent features (Fig. 12-1) (see Chapter 2). We found that the substitutions of conduction aphasics showed a relative predominance of [voiced]→[voiceless] and [fricative]→[stop] transformations; in contrast, we did not observe any particular trends in deviations involving place of articulation. After a series of computerized simulations[30], we suggested that phonemic paraphasias and formal verbal paraphasias resulted from a dysfunction of the same mechanism (see Insertion 8.4). Finally, we emphasized the fact that the phonemic deviations do not contravene the phonological rules of the speaker's language (or of a language which he has mastered).

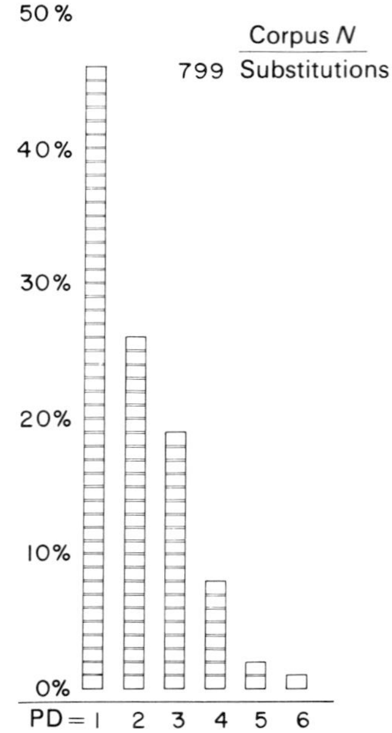

Fig. 12-1 *Analysis of 799 interphonemic substitutions produced during repetition and oral reading (of isolated, three- and four-syllable words) by eight subjects with conduction aphasia. PD (paradigmatic distance) = the number of features which were not shared by the replaced and replacing phonemes. In nearly 50 per cent of the cases, they differed by only a single feature. From Lecours, Deloche and Lhermitte[30].*

In 1973, Blumstein[35-37] published a book[37] devoted entirely to the phonological deviations of aphasics and based on the study of language samples obtained during interviews with Broca's aphasics, conduction aphasics, and Type I Wernicke's aphasics (see Chapter 4). After suggesting a classification of her patient's phonemic deviations, Blumstein reported several interesting lin-

* Other neurolinguistic studies by Hécaen have been discussed elsewhere in this text (see Chapter 10).

guistic findings: the relative frequency of the different phonemes was approximately the same in the three aphasic groups as in normal speakers; interphonemic substitutions were more frequent than any other type of deviation, transformations of the type [marked phoneme]→[unmarked phoneme] were more frequent than those in the opposite direction (a finding which Blumstein considered to be of major theoretical importance[38]); substitutions in which the replaced and replacing phonemes differed by a single feature were more frequent than substitutions in which the replaced and replacing phonemes differed by several features; substitutions affected isolated consonants more often than consonants within clusters; on the other hand, consonant omissions were more frequent within clusters; consonant additions, particularly in Broca's aphasia, sometimes resulted in the creation of consonant clusters, that is, in a deviant production of greater structural complexity than the target segment [which provides a convincing contradiction of a classical notion (see Chapter 3)]; retrograde assimilation was more frequent than anterograde assimilation. On the whole, Blumstein's data did not demonstrate clear linguistic differences in the phonemic deviations of her three groups of patients. On the other hand, her study allowed her to rank the constituent features of English phonemes in order of difficulty and to suggest certain modifications in the phonological systems of the Chomsky school.

Having observed that Broca's aphasics produced more phonemic deviations per syllable as word length increased on a repetition task (one deviation per seven syllables for monosyllable words; one deviation per 4.5 syllables for two-syllable words; one deviation per four syllables for three-syllable words), Lebrun (1967)[39] concluded that phonemes are not 'programmed as successive units': were this the case, 'the polysyllables would not have been proportionately more affected'. According to Lebrun, this finding, as well as others, provides support for his hypothesis that the phoneme 'is not a unit of use but [rather] a unit of description'.

Wondering whether aphasia impaired the perception of stress as a semantic indicator, Blumstein and Goodglass (1972)[40] examined this question using an identification task (which, for example, required discrimination between 'redcoat', with stress on the first syllable, and 'red coat', with stress on both syllables). They concluded that comprehension based solely on stress is difficult for normal subjects and even more difficult for aphasics, but that it was not specifically affected by aphasia (regardless of the clinical type).

FIRST LINGUISTIC PHASE: MORPHOSYNTACTICAL, LEXICAL AND SEMANTIC ASPECTS

Having discussed aphasic disturbances of the third and second linguistic phases, we shall now consider certain findings related to the first linguistic phase (see Chapter 2). Here again, we shall not attempt an exhaustive review of all available publications, an endeavour which would far exceed the aims of this text. We shall simply try to illustrate contemporary relationships between syntactic and semantic research and aphasiology by presenting an almost random selection of examples from an extensive body of literature. Since the Boston school has been particularly productive in this area, we shall consider several examples of their work.

Since 1963, Sabouraud and his collaborators have carried out neurolinguistic studies of aphasia[41-43] from a theoretical perspective which is both Saussureian and Jakobsonian. Thus they were based on a distinction between the 'semiotic level' and the 'phonological level', as well as on a distinction between the axes of 'similarity' and 'contiguity' (see Chapter 10). Different manifestations of Broca's aphasias and Wernicke's aphasias (see Chapter 4) were analysed in terms of these two dichotomies. On the 'semiological level', the expressive and receptive disturbances of Wernicke's aphasics were found to have 'in common a difficulty or inability to assign to words their place in the lexicon, to define them and to fix their limits through mutual opposition, to choose them in placing them in a structured whole; those of Broca's aphasics have in common a permanent and maximally extensive recourse to preserved lexical precision when the use of textual relations is abolished or very reduced'. On the 'phonological level', interphonemic oppositions (and thus phonemic choices) are uncertain in Wernicke's aphasia whereas, in Broca's aphasia, 'the inclusion in the same [phonemic] chain of all of the contrasts is impossible, reduced, incomplete'. When considering the most severe forms of aphasia, Sabouraud added 'that the complete suppression of activity along one of the two axes [may] render the other unusable', a statement which, in our opinion, should not be given too much emphasis.

Beginning in 1956, Wepman, Jones and their collaborators[44-48] adopted a taxonomic point of view in comparing normal discourse with several forms of aphasic discourse. They were particularly interested in the frequency of word usage within various grammatical categories and their investigations led them to identify three clinical varieties of aphasia. One form, called *semantic aphasia** is characterized by a particular reduction in the availability of semantically very precise low-frequency lexical words; this clinical picture corresponds to a similarity disorder in Jakobson's terminology. On the other hand, another form, called *syntactic aphasia,** is characterized by a particular reduction in the availability of grammatical words and, consequently, by a limited number of available grammatical structures; this clinical picture corresponds to Jakobson's contiguity disorder (see Chapter 10). The remaining form, or *pragmatic aphasia*, is not characterized by an obvious disturbance of a particular verbal class or axis of language production but rather by the absence of comprehensible messages (there may not be any reduction of the speech flow or of word variety); this clinical picture appears to correspond approximately to that which we described under the name of Type II Wernicke's aphasia (see Chapter 4).

During the 1960s, Howes[49-51] also studied the relative frequency of lexical and grammatical units in normal discourse and in different forms of aphasic discourse. His findings were consistent with those of Wepman and Jones: grammatical units were found to be much less frequent in the productions of Broca's aphasics (agrammatic) than in those of (jargoning) Wernicke's aphasics or those of normal speakers.

In 1964, Goodglass et al[52] characterized the aphasias according to the patient's flow of speech. They measured conversational phrase length (number of words between two pauses) in Broca's aphasia, Wernicke's aphasia and (Pitres') amnesic aphasia. They found that most of the utterances produced by Broca's aphasics included only one or two words (their conversation was mainly composed of short juxtaposed units; coordinating and subordinating conjunctions were very rare); in contrast, in the other two forms of aphasia, a large proportion of the utterances included five words or more. On the basis of these findings, these investigators suggested a basic dichotomy in the aphasic population: on the one hand there were subjects who spoke little (*non-fluent aphasics*) and, on the other hand, subjects whose speech flow was normal or nearly so (*fluent aphasics*).†

Spreen and Wachal (1973)[53, 54] carried out computerized analyses of a large number of descriptive psycholinguistic variables of aphasic discourse. Their analyses included traditional measures (for example, counts of various normal and deviant linguistic segments, different types of pauses, repetitions, etc., and different mathematical analyses of these counts) as well as measures related to contemporary theories of generative grammar (for example, counts of syntagms and sentences according to their level of 'transformational' complexity). Sixty-nine variables were thus studied and then reduced to a non-redundant group of 48. This research is ultimately aimed at the formulation of a quantitative, linguistic definition of different aphasic populations in reference to that of normal speakers. Spreen and Wachal have already taken a first step in this direction: from a total of 38 measures of lexical diversity in spontaneous discourse, they retained a non-redundant group of 20; a combination of eight of these measures permitted adequate separation of normal and aphasic samples.

After having studied morphosyntactical performance on several different metalinguistic tasks in a large number of agrammatics and Wernicke's aphasics, Tissot, Mounin and one of us (F.L.), with Dordain's collaboration[55], reported

---

* Wepman et al used the terms 'semantic aphasia' and 'syntactic aphasia' in a very logical manner and their meaning does not correspond to that which was given to the same terms by Head (see Chapter 10).

† This represents a quantitatively more precise reformulation of a classical dichotomy.

the findings in a monograph too substantial to be summarized here. Hence we shall mention only the conclusions that the agrammatic subject does not utilize grammar, but recognizes correct grammatical forms and is aware of his impairment while the paragrammatic subject utilizes grammar inappropriately, often fails to recognize correct forms and is unaware of his impairment.* The results also suggested a possible dissociation, in agrammatism, between a morphological disturbance and a syntactical disturbance. Tissot's testing procedures were also used in another study by Rouillon (1971)[57], who examined the syntactical performance of four agrammatic and four paragrammatic patients. Her conclusions were consistent with those reported above; she also added that, on structured tasks, agrammatics could produce syntactical forms which they did not use spontaneously while the syntactical performance of the paragrammatics on structured tasks was the same as in spontaneous language.

Wishing to define certain aspects of agrammatism more precisely, Goodglass and his collaborators[58-61] have studied, beginning in 1958, the production and recognition of different English morphological markers by Broca's aphasics. They thus compared, for example, the homophone morphological markers indicating the third person singular in the present tense, plurality, and the singular possessive. Their results led them to recognize various levels of morphological complexity. On the expressive level, certain findings were interpreted in terms of 'transformational' hypotheses: thus the greater difficulty found for the possessive than for the phonologically identical plural could be attributed to the transformation involved in the former (e.g., 'John's hat'='John has a hat'). However this interpretation was not supported, or was even contradicted, by other findings observed at the receptive level. Thus, when subjects were required to judge the morphological appropriateness of stimuli which they heard (and in which the verb, possessive or plural marker was present or omitted), Broca's aphasics were found to report omission of the plural marker three times more often than that of the phonologically identical verb inflection. They then attempted an explanation in terms of frequency (the plural marker has a high frequency of occurrence) or redundancy (the sentences used as stimuli could be readily understood despite the omission of the verb or possessive marker but this was not the case when the plural marker was omitted). Goodglass and Berko-Gleason[60] also presented phonological arguments in interpreting certain of their findings: thus they proposed that it was because of its greater *saliency* that the syllabic plural inflection /əz/ (as in horses) was more easily produced than the plural inflections /z/ (as in dogs) or /s/ (as in cats) [this finding can be related to previous observations of the particular difficulty of consonant clusters and affricates in phonetic disintegration (cf. pp. 60–64)]. Finally, Goodglass and Berko-Gleason pointed out that aphasics' difficulties with the morphological markers included in their study did not correspond closely to those observed in children during language acquisition.

After noting that prosodic *salience* could be related to intonational, phonological, semantic or emotional factors, Goodglass, Fodor and Schulhoff (1967)[62] suggested that the omission of grammatical words, that is, the deviations most characteristic of agrammatic discourse (telegraphic style), was related to their saliency or non-saliency and to their position in the sentence rather than to their functional qualities. This conclusion was supported by the finding that, during sentence repetition, Broca's aphasics showed a particular tendency to omit the initial non-stressed grammatical word.

Beginning in 1972, Goodglass and his collaborators[63] also studied the linguistic capacities of agrammatic Broca's aphasics by use of a Story Completion Test. In this procedure, the subject must produce the sentence required to complete each of a series of brief stories presented by the examiner. Each of the stories included in the test was designed to elicit a particular grammatical form (e.g., 'Dogs always chase cats. A dog is in the street. A cat comes along. What happens?'). Results from this test indicated that the most easily elicited structures were imperatives (transitive and intransitive), WH questions† and the sequence: adjective + noun; the most difficult were the other interrogatives, the future tense,

* Dordain[55] added that the agrammatic is usually younger than the paragrammatic: the average age of the agrammatic patients was 36 years while that of the Wernicke's aphasics was 50 years.

† Questions beginning with what, which, who, etc.

passives and embedded sentences. In general, the sequence verb + NS object was more available than the sequence NS subject + verb. Goodglass et al pointed out that agrammatism was not the result of 'a new grammar' because the utterances did not follow a constant model, and the speakers, dissatisfied with their inadequate productions, attempted to correct them in accordance with the conventional model. They added that agrammatics prefer the most frequent and unmarked lexical and syntactical forms ('boy' rather than 'son'). Finally, they stressed the extreme fragility of the auxiliary 'do' which they attributed to its lack of semantic content. These findings were confirmed by a similar study of eight Broca's aphasics carried out by Berko-Gleason et al in 1975[64]. The particular vulnerability of initial non-stressed grammatical words was again observed; it was also found that in contexts where normal speakers would begin a sentence with a pronoun, Broca's aphasics tended to begin with a salient word (vocative or substantive).

A French version of the Story Completion Test was developed by Lavalée-Huynh (1975)[65] who presented it to three agrammatics, six Broca's aphasics without agrammatism and 18 control subjects. The main findings for the asphasic patients were as follows: all subjects were more successful in producing affirmative sentences* than sentences which had undergone 'transformations' (negative, imperative, interrogative, negative imperative, passive, subordination). In affirmative sentences, the syntactic structure was preserved but certain obligatory elements (marking subject–verb agreement, tense, etc.) were omitted by Broca's aphasics without agrammatism. In contrast, the agrammatics sometimes omitted subjects, verbs or both elements, omissions which affected the entire syntagm (and not only determiners and grammatical words). Among sentences of the second type (those which had undergone 'transformations'), the imperative and negative were very well preserved in Broca's aphasics without agrammatism while the agrammatics were distinguished by extreme difficulty in the production of passives and sentences with a subordinate clause. The study of certain verb forms (present, future, imperfect, past perfect) revealed that all aphasic subjects used mainly the present tense, even as a replacement for other tenses; Broca's aphasics without agrammatism preferred the analytic verb form, as in '*Il va sortir*' (He is going to go out), to the synthetic form, as in '*Il sortira*' (He will go out); the agrammatic patients did not use the imperfect or past perfect forms. In conclusion, the scale of syntactic complexity, as defined by the performance of aphasics, appeared to be a cumulative scale, that is, the aphasics' productions were usually deviant whenever they were required to produce a sentence with more than a certain number of elements (generally two syntagms).

Hunter and Goodglass (1970)[66] compared oral and written spontaneous productions of a Broca's aphasic with those of a Wernicke's aphasic. Their main observations were as follows: in both expressive modalities, grammatical structures were more available to the Wernicke's aphasic than to the Broca's aphasic and the latter produced fewer non-picturable substantives and verbs than the former; although differing quantitatively between the different forms of aphasia, the syntactic deviations were qualitatively similar in the oral and written productions of the same subject; in both expressive modalities, the Wernicke's aphasic produced more semantically based deviations than the Broca's aphasic; and in both forms of aphasia, there was a relatively lower proportion of verbs in written expression than in oral expression.

With Rouillon and Vanier, we ourselves have studied, since 1970, the different types of deviant segments occurring in various forms of normal and pathological discourse[9, 10, 29, 31, 32]. With the exception of phonetic deviations observed in the dysarthrias and in syndromes including phonetic disintegration, the differences observed from a linguistic point of view were not, in general, qualitative. They were instead related to a quantitative predominance of one or of many types of deviant segments as well as to the speaker's awareness or lack of awareness of his deviant productions and the correspondence or lack of correspondence between thought and linguistic production. Most of the facts thus observed in normal discourse [see (14.21)], conduction aphasia [see (2.24) and (4.5)], Wernicke's aphasia proper [see (4.20) and (4.21)], transcortical sensory aphasia (Type II Wernicke's

* NS + VS; NS + VS + NS; NS + VS + PS; NS + VS + NS + PS (see Chapters 2 and 17).

aphasia) [see (4.28)] and schizophasia [see (13.1) to (13.20)] have been summarized elsewhere in this text (see Fig. 14–1). We have also pointed out the occurrence of rare cases of aphasic jargon including many derived monemic paraphasias[67] [see (2.25) to (2.32) and (13.39) to (13.46)] and discussed certain similarities between the oral and written productions of Broca's aphasics and Wernicke's aphasics[32] (the written productions of certain Broca's aphasics consist of genuine jargon) (see Chapter 4).

Kertesz and Benson (1970)[68] studied deviant segments in the jargon of Wernicke's aphasics (with vascular lesions) in relation to the course of evolution (see Chapter 4). During the initial phase, they observed the production of neologisms and phonemic and verbal deviations; this was followed by a phase in which the deviant productions consisted mainly of semantic paraphasias; if the aphasia continued to evolve favourably, manifestations of word-finding difficulty (circumlocutions, aborted sentences, etc.) finally became the predominant characteristic of the patient's discourse (evolution of a Wernicke's aphasia proper towards the clinical picture of Pitres' amnesic aphasia).

Goodglass, Berko-Gleason and Hyde (1970)[69] studied different aspects of oral language comprehension in normal speakers (children and adults) and in different clinical forms of aphasia. They examined, for example, the comprehension of (English) prepositions and found that some Broca's aphasics who were unable to produce them [particularly in non-stressed positions (cf. p. 299)] could nevertheless understand them fairly well; the opposite dissociation was observed in Wernicke's aphasics. Two general conclusions follow from this study: first, comprehension cannot be considered as a unitary phenomenon, that is, comprehension deficits were found in all types of aphasia studied but they differed qualitatively (and quantitatively) among the different types; second, the performance of aphasics (regardless of the clinical form of aphasia) is not assimilable to that of children. These conclusions appear to conflict with that of Parisi and Pizzamiglio[70]. Using a test which required the identification of syntactic structures by pointing to appropriate pictures, these investigators observed (1970) the same order of difficulty in Broca's aphasics, Wernicke's aphasics and a group of children between the ages of three and six years,* a finding which appears to support Jakobson's regression hypothesis. In our opinion, the conflicting results obtained in these two studies might be especially related to the nature of the tests presented.

In 1972, Von Stockert[71] used an experimental task in which subjects formed sentences by arranging segments which had been printed on separate cards. In some cases, the segment printed on each card corresponded to a syntagmatic constituent (see Chapter 2, concepts of syntagms I, II and III), that is, the printed sentence was divided at the boundaries of its constituents ('The girl / from Boston / is pretty'); in other cases the segments printed on the cards did not correspond to a syntagmatic constituent, that is, the printed sentence was divided within the boundaries of its constituents ('The / girl from / Boston is pretty'). Von Stockert presented this task to a Broca's aphasic whose lexical comprehension was not severely disturbed (as indicated by successful word–picture matching) and to a Wernicke's aphasic with severe alexia (as indicated by failure on the matching tasks). He observed that the Wernicke's aphasic was more successful than the Broca's aphasic in ordering the constituents of simple declaratives. He suggested, in conclusion, that syntagmatic constituents are 'real entities in human language'; that there is a level of cerebral activity at which lexical meaning and syntactical structure are treated separately; and that the Broca's aphasic understands the meaning of lexical words but does not fully understand sentence structure.

Dissociations between production and comprehension were also investigated by Zurif et al (1972)[72]. They compared the behaviour of normal and agrammatic speakers during a test requiring judgements of the links between constituent words of (visually presented) stimulus sentences. In considering their data in a 'transformational' perspective, these investigators observed that the normal speakers' judgements on words reflected consideration of surface syntactical properties whereas the agrammatics' judgements were based on a hierarchical scheme excluding facts which were not essential to the

* There were, however, certain quantitative differences among the subject groups, with Wernicke's aphasics obtaining lower scores than Broca's aphasics.

intrinsic meaning of the sentences. For Zurif et al, these results indicate that the expressive behaviour of agrammatism is only one aspect of a disturbance which also affects other language modalities.

Observations reported long ago by Dejerine[73] and Pitres[74] may have inspired Barton's (1971)[75] demonstration that aphasics can sometimes specify certain characteristics (the initial letter, number of syllables) of words giving rise to manifestations of word-finding difficulty (see Chapter 4) during a naming test. Barton studied eight Wernicke's aphasics and eight Broca's aphasics: the former presented less severe word-finding difficulty than the latter and were found to be superior to the Broca's aphasics in specifying the first letter and the number of syllables in words which they were unable to evoke. Although this finding is consistent with the impression which patients with (mild) Wernicke's aphasia often have of 'knowing' the word which they cannot produce, the superiority of the Wernicke's aphasics is surprising in view of the facilitating effect which phonemic cues often have on Broca's aphasics (see Chapter 4). One wonders whether the findings of this study would be replicated in a comparison of Wernicke's aphasics and Broca's aphasics who are more equally impaired in word finding.

Goodglass et al (1966)[76] noted that some of their aphasic patients presented a disturbance of oral comprehension and word-finding difficulty which were especially, or even specifically, related to certain semantic categories. They studied this question in a large group of aphasics and reported several interesting findings: for patients with Wernicke's aphasia and (Pitres') amnesic aphasia, 'objects' were the most difficult stimuli to name but among the easiest to identify (by pointing in response to the spoken name) while 'letters' were among the easiest to name but the most difficult to identify; the identification of 'body parts' was more difficult for Wernicke's aphasics than for Broca's aphasics and amnesic aphasics; word-finding difficulty did not vary with conceptual fields in Broca's aphasics. Related findings for a smaller number of cases were reported by Ali Cherif (1972)[77], who pointed out that the comprehension disturbance may not only be limited to certain categories (names of colours, body parts, parts of a 'whole') but that it may also be limited to spoken language comprehension, that is, it may not be evident when the stimuli to be identified (by a matching response) are presented in writing.

In 1966, Marshall and Newcombe[78] were particularly interested in certain semantic aspects of aphasia. They analysed a large corpus of verbal paralexias produced, during oral reading of single words, by a young aphasic with a left temporoparietal lesion (from gunshot injury). They found that substantives elicited fewer paralexias than adjectives and verbs; that semantic verbal paraphasias [example (12.7) 'liberty'→'freedom'] predominated in the reading of substantives while formal verbal paraphasias [(12.8) 'next'→'exit'] (see Chapter 2) predominated in the case of adjectives and verbs; and that grammatical words were a particular source of reading difficulty (which was more often manifested by a failure to respond than by a paralexic response). In discussing semantic paraphasias, they noted that the substituted word may range from a quasi-synonym [(12.9) 'ill'→'sick'] to a word which shared 'only one or two semantic markers' with the target word, and suggested, in this regard, the possibility of analyses consistent with the theories of Fodor and Katz[79]].

While at the *Hôpital Hôtel-Dieu de Montréal*, Trépagnier obtained evidence that aphasic patients' understanding of grammatical words may be related to their semantic load She presented experimental tasks in which the semantic load was varied (for a particular segment) in terms of the situational context. For example, a red fork and a red knife were placed in front of the patient who was asked to '*Touchez la rouge*' (touch the red), a command which requires comprehension of the feminine article *la* indicating the fork (as opposed to the masculine *le* which would indicate the knife). When presented with a red fork and a black spoon (both are feminine and take the article *la* in French), correct execution of the same command '*Touchez la rouge*' (touch the red) requires comprehension of the colour name. Finally, when presented with a red fork (feminine) and a black knife (masculine), the command '*Touchez la rouge*' may be correctly executed if the patient understands the meaning of the article and/or the meaning of the colour name.

Working in collaboration with Derouesné (1970–1972)[80–82], we tested a group of control subjects and 50 aphasics with different clinical forms of aphasia on a task requiring that words be classified according to the strength of their semantic association with a specified word heading (for example, 'salmon' is semantically closer to the heading 'fish' than is 'kitchen' which, in turn, is closer than 'brick'). Compared with the control subjects, and with due regard given to the sociocultural level of the aphasic patients, the results of this study indicated that the severity of 'errors' could be judged, to a certain degree, by an analysis of the stimuli in terms of semantic features[79]; that the 'comprehension' disturbance, demonstrated through procedures based on the concept of semantic fields (see Chapter 2), was present in all of the clinical forms of aphasia which were studied [this excluded the so-called pure aphasias (see Chapter 10)]; and that three degrees of disorganization could be identified (mainly on a quantitative basis) which reflected, in order of increasing severity 'defective hierarchization', 'narrowing', and 'widening' of the semantic fields* (Fig. 12–2). Other findings were that the observed disturbances were more dependent on the severity of the aphasia than on the clinical form; that conduction aphasics and Broca's aphasics with a predominant articulatory disturbance tended to be among the least impaired patients whereas Wernicke's aphasics and, it should be noted (Pitres') amnesic aphasics, tended to be among the most impaired; and that the semantic disturbance was not directly dependent on a 'deterioration of general intelligence'.

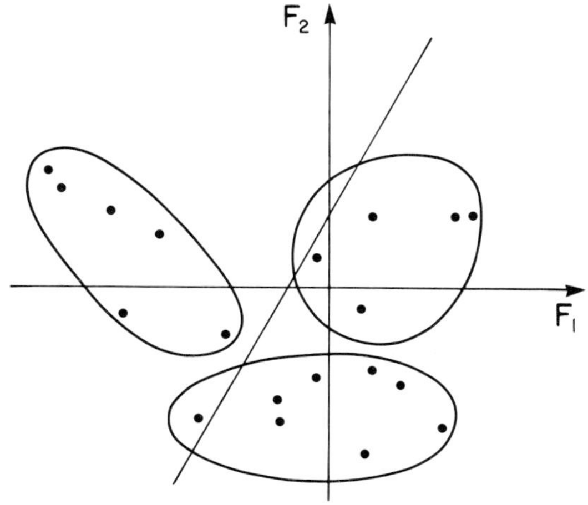

Fig. 12–2 *Semantic fields of Broca's aphasics (see Chapter 4) studied by means of semantic classification tasks*[81]. *All patients represented here had a semantic disturbance and its severity was proportional to that of their aphasia. From the least to the most severe: upper left, defective hierarchization (six subjects whose aphasia was dominated by phonetic disintegration; eventual evolution towards the picture of quasi-pure anarthria); bottom, narrowing of the semantic fields (eight subjects, most of whom presented a common form of Broca's aphasia); upper right, widening of the semantic fields (five subjects who initially presented a global aphasia with subsequent evolution towards the picture of Broca's aphasia, that is, with gradual recovery from a severe comprehension disturbance). From Derouesné*[80].

Having presented several examples of the fruitful interaction between linguistics and aphasiology, we shall close this chapter with a quotation from Whitaker[83], which was selected because of its evident, and perhaps justified, optism: 'I think it has been demonstrated that independent empirical support for linguistic hypotheses can be obtained from aphasia research; when such research is integrated into neurological theory, a reasonably coherent model of human language may be outlined. With luck, filling in the details of the outline will not be long forthcoming.'

REFERENCES

1. Lordat, J. (1843) Analyse de la parole pour servir à la théorie de divers cas d'alalie et de paralalie (de mutisme et d'imperfection de parler) que les neurologistes ont mal connus. *Journal de la Société pratique de Montpellier*, **7**, 333 and 417; **8**, 1.
2. Lordat, J. (1969) Analyse de la parole pour servir à la théorie de divers cas d'alalie et de paralalie (de mutisme et d'imperfection de parler) que les neurologistes ont mal connus. In *La Naissance de la Neuropsychologie du Langage* (Ed.) Hécaen, H. & Dubois, J. p. 130. Paris: Flammarion.
3. Freud, S. (1891) *Zur Auffasung der Aphasien*. Vienna: Deuticke.
4. Freud, S. (1953) *On Aphasia; a Critical Study*. New York: International Universities Press.
5. Alajouanine, Th., Ombredane, A. & Durand, M. (1939) *Le syndrome de désintégration phonétique dans l'aphasie*. Paris: Masson.

* *Narrowing* was manifested by difficulty in forming semantic links which were easily formed by normal subjects. *Widening* does not mean that the patients formed new links but, on the contrary, that they linked words indiscriminately and in such a chaotic fashion that a logical structure could no longer be inferred or even supposed.

6. Martinet, A. (1967) *Eléments de linguistique générale*. Paris: Colin.
7. Buyssens, E. (1967) *La communication et l'articulation linguistique*. Paris: Presses Universitaires de France.
8. Lecours, A.R., Dordain, G. & Lhermitte, F. (1970) Recherches sur le langage des aphasiques: 1. Terminologie neurolinguistique. *Encéphale*, **6,** 520.
9. Lecours, A.R. & Vanier-Clément, M. (1976) Schizophasia and jargonaphasia. A comparative description with comments on Chaika's and Fromkin's respective looks at 'schizophrenic' language. *Brain and Language*, **3,** 516.
10. Lecours, A.R. (1975) Methods for the description of aphasic transformations of language. In *Foundations of Language Development: a Multidisciplinary Approach* (Ed.) Lenneberg, E. & Lenneberg, E. Vol. 2, p. 75. New York: Academic Press.
11. Head, H. (1926) *Aphasia and Kindred Disorders of Speech*. London: Cambridge University Press.
12. Jakobson, R. (1956) Two aspects of language and two types of aphasic disturbances. In *Fundamentals of Language* (Ed.) Jakobson, R. & Halle, M. p. 55. The Hague: Mouton.
13. Jakobson, R. (1964) Towards a linguistic typology of aphasic impairments. In *Disorders of Language* (Ed.) de Reuck, A.V.S. & O'Connor, M. p. 21. London: Churchill.
14. Hécaen, H. (1972) *Introduction á la neuropsychologie*. Paris: Larousse.
15. Alajouanine, Th., Pichot, P. & Durand, M. (1949) Dissociation des altérations phonétiques avec conservation relative de la langue la plus ancienne dans un cas d'anarthrie pure chez un sujet français bilingue. *Encéphale*, **28,** 245.
16. Marcie, P., Hécaen, H., Constans, J.P. & Chodkiewicz, J.P. (1969) Etude spectrographique de la parole chez deux malades après ablation de méningiome de la région du pied de la troisième circonvolution frontale gauche. *Revue neurologique*, **120,** 350.
17. Fry, D.B. (1959) Phonemic substitutions in an aphasic patient. *Language and Speech*, **2,** 52.
18. Jakobson, R. (1968) *Child Language, Aphasia and Phonological Universals*. The Hague: Mouton.
19. Jakobson, R. (1969) *Langage enfantin et aphasie*. Paris: Editions de Minuit.
20. Shankweiler, D.P. & Harris, K. (1966) An experimental approach to the problem of articulation in aphasia. *Cortex*, **2,** 277.
21. Alajouanine, Th., Lhermitte, F., Ledoux, Renaud, D. & Vignolo, L.A. (1964) Les composantes phonémiques et sémantiques de la jargonaphasie. *Revue neurologique*, **110,** 5.
22. Alajouanine, Th. & Lhermitte, F. (1973) The phonemic and semantic components of jargon aphasia. In *Psycholinguistics and Aphasia* (Ed.) Goodglass, H. & Blumstein, S. p. 318. Baltimore, MD: Johns Hopkins.
23. Hécaen, H., Dubois, J., Angelergues, R., Vedrennes, C. & Marcie, P. (1964) Comparaison neurolinguistique et neuropsychologique de deux observations anatomocliniques d'aphasie. *Revue neurologique*, **3,** 401.
24. Renzi, E. (de), Pieczuro, A. & Vignolo, L.A. (1966) Oral apraxia and aphasia. *Cortex*, **2,** 50.
25. Lecours, A.R. & Lhermitte, F. (1969) Phonemic paraphasias; linguistic structures and tentative hypotheses. *Cortex*, **5,** 193.
26. Lecours, A.R. & Lhermitte, F. (1973) Phonemic paraphasias; linguistic structures and tentative hypotheses. In *Psycholinguistics and Aphasia* (Ed.) Goodglass, H. & Blumstein, S. p. 69. Baltimore, MD: Johns Hopkins Press.
27. Poncet, M., Degos, C., Deloche, G. & Lecours, A.R. (1972) Phonetic and phonemic transformations in aphasia. *International Journal of Mental Health*, **1,** 46.
28. Johns, D.F. & Darley, F.L. (1970) Phonemic variability in apraxia of speech. *Journal of Speech Research*, **13,** 556.
29. Lecours, A.R. & Lhermitte, F. (1970) Recherches sur le langage des aphasiques: 2. Mesure des relations de similarité entre unités linguistiques et modèle de référence pour la description des transformations aphasiques. *Encéphale*, **6,** 547.
30. Lecours, A.R., Deloche, G. & Lhermitte, F. (1973) Paraphasies phonémiques; description et stimulation sur ordinateur. In *Colloques IRIA—Informatique médicale*, p. 311. Rocquencourt: Institut de recherche d'informatique et d'automatique.
31. Lecours, A.R. (1974) Linguistic analysis of paraphasias. *Neurosciences Research Program Bulletin*, **12,** 555.
32. Lecours, A.R. & Rouillon, F. (1976) Neurolinguistic analysis of jargonaphasia and jargonagraphia. In *Studies in Neurolinguistics* (Ed.) Avakian-Whitaker, H. & Whitaker, H. Vol. 2, p. 95. New York: Academic Press.
33. Lecours, A.R. (1966) Serial order in writing—a study of misspelled words in development dysgraphia. *Neuropsychologia*, **4,** 221.
34. Lhermitte, F., Lecours, A.R. & Ouvry, B. (1967) Essai d'analyse structurale des paralexies et des paragraphies. *Acta Neurologica Belgica*, **11,** 1021.
35. Blumstein, S. (1968) Phonological aspects of aphasic speech. In *Studies Presented to Professor R. Jakobson by His Students* (Ed.) Gribble, C. p. 39. Cambridge: Slavica.
36. Blumstein, S. (1973) Some phonological implications of aphasic speech. In *Psycholinguistics and Aphasia* (Ed.) Goodglass, H. & Blumstein, S. p. 123. Baltimore, MD: Johns Hopkins.
37. Blumstein, S.E. (1973) *A Phonological Investigation of Aphasic Speech*. The Hague: Mouton.
38. Lecours, A.R. & Caplan, D. (1975) Blumstein's phonological investigation of aphasic speech. *Brain and Language*, **2,** 237.
39. Lebrun, Y. (1967) Le phonème, unité d'emploi ou unité de description? *Revue Belge de Philologie et d'Histoire*, **45,** 761.
40. Blumstein, S. & Goodglass, H. (1972) The perception of stress as a semantic cue in aphasia. *Journal of Speech Research*, **15,** 800.
41. Sabouraud, O., Gagnepain, J. & Sabouraud, A. (1963) Vers une approche linguistique des problèmes de l'aphasie. *Revue de Neuropsychiatrie de l'Ouest*, **1; 2; 3; 4,** 6, 3; 3; 3.

42. Sabouraud, O., Gagnepain, J. & Sabouraud, A. (1965) Aphasie et linguistique. *Revue pratique* (Paris), **15**, 2335.
43. Sabouraud, O. (1974) Bilan d'une collaboration neurologique dans l'approche des aphasies *Le Langage et l'Homme*, **24**, 30.
44. Wepman, J.M., Bock, R.D., Jones, L.V. & Pelt, D. (van) (1956) Psycholinguistic study of aphasia: a revision of the concept of anomia. *Journal of Speech Disorders*, **21**, 468.
45. Wepman, J. & Jones, L.V. (1961) Dimensions of language performance in aphasia. *Journal of Speech Research*, **4**, 220.
46. Wepman, J.M. & Jones, L.V. (1964) Five aphasias: a commentary on aphasia as a regressive linguistic phenomenon. In *Disorders of Communication* (Ed.) Rioch, D. & Weinstein, E. p. 190. Baltimore, MD: Williams and Wilkins.
47. Wepman, J. & Jones, L.V. (1964) The brain and disorders of communication in five aphasics: a commentary of aphasia as a regressive linguistic phenomenon. *Research Publications, Association for Research in Nervous and Mental Diseases*, **42**, 190.
48. Wepman, J. & Jones, L.V. (1966) Studies in aphasia; classification of aphasic speech by the noun-pronoun ratio. *British Journal of Disorders of Communication*, **1**, 46.
49. Howes, D.H. & Geschwind, N. (1960) *Statistical Properties of Aphasic Language*. Progress report NIH grant M-1802.
50. Howes, D.H. (1964) Application of the word-frequency concept to aphasia. In *Disorders of Language* (Ed.) de Reuck, A.V.S. & O'Connor, M. p. 47. London: Churchill.
51. Howes, D. (1967) Some experimental investigations of language in aphasia. In *Research in Verbal Behavior and Some Neurophysiological Implications* (Ed.) Salzinger, K. & Salzinger, S. p. 181. New York: Academic Press.
52. Goodglass, H., Quadfasel, F.A. & Timberlake, W.H. (1964) Phrase length and the type and severity of aphasia. *Cortex*, **1**, 133.
53. Spreen, O. & Wachal, R.S. (1973) Psycholinguistic analysis of aphasic language: theoretical formulations and procedures. *Language and Speech*, **16**, 130.
54. Wachal, R.S. & Spreen, O. (1973) Some measures of lexical diversity in aphasic and normal language performance. *Language and Speech*, **16**, 169.
55. Dordain, G. (1968) *Contribution á l'étude neurolinguistique de l'aphasie. Analyse comparative des performances grammaticales de 28 aphasiques dont 14 agrammatiques.* Medical thesis, Paris.
56. Tissot, R., Mounin, G. & Lhermitte, F. (1973) *L'agrammatisme. Etude neuropsycholinguistique*. Bruxelles: Dessart.
57. Bouillon, F. (1971) *A propos de quelques observations d'agrammatiques et de dyssyntaxiques; essai d'analyse comparative de certaines de leurs performances grammaticales*. Medical thesis, Paris.
58. Goodglass, H. & Mayer, J. (1958) Agrammatism in aphasia. *Journal of Speech Research*, **23**, 99.
59. Goodglass, H. & Hunt, J. (1958) Grammatical complexity and aphasic speech. *Word*, **14**, 197.
60. Goodglass, H. & Berko-Gleason, J. (1960) Agrammatism and inflectional morphology in English. *Journal of Speech Research*, **3**, 257.
61. Goodglass, H. (1968) Studies on the grammar of aphasics. In *Developments in Applied Psycholinguistics Research* (Ed.) Rosenberg, S. & Koplin, J. p. 177. New York: Macmillan.
62. Goodglass, H., Fodor, I.G. & Schulhoff, C. (1967) Prosodic factors in grammar—evidence from aphasia. *Journal of Speech Research*, **10**, 5.
63. Goodglass, H., Berko-Gleason, J., Bernholz, N.A. & Hyde, M.R. (1972) Some linguistic structures in the speech of a Broca's aphasic. *Cortex*, **8**, 191.
64. Berko-Gleason, J., Goodglass, H., Green, E., Ackerman, N. & Hyde, M.R. (1975) The retrieval of syntax in Broca's aphasia. *Brain and Language*, **2**, 451.
65. Lavallée-Huynh, G. (1975) *Echelle de complexité syntaxique établie expérimentalement à partir d'épreuves de mise en phrase chez des aphasiques de Broca*. Montreal: Mémoire, Faculté de Linguistique.
66. Goodglass, H. & Hunter, M. (1970) A linguistic comparison of speech and writing in two types of aphasia. *Journal of Communication Disorders*, **3**, 28.
67. Lecours, A.R. & Lhermitte, F. (1972) Recherches sur le langage des aphasiques: 4. Analyse d'un corpus de néologismes; notion de paraphasie monémique. *Encéphale*, **4**, 295.
68. Kertesz, A. & Benson, D. F. (1970) Neologistic jargon: a clinicopathological study. *Cortex*, **6**, 362.
69. Goodglass, H., Berko-Gleason, J. & Hyde, M.R. (1970) Some dimensions of auditory language comprehension in aphasia. *Journal of Speech Research*, **13**, 595.
70. Parisi, D. & Pizzamiglio, L. (1970) Syntactic comprehension in aphasia. *Cortex*, **6**, 204.
71. Stockert, T.R. (von) (1972) Recognition of syntactic structure in aphasic patients. *Cortex*, **8**, 323.
72. Zurif, E.B., Caramazza, A. & Myerson, R. (1972) Grammatical judgments of agrammatic aphasics. *Neuropsychologia*, **10**, 405.
73. Dejerine, J. (1914) *Séméiologie des affections du système nerveux*. Paris: Masson.
74. Pitres, A. (1898) L'aphasie amnésique et ses variétés cliniques. *Progrès médicale* (Paris), **7**, 321, 337, 369 and 401.
75. Barton, M.I. (1971) Recall of generic properties of words in aphasic patients. *Cortex*, **7**, 73.
76. Goodglass, H., Klein, B., Carey, P. & Jones, K. (1966) Specific semantic word categories in aphasia. *Cortex*, **2**, 74.
77. Ali Cherif, A. (1972) *Considérations sur les troubles de l'expression orale et de la compréhension verbale présentés par deux malades aphasiques*. Medical thesis, Marseilles.
78. Marshall, J.C. & Newcombe, F. (1966) Syntactic and semantic errors in paralexia. *Neuropsychologia*, **4**, 169.
79. Fodor, J.A. & Katz, J.J. (Ed.) (1964) *The Structure of Language*. Englewood Cliffs, NJ: Prentice-Hall.

80. Derouesné, J. (1970) *Contribution á l'étude des troubles sémantiques chez les aphasiques*. Thesis, Faculté des lettres, Paris.
81. Lhermitte, F., Derouesné, J. & Lecours, A.R. (1971) Contribution à l'étude des troubles sémantiques dans l'aphasie. *Revue neurologique*, **125,** 81.
82. Derouesné, J. & Lecours, A.R. (1972) Two tests for the study of semantic deficits in aphasia. *International Journal of Mental Health*, **1,** 14.
83. Whitaker, H. A. (1972) Unsolicited nominalizations by aphasics: the plausibility of the lexicalist model. *Linguistics*, **78,** 62.

BIBLIOGRAPHY

Alajouanine, Th. (1956) Verbal realization in aphasia. *Brain*, **79,** 1.

Alajouanine, Th. (1966) Remarques sur le langage normal suggérées par l'étude de l'aphasie. *Revue neurologique*, **115,** 613–623.

Alajouanine, Th., Cathala, H.P., Métellus, J. & Mlle Siksou (1973) La problématique de l'aphasie dans les langues à écriture non alphabétique. *Revue neurologique*, **128,** 229.

Alajouanine, Th. & Mozziconacci, P. (1948) *L'aphasie et la désintégration fonctionnelle du langage*. Paris: Expansion scientifique française.

Anderson, J.O. (1946) Is not the verb for aphasia? *Journal of Speech Disorders*, **11,** 135.

Anderson, J.O. (1946) Is there a word for aphasics? *Quarterly Journal of Speech*, **32,** 485.

Andreewsky, E. (1972) Informatique et recherche en neuropsychologie. *Encéphale*, **61,** 1.

Barbizet, J. & Lenoir, G. (1968) Etude dynamique d'échantillons verbaux chez des sujets normaux et chez des malades atteints de lésions cérébrales. *Annales psychologiques*, **68,** 431.

Benveniste, E. (1954) Tendances récentes en linguistique générale. *Journal de Psychologie normale et pathologique*, **1–2,** 130.

Bertaux, D., Lecours, A.R. & Lhermitte, F. (1970) Analogy between sequential errors in aphasia and the behavior of a cybernetic system (SARF). In *Technical and Biological Problems of Control—A Cybernetic View* (Ed.) Iberall, A.S. & Reswick, J.B. p. 371. Pittsburgh, PA: Instrument Society of America.

Bijou, S. & Werner, H. (1945) Language analysis in brain-injured and non-brain-injured children mentally deficient. *Journal of Genetic Psychology*, **66,** 239.

Bliss, L.S., Tikofsky, R.S. & Guilford, A.M. (1976) Aphasic's sentence repetition behavior as a function of grammaticality. *Cortex*, **12,** 113.

Borkowski, J.G., Benton, A.L. & Spreen, O. (1967) Word fluency and brain damage. *Neuropsychologia*, **5,** 135.

Borrell, A. & Nespoulous, J.L. (1975) La linguistique à la croisée des chemins: de la neurolinguistique à la psycholinguistique. *Annales*, **11,** 91.

Bouman, L. & Grunbaum, A.A. (1925) Experimental-psychologische Untersuchungen zur Aphasie und Paraphasic. *Zentralblatt für die gesamte Neurologie und Psychologie*, **96,** 481.

Bresson, F. (1953) Langage et communication. *Annales psychologiques*, **53,** 477.

Bricker, A.L., Schuell, H.M. & Jenkins, J.J. (1964) Effect of word frequency and word length on aphasics, spelling errors. *Journal of Speech Research*, **7,** 183.

Bryan, E.L. (1933) Study of 40 cases exhibiting neologisms. *American Journal of Psychiatry*, **13,** 579.

Buckingham, H.W. (1975) The conduction theory and neologistic jargon. *Quarterly Progress Report Communication Sciences Laboratory, University of Florida*, **13.**

Buckingham, H.W., Whitaker, H. & Whitaker, H. (1975) Linguistic structures in stereotyped aphasic speech. *Linguistics*, **154–155,** 5.

Buckingham, H.W. & Kertesz, A. (1976) *Neurolinguistics 3: Neologistic Jargon Aphasia*. Amsterdam: Swets and Zeitlinger.

Caplan, D., Kellar, L. & Locke, S. (1972) Inflection of neologisms in aphasia. *Brain*, **95,** 169.

Caramazza, A. & Zurif, E.B. (1976) Dissociation of algorithmic and heuristic processes in language comprehension: evidence from aphasia. *Brain and Language*, **3,** 572.

Castle, W. (1966) Some linguistic explanations of adult aphasia. *Linguistics*, **24,** 3.

Cherry, E.C., Halle, M. & Jakobson, R. (1953) Toward the logical description of languages in their phonemic aspects. *Language*, **29,** 34.

Clarke, B. (1955) Lexical and grammatical impairment in dysphasia. *Language and Speech*, **9,** 28.

Cohen, D., Dubois, J., Gauthier, M., Hécaen, H. & Angelergues, R. (1963) Aspects du fonctionnement du code linguistique chez les aphasiques moteurs. *Neuropsychologia*, **1,** 165.

Cohen, D. & Hécaen, H. (1965) Remarques neurolinguistiques sur un cas d'agrammatisme. *Journal de Psychologie*, **3,** 273.

Cohen, J.G. & Edwards, A.E. (1964) Word length and discrimination behavior of aphasia. *Journal of Speech Research*, **7,** 343.

Deal, J.L. & Darley, F.L. (1972) The influence of linguistic and situational variables on phonemic accuracy in apraxia of speech. *Journal of Speech Research*, **15,** 639.

Degos, C.F. (1970) *Etude des transformations phonémiques et phonétiques dans l'aphasie* (*essai de comparaison entre le jargon phonémique et le syndrome de désintégration phonétique*). Medical thesis, Paris.

Dingwall, W.O. & Whitaker, H.A. (1974) Neurolinguistics. *Annual Review of Anthropology*, **3,** 323.

Dubois, J. (1967) La neurolinguistique. *Langages*, **5,** 6.

Dubois, J., Hécaen, H., Angelergues, R., Maufras du Chatelier, A. & Marcie, P. (1964) Etude neurolinguistique de l'aphasie de conduction. *Neuropsychologia*, **2,** 9.

Dubois, J., Irigaray, L., Marcie, P. & Hécaen, H. (Ed.) (1967) *Langages 5: Pathologie du langage*. Paris: Didier and Larousse.

Dubois, J., Mazars, G., Marcie, P. & Hécaen, H. (1966) Etude des performances aux épreuves linguistiques des sujets atteints de syndromes parkinsoniens. *Encéphale*, **6,** 496.

Ebbin, J.B. & Edwards, A.E. (1967) Speech sound discrimination of aphasics when intersound interval is varied. *Journal of Speech Research*, **10,** 120.

Fairbanks, G. (1954) Systematic research in experimental phonetics: speech mechanism as a servosystem. *Journal of Speech Disorders*, **19,** 133.

Filby, Y., Edwards, A.E. & Seacat, G.F. (1963) Word length, frequency and similarity in the discrimination behavior of aphasics. *Journal of Speech Research*, **6,** 255.

Fillenbaum, S., Jones, L.V. & Wepman, J.M. (1961) Some linguistic features of speech from aphasic patients. *Language and Speech*, **4,** 91.

Fodor, J.A. & Bever, T. (1965) The psychological reality of linguistic segments. *Journal of Verbal Learning and Verbal Behavior*, **4,** 414.

Fraser, C., Bellugi, U. & Brown, R. (1963) Control of grammar in imitation, comprehension and production. *Journal of Verbal Learning and Verbal Behavior*, **2,** 121.

Freund, D.D. (1973) Recent trends in aphasia research. *American Journal of Psychiatry*, **110,** 186.

Gainotti, G., Caltagirone, C. & Ibba, A. (1975) Semantic and phonemic aspects of auditory language comprehension in aphasia. *Linguistics*, **154–155,** 15.

Gainotti, G., Ibba, A. & Caltagirone, C. (1975) Perturbations acoustiques et sémantiques de la comprehension dans l'aphasie. *Revue neurologique*, **131,** 645.

Gardner, H. & Zurif, E. (1976) Critical reading of words and phrases in aphasia. *Brain and Language*, **3,** 173.

Gloning, K., Haub, G. & Quatember, R. (1967) Speech features in aphasics—a factorial study. *Neuropsychologia*, **5,** 165.

Goldstein, K. (1936) The problem of the meaning of words based upon observations of aphasia patients. *Journal of Psychology*, **2,** 306.

Goren, Y. (1968) Does vocabulary resist mental deterioration? *Journal of Clinical Psychology*, **24,** 341.

Goodglass, H. & Baker, E. (1976) Semantic field, naming and auditory comprehension in aphasia. *Brain and Language*, **3,** 359.

Goodglass, H., Barton, M.I. & Kaplan, E.F. (1968) Sensory modality and object-naming in aphasia. *Journal of Speech Research*, **2,** 488.

Goodglass, H. & Blumstein, S. (Ed.) (1973) *Psycholinguistics and Aphasia*. Baltimore, MD: Johns Hopkins Press.

Gough, P.B. (1965) Grammatical transformations and speed of understanding. *Journal of Verbal Learning and Verbal Behavior*, **4,** 107.

Green, E. (1969) Phonological and grammatical aspects of jargon in an aphasic patient: a case study. *Language and Speech*, **12,** 103.

Green, E. (1969) Psycholinguistic approaches to aphasia. *Linguistics*, **53,** 30.

Green, E. (1970) On the contribution of studies in aphasia to psycholinguistics. *Cortex*, **6,** 216.

Green, E. & Boller, F. (1974) Features of auditory comprehension in severely impaired aphasics. *Cortex*, **10,** 133.

Grégoire, A. (1968) Jakobson's theories and aphasia. *Le Langage et l'Homme*, **6,** 192.

Grewel, F. (1949) Aphasia as linguistic disorder. *Nederlandse Tijdschrift voor Geneeskunde*, **93,** 726.

Grewel, F. (1951) Aphasia and linguistics. *Folia phoniatrica* (Basel), **3,** 100.

Grewel, F. (1962) Disorders in the use of semiotic systems. *Logos*, **5,** 43.

Grewel, F. (1963) Prolegomena to patholinguistics In *Problems of Dynamic Neurology* (Ed.) Halpern, H. p. 71. Jerusalem: Jerusalem Post Press.

Halpern, H., Keith, R.L. & Darley, F.L. (1976) Phonemic behavior of aphasic subjects without dysarthria or apraxia of speech. *Cortex*, **12,** 365.

Hécaen, H. & Consoli, S. (1973) Analyse des troubles du langage au cours des lésions de l'aire de Broca. *Neuropsychologia*, **11,** 377.

Hécaen, H., Dubois, J. & Marcie, P. (1967) Mécanismes de l'aphasie et apport de la neurolinguistique à l'aphasiologie. *Acta Neurologica Belgica*, **67,** 959.

Hécaen, H. & Kremin, H. (1976) Neurolinguistic research on reading disorders resulting from left hemisphere lesions: aphasic and 'pure' alexia. In *Studies in Neurolinguistics* (Ed.) Whitaker, H. & Whitaker, H.A. Vol II, p. 269. New York: Academic Press.

Hécaen, H. & Marcie, P. (1967) L'agraphie au cours de l'aphasie de conduction. In *Wiener Zeitschrift für Nervenheilkunde und Deren Grenzgebiete* (Ed.) Hoff, H. & Reisner, H. p. 193. Vienna and New York: Springer-Verlag.

Holmes, J.A. & Hyman, W. (1957) Spelling disability and asyntaxia in a case involving injury to the language formulation area of the brain. *Journal of Educational Psychology*, **48,** 542.

Huber, M. (1944) A phonetic approach to the problem of perception in a case of Wernicke's aphasia. *Journal of Speech Disorders*, **9,** 227.

Huber, M. (1946) Linguistic problems of brain-injured servicemen. *Journal of Speech Disorders*, **11,** 143.

Imura, T., Nogami, Y. & Asakawa, K. (1971) Aphasia in Japanese language. *Nihon University Journal of Medicine*, **13,** 69.

Jarvella, R.J. & Herman, S.J. (1973) Speed and accuracy of sentence recall: effects of ear of presentation, semantics and grammar. *Journal of Experimental Psychology*, **97,** 108.

Jones, L.V. & Wepman, J.M. (1967) Grammatical indicants of speaking style in normal and aphasic speakers. In *Research in Verbal Behavior and Some Neurophysiological Implications* (Ed.) Salzinger, K. & Salzinger, S. p. 169. New York: Academic Press.

Jones, L.V., Goodman, M.F. & Wepman, J.M. (1963) The classification of parts of speech for the characterization of aphasia. *Language and Speech*, **6,** 94.

Jones, L.V. & Wepman, J.M. (1961) Dimensions of language performance in aphasia. *Journal of Speech Research*, **4,** 220.

Kania, J. & Klimkowski, M. (1967) An attempt to describe aphasia in linguistic terms. *Logopedia*, **7,** 41.

Kaplan, L.T. (1959) A descriptive continuum of language response in aphasia. *Journal of Speech Disorders*, **25,** 410.

Karlin, I.W., Eisenson, J., Hirschenfang, S. & Miller, M.H. (1959) A multi-evaluational study of aphasia and non-aphasic right hemiplegic patients. *Journal of Speech Disorders*, **24,** 369.

Keller, E. (1975) *Vowel Errors in Aphasia*. Dissertation, Department of linguistics, University of Toronto.

Kean, M.-L. (1977) The linguistic interpretation of aphasic syndromes: agrammatism in Broca's aphasia, an example. *Cognition*, **5,** 9.

Kinsbourne, M. & Warrington, E.K. (1964) Disorders of spelling. *Journal of Neurology, Neurosurgery and Psychiatry*, **27,** 296.

Kreindler, A., Gheorghita, N. & Voinescu, I. (1971) Analysis of verbal reception of a complex order with three elements in aphasics. *Brain*, **94,** 375.

Krise, M. (1952) An experimental investigation of theories of reversals in reading. *Journal of Educational Psychology*, **43,** 408.

Lane, H.L. & Moore, D.J. (1962) Reconditioning a consonant discrimination in an aphasic: an experimental case history. *Journal of Speech Disorders*, **27,** 232.

Lansdell, H., Purnell, J.K. & Laskowski, E.J. (1963) The relation of induced dysnomia to phoneme frequency. *Language and Speech*, **6,** 88.

Lasky, E.Z., Weidner, W.E. & Johnson, J.P. (1976) Influence of linguistic complexity, rate of presentation and interphrase pause time on auditory verbal comprehension of adult aphasic patients. *Brain and Language*, **3,** 386.

Leach, E. (1972) Interrogation: a model and some implications. *Journal of Speech Disorders*, **37,** 33.

Lebrun, Y. (1967) Le phonème, unité d'emploi ou unité de description? *Revue Belge de Philologie et d'Histoire*, **45,** 761.

Lebrun, Y. (1967) Linguistic analysis of two cases of emissive aphasia. *Journal of the Neurological Sciences*, **4,** 271.

Lebrun, Y. (1972) La neurolinguistique. *Revue médicale Bruxelles*, **28,** 177.

Lecours, A.R. & Caplan, D. (1983) Recherches neurolinguistiques au Canada. In *Linguistics in Canada—La Linguistique au Canada* (Ed.) Collinge, N.E. Montreal: Centre éducatif et culturel.

Lee, L.L. (1958) Two kinds of disturbed communication. *General Semantics Bulletin*, **22-23,** 47.

Leiber, L. (1976) Lexical decisions in the right and left cerebral hemispheres. *Brain and Language*, **3,** 443.

Lesser, R. (1973) Word association and availability of response in an aphasic subject. *Journal of Psycholinguistic Research*, **2,** 355.

Lesser, R. (1974) Verbal comprehension in aphasia: an English version of three Italian tests. *Cortex*, **10,** 247.

Linsky, L. (Ed.) (1952) *Semantics and the Philosophy of Language*. Urbana, IL: University of Illinois Press.

Locke, S., Caplan, D. & Kellar, L. (1973) *A Study in Neurolinguistics*. Springfield, IL: Thomas.

Luria, A.R. (1958) Brain disorders and language analysis. *Language and Speech*, **1,** 14.

Marcie, P. (1967) Analyses de la structure des phrases dans des énoncés d'aphasiques de conduction. *Langages*, **5,** 37.

Marshall, M., Newcombe, F. & Marshall, J.C. (1971) The microstructure of word-finding difficulties in a dysphasic subject. In *Advances in Psycholinguistics* (Ed.) Flores d'Arcais, G.B. & Levelt, N.J.M. p. 416. Amsterdam: North-Holland.

Martin, A.D., Wasserman, N.H., Gilden, L., Gerstman, L. & West, J.A. (1975) A process model of repetition in aphasia: an investigation of phonological and morphological interactions in aphasic error performance. *Brain and Language*, **2,** 434.

Mehler, J. (1973) Some remarks on psycholinguistic studies. In *The Formal Analysis of Natural Languages—Proceedings of the First International Conference* (Ed.) Gross, M. et al. p. 296. The Hague: Mouton.

Mehler, J. & de Boysson-Bardies. B. (1971) Psycholinguistique—messages et codage verbal. *Annales psychologiques*, **71,** 547.

Mehler, J. & Carey, P. (1969) Rôle de la structure profonde et de la structure de surface dans la perception des phrases. *Langages*, **4,** 106.

Métellus, J. (1970) *Contribution à l'étude du jargon phonémique et de la désintégration phonétique dans l'aphasie*. Medical thesis, Paris.

Michel, F. (1976) Méthode de recueil et d'exploitation quantitative de paramètres temporospatiaux du geste graphique. *Cahiers de Psychologie*, **19,** 39.

Mihailescu, L., Botez, M.I. & Kreindler, A. (1970) Décodage du stress correct et erroné du mot chez le sujet aphasique. *Revue roumaine de Neurologie*, **7,** 65.

Mihailescu, L., Weigl, I., Weigl, E. & Kreindler, A. (1972) Performance chez l'aphasique avec les mots conceptuels et opérationnels utilisés isolément ou dans des phrases. *Revue roumaine de Neurologie*, **9,** 181.

Miller, G.A. & Nicely, P.E. (1955) An analysis of perceptual confusions among some English consonants. *Journal of the Acoustical Society of America*, **27,** 338.

Moore, W.H. Jr & Weidner, W.E. (1974) Bilateral tachistoscopic word perception in aphasic and normal subjects. *Perceptual and Motor Skills*, **38,** 1003.

Mounin, G. (1967) Les caractères linguistiques de l'agrammatisme. *La linguistique*, **2,** 15.

Myerson, R. & Goodglass, H. (1972) Transformational grammars of three agrammatic patients. *Language and Speech*, **15,** 40.

Nespoulous, J.L. (1976) Validité du modèle de Markov pour l'analyse linguistique et psycholinguistique. *La linguistique*, **10,** 71.

Nespoulous, J.L. (1975) *Approche linguistique de divers*

phénomènes d'agrammatisme. Thesis, Département de Linguistique, Université de Toulouse-le-Mirail, Toulouse.

Newcombe, F. & Marshall, J.C. (1967) Immediate recall of 'sentences' by subjects with unilateral cerebral lesions. *Neuropsychologia*, **5**, 329.

Newcombe, F., Olfield, R.C., Ratcliff, G.G. & Wingfield. A. (1971) Recognition and naming of object-drawings by men with focal brain wounds. *Journal of Neurology, Neurosurgery and Psychiatry*, **34**, 329.

Newcombe, F., Olfield, R.C. & Wingfield, A. (1965) Object-naming by dysphasic patients. *Nature*, **207**, 1217.

Olfield, R.C. & Wingfield, A. (1964) The time it takes to name an object. *Nature*, **202**, 1031.

Olfield, R.C. & Wingfield, A. (1965) Response latencies in naming objects. *Quarterly Journal of Experimental Psychology*, **17**, 273.

Oscar-Berman, M., Zurif, E.B. & Blumstein, S. (1975) Effects of unilateral brain damage on the processing of speech sounds. *Brain and Language*, **2**, 345.

Osgood, C.E. & Miron, M. (1963) *Approaches to the Study of Aphasia*. Urbana, IL: University of Illinois.

Panse, F. & Shimoyama, T. (1955) Zur Auswirkung-Aphasischer Störungen im Japanischen. *Arch. Psychol. Z. Neurol.* **193**, 139.

Parisi, D. & Pizzamiglio, L. (1970) Syntactic comprehension in aphasia. *Cortex*, **6**, 204.

Penser G. & Fittschen, M. (1977) On the universality of language dissolution: the case of a Turkish aphasic. *Brain and Language*, **4**, 196.

Pillon B. & Lhermitte, F. (1974) Désignation et dénomination à différents rythmes chez des patients atteints de lesions cérébrales. *Neuropsychologia*, **12**, 55.

Pincas, A. (1965) Linguistics and aphasia. *Journal of the Australian College of Speech Therapy*, **15**, 20.

Pisoni, D.B. (1973) Auditory and phonetic memory codes in the discrimination of consonants and vowels. *Perception and Psychophysics*, **13**, 253.

Pizzamiglio, L. & Appicciafuoco, A. (1971) Semantic comprehension in aphasia. *Journal of Communication Disorders*, **3**, 280.

Pizzamiglio, L. & Black, J.W. (1968) Phonic trends in the writing of aphasic patients. *Journal of Speech Research*, **11**, 77.

Ranschburg, P. (1928) *Die Lese- und Schreibstörungen des Kindesalters*. Halle: Verlagsbuchhandlung.

Reiff, D.G. & Tikogsky, R.S. (1968) Aphasia and linguistic competence. *Studies in Language and Language Behavior*, **6**, 50.

Rinnert, C. & Whitaker, H.A. (1973) Semantic confusions by aphasic patients. *Cortex*, **9**, 56.

Rips, L.J., Shoben, E.J. & Smith, E.E. (1973) Semantic distance and the verification of semantic relations. *Journal of Verbal Learning and Verbal Behavior*, **12**, 1.

Ritter, T., von Stockert, Th. & Heeschen, C. (1971) Eine linguistische Methode zu Untersuchung von Aphasien. *Nervenartz*, **42**, 305.

Rivenc, P. (1968) Lexique et langue parlée. *Le Français dans le Monde*, **57**, 25.

Rochford, G. (1963) Studies in the development and breakdown of the use of names: recovery from nominal aphasia. *Journal of Neurology, Neurosurgery and Psychiatry*, **26**, 377.

Rochford, G. & Williams, M. (1962) Studies in the development and breakdown of the use of names. *Journal of Neurology, Neurosurgery and Psychiatry*, **25**, 222.

Rollin, W. (1964) Oral responses of aphasics under different syntactic conditions. *Language and Speech*, **7**, 167.

Rosolato, G. (1956) Sémantique et altération du langage. *Evolution psychiatrique*, **4**, 865.

Sadock, J.M. (1974) *Toward a Linguistic Theory of Speech Acts*. New York: Academic Press.

Saffran, E.M., Marin, O.S.M. & Yeni-Komshian, G.H. (1976) An analysis of speech perception in word deafness. *Brain and Language*, **3**, 209.

Saffran, E.M., Schwartz, M.F. & Marin, O.S.M. (1976) Semantic mechanisms in paralexia. *Brain and Language*, **3**, 255.

Sakamoto, S. (1940) Contribution à l'étude des atteintes respectives du Kanji et du Kana dans l'aphasie. *Osaka Nisseki*, **4**, 185. (In Japanese.)

Sasanuma, S. (1975) Kana and kanji processing in Japanese aphasics. *Brain and Language*, **2**, 369.

Sasanuma, S. & Fujimura, O. (1971) Selective impairment of phonetic and non-phonetic transcriptions of words in Japanese aphasic patients: kana vs kanji in visual recognition and writing. *Cortex*, **7**, 1.

Sasanuma, S. & Fujimura, O. (1972) An analysis of writing errors in Japanese aphasic patients: kanji versus kana words. *Cortex*, **8**, 265.

Sasanuma, S. & Kamio, A. (1976) Aphasic's comprehension of sentences expressing temporal order of events. *Brain and Language*, **3**, 495.

Schenk, V.W.D. (1953) Troubles des phonèmes en cas d'aphasie sensorielle. *Encéphale*, **42**, 158.

Schlanger, B.B. (1973) Identification by normal and aphasic subjects of semantically meaningful and meaningless emotional toned sentences. *Acta Symbolica*, **4**, 30.

Schlanger, B., Schlanger, P. & Gerstman, J.L. (1976) The perception of emotionally toned sentences by right hemisphere-damaged and aphasic subjects. *Brain and Language*, **3**, 396.

Schnitzer, M.L. & Martin, J.E. (1974) Sequential constraint impairment in aphasia: a case study. *Brain and Language*, **1**, 283.

Schuell, H. (1950) Paraphasia and paralexia. *Journal of Speech Disorders*, **15**, 291.

Schuell, H. & Jenkins, J.J. (1961) Reduction of vocabulary in aphasia. *Brain*, **84**, 243.

Schuell, H., Jenkins, J. & Landis, L. (1961) Relationships between auditory comprehension and word frequency in aphasia. *Journal of Speech Research*, **4**, 30.

Sefer, J.W. & Henrikson, E.H. (1966) The relationship between word association and grammatical classes in aphasia. *Journal of Speech Research*, **9**, 529.

Shanks, J. & Ryan, W. (1976) A comparison of aphasic and non brain-injured adults on a dichotic CV-syllable listening task. *Cortex*, **12**, 100.

Shewan, C.M. (1976) Error patterns in auditory comprehension of adult aphasics. *Cortex*, **12,** 325.

Shewan, C.M. & Canter, G.J. (1971) Effects of vocabulary, syntax, and sentence length on auditory comprehension in aphasic patients. *Cortex*, **7,** 209.

Siegel, G. (1959) Dysphasic speech responses to visual word stimuli. *Journal of Speech Research*, **2,** 152.

Slobin, D.I. (1971) *Psycholinguistics*. Glenview, IL: Scott and Foresman.

Spellacy, F. & Blumstein, S. (1970) The influence of language set on ear preference in phoneme recognition. *Cortex*, **6,** 430.

Spreen, O. (1968) Psycholinguistic aspects of aphasia. *Journal of Speech Research*, **11,** 467.

Starr, A. (1970) Verbal and motor memory in the amnestic syndrome. *Neuropsychologia*, **8,** 75.

Summers, R. (1953) Perceptive vs productive skill in analysing speech sounds from words. *Journal of Speech Disorders*, **18,** 140.

Tikofsky, R.S. (1966) Listener confusions in response to dysarthric speech. *Folia phoniatica*, **18,** 280.

Timmermans, B. & Kumin, L. (1974) Free word association of adult aphasics. *Psychological Reports*, **34,** 389.

Trost, J. & Canter, G.J. (1974) Apraxia of speech in patients with Broca's aphasia: a study of phoneme production accuracy and error patterns. *Brain and Language*, **1,** 63.

Verzeano, M. (1950) Time patterns of speech in normal subjects. *Journal of Speech Disorders*, **15,** 197.

Villiers, J. (de) (1974) Quantitative aspects of agrammatism in aphasia. *Cortex*, **10,** 36.

Wagenaar, E., Snow, C. & Prins, R. (1975) Spontaneous speech of aphasic patients: a psycholinguistic analysis. *Brain and Language*, **2,** 281.

Weigl, E. (1974) Neuropsychological experiments on transcoding between spoken and written language structures. *Brain and Language*, **1,** 227.

Weigl, E. & Bierwisch, M. (1970) Neuropsychology and linguistics: topics of common research. *Foundations of Language*, **6,** 1.

Weigl, E. & Fradis, A. (1977) The transcoding processes in patients with agraphia to dictation. *Brain and Language*, **1,** 11.

Weigl, E. & Mihailescu, L. (1973) Interdépendance entre le contexte syntaxique et ses constituants dans l'aphasie. *Revue roumaine de Neurologie*, **2,** 123.

Weinstein, E.A. & Keller, N.J.A. (1963) Linguistic patterns of misnaming in brain injury. *Neuropsychologia*, **1,** 79.

Wepman, J.M., Bock, R.D., Jones, L.V. & van Pelt, D. (1956) Psycholinguistic study of aphasia: a revision of the concept of anomia. *Journal of Speech Disorders*, **21,** 468.

Wepman, J. & Jones, L. (1961) Dimensions of language performance in aphasia. *Journal of Speech Research*, **4,** 220.

Wepman, J. & Jones, L. (1966) Studies in aphasia—classification of aphasic speech by the noun-pronoun ratio. *British Journal of Disorders of Communication*, **1,** 46.

Werner, H. (Ed.) (1955) *On Expressive Language*. Worcester: Clark University Press.

Whitaker, H.A. (1970) Linguistic competence: evidence from aphasia. *Glossa*, **4,** 46.

Whitaker, H.A. (1971) *On the Representation of Language in the Human Brain*. Edmonton: Linguistic Research.

Whitaker, H.A. (1973) Comments on the innateness of language. In *Some New Directions in Linguistics* (Ed.) Shuy, R.W. p. 95. Georgetown: Georgetown University Press.

Whitaker, H. & Whitaker, H.A. (1983) Language disorders. In *A Survey of Applied Linguistics* (Ed.) Brown, H.D. & Wardhaug, R. Ann Arbor: University of Michigan Press.

Whitaker, H. & Whitaker, H.A. (1976, 1977) *Studies in Neurolinguistics*. Vol. I, II, III. New York: Academic Press.

Wickens, D.D. (1970) Encoding categories of words: an empirical approach to meaning. *Psychological Review*, **77,** 1.

Wyke, M. (1966) Experimental study of verbal association learning in patients with severe dysphasia. *Journal of Neurology, Neurosurgery and Psychiatry*, **29,** 171.

Yacorzynski, G.K. (1943) Modern approach in the study of aphasia. *Journal of Speech Disorders*, **8,** 349.

Yamadori, A. & Albert, M.L. (1973) Word category aphasia. *Cortex*, **9,** 112.

Yasuko, F., Edwards, A.E. & Seacat, G.F. (1963) Word length, frequency and similarity in the discrimination behavior of aphasics. *Journal of Speech Research*, **3,** 255.

Zurif, E.B. & Caramazza, A. (1976) Psycholinguistic structures in aphasia: studies in syntax and semantics. In *Studies in Neurolinguistics* (Ed.) Avakian-Whitaker, H. & Whitaker, H.A. Vol. I, p. 261. New York: Academic Press.

Zurif, E.B., Caramazza, A., Myerson, R. & Galvin, J. (1974) Semantic feature representations for normal and aphasic language. *Brain and Language*, **1,** 167.

Zurif, E.B., Green, E., Caramazza, A. & Goodenough, C. (1976) Grammatical intuitions of aphasic patients: sensitivity to functors. *Cortex*, **12,** 183.

Zurif, E.B. & Ramier, A.M. (1972) Some effects of unilateral brain damage on the perception of dichotically presented phoneme sequences and digits. *Neuropsychologia*, **10,** 103.

Zurif, E.B. & Sait, P.E. (1970) The role of syntax in dichotic listening. *Neuropsychologia*, **8,** 239.

Deviations in Non-aphasic Language

13. The Language of Psychotics and Neurotics

101. Transcendence.

A fan of many spirits in one person or else an accordion in taking these two aforesaid things as an example.

The open fan there are several persons. The closed fan there is only one of them.

—Very important.

102. It is forbidden to allow oneself to be carried in the uterus or the belly of a woman as in a skiff in turning up the volume.

Do not confuse:

—the swelling as a Michelin bibindome
—the occupation
—and the pregnant women

Banish the spirit which wishes to give demonstrations that these things may be. We have enough examples.

103. Do not allow horns or masses of flesh to grow on human heads for the subsequent pleasure of having them operated on.

104. Do not misuse the abuse of the toothache. It may be that in a time to come human beings will have more solid and stronger teeth. Perhaps at that time they will be better and will no longer have recourse to the acts of clawing, slapping, biting.

(*Notebooks; Miss Nis.; 1970*)

Language, at least its spoken form with its subtle interplay of sounds and rhythms, is perhaps the most specifically human of all behaviours and is certainly one of the most complex. Language is the most universal and the most explicit mode for the expression of each individual's thoughts, and their elaboration is reciprocally related to that of language; it also provides the most direct mode of access to the thoughts of others. Thus the principal functions of language are to contribute to the thinking process and permit communication of its contents (see Chapter 2).

Language and disease are entities which interact at several points:

(a) The physician's initial entry into the patient's world is generally accomplished through their common language. All the latter's non-verbal gestures and particularly his/her facial expressions are of course of value, but in most cases, it is the patient's articulated language which orients the medical examination and thus leads directly or indirectly to a diagnosis and, where indicated, to treatment.

(b) Many tests used in psychology and psychiatry to assess intelligence, or to identify mental disturbances or acquired intellectual deterioration, are based on the analysis of linguistic productions in a standardized context (see Chapters 15 and 16).

(c) Although certain diseases may not specifically affect language, they may nevertheless be reflected in its structures (whether it be in terms of meaning which appears—but only appears—to be more immediately accessible, or in terms of form, an indicator of high validity because it is less subject to the speaker's conscious control). For example, clinical observations have led Saint-

Laurent[1] to postulate that the language of coronary patients, which is sometimes of a pseudo-agrammatic nature, generally reflects a trend towards reduced expenditure of energy. It can be easily conceived that psychoses and neuroses, which again are not specifically linguistic disorders, would also lend a particular colour to language or even, in some cases, result in some degree of disorganization: it is these linguistic aspects which are the topic of the present chapter.

(d) Finally, organic disease, when it damages certain cerebral structures, may specifically affect speech and language and sometimes, depending on the case, in a more or less isolated manner. The different clinical pictures which may then result, that is, the dysarthrias and aphasias, were the topic of several previous chapters (see Chapters 3 to 9).

The French psychiatrist Jules-Ernest Séglas (1856–1939) was probably the first to attempt to define a taxonomy of the linguistic disorders observed in various neurological and psychiatric diseases[2]. In 1892, that is, the year before Freud's monograph on aphasia[3,4] was available in Leipzig and Vienna, Séglas classified spoken language disorders under three headings: *dyslogias*, *dysphasias* and *dyslalias*:

(a) The *dyslogias* are language disturbances resulting from intellectual disorders, without impairment of the linguistic function proper: several of those discussed below would belong to this class [they might also be said to include the aspontaneity observed in the linguistic behaviour of certain patients with a lesion of the prefrontal convexity, usually on the left side (see Chapter 6)].

(b) The *dysphasias*, on the other hand, are disturbances of language proper. According to Séglas, the dysphasias include: (i) disorders of organic origin: most of the clinical forms of aphasia discussed elsewhere in this book (see Chapters 3 to 5) would belong to this class [it should be noted that Séglas worked in mental hospitals and mainly observed aphasias occurring in the context of different degenerative diseases (see Chapter 9)]; (ii) disorders of functional origin: with regard to this type, Séglas particularly emphasized a class of behaviours which he named verbal amnesia.

(c) The *dyslalias* correspond to speech disorders. Séglas observed that certain ones were related to organic malformations, for example, a cleft palate, and attributed others, such as stuttering, to poor teaching of speech.

Although the divisions of Séglas' classification are rather superficial, they bear a certain resemblance to the Sausureian's later definitions (1906) of *langue* (Chomsky's competence) and *langage* (language and speech)[5].

In the remaining pages of this chapter we shall first provide brief definitions of the clinical entities to be discussed. These definitions are intended to facilitate understanding of the material which follows and not to imply that these different states are unrelated nor of a static and immutable nature. We shall then list the major characteristics of the language of the mentally disturbed, remaining within the classical framework rather than adopting Séglas' scheme (which is logical in conception and coherent in the etymology of its terms but not easily aligned with empirical observations), and subsequently discuss anomalies of prosody and fluency, anomalies of syntax and anomalies affecting the semantic values of language. Finally we shall consider, without presenting an exhaustive review, certain phenomena observed in psychiatric patients by the use of methods from contemporary psycholinguistics.

CLINICAL DEFINITIONS OF SOME PSYCHIATRIC DISORDERS

SCHIZOPHRENIA

The term *schizophrenia* (*dementia praecox*) refers to a group of psychiatric disorders manifested by characteristic disturbances of thought, affect and behaviour. The Swiss psychiatrist Eugen Bleuler (1857–1939), who first described schizophrenic syndromes, recognized the following four major syndromes[6]:

(a) A dissociation of affect, which was the basis for the name of the disorder [σχιζω (to split) and φρηγ (mind)]; in the prototypic phase, affect may be dulled, flattened.

(b) Ambivalence of feelings and paradoxical behaviour; the patient may have a tendency to behave in regressive, infantile and bizarre ways.
(c) Autism (introversion of interest, i.e., self-centred withdrawal and loss of motivation oriented towards the external world).
(d) Thought disturbances related, according to Bleuler, to the loose association of ideas and generally leading to inadequate, or at least to unusual, interpretations of the facts of external reality.

In the hebephrenic type of schizophrenia, there is a severe disturbance of thought, a discord between thought and emotion, and a superficial, infantile and even absurd affect often manifested by silly laughs; a long string of hypochondriacal complaints is usual in these cases. On the other hand, in the paranoid type of schizophrenia, the clinical picture is dominated by delusions of persecution or, less frequently, of grandeur; the patient is distrustful, suspicious and hostile to those around him; auditory hallucinations are common. In the catatonic type of schizophrenia, behaviour may be completely suppressed (a complete rupture of relations with others and with the milieu, stupor); at the other extreme, extremely violent clastic episodes may occur, supposedly in response to hallucinatory and delusional internal stimuli.

AFFECTIVE PSYCHOSES

The term *affective psychoses* refers to a group of mental disorders marked by a predominant disturbance of mood. This may take the form of depression or of boundless elation, with both affecting the patient's contact with his environment. One speaks of *manic-depressive psychosis*, a disorder which includes a genetic component, when there are alternations between phases dominated by depression and phases dominated by emotional elation. In the *manic phase* (*mania*) the patient is elated, enterprising, loquacious and shows accelerated psychomotor activity which, in some cases, is much exaggerated. In the *depressive phase* (*melancholia*), the emotional state is characterized by sadness, self-depreciation, worry and anxiety; insomnia and anorexia are common; there is generally a slowing of mental and bodily activity, sometimes to a point of stupor; there may be illusions, hallucinations and delusions involving feelings of sadness and guilt.

One type of affective psychosis is manifested only by depression. It typically occurs as a reaction (*reactive depression*) to a particular event such as a loss or death (*pathological mourning*).

NEUROSES

The main clinical pictures to which we shall refer are as follows:

(a) *Anxiety neurosis* is dominated by a feeling of great apprehension, dread or even panic. The subject usually presents symptoms of anxiety such as palpitations, excessive sudation and insomnia (initial insomnia rather than the early-morning insomnia which is typical of depression). As a general rule, the fears are unrelated to specific objects or situations but there are cases in which the symptoms are almost *phobic* in nature (the anxiety attacks are then triggered by one or more precise factors).
(b) *Hysterical neurosis* is characterized by the presence of physical symptoms of functional origin, that is, symptoms with no organic cause. They generally appear and disappear in relation to occurrences which are symbolic of the original psychological conflict. Emotionally unstable, easily influenced and having a tendency to dramatize, the hysteric typically establishes contacts through a seductive approach but is egocentric and lacks emotional maturity.
(c) *Obsessional neurosis* is characterized by the persistent and involuntary intrusion of thoughts or chains of thought (usually completely abstract, sometimes mathematical), of impulses or acts (compulsive gestures) which the subject is unable to control. The compulsive gestures are structured into rituals which are often very complex and follow an immutable course; in typical cases, performance of the ritual allows the patient to avoid an attack of anxiety. Individuals having this type of neurosis usually have a rigid personality and are inhibited, meticulous and conformist.

CLASSICAL CONCEPTION OF THE LANGUAGE OF THE MENTALLY DISTURBED

ANOMALIES OF FLUENCY AND PROSODY

Verbal activity, or its absence, is often a good indicator of psychiatric pathology. We shall here discuss *mutism*, *aphemia*, *bradyphemia* and *logorrhoea*:

(a) Several psychiatric disturbances may be accompanied by total or near total *mutism*:
  (i) The state of profound *melancholia* observed in severe depression is often manifested by mutism. The effort of speaking appears to be an insurmountable obstacle for the patient. The mutism is then accompanied by a general reduction of activity; in differential diagnosis, it must be distinguished from the forms of akinetic mutism associated with the presence of frontal lesions, particularly tumours (see Chapters 6 and 9).
  (ii) The catatonic schizophrenic often takes refuge in the negativism of silence. This must be differentiated diagnostically from different forms of organic dementia (senile, arterosclerotic) accompanied by mental confusion and which may evolve towards mutism (see Chapter 9).
  (iii) The paranoid schizophrenic may voluntarily sever linguistic relations with an entourage which he perceives as threatening.
  (iv) The clinical picture of *infantile autism*, identified by Kanner[7-10] often includes total mutism or, less frequently, a severe reduction of verbal expression.

  The case history, the findings of the neurological examination and the mode of evolution make it easy to distinguish between the suppression initially observed in several clinical forms of aphasia, in both adults and children, and the mutism which occurs in the context of different psychiatric disorders.

(b) Broca[11, 12] used the name *aphemia* to designate the clinical pictures now known by the name of Broca's aphasia (see Chapters 1 and 4). The same term was used by Dejerine[13] to designate pure anarthria, and Goodglass and Kaplan[14] continue to use it in this way (see Chapter 10). In psychiatry, the name *aphemia* (or else *aphonia*) is used to designate a condition which is especially observed in hysteria and in war neuroses: it is generally said that the subject proves unable to emit sounds or to speak although the labial movements of speech are preserved. There is a problem in the differential diagnosis of these cases and those of *arrest of speech* (usually transient, lasting from two to seven days) occurring after cerebral lesions affecting Penfield's supplementary motor area (see Chapter 6); moreover, in several neurological centres, arrest of speech is also called *aphemia*.

(c) *Bradyphemia*, that is, a more or less severe slowing of speech, is common in most of the clinical pictures of depression. It is usually accompanied by attenuated prosody. Research has shown that there is no particular difficulty in initiating speech[15, 16], in contrast to what is observed in most aphasias associated with prerolandic lesions (see Chapters 4 and 8), but rather a uniform slowing in the production of phonemic chains. If this were necessary, the bradyphemia of the depressed can be easily distinguished from that of anarthrics and Broca's aphasics on the basis of purely linguistic criteria: besides difficulty in initiating speech, phonetic approximations and transformations are the rule in the latter case (see Chapters 2 and 4). On the other hand, bradyphemia which is quite similar to that observed in depression may be present in linguistic aspontaneity associated with certain lesions of the left prefrontal convexity (see Chapter 6).

(d) *Logorrhoea* represents the opposite extreme of the speech flow anomalies. In psychiatry, it is observed during the manic phase of manic-depressive psychosis [less frequently, in schizophasia (cf. pp. 317–327)]; and also in *hypomania*, a state of excitation (almost permanent in some cases) which is qualitatively similar to that of the manic phase but is quantitatively attenuated. The inexhaustible nature of the speech flow, as well as its apparent acceleration,* resemble aspects of

* As far as we know, this assumed component of logorrhea (abnormally rapid speech) has never been the subject of systematic study (in terms of the number of segments per unit time) in either aphasia or mania.

the logorrhoea which is observed, especially soon after onset, in certain forms of Wernicke's aphasia (see Chapter 4). However, certain differential characteristics are usually easy to identify: the logorrhoeic discourse of Wernicke's aphasics generally includes many neologisms, some degree of lexical poverty is a rule, and word-finding difficulty is always obvious (aborted sentences, repetition of determiners, prepositions, hesitations, etc.); in contrast, the logorrhoeic discourse of maniacs or hypomaniacs is often striking in terms of its lexical diversity, the numerous instances of word play and the richness of associations which seem to scramble in search of expression (one often has the impression that the subject wishes to amuse his listener). When neologisms do occur in maniacs' productions, they are less frequent than in those of jargonaphasics (soon after onset of the aphasia). In hypomania, the logico-grammatical structure of discourse is preserved and its meaning is coherent and easily identified; on the other hand, in the manic phase of manic-depressive psychosis, discourse is fragmented, incomplete [many sentences may be aborted, reflecting a *flight of ideas*, but they are not, as in aphasia, systematically broken because of failure in retrieving lexical words], and interspersed with cries or laughter.

Other suprasegmental characteristics, especially those related to timbre and vocal tone and quality, merit investigation when assessing the linguistic behaviour of psychiatric patients. They include monotone voice, whispering, cries, affected or mannered language, etc. While they may not necessarily be pathological in themselves, these characteristics may be present in the symptomatological context of different mental disorders. Thus one may see, for example, cases of severe psychotic regression in which verbal activity is progressively transformed into an indistinct, undifferentiated *mumbling* (or *muttering*) in which the phonemic segments themselves cannot be recognized (although rare and atypical, this same phenomenon also occurs in certain aphasics): there is then a total rupture of communication.

SYNTACTICAL ANOMALIES

Agrammatism and *paragrammatism* were defined elsewhere in this text (see Chapter 2). We said that agrammatism corresponds to one of the possible forms of evolution from a Broca's aphasia[17] (Hécaen[18] speaks in certain cases of *agrammatic aphasia*) and that it represents a specific (but never or almost never isolated) disorganization of syntax; we also said that paragrammatism (or dyssyntaxia) is included in the clinical picture of certain Wernicke's aphasias and that it constitutes a particular aspect of paraphasic production, that is, it does not in any way represent a specific disorganization of syntax[19] (see Chapters 4 and 10). When agrammatism is observed as a stable acquired behavioural disorganization of the maternal language [more or less severe bradyphemia; a general reduction of available vocabulary; a reduction in the number and a simplification of available syntactic structures; short sentences and a tendency to juxtaposition; omissions and substitutions specifically centred on grammatical words (see Chapter 12)], it is always, in our opinion, the manifestation of a cerebral lesion (in certain cases of depression, expression may tend towards the juxtaposition of short segments but this is intermittent and cannot be likened to agrammatism). On the other hand, paragrammatism is no doubt less pathognomonic of organic cerebral involvement. Normal discourse is not exempt from paragrammatism[20] and it is likely that the discourse of certain psychotics, particularly that of schizophrenics (inadequate selections from the inventories of prepositions and all types of conjunctions) and maniacs, includes an element of paragrammatism which is quantitatively as important as that of much jargonaphasic discourse (see Fig. 14-1). If such is the case, there would be no more reason to consider the paragrammatism of the mentally disturbed as a specific disorganization of syntax than there is to consider that of Wernicke's aphasics as a specific disorganization of syntax.

Disregarding the notions of agrammatism and paragrammatism and considering the cultural background of different individuals, it can easily be conceived how mental disorders could influence, in the same way as 'personality', the syntactical choices of different speakers. In the last section of this chapter, we shall briefly return to this aspect, still very poorly understood, of language structures in different psychiatric syndromes.

SEMANTIC DISTURBANCES

In his classification of the *dementias praecox*, the Bavarian psychiatrist Emil Kraeplin (1856–

1926)[21] used the term 'schizophasia' to designate the profound dissociation which may be indicated by the linguistic production of certain mental patients. In many respects, schizophasia appears to be the reflection, in linguistic behaviour, of the thought disturbances identified by Bleuler[6] in schizophrenia (cf. p. 315). At least on the surface—and this may be inherent in the structure of the language—the linguistic characteristics of schizophasic discourse are similar in many respects to those of jargonaphasic discourse which were described elsewhere (see Chapter 2 and Fig. 14-1). Thus differential diagnosis may sometimes be difficult from an analysis of linguistic deviations alone. However, schizophasic discourse is much more obviously episodic than jargonaphasic discourse. Furthermore, the case history and results of neurological and psychiatric examinations will permit differential diagnosis in the vast majority of cases, except perhaps in gerontology where it is often impossible to define precisely the border between psychogenic disorders and diseases of organic origin.

Using a tape-recorded sample graciously provided by Professor Gilbert Assal of the *Hôpital Cantonal Universitaire de Lausanne*, one of us (A.R.L.) attempted to describe schizophrenic discourse by comparing it to the characteristic jargon of Wernicke's aphasia proper[20]. We shall now discuss the main points of this analysis.

A *preferred theme* (see Chapter 2) is usually evident in schizophasic discourse and generally remains perceptible throughout the entire schizophasic episode: the vocabulary associated with the preferred theme is typically abstract, varied, selective and includes words belonging to all lexical inventories. The listener has the impression that the theme represents the speaker's particular concern; that words are used intentionally (i.e., that the utterances are not paraphasic) and that the schizophasic patient is satisfied with his or her use of the preferred words (s/he does not criticize them). The schizophasic theme may be delerious but it is expressed in a coherent form. It is the message. Taken from the same interview, utterances (1) to (9) illustrate the notion of a preferred theme in schizophasia:

(13.1) *'L'essentiel de tout travail à accomplir est un classement de travail correspondant à ↓au physique humain. C'est-à-dire que le physique humain, euh animal et végétal est classé d'abord, naturellement, par l'astre. Et l'humain classe l'astre également. Ce sont des classements continuels.'*

(13.2) *'Les yeux sont des appareils de photo qui classent le visuel.'*

(13.3) *'Pour occuper cette étendue de territoire, il faut faire plusieurs classements possibles ... Ça vous classe ... une base classificatrice équilibrée.'*

(13.4) *'Alors, à cette classification—si vous allez à un bord—vous classez un classement d'équilibre, puisque la base est d'équilibre. Toujours à capitale, n'est-ce pas? Vous le reposez et, au casier de classement, il y a une jauge physique, un jaugeage—n'est-ce pas?—une jauge de classement pour vérifier si on est l'équilibre ... Et je me reclasse; et je me jauge.'*

(13.5) *'L'équilibre est lu au mélangé des classements d'équilibre.'*

(13.6) *'Au total du quinzième classement, le premier est au deux, le deux est au premier.'*

(13.7) *'La guerre se prépare à classification de soldats.'*

(13.8) *'Pour dire ça en gros: le premier de l'année, je suis à début-fin; à un quinze d'un mois, je suis au milieu; et, au trente et un de fin d'année, je suis à fin-début. Et alors, le trente et un de fin-début me classe le début-fin, fin-début à milieu d'année, de début et de fin.'*

(13.9) *'Alors, c'est comme ça: on équilibre et on a charge d'équilibrer le troupeau. Et on deviant, à psychiatrie analytique, des psychiatres humano-animaliers-végétariens.'*

(13.1) 'The essential of all work to be completed is a classification of work corresponding to ↓ to the human physique. That's to say that the human physique, uh animal and vegetal is first classified, naturally by the heavenly body. And the human classifies the heavenly body as well. They are continual classifications.'

(13.2) 'The eyes are cameras which classify the visual.'

(13.3) 'To fill this stretch of territory, several possible classifications must be done ... It classifies you ... an equilibriated classificatory basis.'

(13.4) 'So, to this classification—if you go to a periphery—you classify a classification of equilibrium, then the basis is of equilibrium. Always in capital isn't it? You place it and, at the rack of classifications, there is a physical gauge, a gauging—isn't it?—a classification gauge to verify if one is the equilibrium ... And I reclassify myself, and I gauge myself.'

(13.5) 'The equilibrium is read in the blend of the classifications of equilibrium.'

(13.6) 'At the total of the fifteenth classification, the first is to the second and the second is to the first.'

(13.7) 'The war is preparing for classification of soldiers.'

(13.8) 'To state it roughly, the first of the year, I'm at beginning-end; on the fifteenth of a month, I'm in the middle; and, and on the thirty-first of the end of a year, I'm at end-beginning. And so, the thirty-first of end-beginning classifies me the beginning-end, end-beginning in the middle of the year, of beginning and of end.'

(13.9) 'So it's like that: one equilibriates and one is in charge of equilibriating the herd. And one becomes, to analytic psychiatry, some humano-animalist-vegetarian psychiatrists.'

The use of *preferred words*, or even the presence of a preferred theme, is not exceptional in the jargon of Wernicke's aphasia proper [when it is of vascular or traumatic aetiology (see Chapter 9)]. In these cases, it is almost always a transient phenomenon occurring in the initial stage of excitation and logorrhoea. The vocabulary associated with the preferred theme is typically concrete, relatively restricted and composed primarily of substantives. Despite the anosognosia (see Chapter 4), the patient may sometimes criticize, either verbally or through gestures, the ways in which he has used his preferred words: they do not correspond to his intentions and are of a paraphasic nature. The paraphasic theme is not the message but rather replaces it (one could speak of a pseudo-theme). The utterances (10) to (18) illustrate the idea of a preferred theme in jargonaphasia [the speaker's criticisms are particularly evident in (16) and (18)]158.

(13.10) '*Il y a des fois que j'*/âtʀãp/. *Mais alors, il y a des histoires: "CURÉ", par exemple: je ne comprends pas!*'

(13.11) '*Mais aucun PRÊTRE ne peut arriver à me payer.*'

(13.12) '*Il m'a été impossible de ne plus rien entendre, personne—vous voyez—de causer, de ne rien comprendre de ce que le CURÉ a dit.*'

(13.13) '*Voilà. C'est chez le PRÊTRE. Il m'a tout pris. On m'a tout pris en sortant de L'ÉGLISE, à cause de cela, justement.*'

(13.14) '*En étant chez l'ABBÉ, chez le CURÉ que j'avais là-bas, là où j'étais.*'

(2.48) '*Comment on appelle ça? un CURÉ qui cherche tous les crochets qu'il trouve?*'

(13.15) '*J'ai juste le↓ le CURÉ, en somme, presque, qui sort seulement de mes affaires, qui vient chez le PÈRE qui se sert justement quelques affaires avec des ↓ des bois que j'ai.*'

(13.16) '*Puisque tout le monde essaie, maintenant, à être PRETRE,* /di/↓ *comme mon CURÉ, tout partout dans les↓ Vous voyez: c'est ↓ c'est la parole en question, que je suis toujours en train de dire, qui m'énerve assez, que cette réponse, que la "CURÉ". Cette observation est toujours↓ Pourquoi une réponse dans↓comme ça? Vous voulez me dire? Bien! Et, à chaque fois! à chaque fois! j'ai cette parole dans la marque. Et alors, c'est celle-ci qui↓ qui↓qui a marqué. Et elle peut pas s'* /ɔbsi/↓ /ɔbsi/↓ *Rien du tout! Du tout! Rien! Rien! Rien! Non, rien! Et je* /tʀu/↓ *Et j'ai essayé, justement, le plus que je possible, sur le↓ le "CURÉ" que je dis là. Vous comprenez? Vous voyez: ce "CURÉ", il* /Raplisi/. *Toujours ce↓ Et je me demande pourquoi cet existe, pourquoi me résiste tout le temps. Mais enfin! Et alors, il y a ce* /k/↓ *ce monsieur qui est* /k/↓ *qui explique ça au* /k/↓ *au CURÉ. Il peut rien faire! Rien! Rien! Absolument rien!*'

(2.49) '*Ma soeur, elle s'est* /ãfiʀme/, *justement, dans une maladie terrible par un CURÉ qui l'a soignée justement aussi terriblement.*'

(13.17) '*Tandis que le CURÉ, lui alors je suis↓ je suis sûre que, lui, il a été tué par* /akʀ/↓ /aʀtikã/ *dans cette église-là.*'

(13.18) '*Lui, il a été soigné parce que, justement, il a été malade à cette* ÉGLISE, *parce qu'il↓ Vous voyez: c'est ça qui* /ta/ ↓ *m'agace! C'est toujours cette histoire, ce parler qui cause toujours en route. C'est↓ c'est extraordinaire! Je sais pas pourquoi!*'

(13.10) 'There are times that I /ãtrãp/. But then there are troubles: "VICAR", for example: I don't understand!'

(13.11) 'But no PRIEST will be able to pay me.'

(13.12) 'It was impossible for me to hear anything any more nobody—you see—to chat, to understand nothing of what the VICAR said.'

(13.13) 'There you are. It's at the PRIEST'S. He's taken everything from me. One took everything from me in coming out of the CHURCH, because of that exactly.'

(13.14) 'While being at the ABBOTT'S, at the VICAR'S that I had over there, there where I was.'

(2.48) 'What's it called?—a VICAR who looks for all the hooks that he finds.'

(13.15) 'I've just the↓ the VICAR, in summary, almost, who goes out only of my business, who comes to the PRIEST'S, who uses exactly some business with some ↓ some wood that I have.'

(13.16) 'Since everyone tries, now, to be a PRIEST /di/ ↓ like my VICAR all everywhere in the↓ you see: it's ↓ it's the word in question, that I'm always saying, which gets on my nerves, that this response, that the "VICAR". This observation is always ↓ Why a response in↓ like that? Do you want to tell me? Good! And, each time! each time! I have this word in the mark. And then, it's this one which↓ which↓ which has marked. And it can't /ɔbsi/↓ /ɔbsi/↓ Nothing at all! At all! Nothing! Nothing! Nothing! No, nothing! And I /tʀu/↓ And I attempted, precisely, as much as possible on the↓ the "VICAR" that I say there. You understand? You see this "VICAR" he /ʀaplisi/. Always this↓ And I wonder why this exists, why it resists me all the time. But finally! And then, there is this /k/

↓ this man who is /k/↓ who explains that to the /k/ ↓ to the VICAR. He can do nothing! Nothing! Nothing! Absolutely nothing!'

(2.49) 'My sister, she was /ɑ̃fiʀme/, exactly, in a terrible disease by a VICAR who treated her exactly as terribly.'

(13.17)'Whereas the VICAR, him, while I'm↓ I'm sure that, him, he was killed by /akʀ/↓ /aʀtikɑ̃/ in this CHURCH there.'

(13.18)'Him, he was treated because, exactly, he had been ill at this CHURCH because he↓ you see: It's that which /ta/↓ annoys me↓ It's always the same story, this talk that always chats on the way. It's ↓ it's extraordinary! I don't know why!'

Schizophasic discourse includes passages in which semantic information is reduced because of chaining based on alliteration, assonance, rhythm and formal associations [this behaviour is known as *glossomania* (Insertion 13.1)]. Denotative meaning is weakened in favour of word play and puns. Utterances (19) to (21) and (2.86) are good illustrations of this mode of expression.

(13.19)'*Et je le pose de l'autre côté de reprise; je reprends mes poids, comme ci, comme ça, et je repose les deux en même temps.*'

'And I place it on the other side of mending; I put on weight again, like this, like that, and I replace both at the same time.'

(13.20)'*Et alors, on situe le quinze avril: de début, de bout de milieu, des beaux de milieu.*'

'And then one situates the fifteenth of April: from beginning, from end of middle, of the beautiful of middle.'

(13.21)'*Mais vous commencez la nuit à six heures du soir, de minuit à six heures du matin, d'eau crépusculaire et du crépuscule d'eau.*'

'But you begin the night at six o'clock in the evening, from midnight to six o'clock in the morning, of twilight water and of the twilight of water.'

(2.86) '*Mais oui! A cette organisation de travail, il y a donc des plans d'heures et un calendrier du plan de secondes, de minutes, d'heures, d'horlogerie et d'orage. Vous appelez ça des heures-âge, des ors-âge, d'ou des tonnes-âge qui, de l'âge du début d'un certain âge par rapport au calendrier ↓ C'est-à-dire, vous savez: le calendrier possède des↓ des époques d'ères, déserts d'époque.*'

'But yes! To this organization of work there are thus some plans of hours and a calendar of the plan of seconds, of minutes, of hours, of clock-making and of storm. You call that the hours-age, the nows-age, from which the tons-age which, of the age of the beginning of a certain age compared to the calendar↓ That's to say, you know: the calendar possesses↓ [*des*] epochs [*d*] eras, deserts of epochs.'

This type of production is scarcely observed in jargonaphasia:* it requires lexical mastery well beyond that of most aphasics, as well as remarkable control of prosody. Nevertheless, the jargonaphasic may occasionally engage in this type of behaviour in long utterances—usually correct syntactically—in which the repeated use of the same word notably reduces the meaning of the sentences. As seen in the following examples, these utterances have none of the virtuosity of glossomania but do share with it the phenomenon of recurring forms:

(4.28) '*Mais malgré tout, j'arrive à faire↓—euh—à faire—euh—que le↓ que le total arrive à faire un certain bien—ah la! la! la! la!—un certain bien, et qu'on arrive à arriver à↓ à avoir des↓ . . . Il est certain que j'arrive à faire quelque chose de bien parce que j'arrive à obtenir que le raisonnement—euh—soit convenable. On arrive déjà à avoir ça . . . Enfin, on arrive quand même à arriver.*'

'But despite everything, I manage to do↓—uh—to do—uh—that the↓ that the total manages to do something good↓—ah Oh Dear!—something good and that we manage to manage to↓ to have some↓ . . . It's sure that I manage to do something good because I manage to get that the thinking—uh—is appropriate. We have already managed to have that . . . Well, one manages all the same to manage.'

(2.90) '*Mais un jour, euh, vous aurez, dans la France entière, réparti dans la France↓ Vous aurez, dans la France↓ Vous aurez la France. Vous aurez Paris qui sera, vraisemblablement, euh, une partie qui sera difficile à tenir, puis tout le reste sera↓—Je ne veux pas dire tout—dans l'ensemble, sera l'ensemble de la France, mais l'ensemble de la France sera à peu près convenable.*'

'But some day, uh, you will have, in the whole of France spread through France↓ You will have, in France↓ you will have France. You will have Paris which will be, probably, uh, a part which will be difficult to hold, then all the rest will be↓—I don't mean all—on the whole, will be the whole of France, but the whole of France will be about normal.'

In schizophasia, seemingly free chaining of phrases may also be based on conceptual rela-

* Although it may be suggested by certain utterances of conduction aphasics in which the same segment is transformed several times [see example (4.5)].

tionships* rather than on ones of form (see Chapter 2, formal glossomania and semantic glossomania):

(13.22) '*Au TERMINAL de l'année, je suis à DÉBUT de COMMENCEMENT; donc le↓ le PREMIER de l'an↓ d'un↓ d'une année↓ d'un↓ d'un calendrier est à la FIN de l'année, et l'année* [*est*] *au DÉBUT par rapport au MILIEU de l'année, qui est le CENTRE également—n'est-ce pas?—de l'année.*'

'At the TERMINAL of the year, I am at BEGINNING of the COMMENCEMENT; thus the↓ the FIRST of the year↓ of a ↓ of a year↓ of a↓ of a calendar is to the END of the year, and the year [is] to the BEGINNING compared with the MIDDLE of the year, which is the CENTRE—isn't it?—of the year.'

An analogous phenomenon, having an equally debilitating effect on sentence meaning, is sometimes observed in jargonaphasia:

(2.44) '*On s'est aperçu que, partout ailleurs, ils ont mis de PETITS COLPORTEURS et ils ont pu, avec un VESTON ... —Non! C'est pas un "VESTON"—avec de la POUDRE ... — "des POUDRES et du VESTON", j'aillais dire—avec un MANTEAU COLPORTÉ de la MEILLEURE POUDRE pour former de SUPRÊMES JUGEMENTS.*'

'We realized that, everywhere else they put LITTLE PEDLARS and they were able, with a JACKET ... No! It's not a "JACKET"—with POWDER ... — "POWDERS and a JACKET", I was going to say—with a PEDDLED JACKET of the BEST POWDER in order to form SUPREME JUDGEMENTS.'

Schizophasic production typically includes relatively rare words (in the language of the linguistic community) [see utterances (4), (21), (24), etc.]. In jargonaphasia, this phenomenon is observed only in individuals who received intensive therapy over a long period (see Chapter 17) or in those whose premorbid vocabulary was exceptionally rich (or who had a mannered style of speech).

Substitutions between conceptually related words [known as semantic paraphasias in aphasiology (see Chapter 2)] are probably just as frequent in schizophasic discourse (Insertion 13.2) as in jargonaphasic discourse. The meaning of a paraphasic segment is typically weakened but is still related to the semantic system of the linguistic community: when an aphasic says 'apple' instead of 'banana' it may be because the meanings of these two forms have become blurred so that, for the aphasic, they both refer only to 'fruit'. Although they are not usually as humorous, semantic paraphasias are thus related to the *malapropisms* of Sheridan's well-known character, Mrs Malaprop. On the other hand, the listener has the clear impression that the schizophasic's verbal substitutions are invested, either consciously or unconsciously, with highly individualized meanings which deviate from the common semantic convention and are intended—as in children's use of pig Latin—to hide the message from outsiders and to prevent linguistic sharing (*cryptophasia*). This is, for example, suggested by the choice of the two nominal syntagms in the beginning of utterance (23):

(13.23) '*Un bureau ambulant, un cadavre vivant—bureau ambulant pour certains—ou de la↓ de la terre glaise a* /fɔ/ *↓ formé, de dessus aux bases classificatrices de dessous ... un classement continuel.*'†

'An itinerant bureau, a living corpse—itinerant bureau for some—where some↓ some clay earth /fɔ/ formed, from above to the classifying bases from below ... a continual classification.'†

Using words which will be sought in vain in dictionaries of the linguistic community, certain schizophasics produce, sometimes with virtuosity, both derived and compound forms (see Chapter 2, derived monemic paraphasias, compound monemic paraphasias). The three following utterances clearly illustrate this compounding behaviour (which, in the present case, is almost always antonymic):

(2.38) '*Et alors, le vrai calendrier est différent du faux. Et le*

* As in example (2.87) it sometimes happens that within the same sentence, a word having a potential for homonymy generates associations related to more than one of its possible meanings [(2.87) '*Ce sont des campagnes. On appele ça des campagnes. C'est appelé ainsi: des villes, des villas-campagnes. Des villas-campagnes sont les fermes d'ouvre-ferme. Le vrai nom de ferme: ce sont des j'ouvre-ferme*' ('They are countries. One calls that countries. It is named thus: some cities, some country-houses. Some country-houses are farms of open-close. The real name of farm: they are some I open-close')].

† The discourse of certain schizophasic subjects contains many antonymic associations (opposite speech): as here and in (22) they may take the form of bizarre lexical choices; in certain cases they may occur in a spectacular fashion in the form of compound monemic paraphasias [see examples (8), (2.38) and (2.87)]. In this regard, the text cited at the start of this chapter includes a remarkable example: '103. Do not allow ...', etc.

calendrier georgien a été créé ainsi: ils l'ont fait d'un premier à un trente et un, et à euh plusieurs jours de↓ euh de mois—n'est-ce pas?—de /ʒ/↓ nuit et jour, et de jour-nuit. Et le quinze avril est au quinze octobre, pour l'été-hiver, et le quinze octobre est au quinze avril-ré-avril pour l'hiver-été. De telle sorte qu'on passe un été-hiver et un hiver-été, d'hiver-été ou d'été-hiver. De froid-chaud ou de chaud-froid.'

'And then, the true calendar is different from the false. And the Georgian calendar was thus created: they made it from a first to a thirty first and to uh several days of↓ uh of month—didn't they?—from /ʒ/↓ night and day and from day-night. And the fifteenth of April is on the fifteenth of October, for the summer-winter and the fifteenth of October is on the fifteenth of April-re-April for the winter-summer. In such a way that you spend a summer-winter and a winter-summer, of winter-summer or of summer-winter. Of cold-hot or of hot-cold.'

(2.87) '*Ce sont des campagnes. On appelle ça des campagnes. C'est appelé ainsi: des villes, des villas-campagnes. Des villas-campagnes sont les fermes d'ouvre-ferme. Le vrai nom de ferme: ce sont des j'ouvre-ferme ... Puis après une j'ouvre-ferme, une ferme c'est une ferme. C'est comme ça: une ferme. Vous comprenez? Et alors, il y a des joues, jours, des j'ouvre-ferme qui sont des fermes de campagne ... Alors, quand on est à ferme, on doit s'occuper de la petite santé psychique de ses animaux. Alors, évidemment, ça va pas tout seul.*'

'They are countries. One calls that countries. It is named thus: some cities, some country-houses. Some country-houses are farms of open-close. The real name of farm: they are some I open-close ... Then, after an I open-close, a farm is a farm. It's like that: a farm. You understand? And then, there are the cheeks, days, of the I open-close which are the farms of country ... Then, when one is at farm, one must take care of the small psychic health of its animals. So obviously it's not all that easy.'

(13.24)'*Je me fais ce qu'on appelle la méthode couée: couée de côté-devant-gauche ou couée de côté-devant-droite ... comme un espèce de coup de poing.*'

'I'm doing for myself what one calls the couée method: couée from the side-in front of-left or couée from the side-in front of-right ... like a sort of punch.'

Utterances (25) to (30) illustrate schizophasic derivation behaviour (which is, moreover, exemplary in terms of its morphological rigour):

(13.25)'*Tandis que, lorsqu'il commence et qu'il entre, de la vallée dans la plaine, il est à porte de communale↓ de communale↓ de↓ de* /duanʀi akapital/ (*DOUANERIE ACAPITAL*) *mais porte toujours avec lui le communal-capitale.*'

'Whereas, when he begins and he enters, from the valley in the plain, he is at door of communal↓ of communal↓ of↓ of /duanʀi akapital/ (ACAPITAL CUSTOMSRIE) but always brings with him the communal-capital.'

(13.26)'*Et ça fait quatre petits communaux à cinq. C'est à* /lɔgaʀitmi/ (*LOGARITHMIE*), *un quart d'un cinquième. Vous comprenez? ... Alors, lorsque vous êtes arrivé à capitale, d'un quart-cinquième* /lɔgaʀitmi/, *vous avez↓vous êtes d'impair-pair.*'

'And that makes four little communes to five. That is, to /lɔgaʀitmi/ (LOGARITHMIA), a fourth of a fifth. You understand? ... Then, when you arrived in capital, of a fourth-fifth /lɔgaʀitmi/, you have↓ you are of odd-even.'

(13.27)'*Àlors, lorsque je commence une année, je suis à* /fi/↓ *à* /*finitif*/ (*FINITIF*) *d'année également. Et, lorsque je suis au* /finitif/—*ou terminal—d'* /aʀ/↓ *e l'* /a/↓ *de l'année, je suis à début de commencement.*'

'So, when I begin a year, I am at /fi/↓ at /finitif/ (FINITIVE) of the year also. And, when I am at the /finitif/—terminal—of /aʀ/↓ of the /a/↓ of the year, I am at beginning of commencement.'

(13.28)'*qui est le premier* /apaʒe/ (*APPAGÉ*), *ou premier page-commis de bureau. Mais un clerc d'*/apaʒmɑ̃/ (*APPAGEMENT*) *du métier↓ c'est-à-dire qu'un* /apaʒɑ̃/ (*APPAGEANT*) *lui met l'abécédaire dans les mains. Et il commencera.*'

'who is the first /apaʒe/ (APPAGED), or first page-clerk of the office. But a clerk of /apaʒmɑ̃/ (APPAGEMENT) of the trade↓ that's to say that an /apaʒɑ̃/ (APPAGER) puts the spelling-book in his hands. And he will begin.'

(13.29)'*Il sent les* /pʀɛsyʀ/ (*PRESSURES*) *d'autour—n'est-ce pas?—et là, pose, en somme, à pas de marche, une classification* /lytyʀɛlmɑ̃/ (*LUTTURELLEMENT*) *comprise.*'

'He feels the /pʀɛsyʀ/ (PRESSATION) from around—doesn't he?—and there, places, in summary, at a walking pace, a classification /lytyʀɛlmɑ̃/ (WRESTLEY) included.'

(13.30)'*À ce milieu, on classe un quart-cinquième ... Et alors, si vous allez en communale de nouveau↓ Mais vous quittez le milieu pour regagner un des bords d'un* /kaʀtʀiɛm/ (*QUARTRIÈME*), *c'est-à-dire que vous entrez dans une commune, un* /kaʀtriɛm/ *de ce↓ d'un cinquième ... Ça nous fait un quart d'un cinquième.*'

'To this middle, one classifies a fourth-fifth ... And then, if you go in communal again↓ But you will leave the middle to recover one of the borders of a /kaʀtʀiɛm/ (QUARTRERLY), that's to say that you enter in a commune, a /kaʀtriɛm/ of this↓ of a fifth ... That makes a quarter of a fifth.'

In addition to their morphological rigour, the segments compounded and derived by schizophasics are characterized by repeated use, apparently always with the same meaning. Even if the general message remains obscure, it is clear that the compounding and derivation occurs on lexical selections which are semantically determined. As in the examples presented, they almost always belong to the same semantic fields (see Chapter 2) as the more conventional segments of the utterance in which they occur. Moreover, the schizophasic willingly justifies his lexical selections. These characteristics permit schizophasic behaviour to be distinguished from that of jargonaphasia. In addition, compound monemic paraphasias are very rare in the latter case (and never have the systematic character easily identified in those of certain schizophasics). As a general rule, derived monemic paraphasias are only slightly less uncommon. Nevertheless, there are certain cases in which they may be very numerous (in spontaneous discourse). This is illustrated by utterances (31) to (35) which were excerpted from a conversation with a Wernicke's aphasic[24]:

(13.31) '*Mais ça n'intéresse personne, les* /blɑ̃ʃaʒ/ (*BLANCHAGES*/ *avec des gens du Sud.*'

'But that does not interest anyone, the /blɑ̃ʃaʒ/ with the people of the South' (lexical component as in *BLANCH* /blɑ̃ʃ/ [white]).

(13.32) '*Dès que j'aurai des* /prɔmnaʒ/ (*PROMENAGES*), *je m'y remetterai.*'

'As soon as I will have some /prɔmnaʒ/, I will get back to it' (lexical component as in *PROMENER* /prɔmne/ [to walk]).

(2.28) '*Nous voulons avoir deux fois moins de* /fɔʀsaj/ (*FORÇAILLES*).'

'We want to have twice as little /fɔʀsaj/' (lexical component as in *FORCE* /fɔʀs/).

(13.33) '*Le* /flɑ̃byʒ/ (*FLAMBUGE*) *est complètement modifiant.*'

'The /flɑ̃byʒ/ is completely modifying' (lexical component as in *FLAMBER* (flɑ̃be/ [to burn]).

(2.30) '*Je n'ai pas voyagé en* /alʒeʀik/ (*ALGÉRIQUE*).'

'I haven't travelled in /alʒeʀik/' (lexical component as in *ALGERIEN* /alʒeʀjɛ̃/).

(2.31) '*Mon* /sɔldaʒ/ (*SOLDAGE*)—*si vous voulez—s'emploie différemment.*'

'My /sɔldaʒ/—if you like—is used differently' (lexical component as in *SOLDAT* /sɔlda/ [soldier]).

(13.34) '*C'est très* /fʀɑ̃sjɛl/ (*FRANCIEL*) *des Français, ça.*'

'That's very /frɑ̃sjɛl/ of the French' (lexical component as in *FRANÇAIS* /frɑ̃se/ [French]).

(13.35) '*On remballait à l'arrière; c'était un* /balaʒ/ (*BALLAGE*) *assez dur.*'

'They repacked at the back; it was a pretty tough /balaʒ/' (lexical component as in *REMBALLER* /rɑmbale/ [to pack up]).

As in examples (34) and (35), the lexical component of monemic paraphasias may be borrowed from the immediate context.

Some of the neologistic segments of schizophasic discourse (Insertion 13.3) are structurally similar to the phonemic paraphasias (see Chapter 2) of Wernicke's aphasics but they are, in general, relatively few in number. In contrast to their production by aphasics, neologistic segments are used intentionally by schizophasics who—despite claims to the contrary[25]—are not unwilling to give justifying explanations:

(13.36) '*Il est ambulatoire, se fait ambulatoire. Si vous marchez, vous allez comme ceci: c'est un classement de* /pa/. *Et à l'origine, le vieux dialecte de* /bo/ *s'appelle↓ C'est un* /pʀa/; *et non pas un* /pa/. *Pourquoi un* /pʀa/? *Parce que le 'P' onomatopique hiéroglyphique est à 'R'. Il est à 'R': un* /pʀa/. *Pourquoi un* /pʀa/? Parce que euh les↓ *les↓ les définitions du nom↓ des noms furent faites ainsi, pour le laïc, l'ecclésiastique ... Alors, on marche à* /pʀa/, *de* /pʀɔʃ/ *et de* /pʀɔʀʃ/. *Mais le "P" est à "R" le "R" est à "P", donc à* /pʀa/ *de* /pʀɔʀʃ/. *Et ce sont des primes. Vous comprenez? ... Et voilà ce qu'on appelle l'ambulatoire à* /pa/ *de prime, d'abord, de* /pʀɔʀʃ/, *de* /pa/ *et de roi, de roue puisqu'il a dit découvrir la roue qui↓ La première roue fut découverte au bout d'un certain temps et ils commencèrent à faire une espèce de berline-brouette.*'

'He is ambulatory, makes himself ambulatory. If you walk, you go like this: It's a classification of /pa/. And, at the origin, the old dialect of /bo/ is called↓ It's a /pʀa/; and not a /pa/. Why a /pʀa/? Because the "P" onomatopic hieroglyphic is to "R". It is to "R": a /pʀa/. Why a /pʀa/? Because uh the↓ the↓ the definitions of the name↓ the names were made thus, for the laic, the ecclesiastic ... So one walks to /pʀa/, from /pʀɔʃ/ and from /pʀɔʀʃ/. But the "P" is to "R", the "R" is to "P", thus to /pʀa/ from /pʀɔʀʃ/. And they are bonuses. You understand? ... And there is what is called the ambulatory to /pa/ at the outset, at first, from /pRɔRʃ/, from /pa/ and from king, from wheel since he said to discover the wheel which↓ The first wheel was discovered at the end of a certain time and they began to make a type of sedan-wheelbarrow.'

(13.37)'*De* /fRwa-ʃo/ *ou de* /ʃo-fRwa/. *De* /fʃowa/. *Ils↓ Ils parlaient comme ça, les anciens. Ils disaient: un* /fRʃowa/. *C'était les anciens qui parlaient ainsi.*'

'From /fRwa-ʃo/ (cold-hot) or from /ʃo-fRwa/ (hot-cold). From /fʃowa/. They↓ They spoke like that, the ancients. They said: a /fRʃowa/. It was the ancients who spoke like that.'

Utterance (37) illustrates a type of performance almost never observed in aphasics, namely, the production of phonemic sequences which violate the phonological convention of the linguistic community* (see Chapters 2 and 4). It also illustrates the structure of a particular type of phonemic paraphasia resulting from the telescoping of several words (see Chapter 14). This type of transformation is also observed in jargonaphasia [wishing a cigarette, one of our patients asked for (2.81) an /afymɛt/ which is presumably a telescopage of *fumée* (smoke), *allumette* (match) and *cigarette*]; it nevertheless seems to be proportionately more frequent in schizophasia, perhaps because it is particularly well-suited to games of semantic distortion. On the other hand, it should be noted that structurally complex phonemic transformations [(2.23) /inabituɛl/→/ɛanitabjebitil/, (13.38) /dekalœRɔ̃/→/keRadœlRɔ̃/, (2.21) /aʒɑ̃dœpɔlis/→/aplaʒɑ̃dœplɔtis/] are generally much more frequent in jargonaphasia than in schizophasia.

When Wernicke's aphasia proper results from trauma or a cerebral vascular accident, the jargon produced during the initial phases of evolution typically includes a large number of neologisms which do not meet the definition of a phonemic paraphasia nor that of a derived monemic paraphasia (see Chapters 2, 4 and 9). This is well illustrated in example (4.20).

(4.20) '*Je l'avais envoyée à école puisque, moi, je travaillais bien ... à la* /faRmid/ *de↓ de↓ de* /syz/, *n'est-ce pas, de deux* /ɛtmiR/. *Et alors, je↓. Cette* /mwazɛ/*—là—euh, GINETTE, elle s'appelle—elle↓ elle* |abil|. *Tous les jours, elle venait à Paris pour* /pale/ *dans les* /kɔsig/ *parce qu'elle prenait pour aussi↓ pour entrer, le↓ le PALAIS—le PALAIS normal, bien entendu—le* /namytyR/, *la* /tɔktœR/ *et l'*/ɑ̃bœtjɛR/, *pour qu'elle sache tous ces↓ ces CHOSES, pour qu'elle sache à bien s'*/ɛ̃skRyme/ *à bien↓ bien s'*/ɛ̃/↓ *s'*/ɛ̃kyme/.'

'I had sent her to school since I myself was indeed working ... at the /faRmid/ of ↓ of↓ of /syz/ isn't it, of two /ɛtmiR/. And then, I↓. This /mwazɛ/—there—uh, GINETTE is her name—she↓ she |abil|. Each day, she came to Paris to /pale/ in the /kɔsig/ because she was taking in order to also↓ in order to enter the↓ the PALACE—the normal PALACE of course—the /namytyR/, the /tɔktœR/ and the /ɑ̃bœtjɛR/, in order that she would know all these↓ these THINGS, in order that she would know to /ɛ̃skRyme/ herself well, to↓ to↓ /ɛ̃/↓ /ɛ̃kyme/ herself well.'

Prototypical schizophasic discourse also includes neologisms which are not assimilable to either phonemic paraphasias or derived monemic paraphasias (Insertion 13.3). Like other schizophasic segments, these neologisms are often used repeatedly, apparently with the same meaning. While the jargonaphasic is rarely able to explain the meaning of his neologisms, the schizophasic sometimes gives immediate explanations:

(13.39)'*ou en perdant la maîtrise de↓ de sa↓ de sa classification, en↓ en allant euh dire des grossièretés ... Puis il se met à engueuler la loi, n'est-ce pas? Je sais pas. C'est une espèce de maladie, de* /gRosjomiʒ/. [*Interlocuteur:* /gRosjomiʒ/?] *Oui c'est une espèce de bête. Voilà. C'est un terme que j'ai créé, que j'ai fait, comme ça pour↓ pour donner une petite base personnelle, privée. Voilà.*'

'or in losing control of↓ of his ↓ of his classification, in↓ in going uh to make rude remarks ... Then he begins to bawl out the law, right? I don't know. It's a kind of disease, of /gRosjomiʒ/. [Interlocutor: /gRosjomiʒ/?] Yes, it's a sort of beast. There you are. It's a term which I created, which I made, like that in order to↓ to give a little personal, private basis. That's that.'

The borrowing of forms from the context (/gRosjomiʒ/ in proximity to '*grossièreté*') may occur in jargonaphasia as well as in schizophasia. On the other hand, a phenomenon is observed in schizophasic discourse which probably never occurs in jargonaphasia: that is, the production of neologistic sequences corresponding to an intentional shift, through successive phonemic modifications, from one word to another word (Insertion 13.1):

* These are exceptional productions, even in schizophasia.

(13.40) '*Et la ville s'appellera euh savoir-voir, à repartition—vous comprenez?—de classement. Pendant qu'on pourra dire un savoir-devoir, un savoir-voyez, on pourra dire: la ville s'appelle "savoir", n'est-ce pas? ... C'est comme ca que les vieux faisaient les fondations. Ou bien cè cause: un* /kozam/, *un* /kozam/, *un* /klozam/, /glozan/. *Vous comprenez? Et, à ce casier, on a un savoir de Lausanne.*'

'And the city will be named uh knowledge-to see, to allotment—you understand? of classification. During which one can say knowledge-duty, a knowledge-see, one can say: the city is called "knowledge" isn't it? That's how the old people made the foundations. Or else on account of: a /kozam/, a /kozam/, a /klozam/, /glozan/. You understand? And, to his rack, one has knowledge of Lausanne.'

(13.41) '*Bien voici: Je travaille pour une firme d'ingénieurs. Vous savez↓ Des Anglais.* Ils passent par-dessus moi. Ils veulent↓ Bon, enfin, je trouve l'électricité pour eux. C'est un↓ Eux, ils exploitent le Québec. Par exemple, le climatiseur a été enlevé de ma fenêtre. On dirait que les Protestants↓ Ils prétendaient que j'arrivais en retard, parfois pire. Eux↓ Mais↓ il faudrait s'affirmer. Les lois sur l'électricité, J'ai étudié vingt ans, moi. Vous me comprenez?*'

'Well here it is: I work for an engineering firm. You know↓ The English.* They walk all over me. They want↓ Good, finally, I find electricity for them. It's a↓ Them, they exploit Quebec. For example, the air conditioner was taken from my window. One would say that the Protestants↓ They claim that I arrive late, sometimes worse. Them↓ But↓ It's necessary to assert one's self. The laws on electricity↓ I studied twenty years. You understand me?'

Insertion 13.1

In *formal glossomania*, utterances are sometimes observed in which the play on linguistic forms includes only associations between words belonging to the language; utterances are also observed in which there is a shift, through successive phonemic transformations, from one conventional word to another one. Both of these types were illustrated in the text of Chapter 13 [see (19) to (2.86) and (40)]. More often, there is a mixture of real words, which are related in form and sometimes semantically [see (22)], and neologisms:† (13.42) '*Docteur Serrano, Cyrano-Serrano, serre anneau olympique,* /pigʀyʀ/, *Rhur, Rhur. La rue Lepic où je ne peux. J'ai p'us de piqûre, de bureau. Je reste. Je pue.*' ('Doctor Serrano, Cyrano-Serrano, clenches olympic ring, /pigʀyʀ/, Rhur, Rhur. Lepic Street where I cannot. I no longer have injections, offices. I stay. I stink.') The example quoted by Chaslin[22] to illustrate the notion of *verbigeration*‡ is clearly of the same type [according to Chaslin's transcription' (13.43) '*Monsieur Vincent cinq ans, Embaude cinq ans, enfer dix ans, Emmarmet dix ans, Emmon dix ans, emcatholique dix ans.*' ('Mr Vincent five years, Embaude five years, hell ten years, Emmarmet ten years, Emmon ten years, emcatholic ten years.')]

---

* '*Quand à Drapeau, il était sorti de l'église en chantant à tue-tête:*
À cheval, gens d'armes!
À pied, Bourguignons!
Montons en Champagne,
Les Anglais y sont!
Le malheureux était devenu fou.'

('As for Drapeau, he came out of the church singing at the top of his voice:
On horse, people of arms!
On foot, Bourguignons!
Let us go to Champagne,
The English are there!
The unfortunate [fellow] had become crazy.')

[Louis Fréchette, *Originaux et Détraqués*, pp. 97–98, Beauchemin, Montréal, 1949.]

† This term is used according to the definition previously provided (see Chapter 2).

‡ A term previously used to designate discourse reduced to a kind of repetitive, anarchical litany composed of words used without meaning, chained in a compulsive manner, and produced in an oratorical tone: it was said to be observed, during the modification of consciousness associated with epileptic or demential processes, in certain toxic psychoses and, less frequently, in schizophrenia which has developed to a stage of severe regression.

We have previously maintained that production of phonemic paraphasias and of formal verbal paraphasias, in conduction aphasia and in Wernicke's aphasia proper, can be attributed to the same physiopathological mechanism (see Chapters 2 and 4, Insertion 8.5). Similarly, it seems logical to hypothesize that the origin of formal glossomaniac utterances can be attributed to a single mechanism regardless of their particular linguistic characteristics; in addition, it could reasonably be suggested that this same mechanism is also the source of other forms of schizophasic utterances [semantic glossomania, derived and compound monemic deviations; see examples (2.87), (24), (25), etc.] However this may be, it can definitely be stated that these various types of deviant segments are mixed, often almost inextricably, in typical utterances of schizophasic discourse.

Insertion 13.2

Following an approach analogous to that of Freudian analysis of slips of the tongue in 'daily life'[23], one can sometimes gain insight into the meaning of verbal substitutions noted in the discourse of psychoneurotics. Thus a French–English bilingual systematically used the word '*bureau*' (desk) to refer to a refrigerator. In this way, she managed to avoid the anxiety reaction triggered whenever she uttered the phonemic chain /fridʒ/ (frig), a slang word meaning fuck.

Schizophasic discourse is not commonly observed in a form as spectacular as that which we compared with jargonaphasia. The alterations observed in schizophrenia are frequently more subtle, with the language becoming unnecessarily detailed, the associations tangential and the themes abstract. The patient has difficulty in conveying his or her thoughts clearly. The message remains incomplete and includes many implications. This is illustrated in example (13.41) where the patient is explaining why he had come to see the physician.

There are certain cases in which the patient's discourse becomes so obscure and elliptical, includes so many blockages and unusual associations, that prosody provides the main semantic cue for the listener: there is no longer any precise message but only a general one (intellectual confusion, excitation, anxiety, aggression) conveyed by the tone.

In certain cases, and especially when glossomania dominates the picture, it may be difficult to distinguish between the discourse of schizophrenics and that of maniacs (many American authors speak of schizo-affective psychosis). The patient's verbal flow may nevertheless elicit an affective response in the listener which influences diagnostic opinions: an inclination to laugh may be experienced when listening to the discourse of maniacs while that of schizophrenics generally leaves the listener feeling perplexed and ill-at-ease.

The linguistic behaviour of the severely psychotic sometimes includes an element of echolalia. This is particularly striking in certain autistic children. We have already indicated that echolalia belongs to the clinical picture of one of the forms of Wernicke's aphasia (Type II) and of linguistic aspontaneity by a prefrontal lesion, that is, to the clinical pictures of the transcortical aphasias (see Chapters 4, 6 and 10).

PSYCHOLINGUISTIC STUDIES OF THE LANGUAGE OF PSYCHOTICS AND NEUROTICS

PSYCHOSES

Reading of contemporary studies of verbal behaviour reveals a striking change of orientation. Descriptions of symptoms and major syndromes, of the type presented in the first part of this chapter, are being replaced by a quantitative approach aimed at the identification of statistically significant differences between various clinical entities.

Insertion 13.3

The discourse of certain delirious patients may be characterized by the recurrence of one or more preferred neologisms. They sometimes refer to the central concept of the delirium: thus one patient reported that he was being persecuted by /vyʀjɛ̃/ (Vurians),* the evil, dishonest and aggressive inhabitants of /Vyʀ/ (Vur).

Taken to the extreme, the process or processes generating neologisms [see utterances (25) to (30), (36) and (37), (39) and (40)] may result in glossolalia[26–31], that is, a new language. Its lexicon, syntax, and phonological system, which are usually very simple, are generally stable and reflect the influence of conventional language. Moreover, conventional language is retained and is used between the glossolalic utterances. The patient is delirious and may contend that he is possessed by beings from a foreign country, or even from another planet, who speak through his mouth:

(13.4) *'Il y a quelqu'un qui me contrôle ... Un gars qui m'a parlé dans la tête: "Tu vas travailler pour moi" ... J'ai senti quelque chose qui rentrait dans mon corps, comme une vision qui rentrait dans mon corps ... Il était en dedans de moi ... J'entendais toujours des voix ... Je parlais comme ça, avec des termes. Ça sort tout seul ... oui, je suis poussé à parler ... La première langue que j'ai commencé à parler, c'est: La* /kɔ̃tʀabyzebiʀjasjɔ̃/ /likɔm/ /banal/ *de* /Rœkɔ̃kœʀjanis/ /ɛ̃tʀabeʀekal/ /bʀakal/ /ʀjanik/ *et* /bineʀɔmenal/ /brakal/ *de* /ʀœkɔ̃kerjasjɔ̃/ /mɑ̃mbʀan/ *d'une* /bʀideʀigasjɔ̃/ /pineʀɔmenal/ bʀaval/. *En* /ʀœkɔ̃pterjanis/ /ɛ̃tʀabeʀegal/ /bʀakal/ /ʀjanik/ *et* /bineʀɔmanal/ /brabal/ *de* /ʀœkɔ̃mdeʀjanis/ /ɛ̃tʀabeʀygal/ /bineʀɔmenal/ /bʀakal/ /ʀjanik/ *et* /bineʀɔmenal/ *donne des* /bʀideʀigasjɔ̃/ /nesɛ̃/ /pampaʀe/ /pteʀi/ /bʀakal/. *La conviction générale de* /bʀazɔm/ /paleteʀe/ /bʀakal/ *de* /ʀœkɔ̃pteʀjanis/ /ɛ̃tʀabeʀegal/ /bʀakal/ /ʀjanik/ *et* /bineʀɔ̃menal/ /bʀakal/ *de* /ʀœkɔ̃pteʀjasjɔ̃/ /lɔm/ /bʀibeʀigasjɔ̃/ /bineʀɔ̃menal/ /bʀabal/ /ʀjanik/ *et* /bineʀɔmenal/ *des* /bʀibeʀgasjɔnis/ /ɛ̃tʀabeʀygal/ /bʀakal/ /ʀjanik/ *et* /pineʀɔmenal/. *La* /bʀakal/ /bineʀɔ̃menal/ /bʀakal/ /ʀjanik/ *et* /bineʀcmenal/ /bʀakal/ *de* /ʀœkɔ̃pteʀjasjɔ̃/ /bineʀɔ̃menal/ /bʀakal/ *de* /ʀœkɔ̃pteʀjanis/ /ɛ̃tʀabeʀekal/. *Là, je parlais comme ça ... Je répète des mots à plusieurs reprises parce que je suis obligé de les employer ... je répète souvent les mêmes mots mais ils veulent pas dire la même chose ... Ce qui m'arrive, faut que ça arrive. Moi, je prétends que tout le monde est contrôlé, tout le monde est TIMÉ.'*

'There's someone who controls me ... A guy who spoke in my head: "You're going to work for me. I kept hearing voices ... I spoke like that, with some terms. It comes out all by itself ... yes, I'm urged to speak ... The first language that I began to speak, it's: the /kɔ̃tʀabyzebiʀjasjɔ̃/ /likɔm/ /banal/ of /ʀœkɔ̃kœʀjanis/ /ɛ̃tʀabeʀekal/ /bʀakal/ /ʀjanik/ and /bineʀɔmenal/ /brakal/ of /ʀœkɔ̃kerjasjɔ̃/ /mɑ̃mbʀan/ of a /bʀideʀigasjɔ̃/ /pineʀɔmenal/ /bʀaval/. In /ʀœkɔ̃pterjanis/ /ɛ̃tʀabeʀegal/ /bʀakal/ /ʀjanik/ and /bineʀɔmanal/ /brabal/ of /ʀœkɔ̃mdeʀjanis/ /ɛ̃tʀabeʀygal/ /bineʀɔmenal/ /bʀakal/ /ʀjanik/ and /bineʀɔmenal/ gives some /bʀideʀigasjɔ̃/ /nesɛ̃/ /pampaʀe/ /pteʀi/ /bʀakal/. The general conviction of /bʀazɔm/ /paleteʀe/ /bʀakal/ of /ʀœkɔ̃pteʀjanis/ /ɛ̃tʀabeʀegal/ /bʀakal/ /ʀjanik/ and /bineʀɔmenal/ /bʀakal/ of /ʀœkɔ̃pteʀjasjɔ̃/ /lɔm/ /bʀibeʀigasjɔ̃/ /bineʀɔmenal/ /bʀabal/ /ʀjanik/ and /bineʀɔmenal/ of the /bʀibeʀgasjɔnis/ /ɛ̃tʀabeʀygal/ /bʀakal/ /ʀjanik/ and /pineʀɔmenal/. The /bʀakal/ /bineʀɔmenal/ /bʀakal/ /ʀjanik/ and /bineʀɔmenal/ /bʀakal/ of /ʀœkɔ̃pteʀjasjɔ̃/ /bineʀɔmenal/ /bʀakal/ of /ʀœkɔ̃pteʀjanis/ /ɛ̃tʀabeʀekal/. There, I spoke like that ... I repeat words several times because I'm bound to use them ... I often repeat the same words but they don't mean the same thing. What happens to me, it must happen. I pretend that every one is controlled, everyone is TIMÉ.'
controlled, everyone is TIMÉ.'

The jargonaphasia of Wernicke's aphasics very rarely occurs in an almost totally neologistic form [see example (2.84)]; when this does occur, conventional language is, of course, no longer available, the patient is completely anosognosic and the phonemic combinations which he produces may be much more varied than in the above sample of glossolalia. To our knowledge, this form of Wernicke's jargonaphasia has a poor prognosis and is only observed among the elderly.

* Perhaps a phonemic transformation of /vɔʀjɛ̃/ vaurien (a worthless individual)?

Schizophrenia, which was of great interest to the early psychiatrists, has particularly attracted the attention of contemporary investigators. The variations in the different clinical pictures, depending on the evaluators, the subjects and the cultures studied, lead us to believe that all of these mental disturbances should preferably be considered in terms of *schizophrenic disorders*. It should also be noted that the actual existence of this psychosis has been challenged by Szasz[32] and other writers. As stated by Lorenz[33], a linguist, 'We are faced with a paradox that while we recognize schizophrenic language when we see it, we cannot define it'.

This chapter does not include an exhaustive review of the available literature. Our intention is rather to provide brief descriptions of the most conclusive studies and information on new techniques employed. We did not consider it worth while, in the present context, to review the many hypotheses on the aetiology of schizophrenia. Readers wishing to pursue this topic should consult the bibliography.

By the use of vocabulary measures such as Type Token Ratio, that is, the relation between the number of different words and the total number of words in a language sample, it has been possible to distinguish between acute schizophrenic reactions, associated with a high ratio, and chronic schizophrenic processes, associated with a low ratio. The vocabulary of chronic schizophrenics is simplified and contracted whereas diversity is retained by acute psychotics. However these data do not permit identification of the degree of non-conformity in the language of these two groups. Similarly, responses on certain tests of distraction appear to be different for hebephrenics and the organically demented, who are both unable to filter pertinent information, and paranoid subjects, who retain the ability to attend selectively[34, 35].

A comparison of patients from different diagnostic categories with normal speakers in a standardized verbal situation indicated that paranoid schizophrenics use fewer pronouns than normal. This global reduction essentially reflected a decrease in the use of 'I'. On the other hand, there was an increase in the use of 'he': projecting his or her phantasies on others, the paranoid refers to them as the subjects of the action[36].

Several investigators have compared the association processes of schizophrenics and normal controls. It should be noted that the obtained results are indicative of a disorder of thought (as described by Bleuler[6]) rather than of language. The schizophrenic tends to make syntagmatic rather than paradigmatic associations [(13.45) '*chaise*' (chair)→'*assis*' (seated), rather than '*table*'; (13.46) '*chat*' (cat)→'*noir*' (black), rather than '*chien*' (dog)]. The words evoked by schizophrenics sometimes appear to be the last link in an associative chain, whereas normal subjects usually say the first word which comes to mind. It is difficult to maintain the schizophrenic's concentration on the task and thus it is often necessary to repeat the stimulus segment. Moreover, the reported associations often refer to the patient's experiences and emotions vis-à-vis the stimulus word. For example, given the word (13.47) '*violin*' (violin), a patient replied '*Je n'aime pas ça*' (I don't like that) rather than saying '*musique*' (music) or '*concert*', the usual responses of normals. In other instances, when the stimulus is a concrete word referring to an object, the schizophrenic often responds according to object use: (13.48) '*table*'→'*manger*' (eat); (13.49) '*soulier*' (shoe)→'*marcher*' (to walk). Less commonly, in cases of severe regression, perseverative phenomena may be observed: (13.50) '*menuiserie*' (carpentry)→'*bois*' (wood), '*chemin de fer*' (railway)→'*bois*', '*budget*'→'*bois*'. Neologisms are also rare:* (13.51) '*femme*' (woman)→/ɔmʀi/.

Chapman's work[37] has been followed by several studies of association processes in schizophrenics. The experimental task usually requires the interpretation of a sentence containing an ambiguous element ('John offered a perch to Jim', a sentence occurring in a context in which it was mentioned that Jim fell in the water while the two friends were fishing). The ambiguous element generally has two possible meanings, with one being much more common than the other. Several variables then affected the patient's choices and distinguished them from those of the control subjects. Indeed, schizophrenics did not appear to consider the context of the sentence and accepted the commonest meaning of the ambiguous word. It was suggested that these results might explain the schizophrenic's difficulty in evaluating reality and in communicating with others. In other studies, schizophrenic patients were given a similar task

---

* In this case, a monemic paraphasia (see Chapter 2), lexical component as in /ɔm/ *HOMME* (man).

but, in addition to being ambiguous, the stimulus words had emotional connotations. The presence of affective stimuli exaggerated the schizophrenic processes and forced the patients to interpret words by avoiding meanings which were disagreeable to them even if this meant accepting the less common association. When stimuli for the interpretation task were presented within a multiword context, schizophrenics had less difficulty in interpreting ambiguous words when the context favoured an immediate interpretation[38]. However, when the cue to the correct interpretation was situated later on in the passage, they were unable to use it. Finally, it should be noted that the schizophrenic's associations are unstable: unlike normal subjects, they tend to produce new associations if the experimental task is repeated after an interval of some weeks[39,40].

In the *cloze procedure*, words within a text are systematically deleted at regular intervals[41] and the subject must then fill in the blanks in the incomplete sentences. This procedure was used in a study of schizophrenics and normal controls who were required to complete texts written by other schizophrenics and by other normal subjects. The schizophrenics not only had difficulty in completing the schizophrenics' texts but also those of normals and, in both cases, were less successful than control subjects[42]. Wishing to evaluate the effects of context on this type of procedure, words were also deleted from texts of different length, namely, 3, 5, 9, 17 and 29 words. In each case, the patient was asked to fill in the word which was missing from the middle of a statement. The results were analysed in terms of the number of correct responses (retrieval of the exact word omitted) and, for the others, in terms of the syntactical class and the semantic characteristics of the suggested words[43]. These tasks revealed systematic differences between chronic and acute schizophrenics. Disorganization and failure on the experimental tasks increased with increasing length of hospitalization. Schizophrenics paid less attention to contextual constraints than normal controls. In addition, schizophrenics made both semantic and syntactical errors whereas normal controls, if they erred at all, made only semantic type errors. It is interesting to note that impaired conservation of syntactical class was observed in all schizophrenics whether their disorder was chronic or acute[44,45].

Using a standardized test, Irigaray[46] asked subjects to complete a sentence in the shortest and simplest way using certain words provided by the examiner. On this test, the performance of demented subjects and schizophrenics could be distinguished from three points of view: syntactical, lexical and semantic. In the demented, the syntagmatic and transformational models remained intact and complex but there was, in contrast, a loss of lexical stability; these patients could not deal with ambiguity and multiple meanings. On the other hand, the schizophrenics used rules for amusement, commented on the test, and played with the semantic values of words. Their compositions included incomplete sentences, sometimes lacking a verb. Substantives and adjectives were emphasized and neologisms were observed occasionally. Schizophrenics sometimes used the words proposed by the examiner to take off on a whim; for example (13.52) when the word '*mère*' (mother) was presented, a patient formed the associations '*maire*' (mayor) and '*mer*' (ocean) and then used these words to complete the test sentences (cf. p. 51; formal glossomania).

Noting that dissociation (*spaltung*, in Bleuler's[6] terminology) remains a rather vague concept for most clinicians, Rochester and her collaborators[47] at the University of Toronto attempted to define it in terms of reduced cohesion in schizophrenic discourse. This was investigated by evaluating interviews with patients and with normal subjects from three points of view: the referential process, the use of conjunctions, and the lexical relations between words as indicated by repetitions or the use of synonyms or words having the same root. The schizophrenics systematically used fewer conjunctions but more lexical relations (especially repetition). The authors considered that the cohesion of these patients' discourse was weakened by the absence of conjunctions indicating the logical connections between sentences and prepositions. Furthermore, the patients often failed to specify the referent for their nominal syntagms which required textual antecedents.

After analysing a conversational speech sample, Chaika[25] suggested that the six following linguistic characteristics are pathognomonic of *schizophrenic language*:

(a) *Sporadic impairment of the ability to match semantic features with phonemic chains corresponding to lexical items in the language.*
(b) *Significance given to too many of the semantic features of particular words in discourse.*
(c) *Inappropriate noting of the phonological features of particular words in discourse.*

(d) *Sentence production which is influenced by the phonological and semantic features of previously uttered words rather than by a conversational topic* (*cf. p. 51, concepts of formal glossomania* and *semantic glossomania*).
(e) *Disturbance of the ability to apply syntactical and discourse rules.*
(f) *Lack of self-monitoring, that is, unawareness of deviant productions.*

With the exception of the last one [see examples (36) (37) and (39)], the characteristics specified by Chaika provide an adequate linguistic definition of schizophasic discourse. They probably also provide, as one of us (A.R.L.) and Vanier[20] have shown, an adequate linguistic definition of several forms of jargonaphasia or even of some deviations observed in normal discourse (see Chapter 14). In other words, from a linguistic point of view, it is quantitative, rather than qualitative, differences which permit distinctions between schizophasic discourse, jargonaphasic discourse and normal discourse (see Fig. 14.1); these distinctions are also based on the listener's interpretations of the relationships between the speaker's thoughts and utterances.

In closing this discussion of language characteristics associated with schizophrenia, mention should be made of studies of interpersonal and familial communication (although they are not, strictly speaking, linguistic). Those who have investigated this subject agree in saying that communication is idiosyncratic within families having a schizophrenic member. The young schizophrenic appears to represent a familial symptom resulting from a linguistic pathology. These investigators have apparently been able to differentiate between control and 'schizophrenigenic' families in terms of their mode of communication. In pathological families, parental styles apparently differ in the sense that the mother conveys apathy and defeat in her messages while the father openly reveals his distrust and suspicion. Because attempts to satisfy the demands of one parent are associated with fears of rejection by the other, the child is often trapped and thus obliged to divide word meanings. Skewed messages, which encourage the child to remain a 'baby' but at the same time require that s/he be emotionally mature, place him or her in an intolerable situation[48]. In the following excerpt from family therapy, a 19-year-old schizophrenic is describing how she is attempting to live alone in an apartment despite her parents' opposition. Her mother is continuing to demand that she return home for regular meals because, in the mother's opinion, her daughter was letting herself starve to death.

(13.53) *La mère: 'Etant malade, tu ne sais pas ce que tu veux.'*
La fille: 'Tu me traites en enfant.'
La mère: 'Mais tu est mon enfant.'

Mother: 'Being sick, you don't know what you want.'
Daughter: 'You treat me like a child.'
Mother: 'But you are my child.'

Although the word 'child' is clearly used by the mother to indicate her maternal relationship, it is also used to deny her daughter's wish for independence and maturity. In this type of situation, communication becomes fragmented, erratic and illogical. The child has difficulty in learning how to focus attention on what is significant and interprets language in more personal, or even hermetic, terms. Thus language loses its importance as an adaptive tool in dealing with new, reality-based situations.

The best-known hypothesis (formulated by the Palo Alto group[49]) is that of double-bind messages. It illustrates how the patient is caught in a linguistic paradox created by his family; s/he is deprived of metalinguistic ability, unable to criticize the communication and, therefore, obliged to support the harmful consequences. The typical double-bind message includes two directly conflicting levels: thus, 'Be spontaneous' becomes 'Control yourself'. It is clearly impossible to respond adequately to such messages.

Language in the affective psychoses has attracted much less attention than in schizophrenia. In mania, flights of ideas, word games and acceleration of the speech flow have been pointed out, as has an increase in the speed of association and a decrease in the selection of ideas and the inhibition of details. This results in aimless language filled with tangential responses which vary in length according to the extent of the speaker's digression from the original stimulus. Except in extreme cases, syntax and prosody retain their richness and diversity. There is no major distortion of language, but words are occasionally slurred because of the very rapid rate of speech. The style is sometimes telegraphic, revealing the patient's desire to report, as concisely as possible, every idea which has come to mind. The maniac has a fondness for extreme terms ('extraordinary', 'terrifying') and his/her

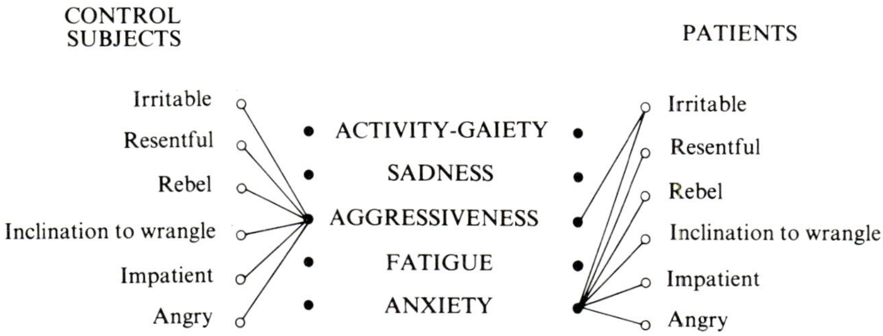

Fig. 13–1 *Misunderstanding of designated emotions: for the control subjects the stimuli 'rebel', 'impatient', 'angry', etc., refer to feelings of aggressiveness; for the depressed subjects, the same stimuli refer to feelings of anxiety. See commentary in the text. Adapted from Roy, Pinard and Tétreault*[52].

style is often affected, pedantic and pretentious[50].

The depressed, on the other hand, have been the subject of a larger number of studies. Certain investigators have attempted to distinguish between language in psychotic versus neurotic depression and it appears that certain physical characteristics of the voice are the most revealing in this regard. In psychotic depression, unlike neurotic depression, the articulation of stops—such as /d/ and /t/—is flaccid and loose. Pitch is modified by a narrowing in the range and by a lack of variation. Stress often disappears and resonance often becomes naso-pharyngeal[51].

In psychotic depression, research done in Montreal indicated the presence of semantic confusion in relation to emotional experiences. The subjects become unable to differentiate words designating sadness, anxiety and fatigue[52]. Moreover, words reflecting feelings of 'anger–aggressiveness' may even disappear from the patients' lexicon. Indeed, words which control subjects judged to connote aggressiveness were considered by patients to refer to anxiety. The emotional semantic field which appeared to be most intact represented gaiety and activity, a more salubrious ground where the judgements of controls and the psychotically depressed overlapped. The results seemed to suggest that, having lived with sadness, anxiety and fatigue simultaneously, the depressed patient referred to this experience as an indivisible whole (rather than to a dictionary) in order to define the stimulus words. The almost complete absence of words signifying 'aggressiveness' may indicate repression of the meaning 'anger' and displacement towards another meaning, namely 'anxiety'[53, 54] (Fig. 13–1).

The content of discourse in psychotic depression has also been studied in two different situations. Compared with that of normal controls, the discourse of the depressed was found to include more self-references, negative syntactical constructions, value judgements and references to the experimental situation. The greater number of references to the experimental situation was interpreted as an attempt to avoid discussion of personal problems. The patients spoke more often than controls about emotional topics, a finding which might be readily explained by supposing that they speak of their sadness and anxiety. Nevertheless, a comparison of a depressed patient's discourse before and after treatment indicated that the number of statements with basic personality than to verbal behaviours which of the patient's state. Thus it may be that the depressed are more aware of their own feelings than are normal subjects. Improvement of the depressive state was also accompanied by the appearance of the ability to express nuances. Similarly, expressions of politeness were used more frequently, suggesting renewed appreciation of the significance of conversational rituals. On the other hand, value judgements, utterances retracting previous affirmations, and negative constructions were unaffected by improvement even though they had been found to be much more frequent in the depressed than in normal controls. It is possible that these criteria correspond more closely to indicators of the patients' basic personality than to verbal behaviours which are specific to the symptomatically depressed[55].

Changes occurring in the syntactical complexity of discourse during recovery from depression have also been analysed[56] in terms of the number of simple sentences (including a nominal syntagm and a verbal syntagm) and complex sentences (including embedding). After treatment, the patient produced more complex sentences but they were of a particular type. While he produced more object subordinates, there was no significant increase in the use of relatives and adverbials. It should be noted that certain linguists consider object subordinates (and not relatives) as a good index of complexity. The former appears later in language development and in second language acquisition. In contrast, relatives may be used to bypass failures in word retrieval: (13.54) '*le monsieur qui fait du pain*' (the man who makes bread) to replace the word '*boulanger*' (baker). Thus the use of relatives would not be a valid indicator of complexity.

In summary, verbal behaviour in psychotic depression appears to differ from that in neurotic depression mainly in terms of physical characteristics of the voice. On the other hand, psychotics differ from normal in speaking more slowly, in speaking on a single theme and in referring more often to themselves or their feelings. They use impoverished syntax and have lost the rituals of communicative exchanges.

NEUROSES

Balkan and Masserman[57] described the verbal behaviour of three groups of neurotic patients when producing phantasies in response to Morgan–Murry Test Cards (Thematic Apperception Test). The cards depicted rather vague characters in ambiguous situations. In this study, the conversion hysterics presented the following characteristics: productions of medium length including much descriptive material but very few actions. These results were confirmed in other studies through calculation of the verb/adjective ratio. It was found to be low in conversion hysterics, leading the authors to conclude that there was little action in the patients' stories. There were few nuances and little ambivalence, as indicated by the certainty–uncertainty quotient, the pro–con quotient and the small number of statements in the form of alternatives. There were few personal references, as indicated by the narrator's identification with a character or by use of the pronoun 'I'[58]. The hysterical patients did not appear anxious and freely questioned the examiner. It was also noted that conflicts were repressed at an unconscious level, that the phantasies showed little aggression or eroticism, and that their affective content focused on organic dysfunctions (which were attributed to the characters shown on the cards).

In contrast, the phantasy descriptions of anxiety state patients were very short and had the highest verb–adjective quotient, reflecting the pre-eminence of action. Alternatives of conation (desire) were evident; hesitations, vagueness and trepidation were frequent. The narrator often identified with characters in his phantasy. The affective symbolism was immediate, and conflicting situations were not resolved.

The language of obsessive–compulsives resembled that of anxiety state patients[57] but the former showed a need to rationalize and elaborate the many ambivalences and uncertainties in their descriptions. These patients were found to have the lowest certainty–uncertainty quotient. Meticulous conversational rituals greatly increased the length of their productions. The obsessive–compulsives had a high verb–adjective quotient which was viewed as a manifestation of the level of anxiety. The narrator often identified with characters in his phantasy.

The above results have been confirmed by other investigators who counted different constituents of discourse[59]. These studies showed that hysterical patients use mainly the second person and the present tense, thus speaking to others of immediate topics, whereas obsessive–compulsives often spoke of the past as it concerned them personally, and used many adverbs and attributive adjectives. Besides using the present tense, hysterical patients often used the imperfect, which creates a greater impression of immediacy than does the past tense. They also showed a fondness for emphasis, spectacular gestures and a theatrical tone; in contrast, obsessive–compulsives took refuge in detailed, intellectual language which contained many comparisons, negations, retractions, measures and quantifications but included few assertions. The few which were made were often qualified in subsequent remarks.

Most of the studies reviewed in the present chapter were undertaken with the aim of interpreting the obtained results in terms of theoretical hypotheses about neurosis and psychosis. Since these considerations are unrelated to the subject of the present book, we have intentionally limited our discussion to the description of language behaviours and avoided drawing conclusions about the extent to which the results agree or conflict with different hypotheses. Our only goal was to emphasize that the verbal behaviour of psychiatric patients may be specific enough to orient the clinician's diagnosis and, when the occasion arises, to permit the description of changes (e.g. changes related to therapy).

REFERENCES

1. Saint-Laurent, C. (1979) *Communication personnelle.*
2. Séglas, J.E. (1892) *Troubles du langage chez les aliénés.* Paris: Rueff.
3. Freud, S. (1891) *Zur Auffasung der Aphasien.* Vienna: Deuticke.
4. Freud, S. (1953) *On Aphasia; a Critical Study.* New York: International Universities Press.
5. Saussure, F. (de) (1967) *Cours de linguistique générale.* Paris: Payot.
6. Bleuler, E. (1966) *Dementia Praecox, or the Group of Schizophrenias.* New York: International Universities Press. (First edition in 1911.)
7. Kanner, L. (1943) Autistic disturbances of affective contact. *Nervous Child,* **2,** 217.
8. Kanner, L. (1944) Early infantile autism. *Journal of Pediatrics* **25,** 211.
9. Kanner, L. (1946) Irrelevant and metaphorical language in early infantile autism. *American Journal of Psychiatry,* **103,** 242.
10. Kanner, L. (1949) Problems of nosology and psychodynamics of early infantile autism. *American Journal of Orthopsychiatry,* **19,** 416.
11. Broca, P. (1865) Du siège de la faculté du langage articulé. *Bulletin de la Société d'Anthropologie,* **7,** 377.
12. Broca, P. (1869) Sur les mots aphémie, aphasie et aphrasie. Lettre à M. le professeur Trousseau. In *La naissance de la neuropsychologie du langage* (Ed.) Hécaen, H. & Dubois, J. p. 267. Paris: Flammarion.
13. Déjerine, J. (1914) *Séméiologie des affections du système nerveux.* Paris: Masson.
14. Goodglass, H. & Kaplan, E. (1972) *The Assessment of Aphasia and Related Disorders.* Philadelphia, PA: Lea and Febiger.
15. Pinard, G., Roy, J.Y. & Tétreault, L. (1972) Etude du comportement verbal dans la dépression psychotique. *Revue de Psychologie appliquée,* **22,** 229.
16. Pinard, G. & Tétreault, L. (1973) Le langage des déprimés psychotiques. *Union médicale du Canada,* **102,** 2282.
17. Alajouanine, Th. & Lhermitte, F. (1960) Les troubles des activités expressives du langage dans l'aphasie; leurs relations avec les apraxies. *Revue neurologique,* **102,** 66.
18. Hécaen, H. (1972) *Introduction à la neuropsychologie.* Paris: Larousse.
19. Lecours, A.R. (1975) Aphasie. *Encyclopédie médico-chirurgie, 17020 A^{10},* 7.
20. Lecours, A.R. & Vanier-Clément, M. (1976) Schizophasia and jargonaphasia. A comparative description with comments on Chaika's and Fromkin's respective looks at 'schizophrenic' language. *Brain and Language,* **3,** 516.
21. Kraepelin, E. (1896) *Psychiatrie, ein Lehrbuch für Studierende und Arzte.* Leipzig: Barth.
22. Chaslin, Ph. (1912) *Eléments de sémiologie et de clinique mentale.* Paris: Asselin-Houzeau.
23. Freud, S. (1967) *Psychopathologie de la vie quotidienne.* Paris: Payot.
24. Lecours, A.R. & Lhermitte, F. (1972) Recherches sur le langage des aphasiques: 4. Analyse d'un corpus de néologismes; notion de paraphasie monémique. *Encéphale,* **61,** 295.
25. Chaika, E.O. (1974) A linguist looks at 'schizophrenic' language. *Brain and Language,* **1,** 257.
26. Flournoy, Th. (1900) *Des Indes à la planète Mars; étude sur un cas de somnambulisme avec glossolalie.* Paris: Alcan.
27. Cénac, M. (1925) *De certains langages créés par les aliénés: contribution à l'étude des 'glossolalies'.* Medical thesis, Paris.
28. Bobon, J. (1952) *Introduction historique à l'étude des néologismes et des glossolalies en psychopathologie.* Paris: Masson.
29. Laurentin, R. (1974) *Pentecôtisme chez les catholiques—risques et avenir.* Paris: Beauchesne.
30. Lecours, A.R. & Kock, J. (de) (1977) Sprachlich Neugebildete Segmente und Glossolalie. *Review of Applied Linguistics,* **37,** 3–17.
31. Lecours, A.R., Lebrun, Y. & Vanier-Clément, M. (1979) La glossolalie. In *Neurolinguistics* (Ed.) Hoops, R. & Lebrun, Y. Amsterdam: Swets and Zeitlinger.
32. Szasz, T. (1961) *The Myth of Mental Illness.* New York: Harper.
33. Lorenz, M. (1968) Problems posed by schizophrenic language. In *Language Behavior in Schizophrenia* (Ed.) Vetter, H.J. Chicago IL: Rand McNally.
34. Maher, B. (1966) *Principles of Psychopathology.* New York: McGraw-Hill.
35. Maher, B. (1972) The language of schizophrenia: a review and interpretation. *British Journal of Psychiatry,* **120,** 3.
36. Lorenz, M. & Cobb, S. (1954) Language patterns in psychotic and psychoneurotic subjects. *Archives of Neurology and Psychiatry* (Chicago), **72,** 665.
37. Chapman, L.J. (1960) Confusion of figurative and literal usages of words by schizophrenics and brain damaged patients. *Journal of Abnormal Social Psychiatry,* **60,** 412.
38. Moran, L.J. (1953) Vocabulary knowledge among normal and schizophrenic subjects. *Psychology Monographs,* **20,** 67.
39. Maltzman, I., Simon, R. & Fecht, K. (1962) Verbal

conditioning by common and uncommon word associations. *Psychology Reports*, **10,** 363.
40. Sommer, R., Whitney, G. & Osmond, H. (1962) Teaching common association to schizophrenics. *Journal of Abnormal Social Psychiatry*, **65,** 58.
41. Taylor, W.L. (1953) Cloze procedure: a new tool for measuring readability. *Journalism Quarterly*, **30,** 415.
42. Honigfeld, G. (1963) The ability of schizophrenics to understand normal, psychotic and pseudo-psychotic speech. *Diseases of the Nervous System*, **24,** 692.
43. Salzinger, K., Portnow, S. & Feldman, R.S. (1963) Verbal behavior of schizophrenic and normal subjects. *Annals of the New York Academy of Sciences*, **105,** 845.
44. Salzinger, K., Portnow, S. & Feldman, R.S. (1960) Verbal behavior in schizophrenics. In *Psychopathology of Schizophrenia* (Ed.) Hock, P.H. & Zubin, J. New York: Grune and Stratton.
45. McGhic, A. (1965) Psychological studies of schizophrenia. In *Studies on Psychoses* (Ed.) Freeman, T., Cameron, J.L. & McGhic, A. London: Tavistock Publications.
46. Irigaray, L. (1968) Epreuve de production de phrases chez les déments et les schizophrènes. *Psychologie française*, **13,** 157.
47. Rochester, S.R., Martin, J.R. & Thurson, S. (1977) Thought-process disorder in schizophrenia: the listener's task. *Brain and Language*, **4,** 95.
48. Lidz, T.H. (1971) Family settings that produced schizophrenic offsprings. In *Problématique de la psychose* (Ed.) Doucet, P. & Laurin, C. P. p. 196. Amsterdam: Excerpta Medica Foundation.
49. Watzlawick, P., Beavin, J.H. & Jackson, D.D. (1967) *Pragmatics of Human Communication*. New York: W.W. Norton.
50. Eisenson, J., Auer, J.J. & Irwin, J.V. (1963) *The Psychology of Communication*. New York: Appleton-Century Crofts.
51. Newman, S. & Mather, V.G. (1938) Analysis of spoken language of patients with affective disorders. *American Journal of Psychiatry*, **94,** 913.
52. Roy, J.Y., Pinard, G. & Tétreault, L. (1971) Adjectif significant et sentiment signifié. *Revue de Psychologie appliquée*, **21,** 133.
53. Pinard, G. & Tétreault, L. (1974) Concerning semantic problems in psychological evaluation. In *Psychological Measurement in Psychopharmacology* (Ed.) Pichot, P. & Oliver-Martin, R. p. 8. Paris: Karger.
54. Pinard, G. & Tétreault, L. (1974) Concerning semantic problems in psychological evaluation. *Modern Problems in Pharmacopsychiatry*, **7,** 8.
55. Pinard, G., Roy, J.Y. & Tétreault, L. (1972) Etude du comportement verbal dans la dépression psychotique. *Revue de Psychologie appliquée*, **22,** 229.
56. Pinard, G. & Tétreault, L. (1974) Evaluation de la complexité syntaxique dans la dépression psychotique. *Revue de Psychologie appliquées*, **24,** 103.
57. Balken, E.R. & Masserman, J.H. (1940) The language of phantasy: patients with conversion hysteria, anxiety state, obsessive-compulsive neuroses. *Journal of Psychology*, **10,** 75.
58. Lorenz, M. (1955) Expressive behavior and language patterns. *Psychiatry*, **18,** 353.
59. Haag, M. & Feline, A. (1968) Une stylistique quantitative du langage oral des hystériques. *Confrontations psychiatriques*, **1,** 119.

BIBLIOGRAPHY

Andreasen, N.J. & Pfohl, B. (1976) Linguistic analysis of speech in affective disorders. *Archives of General Psychiatry*, **33,** 1361.

Andreasen, N.J., Tsuang, M.T. & Canter, A. (1974) The significance of thought disorder in diagnostic evaluations. *Comprehensive Psychiatry*, **15,** 27.

Angyal, L. (von) (1933) Uber den subkortikalen Anteil de schizophrenen Sprachstörungen. *Monatschrift für Psychiatrie und Neurologie*, **86,** 137.

Averback, A. (Ed.) (1959) *Schizophrenia*. New York: Ronald Press.

Bernard, P. & Bobon, J. (1964) Le 'Rinhâûzhâîrhhâûsês: néomorphisme compensatoire chez un paraphrène débile. *Acta Neurologica Belgica*, **64,** 65.

Bianco, P. (del) (1957) Schizophasie et cybernétique. Etude de statistique linguistique. *Acta Neurologica Belgica*, **57,** 937.

Blaney, P.H. (1974) Two studies on the language behavior of schizophrenics. *Journal of Abnormal Psychology*, **1,** 23.

Bleuler, E. (1966) *Dementia Praecox or the Group of the Schizophrenias*. New York: International Universities Press.

Bobon, J. (1952) *Introduction historique à l'étude des néologismes et des glossolalies en psychopathologie*. Paris: Masson.

Bobon, J. (1957) Contribution à la psychopathologie de l'expression plastique, mimique et picturale: les 'néomimismes' et les 'néomorphismes'. *Acta Neurologica Belgica*, **57,** 1031.

Bobon, J., Maccagnani, G. & Piro, S. (1967) Schizophasie et schizoparaphasie: cohérence du dessin spontané; intérêt des épreuves d'anagrammes, de renversement et d'inversion du miroir des mots. *Acta Neurologica Belgica*, **67,** 924.

Brady, J.P. (1958) Language in schizophrenics: review of several approaches to the problem. *American Journal of Psychotherapy*, **12,** 473.

Brown, R. (1972) Schizophrenia, language and reality. *American Psychologist*, **28,** 395.

Chaika, E.O. (1974) A linguist looks at 'schizophrenic' language. *Brain and Language*, **1,** 257.

Chaika, E. (1977) Schizophrenic speech, slips of the tongue and jargonaphasia: a reply to Fromkin and to Lecours and Vanier-Clément. *Brain and Language*, **4**, 464.

Critchley, M. (1964) The neurology of psychotic speech. *British Journal of Psychiatry*, **110**, 353.

Durbin, M. & Martin, R.L. (1977) Speech in mania: syntactic aspects. *Brain and Language*, **4**, 208.

Ferdière, G. ([illegible]954) Notes préliminaires sur les 'portemanteau words' de Lewis Carroll (ou mots-valises) au cours de la schizophrénie. *Acta Neurologica Belgica*, **57**, 993.

Flegel, M. ([illegible]65) *A Linguistic Interpretation of Schizophasia*. Berlin: Springer. (In German.)

Forrest, D.V. (1976) Nonsense and sense in schizophrenic language. *Schizophrenia Bulletin*, **2**, 286.

Forrest, D.V., Hay, A.J. & Kushner, A.W. (1971) Studies in speech disorder in schizophrenia. In *The Schizophrenic Syndrome: an Annual Review* (Ed.) Cancro, R. New York: Brunner-Mazel.

Fromkin, V.[illegible] (1975) A linguist looks at 'A linguist looks at schizophrenic language'. *Brain and Language*, **2**, 498.

Gottschalk, L.A. (Ed.) (1961) *Comparative Psycholinguistic Analysis of Two Psychotherapeutic Interviews*. New York: International University Press.

Grühl (1932) Die Schizophrenie. In *Handbuch des Geistes Krankheiten* (Ed.) Bumke. Berlin: Springer-Verlag.

Haag, M. & Brabant, P. (1963) Le langage de quinze déments séniles dans la perspective de leur perte de l'attitude catégorielle de K. Goldstein. In *Recherches sur les Maladies mentales* (Ed.) Daumézon, G. p. 11. Paris: Imprimerie municipale.

Irigaray, L. ([illegible]57) Approche psycho-linguistique du langage des déments. *Neuropsychologia*, **5**, 25.

Kasanin, J.S. (Ed.) (1944) *Language and Thought in Schizophrenia*. Berkeley and Los Angeles: University of California Press.

Kasanin, J.S. (1964) *Language and Thought in Schizophrenia*. New York: Norton.

Kreitler, M.H. (1957) Les bases psychologiques du langage des schyzophrènes. *Acta Neurologica Belgica*, **57**, 950.

Laffal, J. (196[illegible]) *Pathological and Normal Language*. New York: Atherton Press.

Laplanche, J. & Leclaire, S. (1967) Le langage et l'inconscient. L'inconscient: une étude psychanalytique. *L'inconscient*, **1**, 95.

Lebrun, Y. (1967) Schizophasie et bégaiement. *Acta Neurologica Belgica*, **67**, 939.

Lecours, A.R., Navet, M. & Ross-Chouinard, A. (1981) Langage et pensée du schizophase. *Confrontations psychiatriques*, **19**, 105.

Lecours, A.R. & Vanier-Clément, M. (1976) Schizophasia and jargonaphasia. A comparative description with comments on Chaika's and Fromkin's respective looks at 'schizophrenic' language. *Brain and Language*, **3**, 516.

Martin, J.R. & Rochester, S.R. (1975) Cohesion and reference in schizophrenic speech. In *The First LACUS Forum* (Ed.) Makkai, A. & Makkai, V. p. 302. Columbia, MO: Hornbeam Press.

Milgram, N. (1959) Preference for abstract versus concrete word meanings in schizophrenic and brain-damaged patients. *Journal of Clinical Psychology*, **15**, 207.

Moran, L.J. (1953) Vocabulary knowledge and usage among normals and schizophrenic patients. *Psychological Monographs*, **67**.

Pavy, D. (1968) Verbal behavior in schizophrenia: a review of recent studies. *Psychological Bulletin*, **70**, 164.

Perley, M.B. & Guze, S.B. (1962) Hysteria: the stability and usefulness of clinical criteria. *New England Journal of Medicine*, **266**, 421.

Racamier, P.C. (1955) Troubles de la sémantique (aliénation du langage). In *Encyclopédie médico-chirurgie—Psychiatrie* (Ed.) Ey, H. *37130 C*[10]. Paris: Editions techniques.

Reed, J.L. (1970) Schizophrenic thought disorder: a review and hypothesis. *Comprehensive Psychiatry*, **11**, 403.

Richman, J. (1968) Symbolic distortion in the vocabulary definitions of schizophrenics. In *Language Behavior in Schizophrenia* (Ed.) Vetter, H.J. Chicago, IL: Rand McNally.

Rochester, S.R. (1973) The role of information processing in the sentence decoding of schizophrenic listeners. *Journal of Nervous and Mental Diseases*, **157**, 217.

Rochester, S. & Martin, J.R. (1979) *Crazy Talk*. New York. Plenum Press.

Rochester, S.R., Harris, J. & Seeman, M.V. (1973) Sentence processing in schizophrenic listeners. *Journal of Abnormal Psychology*, **82**, 350.

Shamis, S. (1973) *Linguistic Indices of Schizophrenia*. Thesis, Department of Linguistics, University of California, Berkeley.

Sizaret, P. (1973) Message délirant diffusé par auto-enregistrement magnétophonique. Communication à la *Société française de Psychopathologie de l'Expression*, Tours.

Sizaret, P. & Casanova, B. *L'œuvre d'Alexandre Fortuné Hildevert E.* Editions Sandoz, Rueil-Malmaison, référence 72.058.000.

Somers, H. (1965) Review: a linguistic interpretation of schizophasia by H. Flegel. Berlin: Springer. (*Linguistics*, **34**, 135. 1967.)

Stuchlik, J. (1957) Contribution à la psychopathologie de l'expression verbale: les néophasies et les néographies. *Acta Neurologica Belgica*, **57**, 1004.

Tolentino, I. (1957) Inhibition du langage et mutisme en psychothérapie. Autodescription des motivations du mutisme prolongé par une schizoïde. *Acta Neurologica Belgica*, **57**, 955.

Truscott, I.P. (1970) Contextual constraint and schizophrenic language. *Journal of Consulting and Clinical Psychology*, **35**, 189.

Vetter, H. (Ed.) (1968) *Language Behavior in Schizophrenia*. Springfield, IL: Thomas.

Vetter, H.J. (1969) *Language Behavior and Psychopathology*. Chicago, IL: McNally.

Weintraub, W. & Aronson, H. (1967) The application of verbal behavior analysis to the study of psychological defense mechanisms. IV: speech pattern associated with depressive behavior. *Journal of Nervous and Mental Diseases*, **1**, 144.

14. Deviations in Normal Linguistic Behaviour

'Breeding pheasants? Well, then, uh first of all, must put them in incubator. That's to say, you have the ↓ First of all, you have some hens ↓ some hens and some roosters that you put by pens. You know: you put them in some pens uh a metre and a half by three metres long, approximately. So, there, that's some ↓ For reproduction, you put five hens, one rooster. So there, you↓ you pick up the eggs every night when it's laying time. You pick up the eggs and, every night↓ You put the eggs in the incubator every ten days. The incubators, that's to say↓ that's the↓ the hatchoirs, if you like, the claves. Then, uh, after twenty↓—I mustn't make a mistake—twenty-three days, I believe it is, the pheasant, yes, there, there, yes, there is hatching. You have the little pheasant↓ the little one-day-old pheasant. At the end of a day, you have a one-day-old pheasant. Then, after, you replace it in↓ under some brooders. Brooders, that's a type of↓—How shall I put it?—uh like a lodge on a netla↓ a small↓ an iron gadget which is heated from↓ from the underside what, to give heat uh to the little pheasants which are underneath.'

(*Conversation with Mr Té.; May 1969*)

The *linguistic productions of normal speakers** usually include a certain number of deviant segments.† Deviations affecting the third linguistic phase (articulatory and graphic anomalies) are exceptional but this may not be so for the other types of deviant segments previously discussed (see Chapters 2 to 5, 12 and 13). The number of deviations produced in 'normal' discourse varies widely among different speakers, probably in relation to their individual 'talents' and learning; it may increase with fatigue, distraction, haste, emotion or all other forms of stress.

The following statements are generally true in regard to the deviant productions of normal speakers[3]:

(a) The deviant segments follow the rules of the phonetic and phonological systems of the speaker's language (or of another language which he has acquired); they may also follow the morphosyntactical rules (see Chapter 2). In this respect, there is no qualitative difference between the deviations of normal speakers and pathological deviations.

(b) The deviant productions of normal speakers are usually involuntary. They diverge from the speaker's intention and in this sense, as in aphasia, can be considered to be *minus deviations*[3].

(c) Normal speakers may or may not recognize the nature of a deviant segment which they have just uttered (involuntarily). When they recognize the deviation, or when it is pointed out to them by a listener, normal speakers can almost always identify exactly which segment they had intended to use. Thus there is generally little difficulty in assigning a precise discriptive label to the transformed segment[3–5]. As a consequence, precisely labelled deviations (e.g., phonemic para-

* We shall not include, under this heading, (a) deviant productions related to intoxication (alcoholic or other), (b) improvised or planned deviations deliberately produced by certain speakers in order to amuse or mystify, (c) deviant productions occurring during mystical trances[1].

† Deviations in language reception also occur in normal individuals, who may either notice them or remain unaware. Freud[2] mentioned the occurrence of deviations in written language (mental reading of one word for another) but did not mention those of spoken language comprehension which we believe to be equally frequent (consider, for example, the frequency of comments such as 'He misunderstood'). Lacking a corpus of examples to illustrate these deviations, we shall not discuss them here.

phasias) may appear relatively often in normal linguistic behaviour whereas less precisely labelled forms (e.g., neologisms) appear to be exceptional.

(d) Despite the above, normal speakers are not totally restricted to standard production and involuntary deviations. They have the privilege of producing deviant segments deliberately: this is usually done to convey linguistically a conceptual element for which no conventional linguistic segment is immediately available. For most speakers, this is an exceptional procedure and the segment thus created generally follows the rules of derivation and composition in the speaker's language (see Chapter 2, notions of derived monemic paraphasias and compound monemic paraphasias). Far from opposing the speaker's intention, the deviation is consistent with it and often constitutes a comprehensible message: as in the case of the most characteristic deviations in schizophasia (see Chapter 13), they can thus be referred to as *plus deviations*[3].

The present chapter will be divided into two major sections. In the first, we shall be mainly concerned with deviations observed in the spontaneous discourse of normal speakers: they will be illustrated with examples noted during conversations which, in most cases, were on the subject* of language or diseases which affect it. In the second section, we shall discuss findings observed when normal speakers completed a test of linguistic function which was developed for the assessment of aphasic disturbances (see Chapter 15).

DEVIATIONS IN THE DISCOURSE OF NORMAL SPEAKERS

Under this heading we shall successively discuss the phonemic, monemic and verbal deviations which can be observed, provided that sufficient samples are obtained, in the spontaneous discourse of almost all normal speakers. Although simple omission, addition and displacement may occur at all linguistic phases (see Chapter 2), our discussion will be mainly illustrated by examples of substitutions between linguistic units. In cases where we have particularly clear examples, we shall point out how certain deviations are chiefly determined by formal or conceptual relationships between the replaced and replacing units while other deviations are chiefly determined by formal or conceptual relationships between the replacing unit and another unit in the immediate context (past or future).

PHONEMIC DEVIATIONS

The *phonemic deviations or transformations* observed in the language of normal speakers are qualitatively similar to those which characterize the spontaneous discourse of conduction aphasics[3] (Chapter 4); in regard to the presence of phonemic paraphasias, there is then only a quantitative difference between these two forms of discourse. As previously mentioned, it is possible to speak of phonemic deviations only when the corresponding target segments can be definitely identified. From a purely descriptive point of view, four types of phonemic deviations may be distinguished. Two of them, *phonemic paraphasias* and *formal verbal paraphasias*, have been defined elsewhere (see Chapter 2); both involve the transformation of a single target segment. The other two, *phonemic telescopages* and certain *verbal telescopages*, are characterized by phonemic borrowing from at least two target segments. In the case of phonemic telescopages, the deviant segment is used as a (unique) word even though it is not to be found in dictionaries of the speaker's language; in verbal telescopages, the deviant segment is an actual word in the speaker's language but is not the target segment. These deviations are illustrated by the following examples:

(a) The concept of a phonemic paraphasia [see (2.13) to (2.21), (4.5) to (4.16) and (8.1) and (8.2)] is well illustrated by the transformation of: (14.1) *hypophyse* (hypophysis) '/ipɔfiz/' →'/ipɔtiz/'; (14.2) *morphologie* (morphology) '/mɔʀfɔlɔʒi/'→'/fɔ̃ʀmɔlɔʒi/'; and (14.3) sissure de Sylvius (fissure of Sylvius) '/sisyʀ/ *de* /silvjys/'→ '/sisjyʀ/ *de* /silvjys/'. The influence of units in the immediate context is

* As was probably the case for examples quoted by Fromkin[6–8] in her remarkable works on anomalies in normal discourse.

apparent in each case and it may be that this phenomenon is (relatively) more frequent—at all linguistic phases—in the deviations of normal speakers than in those of aphasics. Normal speakers often have the (introspective) impression that future units exert the greatest influence, as in (3), on clearly programmed productions, that is, when the speaker knows in advance what s/he wants to say, whereas previously produced units have the greatest effect on uncertain utterances which are laboriously programmed during the course of their production.

(b) The concept of a formal verbal paraphasia [see (2.24)] is well illustrated by the transformations (14.4) '*la petite* /fiʃ/'→'*la petite* /fij/' ('the small filing card'→'the small girl') and (14.5) '*une* /bɛl/ /pjɛʀ/'→'une /bɛl/ /bal/' ('a pretty stone'→ 'a pretty ball'). In (4) the replacing word /fij/ incorporates many of the formal characteristics of the replaced word /fiʃ/; in addition, the context ('small') probably favours the deviation. In (5) the form of the replacing word /bal/ is determined by that of another word of the target segment /bɛl/, rather than by that of the word which was replaced (/pjɛʀ/).

(c) The concept of a phonemic telescopage is illustrated by (14.6), competition between *animal* (animal) and *mammifère* /mamifɛʀ/ (mammal) leading to the production of '/maminal/'; (14.7) the transformation of *un tremblement des mains* (tremor of the hands), 'tʀɑ̃blœmɑ̃/ *des* /mɛ̃/'→'/tʀɑ̃blœmɛ̃/'; and (14.8) that of *une bouteille de vin* (bottle of wine), '*une* /butɛj/ *de* /vɛ̃/'→'*une* /vitɛj/'. In phonemic telescopages the deviant production is not a real word. In (6) there is a paradigmatic relationship between the target words, that is, only one of them belongs in the conventional segment; in (7) and (8) there is a syntagmatic relationship between the two target words, that is, both words belong to the conventional segment.

(d) The verbal telescopages considered under the general heading 'phonemic deviations' have the same origin as phonemic telescopages; the verbal telescopages differ from the latter only by the fact that the deviant segment corresponds to a conventional word in the speaker's language. Again, there may be a paradigmatic relationship between the target words [(14.9) '/seri/'+'/kiʀjɛl/'→'/seʀjɛl/' in '*Toute une* /seʀjɛl/ *de symptomes*' ('series'+'string of'→'serial' in 'A whole /seʀjɛl/ of symptoms')]. There may also be a paradigmatic relationship between the target words [(14.10) '*Il est* /suʀ/ *comme un* /po/' ('He is deaf as a pot')→ '*Il est comme un* /purso/' ('He is as a porker')].

MONEMIC DEVIATIONS

Derived and compound monemic paraphasias were defined elsewhere in this text (see Chapter 2) [see examples (2.25) to (2.38) and (13.25) to (13.35)]. With the exception of certain voluntary deviations, such as calling the collaborators of an authoritative department head his [(14.11) /ɛsklavri/ (lexicale element as in *ESCLAVE* /ɛsklav/ [slave])], derived monemic paraphasias usually result from monemic borrowing from two target words. In the examples which we have noted, there was usually a syntagmatic relationship between the targets [(14.12) '*Une* /silab/ *à initial* /fʀicativ/' (a syllable with an initial fricative)→'*une* /silabativ/']; in some cases there was a paradigmatic relationship [(14.13) *isoler* /isɔle/ +*analyser* /analize/ (to isolate+to analyse)→ /izɔlize/ in '*Il faudrait* /izɔlize/ *cette partie de nos résultats*' ('We must /isɔlize/ this part of our results')]. This type of deviation quite often occurs through assimilation [(14.14) 'These fibres perforate the pulvinar'→'These fibres pulvinate the pulvinar'; (14.15) '*S'il y a une lesion du* /sɛʀvo/, *les paraphasies* /vɛrbal/ . . .' ('if there is a lesion of the brain the verbal paraphasias . . .') →'*S'il y a une lesion du* /sɛrvo/, *les paraphasies* /sɛrval/ . . .']; or by mutual replacement [(14.16) 'lexically sophisticated'→'sophistically lexicated'; (14.17) 'foreshortened'→'shortfortened']. As for compound monemic paraphasias, they are rarely produced by normal speakers and the few which occur are almost always deliberate: [(14.18) '*C'est un petit-gros*' ('That's a little-big')].

Certain verbal telescopages, which occur rather frequently in normal language, can also be considered as monemic deviations. In the examples which we have noted, there was a syntagmatic relationship between the target words [(14.9) '*la* /tʀɑ̃smisjɔ̃/ *des* /ɛ̃fʀmasjɔ̃/' ('the transmission of information')→'*la* /tʀɑ̃sfɔʀmasjɔ̃/' ('the transformation'); (4.20) '*les bruits familiers et les cris d'animaux*'→'*les bruits familiaux et les cris d'animaux*' ('familiar noises and animal cries'→'familial noises and animal cries')]. With the exception that the deviant segment is (by definition an actual word in the language, these verbal telescopages are assimilable to derived monemic paraphasias.

NEOLOGISMS

According to the restrictive definition of the term given within the context of this book (see Chapter 2) [see examples (2.39) and (2.83), (4.20) and (13.39) to (13.40)], neologisms are rare in the language of normal speakers. This is true for the following reasons: the target segment is often easily recognized (and one can then speak of phonemic or monemic paraphasias rather than of neologisms); if the listener is unable to recognize the target segment, the speaker can almost always identify it when s/he is made aware of the deviation. Nevertheless, within the context of interviews in which the speaker's deviations are not pointed out, it is not uncommon to note certain segments which must be considered neologisms because the target word (if there was one) cannot be recognized. Thus, when discussing his work a gamekeeper reported

(4.21) '*Des éleveuses, c'est un gendre de↓—Comment je vais vous dire?—euh comme un pavillon sur une* /netla/↓ *un petit↓ un truc en tôle qui est chauffée du↓ du dessous.*'*

'Breeders that's a type of↓—How shall I put it?—uh like a lodge on a /netla/↓ a small↓ an iron gadget which is heated from↓ from the underside.'*

VERBAL DEVIATIONS

Different types of verbal deviations were defined elsewhere (see Chapter 2). They may all occur in the discourse of normal speakers. Verbal paraphasias by simple substitution are among the most frequent. Their occurrence can often be observed to reflect both formal[9] and conceptual influences. Wishing to call a group of female students engaged in protest† (14.22) '*des femmes hystériques*' ('hysterical women'), a politician of May 1968 spoke instead of '*femmes historiques*' ('historical women'). In (22), there is a paradigmatic relationship between the two words. More commonly, the relationship is both paradigmatic and syntagmatic [(14.23) '*un oeillet à la boutonnière*'→'*un oeillet à la bouquetière*' ('a carnation in the buttonhole'→'a carnation in the flower-girl')—a formal relationship on the paradigmatic axis and a conceptual one on the syntagmatic axis—; (14.24) '*prends-le, je t'en prie*'→'*prends-le, je t'en prends*' ('take it, I urge you'→'take it, I will take some from you')—a formal relationship on both axes]. Sometimes there is only (or especially) a syntagmatic relationship [(14.25) '*Méfiez-vous de la première impression, c'est la bonne*'→'*Méfiez-vous de la bonne impression, c'est la bonne*' ('Watch out for your first impression, it's right'→'Watch out for your right impression, it's right'); (14.26) '*comme modèle de la motricité*'→'*comme mouvement de la motricité*' ('as a model of motricity'→'as a movement of motricity')]. These deviations may often involve grammatical words: [14.27) 'needs not be'→'needs but be'] and, in this case, the transformation is usually dyssyntactic. As indicated by examples (23) to (27), the verbal assimilation phenomena may be anterograde as well as retrograde. Like their phonemic paraphasias [14.28) /abʀakadabrɑ̃/→/akʀatakabrɑ̃/; see also (2)], the verbal paraphasias of normal speakers sometimes go well beyond simple substitution [(14.29) '*Je lisais* Le Monde *tranquillement, dans le métro, comme ça*'→'*Je lisais le métro, tranquillement dans* Le Monde *comme ça*' ('I was reading *The World*, quietly, in the subway, like that'→'I was reading the subway, quietly, in *The World*, like that'; (14.30) '*un très court laps de temps*'→'*un très laps* /kur/ *de temps*' ('a very short lapse of time'→'a very lapse short of time')]. As in (29) and (30) (which involve reciprocal displacement), the listener usually has little difficulty in reconstructing the meaning of sentences containing such transformations. Nevertheless, verbal deviations may sometimes result in sentences which exceed the limits of intelligibility: [(14.31) '*Veut-tu que je mette chacune des copies dans une chemise?*'→'*Veut-tu que je mette une chacune dans un copie?*' ('Do you wish me to put each of the copies in a folder'→'Do you wish me to put one each in a copy?')]. When such transformations occur in an aphasic's discourse, one readily speaks of incoherence and it is often maintained, probably incorrectly, that such transformations are secondary to a disturbance of language comprehension.

* In this case, one has the very strong impression that, despite the probable presence of a precise 'idea', the target segment is not immediately available to the speaker.

† During the upheavals in France in May 1968.

WRITTEN EXPRESSION

Different types of deviations may occur in the written productions of normal subjects (particularly in typewritten productions). They include literal paragraphias [(14.32) (*préfabriqué*→) '*préfébraqué*'], graphemic paragraphias [(14.33) (*déjà*→) '*décha*'], literal telescopages [(14.34) (*une lésion hémisphérique gauche*→) '*une l'hésion gauche*': (*a left hemisphere lesion*→) '*a left l'hesion*'], verbal telescopages [(14.35) (*quand un patient se présente*→) '*quand un présent se présente*': (*when a patient is present*→) '*when a present is present*'], monemic paragraphias

(−) No production
(±) Occasional production possible
(<) Occasional production usual
(>) Important production usual
(▲) Exceptional
(■) Usually aware
(×) Occasionally aware
(●) Anosognosia usual
(O) Probably intentional
(*) Belongs with the archetype

		Normal discourse	Broca's aphasia	Jargonaphasic discourse: Conduction aphasia	Jargonaphasic discourse: Wernicke's aphasia (Type I)	Jargonaphasic discourse: Wernicke's aphasia (Type II)	Schizophasic discourse
Phonetic deviations		−	> ■ * 4.4	−	−	−	−
Phonemic deviations		± × 14.1 to 10	< × 3.25 to 28	> ■ * 2.24	> ● * 2.83 and 4.20	<	< × or: < O 13.36 and 37
Monemic deviations	Derived	± × 14.11 to 17	± ×	< ×	< ● 2.25 to 32	< ●	> O * 13.25 to 30
	Compound	± O 14.18	−	± O	±	± ●	> O * 2.38 and 13.24
Neologisms		± ×	< ×	< ×	> ● * 2.39 and 4.20	± ●	< O 13.39
Glossolalia		−	−	−	▲ > ● 2.84	−	▲ > O 13.44
Verbal deviations	Semantic paraphasias	± × 14.23	< ×	< ×	> ● * 2.43	> ● * 4.28	Frequent bizarre words 13.23
	Assimilation and related phenomena	± × 14.24 to 26	< ×	< ×	> ● * 2.71 and 72	> ● * 2.90	± ×
	Dyssyntactic transformations	± × 14.27	Agrammatism possible 2.88	?	< ● or ▲ > ● 2.45 and 78 to 80	< ●	± ×
Preferred words and themes		± ×	± ×	± ×	> × 13.10 to 18	?	> O * 13.1 to 9
Glossomania	Formal	± O	−	± 4.5	±	−	> O * 2.86 and 87 13.19 to 21
	Semantic	± O	−	−	±	± 2.44	> O * 2.86 and 87 13.19 to 21

Fig. 14-1 *Deviant segments in the language of normals, aphasics and schizophasics. The numbers refer to the examples quoted in different chapters. Adapted from Lecours and Vanier-Clément*[3].

[(14.36) (*ces crayons de couleur*→) '*des crayeurs de coleur*' (*coloured crayons*→) '*coloured crayoured*')], and all types of verbal paragraphias [(14.37) (*and remained such for the several months during which* ...→) '*and remained such for the several much during which* ... ',* (14.38) (*a compounded verbal and phonemic transformation*→) '*a compounded and verbal transformation*', (14.39) (*J'aime la compagne parce ce que c'est plus propice à la santé*→) '*J'aime la compagne parce ce que la santé est plus propice*': (*I like the country because it is more propitious for health*→) '*I like the country because health is more propitious*', (14.40) (*même chez les sujets droitiers*→) '*mèche chez les sujets droitiers*': (*even in right-handed subjects*→) '*wick in right-handed subjects*']. The number of deviations varies among subjects and according to the circumstances associated with written composition. It is possible to speak of *dysorthographia* only when there is a constant and abundant production of deviant segments: this fact should be borne in mind when judging whether or not the written productions of aphasics are pathological in nature (see Chapter 15).

The table shown in Fig. 14–1 presents a schematic summary of the (primarily quantitative) characteristics which permit the discourse of normal speakers to be distinguished from various forms of pathological discourse[3].

PERFORMANCE OF NORMAL SUBJECTS ON A TEST FOR THE ASSESSMENT OF APHASIA

Whenever possible, our procedures for the assessment of aphasia include the recording and transcription of a 15-minute sample of conversational language (see Chapter 15). Figure 14–2 (see below) includes a summary of certain general characteristics of the samples obtained from two normal speakers[10] and three aphasics (jargonaphasia in a case of Type I Wernicke's aphasia, jargonaphasia in a case of Type II Wernicke's aphasia, agrammatism in a case of Broca's aphasia). In many respects, the similarities are as striking as the differences. The most noteworthy points are as follows:

(a) The agrammatic patient produced fewer words† than the four other speakers.
(b) The two Wernicke's aphasics produced fewer words than the two normal speakers. In this regard, it should be noted that the patient with Type I Wernicke's aphasia was considered to be logorrhoeic.
(c) Only the Type II Wernicke's aphasics produced relatively few sentences (either simple or complex). This reduction was not immediately apparent when listening to the recorded sample.
(d) Sentence length was characteristically shorter in the agrammatical patient[11].
(e) The proportion of aborted sentences was larger in the Wernicke's aphasics than in the normal controls. In this regard, the difference between the Broca's aphasic and the normal controls was mainly related to the characteristics of agrammatical discourse (high frequency of one-word sentences).
(f) The language of the normal controls could not be distinguished from that of the aphasics in terms of the number of pauses and hesitations ('uh', etc.). On the other hand, the number of words between two consecutive pauses or hesitations[11] was lower in the Broca's aphasic and the Type II Wernicke's aphasic than in the other speakers.
(g) The tendency to repeat segments of all orders of complexity, as indicated here by an *R Index* calculated on the basis of several variables, was more obvious in the three aphasics than in the two control subjects; the R index can be considered an approximate measure of the manifestations of word-finding difficulty in conversation[10].

The following statements summarize certain qualitative findings obtained when our aphasia assessment battery (see Chapter 15) was presented to 25 normal subjects:

(a) Although uncommon, certain subjects nevertheless omitted or repeated items when

* Several factors may have influenced the production of this deviation: the formal syntagmatic relationship between 'such' and 'much'; the formal syntagmatic relationship between 'much' and 'which'; the formal paradigmatic relationship between 'months' and 'much'; and the conceptual syntagmatic relationship between 'several' and 'much'.

† Real words and deviant word-like units.

		Normal control subject 1	Normal control subject 2	Case 1: Wernicke's aphasia (Type I)	Case 2: Wernicke's aphasia (Type II)	Case 3: Agrammatism
Number of words		2653	2674	2238	1676	1227
Number of sentences		353	287	311	196	256
Mean sentence length (in number of words)		7.52	9.31	7.19	8.57	4.79
Number of aborted sentences	Absolute number	43	35	49	42	16
	Percentage of the total number of sentences	12	12	16	21	6
Number of pauses and hesitations		495	330	347	427	402
Mean number of words between two pauses or hesitations		5.36	9.32	6.45	3.93	3.05
R index		0.07	0.03	0.12	0.15	0.13

Fig. 14.2 *Quantitative data on selected characteristics of the conversational language of two normal subjects, a Type I Wernicke's aphasic, a Type II Wernicke's aphasic (transcortical sensory) and an agrammatic aphasic. Language samples were obtained during a 15-minute interview with each subject. Commentary in the text.*

asked to list the days of the week or months of the year.

(b) During an oral naming subtest composed of 30 stimuli (pictures intended to elicit very common words), certain normal speakers produced semantic paraphasias (which were often spontaneously corrected), and one subject produced four. A periphrastic response sometimes preceded production of the target word. Failures were rare and facilitation was immediately effective.

(c) Generally speaking, word fluency was lower in response to a simple formal specification ('words beginning with the letter B': 12 words in one minute) than in response to a simple conceptual specification ('animal names': 15 words in one minute).

(d) A large number of normal speakers produced some inadequate responses on a subtest requiring the production of antonyms. Different types of deviant responses were observed, for example:
   (i) Change of category: (14.41) '*patient*'→'*impatience*'.
   (ii) Negation: (14.42) '*bon*'→'*pas bon*' ('good'→'not good').
   (iii) Periphrase: (14.43) '*patience*'→'*tu n'a pas de patience*' ('patience'→ 'you have no patience').
   (iv) Derived monemic paraphasia: (14.44) '*ordinaire*'→'*incommun*' ('ordinary'→ 'incommon').
   (v) Synonym: (14.45) '*ordinaire*'→'*banal*' ('ordinary'→'banal').
   (vi) Approximate antonym: (14.46) '*capable*'→'*paresseux*' ('capable'→'lazy').

Word definitions given by normal speakers were often vague and imprecise. Definition by usage was common [(14.47) '*fourchette*→'*pour manger*' ('fork'→'in order to eat')], but obviously tautological definitions were rarer [(14.48) '*se déchausser*'→'*quelqu'un qui se déchausse*' ('to take off one's shoes'→'someone who takes off his shoes'); (14.49) '*oublier*'→'*qui oublie quelque chose*' ('to forget'→'who forgets something')].

(e) Formulating sentences using lexical components provided by the examiner proved rather difficult for certain normal speakers. This was especially true when more than two lexical elements were given, particularly when they were relatively abstract words. In this case, the speaker may use only two of the stimulus words, which may or may not be accurately reproduced [(14.50) '*habilité—succès—compétition*'→'*pour avoir du succès, il faut être un peu habile*' ('skilfulness—success—competition—'To be a success, you must be a bit skilful')]. Similarly, the productions quite often included several sentences rather than a single one as specified in the instructions [(14.51) '*habileté—succès—compétition*'→'*Une compétition qui a du succes. Il est habile le gars.*' ('A competition which is a success. He is skilful, the guy'); (14.52) '*pêcheur—appât—poisson*'→'*Mon mari s'est acheté des lignes pour la pêche puis il aime bien aller pêcher mais il n'a pas beaucoup de temps. Il préparait les appâts*' ('fisherman—bait—fish'→'My husband bought himself some fishing lines then he likes to go fishing but he hasn't much time. He prepared the bait')].

(f) The normal speakers occasionally produced phonemic paraphasias during the word repetition subtest. When they occurred, it was almost always on long words having a complex phonological structure and low frequency of usage (they were often perceived as neologisms by the subject). Repetition of three-syllable neologisms was often incorrect, as was the repetition of sentences including many grammatical words [(14.53) '*Quel que soit le temps qu'il fasse mercredi, nous irons à la campagne*' ('Whatever the weather will be like on Wednesday, we will go to the country')→'*Quel que temps qu'il fasse mercredi*'—'*Quel que temps qu'il se fasse mercredi*'—'*Quel que soit le temps qu'il fera mercredi*'].*

(g) In general, deviations in oral reading occurred only at the level of reading textual passages: those which were then produced were usually paradigmatic substitutions between short grammatical words [(14.54) '*endormi dans la voiture*'→'*endormi dans sa voiture*' ('asleep in the car'→'asleep in his car')].

(h) With the exception of the Token Test[12] (see Chapter [illegible]), no errors were made on the subtests of oral and written comprehension. These subtests were clearly less sensitive to individual variations (in education, age, occupation) than were those of oral expression. After listening to a story, all subjects were able to provide an adequate summary, although one or two details were sometimes omitted. Only one of the 25 control subjects made an error on Pierre Marie's Paper Test[13] (the error was one of inversion during the execution of the second and third elements of the command).

(i) No errors occurred in writing numbers and the days of the week in sequential order. On the other hand, subjects with little education sometimes omitted or transposed letters when required to write the alphabet.

(j) Errors in copying (with or without transposition from print to cursives or vice versa) were very rare but a few graphemic paragraphias were noted [(14.55) '*Le* (commandant→) *commandan a quitté le bateau en dernier*'. (*The* commandan *left the ship last*')].

(k) Written compositions and writing to dictation often included literal and graphemic paragraphias whose frequency of occurrence was generally related to educational level. The results indicated that some normal speakers can clearly be considered to present a 'cultural' dysorthographia as illustrated by the following passage which was written to dictation:

(14.56) (Plusieurs→) '*Plusieur* (mineurs→) *mineur sont* (morts→) *mort* (à la→) *à suite d'une explosion* (survenue→) *survenu hier dans une mine de charbon* (aux Etats-Unis→) *au état unis la cause de l'* (explosion→) *expossions* (n'a→) *na pas été determinée. les equipes de* (secours→) *checoure* (ont→) *on perdu toute* (espoir→) *espoirs de* (retrouver→) *retrouvée des* (survivants→) *sur vivants.*'

'Several miners *are* dead after *an explosion that* took place *yesterday in a coal mine* in the *United* State. *the cause of the* expossions has not *been determined. the* emergency *crews* have *lost all* hope *of* finding sur vivors.'

The above findings clearly indicate that the results obtained by a (presumably) aphasic individual on subtests of linguistic performance cannot be interpreted without considering the 'deviations' made by normal individuals of the same age and cultural background. In the vast majority of cases, the aphasia is such that its presence cannot be doubted. Nevertheless, problems sometimes arise in identifying the onset of an insidiously progressive disorder or in identifying the sequelae of a disorder which has

* Differences between grammatical monemes in French and English make these examples nearly impossible to translate.

evolved favourably. The study of expression is then more difficult than that of comprehension. In regard to written expression, there are some cases in which the presence of a possible aphasia can be judged only by comparing the patient's performance to a sample of his or her premorbid production.

REFERENCES

1. Lecours, A.R. & Kock, J. (de) (1977) Sprachlich neugebildete Segmente und Glossolalie. *Review of Applied Linguistics*, **37**, 3–17.
2. Freud, S. (1967) *Psychopathologie de la vie quotidienne*. Paris: Payot.
3. Lecours, A.R. & Vanier-Clément, M. (1976) Schizophasia and jargonaphasia. A comparative description with comments on Chaika's and Fromkin's respective looks at 'schizophrenic' language. *Brain and Language*, **3**, 516.
4. Lecours, A.R. & Rouillon, F. (1976) Neurolinguistic analysis of jargonaphasia and jargonagraphia. In *Studies in Neurolinguistics* (Ed.) Avakian-Whitaker, H. & Whitaker, H. Vol. 2, p. 95. New York: Academic Press.
5. Lecours, A.R., Dordain, G. & Lhermitte, F. (1970) Recherches sur le langage des aphasiques: 1. Terminologie neurolinguistique. *Encéphale*, **59**, 520.
6. Fromkin, V.A. (1971) The non-anomalous nature of anomalous utterances. *Language*, **47**, 27.
7. Fromkin, V.A. (1973) Slips of the tongue. *Scientific American*, **110**, 110.
8. Fromkin, V.A. (1973) *Speech Errors as Linguistic Evidence*. The Hague: Mouton.
9. Major, R. (1969) L'économie de la représentation. *Revue française de Psychanalysé*, **33**, 79.
10. Lecours, A.R., Bérubé, L., Courtois, G. & Lhermitte, F. (1972) Recherches sur le langage des aphasiques: 3, Désorganisation de l'expression orale et désorganisation de l'expression écrite. *Encéphale*, **3**, 1.
11. Goodglass, H., Quadfasel, F.A. & Timberlake, W.H. (1964) Phrase length and the type and severity of aphasia. *Cortex*, **1**, 133.
12. Renzi, E. (de) & Vignolo, L.A. (1962) The token test: a sensitive test to detect receptive disturbances in aphasics. *Brain*, **85**, 665.
13. Marie, P. (1906) Révision de la question de l'aphasie: la troisième circonvolution frontale ne joue aucun rôle spécial dans la fonction du langage. *Semaine médicale* (Paris), **26**, 241.

BIBLIOGRAPHY

Bond, Z.S. (1973) Perceptual errors in ordinary speech. *Zeitschrift für Fonetik*, **26**, 691.

Boomer, D.S. & Laver, J.D.M. (1968) Slips of the tongue. *British Journal of Disorders of Communication*, **3**, 1.

Boudard, A. & Etienne, L. (1974) *Là méthode à Mimile*. Paris: La Jeune Parque.

Etienne, L. (1957) *L'art du contrepet*. Paris: Pauvert.

Etienne, L. (1965) *L'art de la charade à tiroirs*. Paris: Pauvert.

Fréchette, L. (1949) *Originaux et détraqués*. Montreal: Beauchemin.

Freud, S. (1960) Slips of the tongue. In *Psychopathology of Everyday Life* (Ed.) Freud, S. p. 53. London: The Hogarth Press and the Institute of Psychoanalysis.

Freud, S. (1960) Misreading and slips of the pen. In *Psychopathology of Everyday Life* (Ed.) Freud, S. p. 106. London: The Hogarth Press and the Institute of Psychoanalysis.

Freud, S. (1960) Bungled actions. In *Psychopathology of Everyday Life* (Ed.) Freud, S. p. 162. London: The Hogarth Press and the Institute of Psychoanalysis.

Fromkin, V.A. (1973) *Speech Errors as Linguistic Evidence*. The Hague: Mouton.

Guiraud, P. (1976) *Les jeux de mots*. Paris: Presses Universitaires de France.

Comtesse, M. de la F. (1967) *L'album de la Comtesse—Le général est arrivé à pied par la Chine*. Paris: Pauvert.

Pearson, G.H.J., Alpers, B.M. & Weisenburg, T.H. (1928) Aphasia: a study of normal control cases. *Archives of Neurology and Psychiatry* (Chicago), **19**, 281.

Penn, C. (1974) A linguistic approach to the detection of minimal language dysfunction in aphasia. *Journal of the South African Speech Association*, **21**, 3.

Perceau, L. (1963) *La redoute des contrepèteries*. Paris: Briffaut.

Pichot, P. (1955) Language disturbances in cerebral disease. Concept of latent aphasia. *Archives of Neurology and Psychiatry* (Chicago), **74**, 92.

Assessment of the Aphasic Patient

15. The Assessment of Aphasia

'There are things that I ossimilate. But there are some things that I await well. For example, I went to a talkage, there, here, below, on the other side, then where you come to searcher me just now a young bean which had—I don't know—that I am remained perhaps to a vow, about, in her office. But then, she was complent nauseated. She said: "But one doesn't know you anything!" ... She said: "But tell in your metron!" Now I didn't have any glevers. I didn't have any glassens. And then I asked my husband, the evening, who came. I said to him: "Listen! I must go over there now." I said to him: "They are very very very very very acurose." I said to him: "They show me some admired. They show me some hens" ... Then, I was askered exactly the same lebre that I lebed the day before where I was given all the noise ... She says: "I don't know what to peel to her." He says: "I don't know. What do you call that?" ... Well! I say: "A very pretty caressier" ... But then, where I was really correctated it's when I came here, that I had had fallen and that I had broken myself here a bit of sotu.'

(*Conversation with Madame Co.; May 1969*)

The study of aphasia, whether by clinicians or researchers, is based on the development and appropriate use of empirical procedures for the assessment of speech and language behaviours. The primary goals of this assessment are to determine if aphasia is present and, if so, to identify the aphasic syndrome and to permit a detailed description of the disorder. Since these aims will be evident in the nature of the aphasiological assessment, it will differ to some extent from a purely linguistic approach: for example, repetition, oral reading, copying, and writing to dictation—behaviours which are, a priori, of little interest to linguists—are examined and described, and the absence of this information would invalidate an aphasiological assessment. It is thus from observations of all elementary aspects of linguistic functioning that the presence of aphasia and its clinical form (see Chapters 3 to 6) can be identified. Consideration of the results of the aphasiological assessment, in conjunction with those of the neurological and psychological evaluations (see Chapter 16), will permit conclusions regarding the nature and localization of the patient's cerebral lesion(s) (see Chapters 8-2, 8-3, 8-4 and 9).

While the results of an initial medical examination and aphasiological assessment generally permit the physician to make a diagnosis and prognosis concerning the eventual course of the disease causing the aphasia, they often do not permit prognosis concerning the probable degree of recovery from the aphasia itself (this is particularly true in the case of aphasia associated with vascular or traumatic disease). Judgements to this effect can be formulated more easily after a second evaluation of language behaviour. It is carried out, using procedures as similar as possible to those of the initial assessment, after a period of evolution whose exact duration varies among different cases. In addition to the fact that they are often required for prognostic statements about the language disorder, comparisons between at least two sets of clinical data obtained at different times provide guidelines, in cases where the known aetiological factors suggest the utility of such a venture, for the development of a therapy programme (see Chapter 17); the identification of intact (or well preserved) linguistic behaviours and aspects of the disorder showing a tendency towards spontaneous improvement is particularly important in this regard.

Before discussing the various constituent subtests of a basic aphasiological test battery, we shall briefly consider certain generalities of aphasia testing:

1. The importance of certain information to be

obtained from the patient or from a family member or knowledgeable informant cannot be over-emphasized as it is indispensable when interpreting the results of the aphasia test. Which is the patient's preferred hand (for the execution of acts which have not been formally taught as well as for writing), and what are the manual preferences of his/her forebears and descendants (see Chapter 11)? Is there a personal or familial history of stuttering or of developmental dysphasia-dyslexia-dysgraphia[1], etc.? What is the patient's educational and cultural background? What is his/her maternal language and is it the only one which has been acquired? What were the patient's premorbid linguistic habits? Was s/he loquacious or taciturn? Did he do much writing? What did he read? What is the history of the present linguistic disorder? Is it a first episode? How long has the disorder been present? Was the onset sudden or gradual? Was there an initial *suppression* (see Chapter 4)? Has the disorder changed between the time of onset and the date of testing and, if so, how?

2. Results obtained on an aphasia test should not be interpreted with reference to the norms of standard grammar (i.e., of *proper usage*), but rather with reference to the norms of common usage, ones which are generally more poorly defined and influenced by many complex sociocultural factors. These norms do not exclude, within certain quantitative limits, either hesitations, incomplete sentences, the repetition of words or short syntagms, or segments assimilable to aphasic transformations[2–5], including paragrammatic transformations (see Chapter 14). This is usually more evident in the case of written language, especially with regard to orthographic deviations, than in the case of spoken language. Furthermore, within the same linguistic community, the norms of common usage are subject to large geographical variations: thus, when assessing the clinical picture of pure anarthria (see Chapter 3), it would, for example, be wrong to consider that the production of diphthongs and affricates by a patient from Montreal has the same significance as when produced by a patient from Paris.
3. The patient's general state and susceptibility to fatigue may be such that a lengthy assessment is contra-indicated. This is often true, during the acute phase, in cases of vascular or traumatic disease (see Chapter 9). It may then be decided that a thorough assessment will be carried out over several testing sessions in order to obtain systematic quantitative data on the disorder; it is, nevertheless, usually more advantageous to opt for a qualitative assessment aimed at determining whether the primary elements of aphasic symptomatology (see Chapter 4) are present. In the vast majority of cases, a 20- to 30-minute assessment carried out at the patient's bedside will permit answers to the following questions. In the absence of suppression, what are the characteristics of the speech flow (stereotype, reduction, normal fluency, logorrhoea)? Is word-finding difficulty evident and, if so, is there a dissociation between word-finding difficulty in spontaneous language and in naming? Are repetition and oral reading disturbed and, if so, is the impairment of these two behaviours comparable? Is it manifested by an absence of production or by abnormal production? What types of transformations are observed in spontaneous language, repetition, oral reading (phonetic, phonemic, verbal transformations; neologisms)? What are the patient's abilities in spontaneous written language, writing to dictation, copying and, when present, what types of transformations are observed in these behaviours? Does the patient write with the left or right hand? With respect to comprehension, what is the examiner's impression after conversation with the patient? Can the patient's attention be focused? Does s/he consider the interventions of his/her interlocutors? Does s/he appear to understand their meaning, at least in a global way? Is the patient able to follow simple orders and to match some objects or pictures to the corresponding words (spoken stimuli and written stimuli)? Can s/he follow the directions of Pierre Marie's Paper Test[6] or of a task of comparable difficulty? Is there a clear dissociation between oral versus written expression, or between the comprehension of oral versus written language? Are certain phenomena indicative of automatic-voluntary dissociation (see Chapters 1 and 4)? Is the patient anosognosic? Is s/he calm, sad, excited? Are there notable particularities of facial expression or gesture? Is there an associated hemiplegia, hemihypo-aesthesia, or hemianopsia? Is there a buccofacial apraxia or limb apraxia?

4. It is not uncommon that a complete assessment will have to be delayed until a time when the disorder begins to stabilize (in the case of aphasias of sudden onset with subsequent improvement). In order to follow the evolution of the aphasia, it is then useful to carry out several shortened, qualitative assessments on a periodic basis. Progressive changes will often be observed in the clinical form of aphasia: for example, a gradual transition from global aphasia to Broca's aphasia, from the latter to anarthria, from Wernicke's aphasia proper to conduction aphasia, from the latter to amnesic aphasia, etc. (see Chapter 4). In other words, nosological labels will be observed, in many cases, to be applicable only during a given period in the evolution of the aphasic syndrome (see Chapter 10).

5. The time which should be devoted to an aphasiological evaluation depends, to a large extent, on the patient's residual abilities: one would hardly attempt to obtain a large corpus of aphasic transformations from patients who present a suppression of both oral and written language; similarly, one would not present procedures intended to demonstrate mild deficits of comprehension (e.g., impaired comprehension of wholes) to patients who do not understand the meaning of the names of very common objects. Hence there are cases in which a complete aphasiological assessment can be carried out within a period of minutes; in other cases, a complete qualitative and quantitative assessment may require several hours as, for example, when a sufficient sample of spoken language (spontaneous

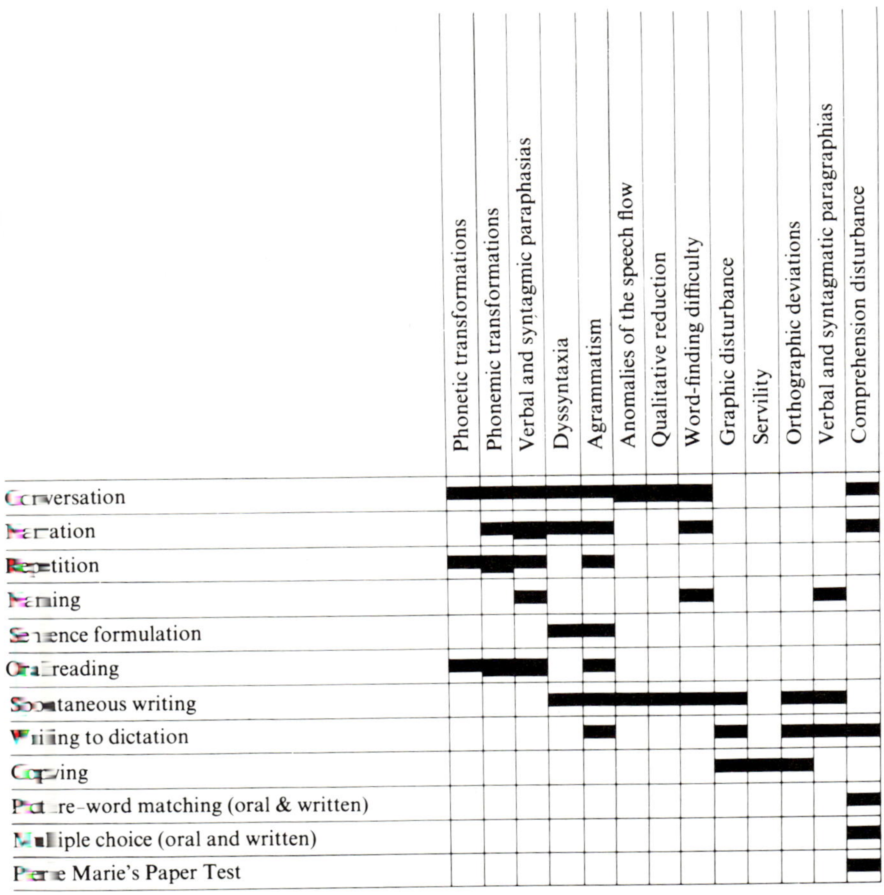

Fig. 15-1 *Relationships between the main subtests of an aphasia assessment (listed horizontally) and the principal features of aphasic symptomatology (listed vertically). The black lines indicate which symptomatological features are most likely to be detected through the presentation of particular subtests; the thicker black lines in certain sections indicate relationships which are particularly clear.*

discourse, repetition, oral reading) must be tape-recorded to permit phonetic disintegration or paraphasic or neologistic production to be adequately described, or when there is a need to clarify the nature of mild deficits of oral or written comprehension, etc.
6. For most patients, and in all cases of an initial complete assessment, the preferred presentation order for items within each subtest is from the most simple to the most complex and from the most elementary to the most elaborated. On the other hand, when the assessment is intended to chart the progress made by the patient whose aphasia has clearly decreased, time may be saved by working from the more complex items to the simpler ones: when responses to the more difficult items are correct, the simpler items may then be omitted.

In the present chapter we shall discuss a group of subtests which, in our opinion, constitute a complete (but elementary) test for the assessment of aphasia. Depending on their particular research or clinical interests, different examiners may, of course, extend certain subtests or present additional ones. For reasons which are primarily didactic, our presentation will follow the classical scheme and we shall discuss the assessment of oral expression, the assessment of spoken language comprehension, the assessment of written expression and the assessment of written language comprehension. These subdivisions are pragmatic and have no necessary functional or physiopathological implications [for example, even though a repetition disturbance is detected in oral expressive behaviour, it may well result from a receptive disorder: such is the case in word deafness (see Chapter 5)].

Although not equally obvious in all cases, each subtest included in the aphasia test is of specific interest. It is nevertheless clear that the same sign of aphasia may be detected on several subtests: thus agrammatism and dyssyntaxia will be observed in conversation, narration and picture description, and even in repetition and oral reading. The figure accompanying the text (Fig. 15-1) schematically presents the commonest relationships between the main subtests of an aphasiological assessment and the principal clinical signs of aphasia; this figure can serve as a guide to the shortened assessment procedure which we have already discussed (cf. pp. 347–348).

ASSESSMENT OF ORAL EXPRESSION

CONVERSATION

Of all the linguistic behaviours observed in aphasia, conversation—when it remains possible—is undoubtedly the richest source of symptomatological information: after having engaged an aphasic patient in conversation for about ten minutes, even a relatively inexperienced observer will usually be able to form a rather clear impression about the clinical form of aphasia which the patient presents (see Chapter 4). In other words, the behaviours observed during conversational exchanges generally allow the examiner to anticipate which tasks of a more constrained nature should be subsequently presented in order to demonstrate specific symptomatological features (word-finding difficulty during naming tasks, phonetic and/or phonological transformations during repetition tasks, deficits in syntactic elaboration during sentence formulation tasks, etc.) which should be examined with particular attention.

Both qualitative and quantitative characteristics of discourse can be judged from a sample of conversational language. Does the patient speak readily, producing long utterances or, on the contrary, does s/he respond in only a minimal way, even to very intense stimulation? Quantitatively, in terms of the number of words per unit time, is his/her production restricted, normal or nearly so, or seemingly more abundant than normal (the presumed characteristic of logorrhoea)? Qualitatively, is a variety of words produced, as by normal speakers, or are the same words or expressions frequently repeated? In the latter case, is the qualitative reduction of such severity that only the production of certain stereotyped segments and ready-made expressions remains possible? Are verbal sequences articulated with normal conversational speed and rhythm or, on the contrary, are words pronounced slowly, laboriously and syllabically? Does the melodic aspect of speech appear normal and appropriate or is prosody attenuated? Are dysprosodic transformations observed? Does the patient tend towards the echolalic repetition of the interlocutor's words and, if so, is this phenomenon more pronounced for the final words of sentences? Is the patient's gestural behaviour, particularly that of the face and upper limbs, abundant or restricted? Are gestures superimposed on ample verbal output or are they intended to replace information which can no longer be conveyed through speech? Are the meanings conveyed by gestures sometimes dissociated from those conveyed by words?

One of the essential signs of aphasia, namely word-finding difficulty, is often revealed in spontaneous discourse. Does it include too many hesitations ('um'), too many incomplete sentences or the continued repetition of determiners, prepositions and other functional units? Are unavailable words usually replaced by periphrases, by words which are related in form or in meaning, by neologisms, by a preferred word or by general multi-purpose words ('thing', 'thingumijig', 'gadget', 'do', 'be', etc.)?

The precise identification of linguistic transformations (see Chapter 2), when they occur in conversation (which is almost always the case), as well as even a gross estimate of their number, allows judgements concerning the linguistic typology of the aphasia. Are phonetic transformations produced and, if so, can a predominantly paretic or dystonic component be discerned[7] (see Chapter 3)? Are the phonetic transformations accompanied by the production of paraphasias and, particularly, by the production of phonemic paraphasias? In cases where the strictly articulatory aspects of production are normal, are various types of transformations produced or is there a predominant or nearly exclusive production of a particular type of transformation? In the latter case, do phonemic paraphasias predominate[8] and, if so, do these transformations particularly affect words from lexical inventories or longer words? Do words evoked with difficulty appear to be more subject to phonemic transformations than words which the patient began to utter without any noticeable delay? If verbal transformations predominate, can they usually be definitely identified as being of a semantic type? Is there a preferred word or theme? Are the verbal and syntagmatic paraphasias so numerous that the patient's language appears very incoherent? Are neologisms produced and, if so, do they especially appear to replace nouns and predicative adjectives[9]? Considered in general, is the patient's discourse so transformed that it meets the definition of jargonaphasia[5, 9]?

The study of the syntactical aspects of the patient's spontaneous language is equally important. Does production consist mainly of short, juxtaposed sentences, which are often reduced to a single word (substantive, infinitive verb form), or does it consist of sentences of varied length, including juxtaposition, coordination and subordination and differing in this regard from normal language only by the greater proportion of syntagms which are faulty in terms of conventional usage? In other words, is there a clear tendency towards agrammatism [see example (4.1)] or towards dyssyntaxia? In the latter case, is it possible to determine whether the dyssyntactic transformations are usually attributable to word-finding difficulty or to the paraphasic usage of grammatical segments?

It is also of interest to note variations in the patient's discourse according to the topics discussed or the characteristics of the conversational context. Is word-finding difficulty less obvious and are transformations less frequent (including phonetic transformations) when the patient speaks about subjects which are personally very familiar, and, as a complement, do the signs of aphasia become more evident when he or she attempts to reply to the examiner's specific questions? Are there times, for example, when the patient is affected by emotion, when s/he easily produces words or sentences which s/he was unable to formulate in a more abstract situation, in a more propositional context (automatic–voluntary dissociation)?

While a conversational language sample is obviously most suited to the study of aphasic disturbances of oral expression, it also allows the examiner to form an initial impression about the possible presence of a disturbance of spoken language comprehension. This impression is generally global and uncertain and pertains only to an elementary and concrete level of comprehension. It may nevertheless be very valuable in certain cases where the nature of the comprehension disturbance is such that more specific tests cannot be completed. Several aspects of the aphasic's behaviour may be of interest in this regard. Does s/he often ask the interlocutor to repeat? Are the aphasic's responses to questions abnormally delayed or, on the contrary, does s/he immediately continue his/her past discussion as soon as the interlocutor has stopped speaking? Does the verbal content of the examiner's questions influence the nature of the patient's responses, and if so, is this a constant phenomenon or evident only in the initial parts of the patient's response to a question? Does the patient generally attend to and consider the interlocutor's interventions or does s/he sometimes continue speaking when someone is talking to him/her? Are certain non-ambiguous responses, such as 'yes' or 'no', or their corresponding gestures, generally appropriate?

Conversation with an aphasic allows judgement concerning the patient's awareness of his impairment. Does s/he acknowledge any difficulties in response to direct questioning by the examiner? Does s/he often allude to them spontaneously? Does s/he continue to converse at length despite occasional allusions to his/her disorder [see examples (13.16) and (13.18)]? In the case of jargonaphasia, does the patient appear to believe that his/her discourse constitutes effective communication. In other words, is the patient anosognosic and, if so, is the anosognosia complete or partial?

Finally, certain general characteristics may be revealed by the patient's attitudes during conversational exchanges, such as a state of excitation or a tendency towards aggressiveness, euphoria or sadness.

The analysis of a spontaneous language sample is the only part of an aphasia assessment which examines language in a natural (or nearly natural) situation. Conversation with the aphasic should thus be as open and as candid as possible. The examiner should nevertheless attempt to orient the patient's productions, although never in an overly rigid way. The examiner's role is that of an interviewer, whose comments and questions should be clearly and completely formulated and, in general, should be provided only when the patient has stopped talking. In such conditions, the number and length of the examiner's interventions, when compared with those of the aphasic, may provide a valuable index to the clinical type of aphasia [see examples (4.5), (4.20) and (6.1)]. In order to obtain adequate samples of language and, especially, to facilitate comparisons among different groups of patients, the conversation should be systematically directed towards certain pre-selected topics—family, work, hobbies, vacations, politics—which most patients will willingly discuss if they are able to do so. Other questions, directed towards less 'programmed' topics, may permit the demonstration of relatively mild word-finding difficulty or some other feature of the aphasia. The language sample should be tape-recorded if the examiner wishes to carry out a detailed study of particular aspects of the patient's production or if s/he simply wishes to obtain an illustration of the patient's productions at a particular time during evolution. The use of a tape recorder is essential for patients presenting an articulatory disturbance or abundant discourse containing paraphasic and neologistic segments. Except in cases presenting a severe reduction or asponaneity, it is nearly impossible to make an immediate and accurate transcription of an aphasic's productions (a fact which can be convincingly illustrated by reading an immediate transcription, even by a very experienced clinician, while listening to the corresponding tape-recorded sample).

NARRATION AND PICTURE DESCRIPTION

When they contain many transformations, samples of conversational language have the disadvantage of not permitting the examiner to identify with reasonable certainty exactly what it was that the patient wished to say (if s/he was, in fact, attempting to say something specific). As a consequence, different transformations, and particularly phonemic and semantic paraphasias, may not be precisely identified. This difficulty may sometimes be overcome by asking the patient to recount a well-known story (Insertion 15.1). In our work, we usually use the story *Little Red Riding Hood* and ask the patient to recount it as if 'telling it to a group of children'. This specification is added in order to alleviate the embarrassment which most adults otherwise feel when given such a task.

It can easily be seen how one or another of the popular versions of this story can serve as a 'norm' and thus provide a basis for comparison of the aphasic's narration: his/her production will provide material especially suited to the study of verbal transformations and the logical sequencing of sentences.*

Picture description tasks are also used to facilitate the identification of verbal transformations and the study of the logic of discourse. In addi-

* After having tape-recorded a production based on the patient's memory, the investigation may be completed by asking the patient to repeat his/her narrative, this time using a sequence of pictures which illustrate the story (see Fig. 15-3) as a guide.

Insertion 15.1

'En définitive, c'était la MÈRE qui s'/de/↓ qui s'débinait, mangée par le↓ par le loup↓ par le loup. Alors↓ Alors donc, avant, c'était un mythe. Ils s'etaient montrés les uns les autres d'une manière /difɛʀ/↓ *sous une forme différente et, en définitive, il y avait des ÂMES↓ des ÂMES, en tout coïncidence↓ enfin toute↓ qui sont arrivées ... Bon, bien, elle a traversé la↓ la↓ elle a traversé la* /fu/↓ /fulɛt/↓ /fu/↓ /fu/↓ forêt. Bon, *elle a été suivie par le↓ le↓ le↓ par le loup et il y a↓ Là, théoriquement, on l'a mangée. Ce loup l'a mangée et a mangé sans doute les↓ les galettes dans le↓ dans le petit↓ dans le petit SAC... Ils sont arrivés, en définitive. Alors là, le↓ le↓ le↓ le loup↓ le loup a SONNÉ: "Tire* /tetavtatavʀa/ /ʃe/↓ *cherra." Là, la vieille grand↓ grand↓ grand-mère est RENTRÉE↓ a été mangée. ELLE↓ ELLE a pris la place. ELLE s'est HABITUÉE comme↓ comme↓ ELLE s'est HABITUÉE avec les mêmes↓ comme une↓ et quand elle↓ la petite est arrivée, elle a dit: "C'est la MÈRE qui rentre." Et la MÈRE, aussi, doit↓ devait rentrer. Elle est rentrée et elle a dit: "Pour avoir des jambes comme↓ sont↓ sont grandes. C'est de ta faute parce que↓ envie de manger. Euh, et les↓ les↓ les pieds sont↓ sont ceci. C'est parce que↓ c'est de ta faute... Les grandes oreilles, par exemple. Alors, les grands oreilles sont↓ sont plus↓ elles sont plus grandes que d'habitude↓ elles sont plus grandes que chez toi↓ que chez la grand-mère." Elle dit: "Oui, oui. Mais c'est pour mieux↓ c'est pour mieux t'entendre, etc., etc." "Vos↓ vos jambes sont↓ sont trop grandes pour↓ pour↓ par rapport↓ parce que ça donne plus de place, etc."... Et en↓ et en↓ la dernière phrase: "Et toi, TU AS DES DENTS LES PLUS LONGUES PARCE QUE C'EST POUR TE MANGER." Et voilà, et hop! Et il y avait théoriquement↓ ça devait être la fin (faim?) qui devait manger le↓ la petite... Le commencement de l'histoire du↓ de la↓ de la VEILLE GRAND-MÈRE. Bien, elle avait l'habitude de se promener dans les↓ dans les↓ dans↓ dans↓ dans LES forêts↓ dans la forêt. Pour commencer↓—hien!—pour porter un* /sa/↓ *un SACHET, un petit↓ un petit SAQUET↓—pas "saquet", c'est pas "saquet"—c'est↓ c'est la BOURSE. Maintenant, c'est dit: Une BOURSE. Mais c'est pas encore ce nom-là. C'est encore un autre. Pour↓ pour apporter la nourriture de la grand-mère. Et, entre temps, elle↓ elle c'est↓ ce qui est↓ ... Tout le long du TROTTOIR↓ du petit↓ du petit TROTTOIR, elle ramassait du↓ des fleurs dans la grand↓ dans la↓ entre les arbres ... Alors donc, voilà le début du commencement, et après la suite.'*

'Finally, it was the MOTHER who /de/↓ made off, eaten by the↓ by the wolf↓ by the wolf. So↓ So therefore, before, it was a myth. They appeared one and all in a manner /difɛʀ/↓ under a different form and, finally, there were some SOULS↓ some SOULS, in all coincidence↓ finally all↓ who arrived. ... Well, then, she crossed the↓ the↓ she crossed the /fu/↓ /fulɛt/↓ /fu/↓ /fu/↓ forest. Well, she had been followed by the↓ the↓ the↓ by the wolf and there is↓ There, theoretically, she was eaten. This wolf ate her and no doubt ate the↓ the cakes in the↓ in the little BAG ... They arrived, finally. So there, the↓ the↓ the↓ the wolf↓ the wolf RANG: "Tire /tetavtatavʀa/ /ʃe/↓ cherra." There, the old grand↓ grand↓ grand-mother RETURNED↓ has been eaten. SHE↓ SHE took the place. SHE was ACCUSTOMED to like↓ like↓ SHE was ACCUSTOMED to with the same↓ like a↓ and when she↓ the little girl arrived, she said: "It's MOTHER who returns." And the MOTHER, too, must↓ had to return. She returned and she said: "To have legs like↓ are↓ are big. It's your fault because↓ want to eat. Uh, and the↓ the↓ the feet are↓ are this. It's because↓ it's your fault ... The big ears, for example. The big ears are↓ are more↓ they're bigger than usual↓ they're bigger than yours↓ than grandmother's." She said: "Yes, yes. But it's to better↓ it's to hear you better, etc. etc." "Your↓ your legs are↓ are too big for↓ for ↓ compared with↓ because that makes more room, etc." ... And in↓ and in↓ the last sentence: "And you, YOU HAVE THE LONGEST TEETH BECAUSE IT'S TO EAT YOU." And there it is, and off with you! And there was theoretically↓ that should have been the end (hunger?) who should have eaten the↓ the little girl ... The beginning of the story of a↓ of the↓ of the OLD GRAND-MOTHER. Well, she had the habit of walking in a↓ in a↓ in↓ in↓ in the FORESTS↓ in the forest. In order to begin↓—eh!—in order to carry a /sa/↓ a SACHET, a little↓ a little SACKETTE↓—not 'sackette', it's not "sackette"—it's↓ it's the PURSE. Now, it's been said: A PURSE. But it's still not that name. It's still another one. To↓ to carry the grandmother's food. And, meanwhile, she↓ she is↓ which is↓ ... All along the SIDEWALK↓ of the little↓ of the little SIDEWALK, she picked of↓ some flowers in the big↓ in the↓ between the trees ... And so, there is the beginning of the commencement, and after the continuation.'

(*Narration by Mr Les.; May 1969*)

tion, they also permit identification of word-finding difficulty. Suitable stimuli include realistic drawings clearly drawn in black ink against a white background and containing illustrations of several common objects. The analysis of the patient's productions is often facilitated by his or her spontaneous pointing to different parts of the picture as s/he carries out the verbal description. The task may provide relevant information about the patient's descriptive strategy. Does s/he proceed by listing details, that is, by the isolated naming of various elements of the picture? Is s/he able to provide a well-organized description? Does s/he spontaneously attempt a synthetic interpretation of the stimulus, as would be indicated by the suggestion of an appropriate title? Descriptions limited to only one half of the picture suggest the possibility of unilateral visual neglect (see Chapters 4 and 16).

AUTOMATIC UTTERANCES

We use the term *automatic utterances* to refer to over-learned verbal responses reproduced from memory, such as counting, reciting the days of the week, months of the year, highly familiar stories, prayers, etc. When necessary, the examiner can attempt to facilitate this type of production by cueing the patient with the first word or words of the utterance or recitation (see Chapter 10, Goldstein's *central motor aphasia*). In certain cases of severe aphasia, automatic utterances may constitute the only form of production which remains possible, besides one or a few verbal stereotypes: such cases then provide a remarkable demonstration of automatic–voluntary dissociation. In other cases, the manifestations of such a dissociation may be more subtle: for example, articulatory production may be normal or nearly normal during the recitation of automatized sequences whereas an articulatory disturbance is clearly evident during the production of more propositional language. The examination of automatic utterances also permits verification of whether the patient is able to produce ordered listings and whether s/he shows a tendency towards perseveration.

WORD EVOCATION

Naming

Naming subtests are among the most important of those comprising an aphasia test. In most cases, naming can be adequately explored through a subtest involving the presentation of around 30 drawings or photographs representing common objects, familiar animals, etc. The stimuli selected should be highly codable in the sense that they would normally elicit only one or a very small number of different responses. During the naming subtest, the examiner notes which stimuli fail to elicit a response, as well as the nature of all abnormal responses, be they in the form of semantic paraphasias [(15.1) '*cheval*'→'*boeuf*' ('horse'→'ox')], formal verbal paraphasias [(15.2) '*cheval*'→'*cheveux*' ('horse'→'hair')], neologisms [(15.3) '*cheval*'→ '/nepɔl/' ('horse'→'/nepɔl/')], periphrasis [(15.4) '*cheval*'→'*c'est pour la ferme*' ('horse'→'it's for the farm')], etc. In mild cases, word-finding difficulty may escape notice unless items are presented which require the retrieval of words which are more specific and have a lower frequency of usage: in such cases the patient will be asked to name not only objects, but also parts of objects (e.g., the face, second-hand, bracelet and buckle of a watch, the stem and veins of a leaf).

Certain aphasics may exhibit word-finding difficulty only, or mainly, in the form of abnormally long response latencies. Since they will be globally reflected in the total duration of the naming test, this measure should be systematically recorded (and compared with figures obtained from normal subjects). The overall severity of word-finding difficulty (in confrontation naming) is probably best estimated by a composite index combining this temporal measure with the proportion of failures to respond and erroneous responses relative to the total number of stimuli. Responses which can be recognized as adequate word selections despite abnormal articulation [(15.5) '*cheval*'→ ≃/tʃœfal/] or production of a phonemic paraphasia [(15.6) '*cheval*'→ ≃/ʒalaval/] would not, of course, be counted as naming errors.

Naming errors may sometimes appear at least partially attributable to the presence of an agnosic, rather than aphasic, impairment [(15.7) '*corde*' → '*serpent*' ('rope' → 'snake'), (15.8) '*accordéon*' → '*radiateur*' ('accordion' → 'radiator'), (15.9) '*champignon*' → '*parapluie*' (mushroom' → 'umbrella') during picture naming]. In these cases, other subtests will be presented to examine naming in different sense modalities, that is, naming of palpated objects, seen objects, sounds made by objects. The presence or absence of a dissociation between different modalities will permit confirmation or refutation of a suspected agnosia.

When the patient is unable to produce the name of a given stimulus, the examiner will try to facilitate its production by the use of different procedures. For example, if the patient is unable to evoke the word 'hammer' in response to the corresponding picture, the examiner will attempt to facilitate production through a phonemic cue (It's a /hæ/ . . . It's a /hæm/ . . .) or a contextual cue (You pound nails with a . . .). Other possible modes of facilitation include the presentation of the first letter of the word or the complete written word, gestural cues, or the pronunciation of a word which is similar in form or in meaning[10]. Depending on the case, the examiner will note that one or more types of facilitation are particularly effective, that all types of facilitation are of approximately equal efficacy or that no form of facilitation has a positive effect [such information is relevant to the planning of an eventual therapy programme (see Chapter 17)].

Evocation of action verbs

Drawings and photographs may also be used as stimuli in a subtest intended to elicit production of certain action verbs (run, write, cry, etc.) (see Fig. 15-4). The examiner notes whether the patient's responses are usually in the form of a short syntagm or the infinitive verb form and, in the latter case, whether this tendency persists regardless of specific instructions ('run', rather than 'A boy is running', and 'write', rather than 'A man is writing', etc. may indicate a tendency towards agrammatism).

Word fluency (evocation of category exemplars)

During this subtest, the examiner designates a particular category and asks the patient to name as many members as possible within a predetermined period. The category may be specified in either semantic (names of animals, vegetables, etc.) or formal (words beginning with a given letter) terms. The patient's productions are recorded and judged with reference to the performance of normal subjects. Unlike confrontation naming, the evocation of category exemplars does not depend on a sensory stimulus specific to each word (the patient must, so to speak, draw upon mnemonic inventories) and, unless otherwise indicated by the instructions, does not limit production solely to concrete substantives. A dissociation is sometimes observed, especially in the case of certain frontal lesions (see Chapter 6), between naming, which is normal or nearly so, and word fluency, which is particularly deficient.

Antonyms

On this subtest, which is particularly well suited to the evocation of adjectives and verbs, the patient is asked to produce a word which is opposite in meaning to each stimulus word spoken successively by the examiner. It is sometimes noted that the evocation of lexical antonyms (e.g., 'thick'↔'thin', 'poor'↔'rich') is easier than that of morphological antonyms (e.g. 'useful'↔'useless', 'lock'↔'unlock') for certain Broca's aphasics, and may then reflect one aspect of agrammatism[11, 12]. In contrast, the evocation of morphological antonyms is sometimes easier than that of lexical antonyms for certain Wernicke's aphasics (since, in the former case, word-finding difficulty is reduced by the provision of the lexical moneme).

Definitions

The patient is asked to define a few words from different lexical inventories. The stimulus words are generally presented in order from the most concrete to the most abstract. For abstract words, which cannot be easily studied on naming tests, this subtest provides one approach to the investigation of the links remaining between word forms and meanings (*liens signifiants—signifiés*). The types of definitions observed during this subtest (repetition of the stimulus, definition by use, description, production of a synonym or antonym, etc.) may indicate whether there is a loss of what Goldstein[13] has called the *categorical attitude* (see Insertion 10.2).

Sentence formulation

It is often useful to extend the investigation of syntactic disturbances beyond the information which can be gained from the study of a conversational language sample, narration and picture description (cf. pp. 350–354). There are cases, for example, in which this will be necessary in order to plan an appropriate therapy programme (see Chapter 17). Many different types of tasks can be used in this regard but we generally ask the patient to 'make a sentence' which includes words specified by the examiner. Here, again, the stimuli are usually presented in order from the most concrete to the most abstract ('Make a sentence with "baker" and "bread"' before 'Make a sentence with "skill", "success" and competition"'). The difficulty of the task can be greatly increased for the aphasic by asking him or her to formulate a sentence using words which bear no obvious conceptual relationship to each other (e.g., 'plumber' and 'squirrel'). Goodglass[14] has proposed the use of a task in which the patient must formulate a sentence to complete a given context ('Peter is in Mary's room. Mary wants Peter to leave her room. She says: " ... ') (see Chapter 12).

REPETITION AND ORAL READING

Audiophonatory transposition (repetition) and visuophonatory transposition (oral reading) are impaired in most aphasics (see Chapters 3 to 5). These impairments may occur in the absence of any auditory or visual perceptual disturbance or, in other instances, reflect an agnosic disturbance. In the latter case, the disorder generally affects perception of both linguistic and non-linguistic stimuli but, exceptionally, may be limited to linguistic stimuli (see Chapter 5). Distinguishing among these different cases is of great importance in aphasiology and requires that repetition and oral reading be very carefully examined.

Repetition and oral reading are particularly well suited to the study of oral language transformations, especially phonetic and phonemic transformations, because the subject's responses can be described with reference to specified stimuli. These behaviours thus merit particular emphasis when studying aphasic disorganizations of the third and second linguistic phases of oral language (see Chapters 2 and 10). In all cases, observations obtained during repetition and oral reading should be carefully compared, both qualitatively and quantitatively, with those obtained during conversation and narration.

Several characteristics of repetition and oral reading should be systematically noted. Is there total or near total impairment, as indicated by the absence of production or minimal production, or is the disturbance manifested by the constant or intermittent production of transformations? Does the disturbance become increasingly evident as the stimuli become longer? Does phonetic complexity affect performance and, if so, does the patient have particular difficulty with stimuli including vocalic groups or consonant clusters, those with an initial vowel, or those with a final consonant? Do the transformations indicate a tendency to simplify the phonological structure of the stimulus or is the phonological structure of the transformation sometimes more complex than that of the stimulus? Does the patient have more or less difficulty with stimuli which have no conventional meaning (e.g., nonsense words such as /pɪvæglo/, /strɛmɪfaθ/, etc.) than with meaningful words or sentences? When the stimuli are single words, is performance affected by their concrete or abstract nature, by the lexical or grammatical inventory to which they belong, or by their frequency of usage in the linguistic community? In the case of sentence stimuli, are those containing many grammatical words more difficult than those of equal length which contain few grammatical words? Is the severity of the disturbance similar for the transposition of single words and for sentences?

When phonetic distintegration (see Chapter 3) is present, the production of individual phonemes will be studied with reference to the position which they occupy in different stimuli [initial, final, intervocalic or interconsonantal, within various vowel or consonant groups; e.g., production of the phoneme /l/ would be studied in contexts such as /lo/ (low), /ɪl/ (ill), /vælɪ/ (valley), /slɪp/ (slip), /klærɪtɪ/ (clarity), /spɛktækl/ (spectacle), etc.]. In most cases, an experienced listener will have relatively little difficulty in distinguishing between paretic and dystonic aspects, or in reaching conclusions about the presence or absence of different abnormalities such as the production of pseudodiphthongs or pseudopolyphthongs or transformations resulting from affrication, glottalization, nasalisation or oralization, voicing or devoicing, etc. (see Chapters 3 and 12). Use of a speech spectrograph will nevertheless be necessary if a more detailed qualitative and quantitative investigation is required.

When phonemic transformations are produced, the examiner will note their frequency, their degree of complexity (i.e., the extent to which their structure differs from that of the stimuli), a possible predominance of selection errors [(15.10) /vɛstiʒ → fɛstiʒ/] or of sequencing errors [(2.74) /pulaje → apulje/, (15.11) /finisɛ → fisinɛ/, (2.14) /deɑ̃bylɑ̃ → debɑ̃bylɑ̃/, (15.12) /fuʀniʀ → fuʀfir/, etc.] (see Chapter 2), the presence of telescopages [(14.6) /animal + mamifɛr → maminal/], responses contaminated by the structure of a preceding response [(15.13) /fʀɔmaʒ → fʀɔmaʒ/ then /ʀado → fʀado/], and perseveration. Comparisons between spontaneous language and transposition activities are of interest in the case of patients who produce numerous phonemic transformations: in conduction aphasia, for example, phonemic paraphasias commonly predominate in repetition whereas spontaneous discourse includes formal verbal paraphasias as well as phonemic paraphasias [see examples (4.5) to (4.16)]. Similarly, in conduction aphasia and Wernicke's aphasia proper, a qualitative and quantitative comparison of audiophonatory and visuophonatory transposition will often reveal the presence of a dissociation [one which has implications for the planning of an eventual programme (see Chapter 17)].

Repetition and oral reading tasks, especially those involving sentences (and passages of text in the latter case) may also be useful in studying certain aspects of aphasic disorganizations affecting the first phase of oral language (see Chapter 2). If present, agrammatism is almost always observed during these subtests. This is less often the case for dyssyntaxia (paragrammatism), although the repetition or reading of grammatical words may be particularly difficult for many Wernicke's aphasics. Semantic paraphasias, which are fairly common in oral reading, are rarely produced in repetition; when they are observed, they are considered to be one of the possible manifestations of a partial rupture of the links between forms and meanings.

Finally, it should be mentioned that sentence repetition may be useful in the study of aphasic disturbances of prosody and that oral reading sometimes leads to a demonstration of unilateral visual field neglect [(15.14) *'chèvre-feuille'* → *'chevre'* or *'feuille'* ('honeysuckle' → 'goat' or 'leaf'), or (15.15) *'formule'* → *' forme'* or *' mule'* ('formula' → 'form' or 'mule')].

In concluding this discussion of oral expression, we note that all observations obtained during an aphasia assessment should be recorded and kept for future reference in the patient's file. In this regard, observed phonetic and phonemic transformations should be transcribed using the symbols of the International Phonetic Alphabet so that they are recorded in a standard manner and one which is meaningful to others. Similarly, if certain subtests were omitted because the examiner judged them to be inappropriate for a particular patient, these omissions should be explicitly mentioned in the patient's file (e.g., the examiner would not ask patients whose oral expression is reduced to a stereotype to attempt to tell the story of *Little Red Riding Hood* but would note the reason for the omission of this subtest).

ASSESSMENT OF ORAL LANGUAGE COMPREHENSION

Certain characteristics of subtests used to assess spoken language comprehension were discussed elsewhere (see Chapter 4, 'Symptomatology of the Aphasias'). Although these subtests are intended to reveal the presence of a comprehension disturbance, their nature is such that performance may also be abnormal for other reasons. Hence a comprehension disturbance can be positively identified only after ruling out the presence of other conditions which could account for the observed abnormalities. They include:

1. Visual impairment if, as is often the case, the tasks used to assess auditory comprehension require that spoken stimuli be identified by pointing to pictures or visually presented objects; in Wernicke's aphasia and global aphasia, caution is particularly necessary in regard to the identification of pictures or objects presented in the right visual field.
2. A praxic disturbance, if the correct responses require relatively complex movements.
3. A memory disturbance affecting linguistic messages[15,16] if the spoken commands are long and include several steps; in this regard it should be borne in mind that impaired auditory comprehension and impaired retention are not mutually exclusive and, in fact, are generally associated.

If it is concluded that a comprehension disturbance is present, the examiner will ask whether or not it is related to word deafness (see Chapter 4, 'Wernicke's aphasia proper', and Chapter 5, 'Word deafness'); in this regard, the comparison of spoken language comprehension and written language comprehension (cf. p. 360) may be extremely significant. In summary, we note that it is relatively easy to reach a definite conclusion about the status of auditory comprehension when the patient successfully completes the tests presented. Failures are more difficult to interpret and, in cases of poor performance, conclusions are sometimes guarded and uncertain.

Answers should be obtained to several questions about the patient's general behaviour during oral comprehension testing. Does the patient respond confidently, regardless of the adequacy of his/her responses, or does s/he frequently hesitate, cup an ear, or ask that stimuli or instructions be repeated? Does the patient spontaneously acknowledge difficulty in understanding or react to the interlocutor's gestures of acquiescence or puzzlement? Does s/he appear particularly attentive to information conveyed by mime or gesture and does performance deteriorate when the examiner's face, and particularly the mouth, is concealed? Is comprehension affected by the presence of background noise? Does it appear to be dependent on the concrete nature of the stimuli or on their insertion in an immediate, pragmatic context? Does the acoustic complexity of the stimuli appear to play a role: are single words better understood than words presented within sentences or vice versa? Are the intervals between stimuli and responses abnormally long, delays which cannot be attributed to the presence of hemiparesis, a hemianopsia, etc.? Generally speaking, does comprehension appear to improve during the course of the different subtests, even during the simplest ones which have no time limits? Does the degree of comprehension vary, from one moment to another, during tasks of equivalent difficulty? Are perseverative phenomena (in the form of identical responses to different, successively presented stimuli) observed as 'fatigue' increases and, if so, is there a return to the initial level of performance after a few minutes of 'rest' or 'distraction'?

With the exception of those cases in which aphasia results from a progressive disease, for example, a malignant tumour or degenerative disease (see Chapter 9), disturbances of oral comprehension are generally most severe at the time of onset. Considerable recovery usually follows, with the patient regaining at least an 'elementary' level of understanding (see Chapters 4 and 10). The extent of such recovery should thus be assessed on several occasions, particularly since it may be of great importance when planning therapy exercises.

COMPREHENSION OF SINGLE WORDS

Substantives

Comprehension of single words is generally tested using word identification tasks. Strictly speaking, the stimuli are not usually presented as isolated words but rather as the final word of a spoken sentence (which is otherwise identical on every trial and whose meaning is made explicit by the test situation: 'Show me the . . .' or 'Where is the . . .?'). In the case of substantives, the identification tasks are usually carried out using a large card showing several pictures (drawings or pho-

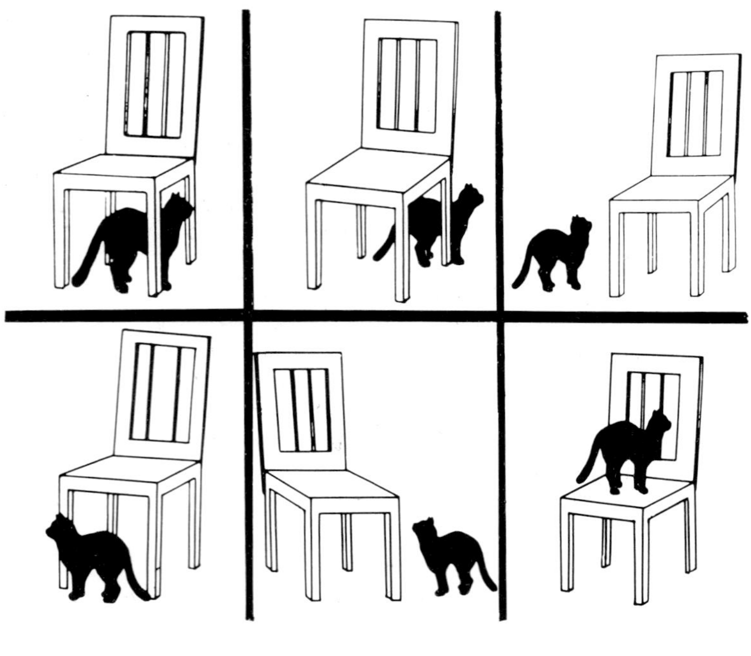

Fig. 15-2 *The assessment of aphasia: André Ombredane's task, known as* 'The Cat and the Chair Test' (*a test examining comprehension of prepositions:* 'on' 'under' 'in front of', etc.). *From Ombredane*[17], *p. 403. Drawings by Laurent Coderre.*

tographs of common objects, fruits or vegetables, animals etc.). It is not unusual, and such an observation should always be recorded, for the identification of spoken words to be normal, or near normal, when the pictures on the response card illustrate words which are unrelated in either meaning or form (orange, razor, button), while many errors occur when the pictures illustrate words which are related in meaning (orange, lemon, apple) or in form [(razor, raisin, raven); /reɪzə/, /rezn/, /revən/]. The former case suggests that the oral comprehension disturbance is primarily of a psycholinguistic type (especially when comprehension of written language is also impaired) whereas the latter suggests a more elementary disturbance related to auditory perception (especially when comprehension of written language is relatively spared) (see Chapters 4, 5 and 17).

Grammatical words

Regardless of the clinical type of aphasia, the comprehension of grammatical words is often relatively more impaired than that of lexical words (or, in any case, than that of concrete lexical words). This point merits the most detailed examination in cases presenting a mild disturbance of oral comprehension and should always be thoroughly explored in those Broca's aphasics who, on first observation, appear to 'understand everything'. Prepositions (and prepositional idioms) are particularly well suited to investigation by use of stimulus sentences which specify the relationship between two common nouns (the examiner ensures that these two words are understood by having the patient point several times to the corresponding pictures or objects). Like Ombredane[17], we use a card illustrating different spatial relationships between a cat and a chair. The patient's task is to point to the cat 'on', 'under', in front of', 'behind', 'beside' the chair (Fig. 15–2).* Errors on this task often reflect confusions between antonyms ('on' versus 'under', 'in front of' versus 'behind')*. When observed, the nature of such confusions should be recorded.

Verbs

The visual illustration of certain action verbs is relatively easy (e.g., 'run', 'cry', 'drink', etc.) so that comprehension may then be tested using an identification-by-pointing procedure analogous to that described for the testing of concrete substantives. For verbs which are less suited to direct illustration, comprehension can sometimes be tested by presenting conceptually related pictures and asking the patient to point to the one which answers a question centred on a verb (for example, the patient is asked 'which one stings?' when presented with a picture of a bee, a butterfly and a dragonfly).

SENTENCE COMPREHENSION

In the investigation of sentence comprehension, the stimuli and required responses should be carefully selected in order to eliminate the effects of possible visual, mnemonic or praxic factors. In this regard, we find it advantageous to present short utterances which require, as the response, the selection of one of the elements of the stimulus sentence. This type of task usually permits the examiner to identify correct responses even when they are only gestured or are verbal but non-specific (e.g., 'Yes!', 'That's it', 'That one', etc.). The difficulty of the test items can be varied in several ways: by distributing the main semantic load over words from different lexical or grammatical inventories; by varying the type of associations required for a correct response (e.g., 'Is a carrot a vegetable, a tool or a piece of furniture?' requires only simple semantic associations but relatively more complex ones are required to answer the question 'Are plans for houses designed by an architect, a carpenter or an electrician?'); and by varying the degree of similarity in meaning or in form among the multiple-choice words ('Is a carrot a vegetable, a tool or a piece of furniture?' or 'Is a tulip a fruit, a flower or a tree?' or 'Do you write with a pan, a pen or a pin?').

Several questions can be asked about the results of these multiple-choice tasks. Were the patient's responses decisive or hesitant? Did s/he often ask that the stimuli be repeated or spoken more slowly? What is the total percentage of errors? Does stimulus complexity appear to affect performance? Is there particular difficulty when the multiple-choice words are related in

* During this task, many normal subjects respond incorrectly to the stimuli 'to the left of' and 'to the right of' (because they refer to their own left or right rather than to the left or right of the chair). Thus, for these stimuli, aphasic errors are significant only when they are not of an antonymic type.

meaning or in form? Is there a dissociation between the comprehension of single words and that of sentences?

PIERRE MARIE'S THREE PAPER TEST

Pierre Marie's Test[6], which is still known as the 'Three Paper Test', is a classical procedure in clinical aphasiology. Numerous equivalents can be easily imagined but the force of tradition is such that the task is usually presented in its original form. It consists of a three-stage command which is presented as a whole before a response is permitted. Three pieces of paper, of different sizes, are placed in front of the patient who is told, for instance, to throw the large one on the floor, to give the small one to the examiner and to put the medium-sized one in his or her pocket. Completely accurate performance indicates the absence of a significant disturbance of oral comprehension. On the other hand, performance which deviates from the instructions does not necessarily indicate a disturbance of oral comprehension (cf. p. 357) and may, in fact, be evidence of an amnesic or praxic impairment.

TOKEN TEST

The Token Test, as originally developed by de Renzi and Vignolo[18], is composed of five series of commands representing five successive levels of complexity. Each command is presented orally and requires the manipulation of one or more tokens from a group of tokens which differ in shape, size or colour (see Chapter 16). Many neuropsychological disorders—such as colour agnosia, unilateral visual neglect apraxia, aphasia, intellectual deterioration, etc.—may impair performance on this test. On the other hand, when an aphasic's performance on the Token Test is comparable with that of normal subjects, it can definitely be concluded that s/he does not present a disturbance of oral language comprehension.

COMPREHENSION OF DISCOURSE

The comprehension of discourse is tested using a relatively concrete descriptive or narrative text which is selected because it includes several distinct facts and can be easily summarized in relatively few words. The passage is read or recited to the patient who is then asked questions regarding specific pieces of information which were presented. To examine overall comprehension of the entire text, which is the major purpose of this subtest, the patient is asked to summarize the passage and to suggest an appropriate title. The inability to do so, despite adequate expressive language and preserved comprehension of specific information, indicates impaired comprehension of wholes, one of the most subtle manifestations of an aphasic disturbance of oral comprehension. As indicated by this statement, performance on this subtest must be interpreted relative to the patient's oral expressive abilities and performance on subtests assessing comprehension at more elementary levels.

ABSURD STORIES

The stimulus for this subtest is a short story which includes an implicit contradiction. We use the following one, selected from those included in Ribaucourt-Ducarne's procedures for the assessment of aphasia[19]: 'Peter met the postman and asked if he had a letter for him. The postman asked for his name. Peter told him to look on the envelope.' This is probably the most sensitive of all the subtests included in our routine aphasiological assessment. Although aphasics with a mild disturbance of oral comprehension, that is, with impaired comprehension of wholes, are able to retell the story in detail and to answer different questions about it, they are unable to appreciate the absurd nature of the stimulus.

Neither the absurd stories subtest nor some of the more difficult ones previously described would be presented to patients who demonstrate severely impaired oral comprehension. In this case again, the examiner would record the reason for these omissions in the patient's file.

ASSESSMENT OF WRITTEN EXPRESSION

We generally have an intuitive appreciation of what is 'normal' spoken language in our mother tongue and (if one is tolerant) can refer to this standard with some confidence. This is not the case for written language which is so subject to socio-cultural variation that 'normal' behaviour varies over a vast range whose limits are ill-defined. From an aphasiological point of view, this is particularly true for the second phase of written language (see Chapter 2); while a severe, acquired dysorthographia can usually be identified without difficulty, and certain milder impairments are sometimes indicated by the particular clarity of the transformations themselves, other mild impairments can only be identified by comparisons with samples of premorbid written production.

The assessment of written expression is frequently difficult or even impracticable because a sensorimotor hemi-deficit is associated with aphasia. This is especially true in cases of Broca's aphasia and global aphasia, particularly in the early post-onset period. The examiner should nevertheless attempt to obtain a sample of left-handed writing as soon as possible and, although it may not be easy or always possible, to distinguish among the effects of aphasia and those related to awkwardness or, especially, to apraxia. To permit preliminary study of residual orthographic skills in right-handed expression, the patient should also be asked to 'write' by arranging mobile letters. Regardless of the presence or absence of associated sensorimotor impairment, the majority of aphasics, including Wernicke's aphasics, show an aversion to writing and do not write spontaneously (see Chapter 4). Although the importance of the patient's educational background and premorbid writing habits should not be underestimated, we do not think that this aversion can be entirely explained by these factors (nor can occasional exceptions to this general rule which include some patients with relatively little education); the methods used in teaching written language when most of the patients were in school may also enter into account. Whatever the case, the evaluation of written expression (when it is, in fact, possible), often requires that the examiner be much more patient and energetic in eliciting production than during the evaluation of oral expression.

Although there are certain cases in which a disturbance of written expression dominates the clinical picture (see Chapters 3, 4 and 6), a disturbance of written language is most frequently paired with a disturbance of oral language and is, to a certain extent, dependent on it. Thus the examiner will carefully compare the results obtained during the assessment of written language with those obtained during the corresponding phases of the oral language assessment.

SPONTANEOUS WRITING AND WRITTEN NARRATION

When written expression is not completely or almost suppressed, every attempt should be made to obtain a sufficient sample of 'spontaneous' writing (see Fig. 4–1 and 4–2). Such a sample will facilitate the study of written language transformations and thereby contribute to the identification of the clinical form of aphasia and to reflection concerning the most advantageous approach to an eventual therapy programme (see Chapter 17). Nevertheless, an adequate sample is seldom easily obtained: the aphasics' aversion to writing, which appears to be shared by an increasing number of literate normals, is particularly marked in situations having few constraints (the interlocutor's interventions, which stimulate conversation, are absent during spontaneous writing). Recognizing that the examiner's approach must not be overly rigid, the following sequence is suggested as a general guideline: the patient is first asked to write about whatever s/he wants or whatever comes to mind; if s/he is then unable to begin writing, the examiner suggests a topic (the commonest ones, such as work, family and vacations, etc., are usually the most productive); finally, the patient is shown a series of pictures and is asked to write the story which they illustrate (Fig. 15–3). If the examiner is patient and ready to provide much encouragement, it will often be possible to obtain about ten lines of written production for both the suggested topic and the pictured story (the examiner notes the time required, which is usually abnormally long). Such a sample is usually adequate, although a longer one would obviously be preferable.

Besides the time required for written production, and the presence (or absence) of aspontaneity in written expression, several other characteristics should be investigated. Are automatisms of writing (see Chapter 4) well preserved? Is there a disturbance of graphism proper (see Fig. 3–1) and, if so, is it of such severity that no conventional alphabetic signs can be recognized? Are perseverative phenomena evident (recurrence of the same letters, syllables, words)? Do the samples contain paragraphic transformations and, if so, are they literal, graphemic [see example (4–19)] or verbal (the possible presence of verbal transformations will be particularly examined in the written narrative since the patient's productions can be compared with the standard version)? Are there several different types of transformations or is there a clear predominance of one particular type? Is there a correspondence or dissociation between written and oral transformations (e.g., literal paragraphias versus phonemic paraphasias)? Do certain segments appear to be neologisms and could production generally be referred to as jargonagraphia (even in the case of Broca's aphasia[9]) [see examples (2–85) and (4–3)]? If the patient speaks while writing, does s/he actually write what s/he says [see example (4–31)]? Is agrammatism or dyssyntaxia apparent and, if so, how does written production compare, in this respect, to the observations obtained during conversation and oral narration? With regard to dyssyntaxia specifically, is it not more evident in written than in oral expression [see example (2–82)]? Do the written language samples indicate lexical poverty or word-finding difficulty? Is the patient aware of having the impairment (refusal to continue writing is often a sign of discouragement, of lucidity)? In written narration, does the sequencing of sentences and the patient's comments indicate that the stimulus was perceived as a whole?

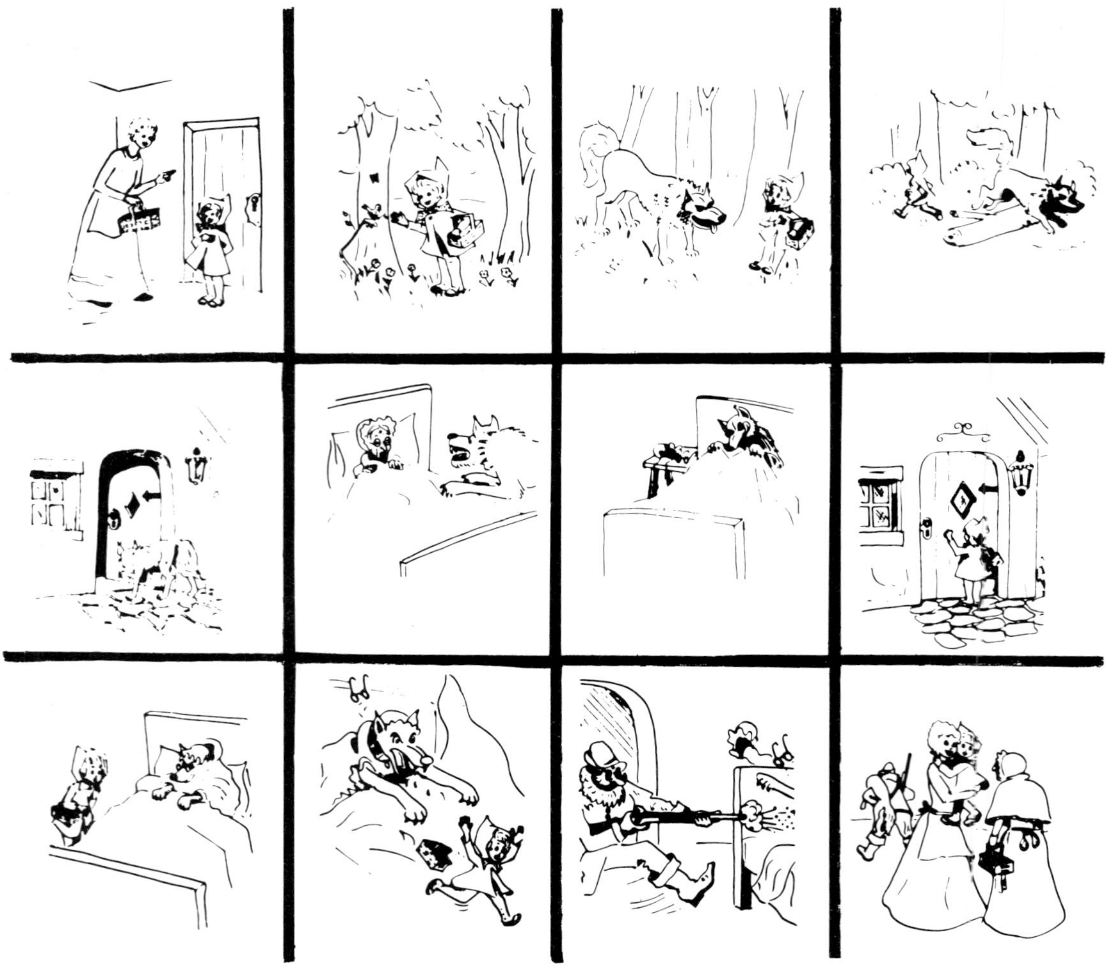

Fig. 15-3 *The assessment of aphasia: picture series* (Little Red Riding Hood) *used as visual support during the oral narration and written narration subtests. Drawings by George Vincelli* (Examen de l'aphasie du Laboratoire Théophile Alajouanine, Centre de Recherche du Centre Hospitalier Côte-des-Neiges, Montreal).

AUTOMATIC PRODUCTIONS

In cases of severely reduced written expression (i.e., cases of near suppression) the patient may retain only the ability to write his or her name or name and address (even this minimal sample can be judged with respect to the presence or absence of a graphic disturbance and, despite the automatized nature of the production, the effects of a dysorthographia may sometimes be observed). When the reduction is less severe, the patients may be willing to try to write numbers, the alphabet, the days of the week and the months of the year (the conventional order may not be followed and perseverative phenomena may be observed). Finally, certain patients will be able to write, with varying degrees of accuracy, memorized texts such as the words of a song, a poem or a prayer (these longer productions will be more useful than other automatic productions in permitting the identification of a possible graphic disturbance, paragraphic transformations, neologisms).

A comparison of the productions observed during this stage of the assessment with less constrained samples, such as written description and narration (cf. above), will ensure recognition of possible automatic–voluntary dissociation phenomena. For example, a patient who has great difficulty in writing propositional statements may nevertheless be able to write (usually with some transformations) a text which s/he has long known by heart. Similarly, in cases where written expression is more abundant, it may be noted that aphasic transformations—affecting one or more linguistic phases (see Chapter 2)—become less obvious as the written productions are less propositional.

WORD EVOCATION

The word evocation subtests discussed with regard to oral expression can, in general, be used in the study of written expression as well. If time is limited, the examiner may decide to restrict this part of the assessment to the evocation of substantives and verbs in response to pictured stimuli (Fig. 15-4). In addition to permitting further study of word-finding difficulty, these subtests, which require a known, predetermined response, often provide the most appropriate material for the identification and description of neologisms and of all types of paragraphias [see examples (4.33) to (4.42)]. For certain patients, written naming will be the part of the aphasia assessment which definitely confirms the production of verbal paragraphias (semantic and/or formal verbal paragraphias); in such cases, the corresponding phenomenon will usually have been observed in oral naming. For other patients, the written naming subtest will reveal the profile of dysorthographia, either with or without a predominance of literal or graphemic paragraphias: in these cases, the orthographic deviations in written naming should be compared with those produced when writing to dictation and, if the patient has undergone a previous assessment, it should be noted whether or not the observed dysorthographia represents a stage in the evolution of production which was initially neologistic [see example (4.27)].

The examiner should bear the following points in mind when presenting the written naming subtests:

1. Certain means of facilitation used in oral naming can also be used in written naming. The examiner may also use other facilitating techniques which are specific to written expression. [For example, the examiner may give the patient, in writing, the first letter of the word which s/he is unable to retrieve. The efficacy of this type of cue should then be noted and compared with that of phonemic cues (cf. p. 354).]
2. If the patient spontaneously speaks while writing, it is interesting to note the relationship between the oral and written productions. When they do not correspond, the examiner will attempt to determine whether one of the two segments produced (oral or written) is systematically closer to the required response. Because they are of obvious theoretical interest, the examiner will note the occurrence of concomitant dissociated responses, that is, responses which are correct in one modality but paraphasic or paragraphic in the other [such responses are especially interesting when the transformation is in the form of a paraphasia or paragraphia; for example (4.41), shown a picture of a *perroquet* (parrot), the patient said the name correctly (/pεRɔkε/) and wrote *hibout* (owl)].
3. If word-finding difficulty itself (i.e., ignoring articulatory and graphic impairment and phonemic and dysorthographic deviations) is

characterized by a clear dissociation between written and oral naming, it can be logically supposed that performance in the impaired modality reflects an 'instrumental' disturbance[13] (see Chapter 10, Kurt Goldstein) rather than a 'psycholinguistic' one. This is not, however, an absolute rule.

4. If the examiner suspects that errors in written naming reflect an agnosic rather than an aphasic disturbance, s/he may follow the same verification procedures as those suggested for oral naming (i.e., compare the ability to write the names of stimuli presented in different sense modalities).

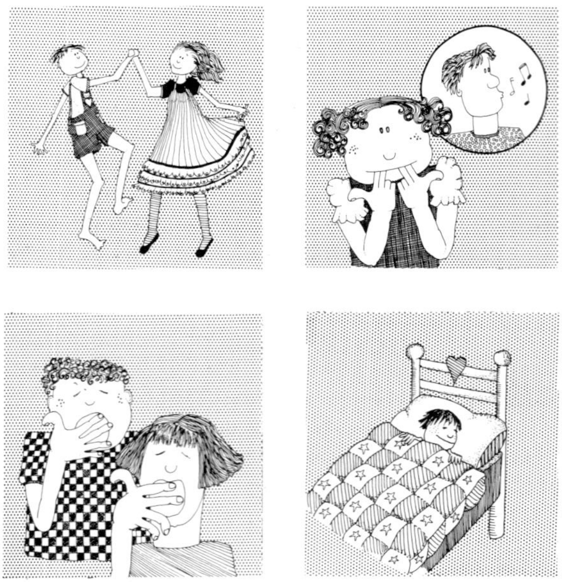

Fig. 15-4 *The assessment of aphasia: naming subtest (action verbs: 'dance', 'whistle', 'yawn', 'sleep'). Drawings by Marie-Josée Lachance* (Examen de l'aphasie du Laboratoire Théophile Alajouanine, Centre de Recherche du Centre Hospitalier Côte-des-Neiges, Montreal).

COPYING AND WRITING TO DICTATION: WRITING WITH MOBILE LETTERS

Being the counterpart, in written expression, of repetition in oral expression, copying or visuomanual transposition is of considerable interest from an aphasiological point of view. The patient will be asked to copy from a model which remains exposed [a situation which is particularly suited to the study of distortions of graphic features (disturbance of graphism)] and, to make the task more comparable to repetition, to reproduce the model after it has been removed. Between the extremes of normal performance and total failure, many forms of deviant behaviour may be observed. Does the patient's copying indicate the presence of a graphic disturbance and, if so, does it appear within the context of an elementary sensorimotor disorder (hemiparesis and/or hemihypo-aesthesia), an apraxia of the upper limbs or a constructional apraxia (see Chapters 3, 4 and 17)? Do the copied productions contain paragraphias and, especially, orthographic deviations? Is the copying servile, a characteristic which might indicate, even in the case of complex symptomatology, the influence of an element of word blindness (see Chapter 5) (in this regard, the examiner will verify whether the patient is able to transpose printed stimuli into cursives and vice versa)? Are phenomena of visual neglect observed when comparing the left and the right sides of the patient's copied productions?

Writing to dictation, or audiomanual transposition, is investigated by successively dictating groups of letters, syllables, single words, isolated sentences and, finally, a short text. This is also an important part of the aphasia examination and, for certain patients, yields the most valuable material for the study of orthographic deviations. Should they be observed, the examiner will verify, as in the case of written naming, whether there is a predominance of either literal or graphemic paragraphias. In the case of follow-up assessments carried out after a certain period of evolution, orthographic deviations may remain evident in material written to dictation but be absent, or much decreased, in less constrained productions. The agrammatism of Broca's aphasics may be manifested, especially by the omission of grammatical words (or monemes), during the dictation of isolated sentences or of a text: on the other hand, for certain Wernicke's aphasics with relatively mild impairment of written expression, it is the lexical constituents of the dictated text, rather than the grammatical ones, which elicit all types of paragraphic transformations.

The behaviours observed during the copying and writing to dictation subtests should be compared with: (a) each other (e.g., normal writing to dictation in association with servile copying is observed only in the presence of pure, or nearly pure, word blindness); (b) other modalities of written expression (e.g., an acquired disturbance of written expression limited solely to writing to dictation is observed only in cases of pure or nearly pure word deafness); (c) other transposition behaviours (e.g., in conduction aphasia, the production of phonemic paraphasias during audiophonatory transposition is often paired with the production of literal paragraphias during audiomanual transposition whereas, in Type III Wernicke's aphasia, writing to dictation is usually far more impaired than repetition) [see examples (4.43) to (4.52)].

Like the other written expression subtests, the copying and writing to dictation tasks may reveal unilateral visual neglect (as in cases where the patient spontaneously writes on only the left or the right half of the page); although far more frequent in right hemisphere lesions (left negligence), the same phenomenon is sometimes observed following a left hemisphere lesion (right negligence) and thus may be associated with aphasia (see Chapter 4).

Many right-handed aphasics have a right hemiparesis of such severity that writing with this hand is no longer possible. Thus, in the early post-onset period, the assessment of written expression must generally be limited. In addition to the production of certain words by the arrangement of mobile letters (cf. below), it is often possible to obtain only a short sample of left-handed writing: if the patient is encouraged and given ample time, s/he may write his/her name and address, copy a few words and write a few words to dictation. Even such a minimal sample will often permit the detection of aphasic elements—dysorthographia and the production of verbal transformations—even though they are masked by the elementary sensorimotor impairment. On the other hand, the natural awkwardness of the left hand makes it difficult to speak of a graphic disturbance on the basis of samples of left-handed writing by a right-handed aphasic [unless there is an obvious apraxia of the left upper limb (see Chapter 4)]. It should nevertheless be remembered that right-handers show varying degrees of awkwardness in left-handed writing (see Chapter 9): thus a note will be made in the patient's file, especially if it is expected that therapy for written expression will be attempted (see Chapter 17), concerning his/her relative proficiency in left-handed writing or an aversion towards it. In the former case, the examiner will later attempt to obtain a more extensive sample of writing.

Attempts to obtain a short sample of left-handed writing will also be made with patients whose right hand is not paralysed. Certain dissociations are possible, such as that observed in one of our patients whose production was characterized by a graphic disturbance and dysorthographia when written with the right hand but only by a dysorthographia when written with the left hand[20] (see Insertion 6.2 and Fig. 3-1 and 4-2). Similarly, Geschwind[21] has reported a patient whose writing indicated only the presence of a paretic graphic disturbance when done with the right hand and only the production of paragraphias when done with the left hand (a case which Geschwind interpreted in terms of a unilateral, left apraxia).

In cases where the characteristics of a dysorthographia require further study, the assessment of written expression will be extended to include the observation of oral spelling and spelling carried out by the arrangement of mobile letters* (these results should be compared with those obtained when writing to dictation). These two means of spelling (and particularly the latter when there is a severe disturbance of articulation) may also prove useful when assessing written language in patients whose graphic disturbance is such that the study of written expression is almost limited to the third linguistic phase; if the patient was a proficient typist, the examiner may also attempt to obtain a typed sample of written language.

ASSESSMENT OF WRITTEN LANGUAGE COMPREHENSION

Certain aspects of the assessment of reading comprehension were discussed elsewhere (see Chapter 4, 'Symptomatology of the Aphasias'). Like the assessment of oral comprehension, that of written language comprehension is based on a group of successive subtests intended to provide information about the comprehension of single words, isolated sentences and sentences

---

* The patient may then be given, in an incorrect sequence, only the letters of the word which are to be produced, or may be presented with a much larger inventory including all the letters of the alphabet.

associated within a text. The patient's performance should be compared with that observed during other subtests, particularly during the oral reading subtests. Does the patient fail to understand segments which s/he reads aloud correctly, as in certain cases of Type II Wernicke's aphasia? Does s/he correctly understand those segments which s/he transforms when attempting to read them aloud, as in certain cases of conduction aphasia? Or does s/he present a disturbance of reading comprehension which is proportional in severity to that of oral reading, as is the rule, for example, in cases of pure word blindness (see Chapters 4 and 5)? Observations of written language comprehension should also be compared with those obtained during the assessment of oral language comprehension. Is comprehension of oral language clearly more disturbed than that of written language (auditory aspect; *versant auditif*), is comprehension of written language clearly more disturbed than that of oral language (visual aspect; *versant visuel*), or is there parallel impairment in the two modalities? This distinction alone will often permit identification of the different common forms of Wernicke's aphasia (see Chapters 4 and 5).

Because the subtests of written language comprehension entail the presentation of visual stimuli, the examiner must distinguish between abnormal behaviours which are related to a hemianopsia and/or unilateral visual neglect and those which are indicative of a true disturbance of written language comprehension. The examiner must also attempt to distinguish, as in the oral comprehension subtests, between the effects of an apraxic impairment and those of an aphasic disturbance (cf. p. 357); since the stimuli included in the subtests of written language comprehension may remain exposed until the subject responds, the effects of a possible memory disturbance are largely eliminated. In cases where the comprehension of written language is found to be impaired, it should be asked whether or not the disturbance is related to word blindness (see Chapter 4, 'Type III Wernicke's Aphasia', and Chapter 5, 'Word Blindness').

The comprehension of single lexical words, either substantives or the infinitive form of verbs, can be tested by subtests requiring the matching of printed words and pictures [which are analogous to the identification subtests used in the assessment of oral comprehension (cf. p. 358)]; each test word is printed on a small card which is to be matched to the corresponding picture presented among a group of pictures on a large card. Here again, the examiner will compare the

Insertion 15.2

If the matching of single written words with pictures, or the identification of single spoken words by pointing to the appropriate picture (cf. p. 358), indicates particularly poor performance when the matching stimuli are from the same field of forms (*champs de signifiants*) or from the same semantic field (*champs de signifiés*) (see Chapter 2), the examiner should present a further subtest in which the patient is given a series of cards, each one showing several words written in a column, and is required to point out (on the response cards) each of the different stimulus words which are spoken by the examiner. If the patient's errors usually seem to reflect difficulty in distinguishing between stimuli which are similar in form (auditory aspect or visual aspect) the patient will also be asked to identify, by pointing to the appropriate item in a group of written letters, a group of written monosyllables, a group of written bisyllables (etc., if appropriate), those letters, monosyllables and bisyllables which are spoken by the examiner. The examiner will verify, for each of these types of stimuli, whether or not difficulty is significantly increased by the presentation of multiple-choice stimuli which are similar in form [i.e., s/he will compare the identification of /bi/ among 'b', 'f', 'n' and 's' versus the identification of /bi/ among 'b', 'd', 'p' and 'g'; the identification of /bæ/ among 'ba', 'fa', 'ka' and 'za' versus the identification of /bæ/ among 'ba', 'ma', 'pa' and 'da'; the identification of /pubu/ among 'poubou', 'nousou', 'routou' and 'voulou' versus the identification of /pubu/ among 'poubou', 'boupou', 'boubou' and 'poupou'][22] (see Chapter 10).

Luria

patient's performance when the group of matching stimuli illustrates words which are unrelated in both meaning and form (daffodil, camel, bottle) with that observed when the matching stimuli illustrate words which are similar in meaning (daffodil, tulip, peony) or in form (beetle, bottle, battle) (Insertion 15.2).

The comprehension of grammatical words (represented in this instance by prepositions and prepositional idioms) may be tested by the use of a written version* of the Cat and the Chair Test[17] (Fig. 15.2). Similarly, the comprehension of certain grammatical words and morphological markers (see Chapter 2) can be examined by presenting verbs written in the past, the present and the future tenses and asking the subject to match each verb form with the appropirate temporal adjective among 'yesterday', 'today' and 'tomorrow'.

Sentence comprehension is initially studied using written multiple-choice questions (to eliminate the effects of possible motor impairment, the response should require only a very simple movement—e.g., pointing to the appropriate answer, underlining it, or marking it with an 'X' or a checkmark). Previous comments concerning the manner in which the linguistic content of the stimuli may be varied when this type of subtest is used to assess oral comprehension (cf. p. 359) are equally valid with regard to written comprehension. Since this is a fairly elementary subtest, it should be supplemented by a more complex one which requires understanding of a sequence of ideas when each is expressed by a sentence written on a separate card. The patient is given all the sentence cards, in a random order, and asked to match each one to its corresponding illustration in a picture sequence (Fig. 15-5).

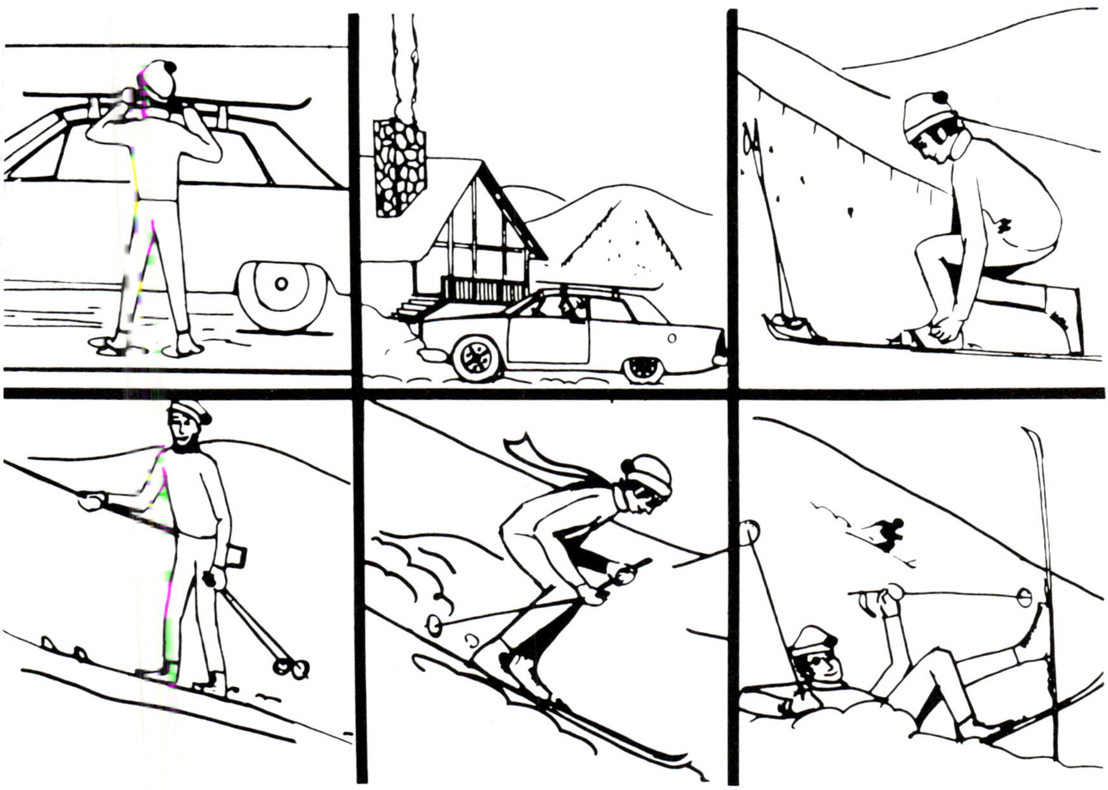

Fig. 15-5 *The assessment of aphasia: picture sequence used in the written sentence-picture matching subtest. Each of six sentences, written on a separate card and presented within a randomly ordered group, must be matched with its corresponding picture. Drawings by George Vincelli* (Examen de l'aphasie du Laboratoire Théophile Alajouanine, Centre de Recherche du Centre Hospitalier Côte-des-Neiges, Montreal).

* In the oral version of this test, the prepositions may be emphasized by increased vocal intensity or by a brief pause: in the written version, they may be emphasized by underlining or by use of larger print.

Even if the patient eventually succeeds on this subtest, the examiner will note hesitations, the time required to complete the task, successive corrections, or uncertainties, suggested by leaving certain cards until the end. Such behaviours are possible signs of a relatively mild disturbance of written language comprehension.

In cases presenting a striking dissociation between oral and written language comprehension, the assessment may sometimes be extended to include the written version of Pierre Marie's Three Paper Test[6] and the Token Test[18] (see Chapter 16).

In the case of written language, the patient's ability to understand a general meaning (comprehension of wholes) is tested by using a fairly simple text selected because it includes several pieces of information, can be easily summarized in a few words and can readily be given an appropriate title. The patient is asked to read the written text silently, taking the time s/he requires. Different questions are asked about specific facts mentioned in the text and then the patient is asked to summarize it and to suggest an appropriate title. Two procedural points should be noted with regard to this subtest: the questions are presented in writing, rather than orally, when oral comprehension is clearly much more impaired than reading comprehension; and the written text remains exposed during the question period in order to eliminate the effects of possible memory impairment (in cases of severe reduction, this also has the advantage of allowing the patient to answer each question by pointing to what s/he considers to be the appropriate line(s) in the text).

During the assessment of written language comprehension the examiner should seek answers to several general questions. Does the patient respond confidently, regardless of the accuracy of his/her responses? Is the patient aware of any difficulty in reading comprehension and, if so, does s/he refer to it spontaneously? Does the patient generally appear to respond randomly or on the basis of partial comprehension? When manipulating stimuli, does s/he place them appropriately relative to the direction in which s/he is looking? Does the patient appear somewhat puzzled by the visual stimuli placed before him/her? Is the patient's behaviour suggestive of a deficit limited only to a visual field? Do the size and clarity of the stimuli seem important? Is performance affected by the complexity of the visual material itself, that is, are words presented in isolation better understood than words presented within the context of a sentence, or vice versa? Are response latencies abnormally long? Does comprehension vary, from one moment to the next, over tasks of similar difficulty? Do perseverative phenomena appear as the patient becomes increasingly fatigued?

SUPPLEMENTARY TESTS

Because aphasia may occur in conjunction with an apraxia, particularly a buccofacial apraxia [especially in patients with the phonetic disintegration syndrome (see Chapters 3 and 4)], an auditory or a visual agnosia (see Chapters 4 and 5), it is important that the effects of these disturbances be identified. Although this point has been mentioned several times in the present chapter, it merits further discussion since an aphasiological assessment would remain incomplete if it did not include at least a few brief subtests for these impairments. A buccofacial apraxia can be readily demonstrated by instructing the patient to carry out different movements such as protruding the tongue, pointing it towards the nose or chin, puffing the cheeks, biting the lower lip, blowing, whistling, etc. (see Chapter 3, 'Buccofacial apraxia'). The patient is required to execute these movements in response to oral or written verbal commands and then on imitation (dissociations are possible, especially in patients with impaired comprehension). The possible presence of upper limb apraxia should be explored, particularly in patients presenting a disturbance of written expression; here again, the patient will be asked to execute different movements in response to verbal commands and on imitation (see Chapter 4). The word deafness component of auditory agnosia and the word blindness component of visual agnosia were discussed in detail elsewhere (see Chapters 4 and 5). The other behaviours associated with auditory agnosia can be assessed by means of tasks requiring the identification of tape-recorded popular melodies, the sounds of different musical instruments, and familiar noises (telephone, train, bell, running water, the sounds produced by different animals, etc.) while the other behaviours associated with visual agnosia can be assessed using tasks requiring the recognition of objects, pictures (which are somewhat similar and/or could easily be confused in terms of visual form), faces, coloured tokens, etc. In both cases, the patient is first asked to name the stimuli (the results will be compared with those obtained when naming stimuli presented through other sensory modalities) and then, if this proves necessary, to carry out different types of matching tasks.

The present chapter was intended to provide general guidelines to the assessment of aphasia by indicating the types of questions which should be asked during an aphasiological assessment and by describing different subtests which yield information pertinent to these questions. We have intentionally limited our discussion* to testing procedures which we ourselves use rather than describing the numerous test batteries for aphasia which are presently available (for reviews see Brookshire[23], Darley[24]). It should be noted, however, that the differences among many of these published tests are often greater with regard to their theoretical bases, procedural aspects (directions for administration, scoring, interpreting results) than with regard to the types of tasks actually presented to the patient.

REFERENCES

1. Critchley, M. (1964) *Developmental Dyslexia*. London: Heinemann Medical Books.
2. Fromkin, V.A. (1971) The non-anomalous nature of anomalous utterances. *Language*, **47**, 27.
3. Fromkin, V.A. (1973) *Speech Errors as Linguistic Evidence*. The Hague: Mouton.
4. Fromkin, V.A. (1973) Slips of the tongue. *Scientific American*, **10**, 110.
5. Lecours, A.R. & Vanier-Clément, M. (1976) Schizophasia and jargonaphasia. A comparative description with comments on Chaika's and Fromkin's respective looks at 'schizophrenic' language. *Brain and Language*, **3**, 516.
6. Marie, P. (1906) Révision de la question de l'aphasie: la troisième circonvolution frontale ne joue aucun rôle spécial dans la fonction du langage. *Semaine médicale* (Paris), **26**, 241.
7. Alajouanine, Th., Ombredane, A. & Durand, M. (1939) *Le syndrome de désintégration phonétique dans l'aphasie*. Paris: Masson.
8. Lecours, A.R. & Lhermitte, F. (1969) Phonemic paraphasias; linguistic structures and tentative hypotheses. *Cortex*, **5**, 193.
9. Lecours, A.R. & Rouillon, F. (1976) Neurolinguistic analysis of jargonaphasia and jargonagraphia. In *Studies in Neurolinguistics* (Ed.) Avakian-Whitaker, H. & Whitaker, H. Vol. 2, p. 95. New York: Academic Press.
10. Bérubé, L. (1972) *Aphasie: le manque du mot et les méthodes de facilitation*. Thesis, Département de psychologie, Université du Québec à Montréal, Montreal.
11. Dordain, M. (1968) *Contribution à l'étude neurolinguistique de l'aphasie. Analyse comparative des performances grammaticales de 28 aphasiques dont 14 agrammatiques*. Medical thesis, Paris.
12. Tissot, R., Mounin, G. & Lhermitte, F. (1973) *L'agrammatisme. Etude neuropsycholinguistique*. Brussels: Dessart.
13. Goldstein, K. (1948) *Language and Language Disturbances*. New York: Grune and Stratton.
14. Goodglass, H., Berko-Gleason, J., Bernholz, N.A. & Hyde, M.R. (1972) Some linguistic structures in the speech of a Broca's aphasic. *Cortex*, **8**, 191.
15. Pitres, A. (1898) L'asphasie ámnésique et ses variétés cliniques. *Progrès médicale* (Paris), **7**, 321, 337, 369 and 401.
16. Lhermitte, F. & Derouesné, J. (1976) L'aphasie amnésique; étude de 25 cas. *Revue neurologique*, **132**, 669.
17. Ombredane, A. (1951) *L'aphasie et l'élaboration de la pensée explicite*. Paris: Presses Universitaires de France.
18. Renzi, E. (de) & Vignolo, L.A. (1962) The token test: a sensitive test to detect receptive disturbances in aphasics. *Brain*, **85**, 665.
19. Lhermitte, F. & Ducarne, B. (1965) Plan de l'examen clinique des aphasiques. *Revue pratique* (Paris), **17**, 2365.
20. Lecours, A.R., Bérubé, L., Courtois, G.A. & Lhermitte, F. (1972) Recherches sur le langage des aphasiques: 3. Désorganisation de l'expression orale et désorganisation de l'expression écrite; une étude comparative de deux cas d'aphasie. *Encéphale*, **61**, 208.
21. Geschwind, N. & Kaplan, E. (1962) A human cerebral deconnection syndrome. *Neurology*, **12**, 675.
22. Luria, A.R. (1964) Factors and forms of aphasia. In *Disorders of Language* (Ed.) de Reuck, A.V.S. & O'Connor, M. p. 143. London: Churchill.
23. Brookshire, R.H. (1878) *An Introduction to Aphasia*. 2nd edition. Nokomis Station: BRK Publishers.
24. Darley, F.L. (Ed.) (1979) *Evaluation of Appraisal Techniques in Speech and Language Pathology*. Reading: Addison-Wesley.

---

* We have also omitted reference to the supplementary examinations required for an aetiological diagnosis, a topic which is clearly beyond the scope of the present text. Considering the major interest of anatomoclinical correlations (see Chapter 8-3), we should nevertheless emphasize the increasing importance of computerized tomography scans (CT scans) in identifying the site of cerebral lesions causing aphasia (see Fig. 9-5).

BIBLIOGRAPHY

Anderson, J.O. (1942) The speech examination of aphasic patients. *Journal of Speech Disorders*, **7,** 361.

Barbizet, J. (1965) Méthode clinique de cotation de l'aphasie. *Revue neurologique*, **112,** 137.

Bay, E. (1960) On the methodology of the study of aphasia. *Nervenartz*, **31,** 145.

Brown, J.R. (1952) A technique for teaching testing for aphasia. *Archives of Neurology and Psychiatry* (Chicago), **67,** 411.

Brown, J.R. & Schuell, H. (1950) Preliminary report of a diagnostic test for aphasia. *Journal of Speech Disorders*, **15,** 21.

Chesher, E.C. (1937) Aphasia; technique of clinical examination. *Bulletin of the Neurological Institute, New York*, **6,** 134.

Delay, J. & Lhermitte, F. Aphasie: examen des aphasiques; sémiologie de l'aphasie. *Système nerveux sémiologie*, 17019, A[10], 1, 4–1963.

Dordain, G. (1970) Aide-mémoire pour l'examen d'un aphasique. *Livrets du Médecin*, **2,** 269.

Draper, I.T. (1958) Aphasia: a problem of clinical assessment. *Surgo*, **25,** 30.

Eisenson, J. (1954) *Examining for Aphasia.* New York: Appleton.

Fog, M. (1961) A quantitative study of the fundamental factors of aphasia. *Proceedings of the VIIth International Congress of Neurology, Rome*, 647.

Fox, C. (1931) Tests of aphasia. *British Journal of Psychology*, **21,** 242.

Fox, C. (1935) Test of aphasia. *British Journal of Educational Psychology*, **33,** 791.

Gaddes, W.H. & Crockett, D.J. (1975) The Spreen–Benton aphasia tests; normative data as a measure of normal language development. *Brain and Language*, **2,** 257.

Goodglass, H. & Kaplan, E. (1972) *The Assessment of Aphasia and Related Disorders*. Philadelphia, PA: Lea and Febiger.

Halstead, W.C. & Wepman, J.M. (1949) The Halstead–Wepman aphasia screening test. *Journal of Speech Disorders*, **14,** 9.

Holland, A.L. (1980) *Communicative Abilities in Daily Living*. Boston, MA: University Park Press.

Keenan, J.S. & Brassel, E.G. (1975) *Aphasia Language Performance Scales*. Murfeessboro: Pinnacle Press.

Kertesz, A. (1980) *Western Aphasia Battery*. London: University of Western Ontario.

Kiml, J. (1961) Phoniatric testing procedure for the aphasic patient. *Czech Otolaryngology*, **10,** 18. (In Czechoslovakian.)

Kiml, J. (1967) La désintégration du langage et la méthode d'examen des aphasiques. *Acta Neurologica Belgica*, **67,** 988.

Lhermitte, F. & Ducarne, D. (1965) Plan de l'examen clinique des aphasiques. *Revue pratique* (Paris), **15,** 2365.

Luria, A.R. & Hutton, J.T. (1977) A modern assessment of the basic forms of aphasia. *Brain and Language*, **4,** 129.

Markel, N. (1960) *Intra-test Relationships in the Language of Aphasic Adults*. Unpublished doctoral thesis, University of Chicago.

Muma, J.R. (1973) Language assessment: some underlying assumptions. *Journal of the American Speech and Hearing Association*, **15,** 331.

Olson, J.A. (1960) *A Comparison of Sensory Aphasia, Expressive Aphasia and Deaf Children on the Illinois Test of Language Ability*. Unpublished doctoral thesis, University of Illinois.

Orgass, B. & Poeck, K. (1966) Clinical validation of a new test for aphasia: an experimental study of the token test. *Cortex*, **2,** 222.

Porch, B.E. (1971) *The Porch Index of Communicative Ability*. Palo Alto, CA: Consulting Psychologists Press.

Riese, W. (1957) Petit traité de l'interrogatoire suivi d'observations faites dans l'interrogatoire des malades privés de l'usage de la parole (aphasie). *Encéphale*, **46,** 347.

Sands, E., Sarno, M.T. & Shankweiler, D. (1969) Long-term assessment of language function in aphasia due to stroke. *Archives of Physical Medicine*, **50,** 202.

Sarno, M.T. (1969) *The Functional Communication Profile*. Institute of Rehabilitation Medicine, New York.

Schuell, H. (1965) *The Minnesota Test for Differential Diagnosis of Aphasia.* University of Minnesota Press, Minneapolis.

Schuell, H. (1957) A short examination for aphasia. *Neurology*, **7,** 625.

Schuell, H. (1966) A re-evaluation of the short examination for aphasia. *Journal of Speech Disorders*, **31,** 137.

Simon, C.T. (1946) Comments on testing aphasics in the speech clinic. *Journal of Speech Disorders*, **11,** 139.

Sklar, M. (1973) *The Sklar Aphasia Scale*. Los Angeles, C.A: Western Psychological Services.

Spreen, O. & Benton, A.L. (1969) *Neurosensory Center Comprehensive Examination for Aphasia.* Victoria: University of Victoria Press.

Sterne, D.M. (1964) Use of a picture vocabulary in evaluating comprehension in residual aphasia after CVA. *Journal of Clinical Psychology*, **20,** 357.

Ustvedt, H.J. (1937) The method of examination in amusia. *Acta Psychiatrica Scandinavica*, **12,** 447.

Wepman, J.M. & Jones, L.V. (1961) *Language Modality Test for Aphasia.* Chicago, IL: Education-Industry Service.

16. Psychological Assessment in Aphasiology

'One day, I had ... I didn't remember ... I didn't remember the ... the the name of the ... of the words, in taking a taxi, which makes a uh strange elect and it's quite curious. And I wasn't able uh, to tell the taxi driver uh, where I ... where I wanted to go. It amazed me that he didn't understand what I told him. And then, uh, he appeared quite normal. I don't know if I appeared norm ... normal to him but finally I had ... that ... and that ret ... that retir ... that recurred with a second taxi, then a third. And then, I said to myself that something was ... something was definitely happening. Well I went to the hospital, you see, it was a good idea, I believe.'

(*Conversation with Mr Spo.; March 1969*)

Is aphasia a form of intellectual deterioration, the result of intellectual deterioration or the cause of intellectual deterioration? Or rather, is it best considered as a specific disturbance of linguistic functioning which should be distinguished from intellectual deterioration?

These questions are not new: they were formulated by the earliest aphasiologists, and the answers which scientists subsequently provided were, in general, both dogmatic and contradictory (see Chapter 1). It was Wernicke's opinion, for example, 'that nothing worse could happen to the study of aphasia than to consider the intellectual disturbances which are present [in aphasics] as belonging to the picture of the disease' (quoted by Hécaen[1]). On the other hand, Marie[2] wrote that 'in aphasics there is something much more important and much more serious than the loss of ... words; there is a very marked decrease of the intellectual capacity in general ... If, for my part, I had to give a definition of aphasia, the fact that I would especially aim to highlight would be the decrease in intelligence.'

Marie[2] believed that the soundness of his view was demonstrated by his clinical observations, which were, indeed, exceptionally rigorous. He described for example, how he went one day to the kitchens of Bicêtre to observe the behaviour of an aphasic who had formerly been a chef. After asking him to fry an egg, Marie noted: 'he begins by breaking the egg in a very awkward way and empties it in the dish without any precaution to avoid breaking the yolk, then he puts some butter in the dish, on top of the egg, sprinkles some salt and some pepper and puts the whole thing in the oven. That was an essential mistake and the nurse pointed out to us that he had done the opposite of what should be done, the butter needing to be heated beforehand and the egg [then] tossed in. There is no need to add that the dish was absolutely unpresentable which, moreover, did not appear to disturb ... our patient.' Marie then concluded: 'Here again it is very evident that it is not a question of a language disturbance, but of an intellectual decline.' According to Marie, this same decline is also obvious in the behaviour of the aphasic musician who can no longer read or compose music and in that of all aphasics who cannot carry out simple arithmetic operations or accurately imitate the examiner's movements. [Nowadays, the observation of such patients would lead to the conclusion that aphasia may be associated with apraxia, amusia, etc., and that it is frequently associated with acalculi (see Chapters 4 and 5)]. Dejerine[3–5], an advocate of Wernicke's views, strongly criticized Marie's[2–5] doctrine, thus obliging him to modify it to a considerable extent: 'Is it therefore necessary to stress this point that the specialized intellectual deficit of the aphasic is in no way comparable with the generalized impairment of certain demented patients or those with advanced general paresis? ... What separates us here, from M. Dejerine, is that my colleague does not seem to want to admit that there can be possible dissociations of intelligence.' If not at the level of words, there was thus clearly some agreement between the positions adopted.

Different and vague notions about the meaning of intelligence appear to explain the many opinions which have been expressed about the intellectual status of aphasics. If their 'intelligence' is measured only by the use of tests which require language comprehension and production, the results will inevitably support the conclusion that aphasia is a form of intellectual deterioration: aphasics have difficulty in understanding and transmitting abstract linguistic material; their comprehension is even more impaired when complete understanding requires that an increasing number of linguistic facts be related; unlike normal subjects, aphasics can no longer rely on inner language to refine their thoughts and their ideational activity is considerably slowed. On the other hand, if 'intelligence' is assessed solely through the use of tests which are minimally affected by the status of language comprehension or production, or tests in which linguistic mediation may be replaced by other forms of mediation, the results will lead to different conclusions, depending upon the cases observed. A fair number of patients, like those whose test results were previously reported (see Chapter 8-4)[6–8], will demonstrate normal performance on such tests: it might then be concluded that aphasia does not imply intellectual deterioration and, as several neurologists of the contemporary French School have maintained[1, 9–11], that the presence of aphasia does not necessarily result in a generalized intellectual deterioration. In many cases, however, aphasics will be found to be impaired even if the tests are mostly non-verbal. Although aphasia might then be considered the cause—or the effect—of generalized intellectual deterioration, few contemporary aphasiologists, other than Bay[12, 13], adopt this point of view. When interpreting poor performance by aphasics on tests with few linguistic requirements, it is in fact more prudent, especially when it has been previously established that some aphasics do perform normally, to ask whether the patients do not present, instead of generalized intellectual deterioration, one or several other deficits associated with an aphasia. If this point of view is adopted, it is apparent that the systematic assessment of aphasia should not only include a detailed study of the patient's linguistic behaviour (see Chapter 15) but also an evaluation of his/her non-verbal gestural behaviours, perceptual capacities, memory, etc. Like Jackson[14], one would then ask, not whether intelligence is disturbed in aphasia but rather which aspects of intelligence are disturbed by the aphasia; and one would attempt to determine, when appropriate, which functions are most often impaired, probably as the result of the usual distribution of lesions, when linguistic functioning is impaired. In other words, when considering the intellectual deterioration present in certain patients, an attempt would be made to distinguish between behaviours which can be attributed to aphasia itself and those which are related to the disorganization of one or more other functions which are relatively independent of language comprehension or production.

A rather large array of examinations and tests must thus be presented in order to obtain a fairly coherent picture of the intellectual status of an aphasic patient, as for any patient with a neuropsychological disorder. A neurological examination and a particularly detailed assessment of language (see Chapter 15) are of course part of this array. The evaluation of the patient will be completed by a psychological assessment incorporating the methodology of psychological testing and emphasizing systematic comparisons and correlations. It is the psychological assessment, which includes—but extends well beyond—the administration of tests measuring perceptual-motor and intellectual abilities, which constitutes the topic of the present chapter. We shall begin by presenting some general ideas about the use of psychological (psychometric) tests in clinical neuropsychology; we shall then briefly describe different psychological tests which we consider particularly well suited to the assessment of aphasic patients and, finally, we shall illustrate the use of psychological testing in clinical aphasiology by presenting four illustrative (and fictitious) case studies.

THE USE OF TESTS IN CLINICAL NEUROPSYCHOLOGY

Certain directions followed in psychology over the last decades are of particular interest in the present context: the development of instruments and tests intended to provide a qualitative and quantitative definition of different behaviours; the standardization of these instruments and the establishment of norms for given populations through the accumulation and analyses of data obtained from large samples; and more recently, the study, although still very fragmentary, of the relationships between different behaviours and the biological substratum of their control, that is, the brain, the organ which analyses information received from the external world and compares it with that already stored in memory and also plans, initiates and controls an organism's responses to the external world. This last direction, at least with regard to investigations of abnormal human behaviour, has brought psychology into closer contact with neurology: this is easily understood since the study of brain behaviour relationships, when founded on organic pathology, must necessarily entail the systematic observation of individuals with natural or therapeutically induced cerebral lesions.

Weisenburg and McBride[54] were the first to apply the methodology of psychological testing to the study of aphasia. During more than 20 years, a group of clinicians and researchers headed by Reitan[15–24] attempted to develop a model of psychological assessment specifically intended for the evaluation of neurological patients. This team's work followed that of Halstead[25] and was in general greatly influenced by his theory of biological intelligence: 'the level of normal efficiency of an organism functioning under the control of a healthy nervous system'. Much of what follows in the remaining pages of this chapter will be concerned with the type of neuropsychological assessment refined by Reitan and with his conception of this assessment.

The use of psychological tests for the purpose of identifying relationships between certain behavioural anomalies and cerebral injuries of varied aetiology and localization is far from straightforward since many factors which do not specifically depend on cerebral lesions—such as age, cultural background, etc.—may nevertheless enter into account by significantly affecting the patient's psychological state and behaviour. Investigators in this area must constantly confront the dual problem raised by the complexity of human behaviour and the complexity of the pathological conditions which may alter normal brain functioning. Hence tests which are to be used in clinical neuropsychology must be selected with care: they must provide, either alone or in combination with others, a certain amount of specific information about the pathological state of the nervous system in the patients observed. With the exception of certain tests which are more a part of a routine neurological examination than of a psychological assessment proper, it cannot in fact be hoped that the administration of any single test will permit a distinction between the presence or absence of a cerebral lesion. A battery of tests must therefore be presented if a sufficiently valid profile is to be obtained of the level of intellectual efficiency in patients with any type of cerebral lesion. This battery should permit the patient's different behaviours to be as exhaustively sampled as possible within a reasonable period of time: the optimal battery would be one composed of tests selected because they are known to detect the presence of brain lesions and one for which intercorrelations among the tests have been established through its administration to subjects with different sites of cerebral pathology. Since knowledge of the correlations between cerebral structures and behaviour is still very limited, the administration of even the best test battery can provide answers to only some of the questions which the psychologist may ask.

It is relatively easy to define the general characteristics of a good test battery and thereby anticipate its eventual constituents. It should evaluate, in terms of behavioural measures, the simplest sensory-perceptual functions in each modality: vision, audition, touch. Similarly, it should provide a measure of elementary motor skills which considers force of movement, speed of execution, etc. At a more complex level of integration, namely that of psychosensory and psychomotor functions, it should permit measurement of the subject's ability to recognize stimuli in different modalities, to associate them, and to plan the execution, in time and in space, of behaviours proceeding from these stimuli. Among the most complex sensory information which will be studied, and among the most complex behaviours whose structure will be analysed, those which are related to language comprehension and verbal expression are of particular importance if the battery is to be used in studying diseases which affect linguistic functioning. Finally, whether or not they involve language, certain tests should be especially focused on the patient's memory and his or her ability to deal with abstractions, to reason, to plan ahead, and to make decisions. It is obviously impossible to design tests which assess only a particular aspect of a given sensory modality or only a single aspect of one higher mental function, etc. Nevertheless, the different tests can be aimed—in terms of their organization, modality of presentation, required response and analysis of observed behaviours—towards the study of more or less precise points: depending on the tests, it can thus be said that particular ones assess a given sensory modality or an elementary motor skill, that others mainly involve the more complex level of recognition and organization of information or the execution of gestures, that certain ones measure intelligence, etc.

These different tests are the working tools of psychologists engaged in clinical work or in neuropsychological research with humans. They allow the psychologist to study certain characteristics of neurological disease using a psychometric and statistical approach, one which is a natural complement to the clinical methods of the neurologist. We shall now briefly discuss, under headings which have mostly been borrowed from Reitan, certain characteristic aspects of the psychologist's approach to the assessment of a patient suspected of having a cerebral lesion.

STUDY OF PERFORMANCE LEVELS

The patient's performance level on a particular test or on an entire battery is compared with norms established through previous research in which normal subjects were compared with subjects who had known cerebral lesions. Although lowered efficiency is unquestionable in regard to groups of brain-damaged patients, the finding of lowered performance in an individual patient does not necessarily imply the presence of an organic lesion: genetic, educational or cultural factors or variables related to the patient's age, to the presence of a coexisting psychiatric disorder or to the type of rapport established between the examiner and the patient, etc., could partially or totally account for the lowered performance observed on particular tests. The presence of such a lesion might exacerbate the effects of some of these factors but they might also be entirely independent from it: however this may be, a finding of lowered performance cannot be related, in certain cases and for certain tests, to a precise site of lesion.

Other factors must also be considered when interpreting performance levels in a subject known to have a cerebral lesion. We shall mention here only the two main ones. First, because there is considerable variation among different individuals in their (premorbid) abilities, lowered performance on a single test, and sometimes even on a group of tests, can, in general, be definitely attributed to the brain lesion only when there is a major deficit. Second, the patient's test results must be carefully considered in relation to the aetiology and the time since onset of the disease (see Chapter 9): in the presence of a stable or reversible lesion, the brain's potential for functional reorganization remains considerable even if it is generally insufficient to permit a complete return to normal; on the other hand, this potential decreases, often in an inexorable manner, in degenerative diseases.

SEEKING PATHOGNOMONIC SIGNS

Certain psychological deficits are recognized to have specific, localizing value; for example, word deafness, an agnosic impairment of reading, constructional apraxia, sensory extinction phenomena, etc. (see Chapters 3 to 8). The identification of these signs not only provides valuable information about lesion localization but also permits a more precise qualitative analysis of the patient's behaviours during the various psychological tests presented. Although we have previously pointed out that the psychologist's testing methods complement those of the neurologist, this is not generally the case with regard to the identification of pathognomonic signs: with only a few exceptions (at least until now), the psychologist's approach, like that of the neurologist, entails qualitative identification rather than quantitative measures. The identification of pathognomonic signs and their classification with respect to their diagnostic significance is usually based on a group of more or less objective factors which cannot be interpreted by reference to pre-established norms. Nevertheless, psychologists do apply their quantitative methods in attempts to establish systematic correlations between the presence of particular (qualitatively identified) pathognomonic signs and certain, more traditional, psychological measures.

RETESTING OF THE SAME PATIENT

It is clear that a systematic behavioural study of the same individual, prior to the onset of disease and again after onset, would be the ideal means of identifying the effects of cerebral damage. It is equally clear that comparisons of premorbid and post-onset measures are only possible in exceptional cases. Thus systematic, pre- and post-operative assessments, particularly in certain types of elective neurosurgery, are of great value in the study of the relationships between behaviour and different constituent structures of the brain (see Chapter 7). Similarly, periodic assessments of the same patient during the evolution of the disease, particularly in cases with reversible diseases (see Chapter 9), may sometimes lead to hypotheses about the effects of focal cerebral lesions and about the mechanisms underlying functional recovery.

Finally, it should be noted that information obtained about the patient's personal and family background may be extremely useful: although clearly less desirable than systematic premorbid testing, such information can nevertheless contribute to a more insightful analysis of the patient's performance on tests presented after the onset of the disease.

DIFFERENTIAL STUDY OF PERFORMANCE SCORES

As we have already pointed out, it is not isolated tests, but rather an entire test battery, which is generally of greatest value in clinical neuropsychology. Two facts should be discussed with regard to this assertion. First, it is true that certain tests are useful in detecting the presence of a cerebral lesion and sometimes even in indicating the (general) site of lesion: nevertheless, the indices which can be inferred from these tests are not completely reliable (with the obvious exception of qualitative tests intended to reveal the presence of pathognomonic signs, the best of numerous tests, when used alone, were found to have a 15 to 20 per cent margin or error[21, 22]). Second, the study of the correlations between normal and abnormal scores on the different tests comprising a battery—regardless of whether each test by itself is sensitive to the presence of brain damage—considerably reduces the margin of error and allows more precise conclusions about the probable localizations of lesions.

COMPARATIVE STUDY OF LEFT AND RIGHT PERFORMANCE

We have previously indicated that the treatment of somaesthetic information coming from one side of the body, as well as motor control of this side, is ensured by the contralateral hemisphere (see Chapter 8-1). We have also pointed out that, in most people, there are natural differences between the sensorimotor capacities of the two halves of the body (see Chapter 11). This knowledge constitutes the basis of the procedure followed by psychologists in comparing a patient's right- versus left-sided performance during certain fairly elementary tests. This procedure has the advantage of permitting comparisons between different performances by the same patient and thus avoiding, at least to a certain point, recourse to the more tenuous comparison of an individual with a group (inferences through intergroup comparisons). Obviously, these comparisons between the patient's own performances, especially when they are studied in relation to his or her results on other tests and the findings from the neurological evaluation, may prove very useful in diagnosing the site of possible cerebral lesions.

PSYCHOMETRIC STUDY OF APHASICS

During the neurological examination of patients with telencephalic lesions and, especially, when evaluating the residual linguistic abilities of an aphasic during an aphasiological assessment proper (see Chapter 15), it is often noted that certain behaviours are much closer to normal when there are no time limits or when the task is such that its performance can be voluntarily slowed. After recovering from aphasia, Lordat[26] noted that his inability to understand the language of others was mainly due to the rapidity of spoken information (see Chapter 1); similarly, it is well known that deviations in the discourse of a conduction aphasic will decrease in number and complexity if the patient can maintain a slower rate of speech (see Chapter 4). These considerations suggest a crude metaphor, namely, that in the same way as a small computer can slowly work through a problem which is rapidly solved by a large computer, there are some circumstances in which a damaged brain can succeed, or nearly succeed, in directing certain behaviours provided that more time is available than would be required by a normal brain to achieve the same result.

Although neurologists and speech pathologists generally note how the patient's performance of assigned tasks is affected by available time, their observations are usually qualitative. In contrast, time is often one of the variables which is systematically measured by the psychologist. Consequently, an abnormally low psychometric score will frequently be a partial reflection of penalties associated with abnormal slowness in performing the required tasks. Hence this factor should be isolated, as far as possible, when interpreting the significance of different psychometric abnormalities which may be observed: this is particularly necessary since the penalized slowness may well be the result of an instrumental impairment. Consider, for example, a right-hander presented a mild residual of a right hemiparesis and whose 'intellectual abilities were measured' by means of graphic production carried out within a limited time period (as an illustration see, below, the Digit Symbol Subtest of the Ottawa-Wechsler Intelligence Scale).

Besides the factor of time, there are other general factors which must be considered when interpreting the significance of certain psychometric scores obtained by an aphasic. Among them is variability of performance, which is probably related to increased susceptibility to fatigue and is characteristic of most of the common neuropsychological disorders (including aphasia). Of the different characteristics which may have a general influence on aphasics' performance during a psychometric evaluation, we shall mention only the patient's premorbid personality and, especially, certain character traits which may have been exaggerated by the onset of the disease. In this regard, Broca's aphasics, who are very aware of their handicap, may become so discouraged and unmotivated during psychometric testing that the validity of the assessment is compromised.

DESCRIPTION OF THE MAJOR TESTS USED IN CLINICAL APHASIOLOGY

With only a few exceptions, the most commonly used psychological tests were not designed for the purpose of assessing brain-damaged patients; rather they are usually used to situate the performance of a normal subject in reference to his or her peers. Thus the psychologist working in clinical neuropsychology has to choose, among the multitude of available tests, those which s/he will use to assess neurological patients. The psychologist does not modify or adapt these tests, since they would then lose their original value, but instead learns to recognize the particular dimension which is added by their use with pathological populations. In this respect, a total score which is significantly below the norm is of much less interest than the identification of factors contributing to the decrease, since the latter may contribute, in certain cases, to the diagnosis of lesion localization or even to an aetiological diagnosis.

Those tests which we have found useful in clinical neuropsychology can be roughly subdivided into the following three categories:

1. *Tests of elementary motor functions* (measures of strength of grasp, of finger tapping, etc.) or of *elementary sensation* (measures of visual acuity, assessment of colour vision by use of Ishihara's* test plates, Farnsworth's† test, etc.
2. *Perceptual-motor tests* (The Complex Figure of Rey,‡ The Bender Motor Gestalt Test,§ Benton's Visual Retention Test,|| etc.

* Tests for Colour Blindness (1972), Kanehara Shuppan and Co. Ltd, Tokyo, Japan.
† Farnsworth-Munsell 100-Hue Test for the Examination of Color Discrimination, Munsell Color Company, Inc., 2441 North Calvert Street, Baltimore, Md 21218, USA.
‡ Figure Complexe de Rey (1959), Centre de psychologie appliquée, 48 avenue Victor-Hugo, 75783, Paris, Cedex 16, France.
§ Bender Motor Gestalt Test (1946) Lauretta Bender, American Orthopsychiatric Association, Inc., New York, USA.
|| The Revised Visual Retention Test, A.L. Benton, Distributor: The Psychological Corporation, 304 East 45th Street, New York, NY 17, USA.

3. *Tests of higher mental functions* which, in addition to testing particular motor or sensory functions, extend beyond this level in requiring more highly integrated activities (Raven's Progressive Matrices,* Halstead Category Test,† etc.); certain scales yielding an intelligence quotient, for example the Wechsler Scale, are included in this category.

We shall now discuss those tests which we have found to be of some value in clinical aphasiology. Since their membership in one or another of the above categories is generally self-evident, we shall not discuss them in order of these categories but rather according to the order in which we usually present them in the course of an assessment.

AUDIOMETRY

Audiometry permits identification of the patient's limits of hearing. Systematic measurements are obtained by using a special instrument (*audiometer*) which allows the examiner to control the frequency and intensity of the stimuli. The threshold levels of hearing for pure tones of different frequencies are identified and mapped out on a *pure tone audiogram* (Fig. 16–1). Lists of single words may also be presented to obtain measures of the intensity at which speech can be heard (*speech reception threshold*) and of the ability to identify words presented at an intensity above the speech reception threshold (*speech discrimination score*). For the tests which involve speech stimuli, the subject's task is usually to repeat each of the stimulus words but aphasics with severely disturbed repetition can be asked to respond to each stimulus by pointing to the appropriate picture or written word among a group of pictures or a list of words. In aphasiology, audiometric testing is especially valuable in cases of temporal lesions, particularly when the patient presents an aphasia which includes a clear component of word deafness[27] (see Chapters 4 and 5). It is then not uncommon, especially in cases of bilateral temporal lesions, to observe a high-frequency hearing loss (Fig. 16–1). It is not, however, sufficient to account for the word deafness, and hearing may eventually improve while the word deafness persists.

PERIMETRY

Perimetry is a technique to determine the limits of the visual field. In its simplest application, it is part of a routine neurological examination. The patient faces the examiner and fixates on a specific immobile point (usually the tip of

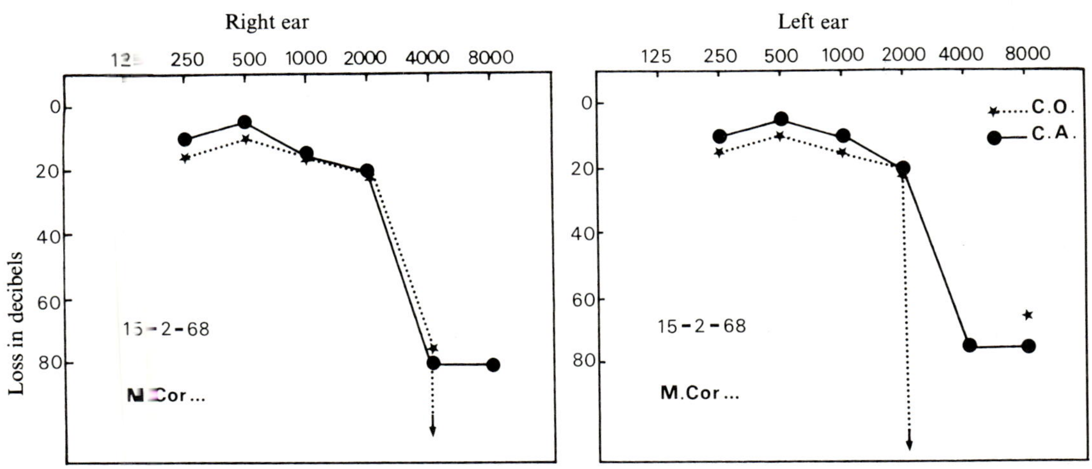

Fig. 16–1 *Pure tone audiogram: high-frequency hearing loss in a case of acquired bilateral temporal lesions. From Lhermitte et al*[27].

* Standard Progressive Matrices (1960), Printed by William Grieve and Sons, Buenfries, Scotland, Published by H. K. Lewis and Co. Ltd, London.

† See Halstead-Reitan Battery.

examiner's nose): the visual field is then explored by asking the patient to report the presence or movement of visual stimuli, usually the examiner's fingers presented either unilaterally or bilaterally. If more precise measurements are desirable, as is generally the rule in global aphasia, Wernicke's aphasia and, especially, in pure word blindness (see Chapters 4 and 5), the examination will be done using a special instrument (*perimeter*). It is then possible to present stimuli differing in number, form, size, brightness and colour as well as in their movements. Such an examination will permit identification of possible defects such as the presence of a relative or absolute hemianopsia (Fig. 16–2) or quadranopsia, or hemiachomatopsia. Aphasias from lesions limited to the parietal lobe are often accompanied by an inferior quadranopsia while aphasias from lesions limited to the temporal lobe are often accompanied by a superior quadranopsia (see Chapter 4). Determination of the presence or absence of these defects is particularly important in aphasics whose symptomatology includes a reading disturbance.

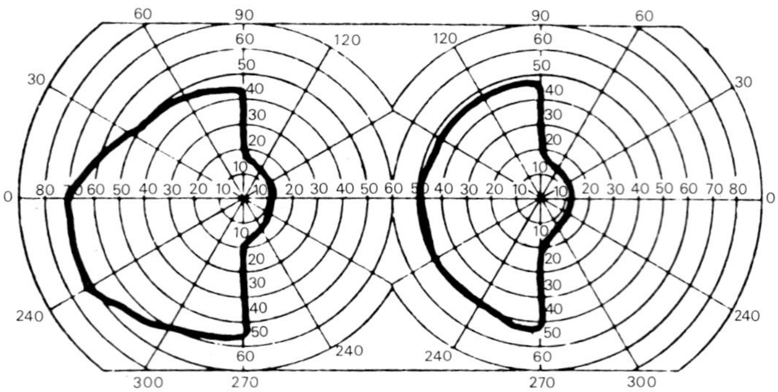

Fig. 16–2 *Perimetry demonstrating the presence of a right homonymous hemianopsia with macular sparing. From Bastron et al*[55].

ROSSANO–WEISS TEST

The Rossano–Weiss Test is an optometric test in which calibrated (progressively smaller) forms are presented instead of the letter stimuli normally used when testing visual acuity. It permits visual acuity to be measured in subjects who have not learned or no longer recognize letters, and may therefore be useful in the examination of aphasics whose symptomatology includes a major component of alexia.

COLOUR VISION

In aphasiology, the examination of colour vision is especially important in patients presenting an isolated or relatively dissociated reading disturbance. This is particularly true in the case of pure word blindness since it is frequently associated with colour agnosia[28]. The examination is carried out by presenting various tests under adequate lighting (a Macbeth lamp or equivalent):

1. *Pseudo-isochromatic charts* require the identification of figures which differ in colour from that of the background and permit the examination of colour perception along the red–green axis (Polak's* test and Ishihara's test) and the blue–yellow axis (Hardy–Rand–Ritter Test*). Patients with language disorders and/or visual field defects are asked to outline the stimulus forms with their finger instead of identifying them by name.
2. *Epreuve des Appariement des Doubles** (Paired Colours Test): this test is composed of bands of equal luminance which differ in colour (hue and saturation). The test includes pairs of identical stimuli and the subject must match each coloured band to the other one of the same colour.
3. *Holmgreen's Colour Sorting test** is composed of an assortment of small skeins of wool. The subject must first sort them according to hue and then serially order those of each hue according to their saturation (i.e., from the lightest to the darkest).
4. *Farnsworth's tests* (*15 Hue and 100 Hue*) are

* Centre de psychologie appliquée, 48 avenue Victor-Hugo, 75783, Paris, Cedex 16, France.

composed of coloured chips which are equal in luminance and saturation and differ only in hue. The subject must gradually classify the chips according to this variable. The high sensitivity of the Farnsworth 100 Hue Tests makes it a choice instrument for the detection of pseudo-dyschromatopsias resulting from certain occipital lesions[28].

The examination of colour vision is completed by tests requiring colour naming and the identification of colours in response to names as well as by tests requiring the recognition and the evocation of object colours (e.g., naming the colour or pointing to a coloured band which corresponds to the object named by the examiner; coloured drawings of objects or selecting the appropriately coloured drawing of different objects).

THE BENDER VISUAL MOTOR GESTALT TEST

Bender's test requires the copying of nine simple drawings (geometric figures, curved or broken lines, series of points differently oriented on the stimulus cards). The subject is asked to copy, successively, each of the nine drawings on a single page of paper and to make his/her reproductions as accurate as possible with regard to the forms, dimensions, proportions and spatial orientation of the stimuli. No time limits are imposed. The test examines the ability to perceive visuospatial information and to reproduce it in the presence of a model. The results are compared with normative data taking account of various aspects of graphic production: an increase or decrease in the size of the stimuli, instances of lateralized neglect, modifications of the model (simplifications, separations, superpositions, omissions), spatial shifts (rotations, increased or decreased proximity, changes of direction or angle), perseveration or contamination from one stimulus to another, graphomotor anomalies, etc. The Bender test is said to be very sensitive to the presence of cerebral lesions, regardless of lateralization, age or intellectual level; if present, a constructional apraxia will be very clearly manifested on this test. Wernicke's aphasics demonstrate particular difficulty on the Bender test[29] but the extent of impairment is not, however, directly proportional to the severity of aphasia.

COMPLEX FIGURE OF REY

The stimulus for this test is a complex geometric figure having a basic framework which delineates several different sectors, each one containing numerous details. The figure is presumably meaningless and its reproduction is not particularly difficult from a strictly graphic point of view. The subject's task is first to copy the figure and, later, to reproduce it from memory. He or she does so using crayons of different colours which are supplied by the examiner in a predetermined sequence in order to facilitate the subsequent study of the drawing. The first part of the test (copying) examines the subject's abilities to perceive and identify the basic framework, and then the more elementary details of a complex visual array, and to organize this information in the form of graphic behaviour executed by the hand under visual control. The subject's drawing constitutes a record of this behaviour. Although this drawing will be the main focus of systematic study, observation of the subject during the test will often permit detection of certain anomalies. The second part of the test entails an additional ability, namely visual memory.

No time limits are imposed. Nevertheless, the time required to complete each drawing is recorded and can be compared with normative data, on copying and on reproduction from memory, for the subject's age group. Several different factors are considered in scoring the drawings, the main ones being: how the basic framework is constructed, that is, drawn completely from the start or drawn in successive fragments; the order in which the different parts of the figure are drawn; the number and position of elements which are correct, deformed, incomplete, unrecognizable, displaced, replaced, added, omitted; the relationships established between different elements; the nature of the intersections between lines forming angles; and graphic skill proper. This scoring procedure allows the patient's production to be classified, when this appears useful, according to a scale of eight types which have been more or less clearly defined: according to Rey and Osterrieth, Type I represents the most rational approach whereas Type VIII can be considered merely as scribbling which bears no apparent relationship to the stimulus.

Besides a quantitative analysis, simple inspection of a copy of the Rey figure will quite often permit the detection of particular

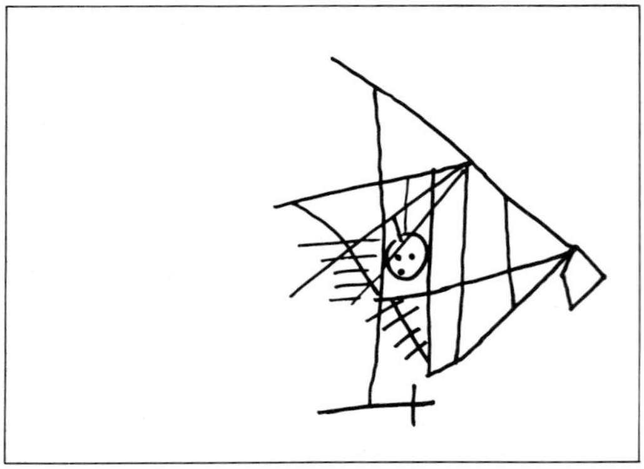

Fig. 16-3 *Copy of the Complex Figure of Rey: left visual neglect and constructional apraxia in a patient with right parietal softening. Courtesy of Mesdames Solange Tremblay and Johanne Dupuis,* Laboratoire Théophile Alajouanine, Centre de Recherche du Centre Hospitalier Côte-des-Neiges, Montreal.

symptomatological elements such as visual neglect (Fig. 16-3) or constructional apraxia[30].

BENTON VISUAL RETENTION TEST

The Benton Visual Retention Test[31] is intended to examine visual perception, visual memory and visuoconstructional abilities. Like the Rey figure, it is useful in aphasiology since various disturbances of visual and praxic functions are often associated with aphasia or may even be the origin of certain aspects of its symptomatology. The test is composed of three series of stimuli (forms C, D and E); each series consists of ten plates with each one displaying between one and three figures (varying in form, size, mutual relationships). The plates are presented one by one and, after each presentation, the patient reproduces the stimulus from memory. Depending on the case, the examiner selects one of four testing procedures. Two different scoring systems are suggested: the first is based on the number of correct drawings and provides a measure of general efficiency: the second one, which is more suited to the particular interests of clinical aphasiology, considers different types of anomalies in form (errors in size and relative position of the figures, particularly overlapping figures; omission of figures on the sides of the plate; errors involving angles, especially acute angles; instances of rotation, fragmentation, perseveration; anomalies of graphism proper, etc.).

Generally speaking, performance on the Benton Visual Retention Test is less affected by frontal lesions than by lesions of other sites, and is more impaired by lesions of the right than of the left hemisphere. The presence of constructional apraxia may nevertheless be manifested by numerous inaccuracies in the case of either a left or right parietal or parieto-occipital lesion. Certain plates from Benton's test are particularly useful in demonstrating phenomena of visual neglect.

STANDARD PROGRESSIVE MATRICES (PM-38)

The Standard Progressive Matrices (or the French edition called the PM-38) is composed of more or less abstract patterns. Each test plate displays a continuous or discontinuous pattern with a piece missing in the lower right segment. Six or eight matching stimuli are shown below the incomplete pattern and the subject's task is to select the one which would best complete it. The test consists of a total of 60 problems grouped into five series of 12. The logical principle underlying the solution of each problem remains constant within each series but the 12 problems become increasingly difficult in terms of the graphic characteristics of the stimulus patterns as well as those of the multiple-choice pieces. The problems are presented in an order which facilitates correct choices if reasoning by an analogy is possible and is extended as each series progresses. At comparable stages in the order of presentation, the problems also become increasingly difficult from one series to the next. The test is administered without time restrictions, a feature which sometimes makes it an instrument of choice in the neuropsychological assessment of patients with cerebral lesions. The raw score on this test is converted to a percentile which may then be considered in relation to results obtained on other tests, for example the Wechsler-Bellevue Test (cf. below).

Complex linguistic mediation is probably not required during completion of the Standard Progressive Matrices. Such a conclusion is, in any case, consistent with two types of evidence:

1. Some severely aphasic individuals, particularly those without major left parietal lesions, may obtain very high scores on this test (see Chapter 8-4). Indeed, the site of

lesion does not seem to be of prime importance with regard to results obtained on the Standard Progressive Matrices: poor performance is, in fact, often associated with the presence of constructional apraxia whether caused by a left or by a right hemisphere lesion.

2. Many normal subjects realize that they solved the various problems without elaborate inner verbalization. This is especially clear in the case of the relatively more complex problems. Although elaborate verbalization (i.e., systematic verbal mediation at every phase of reasoning) is certainly possible, at least in general terms and to a variable extent among different subjects, this strategy seldom appears to be used spontaneously. Furthermore, such verbalization would require more time than most individuals need to discover the solutions to the corresponding problems (see Chapter 19).

It thus appears that language is less essential during the Standard Progressive Matrices than are the abilities to perceive visuospatial organization and to deduce a logical principle and to generalize it through reasoning by analogy. These abilities may be impaired by several types of neuropsychological disorders including different, more or less well-defined types of intellectual impairment and, at a more elementary level, various visual and visuospatial disturbances such as neglect and agnosia (see Chapter 4). In aphasiology, the results obtained on the Standard Progressive Matrices are often in agreement with those obtained on the Performance Scale of the Wechsler Scale (cf. below).

THE OTTAWA-WECHSLER INTELLIGENCE SCALE (15-60 YEARS)

The Ottawa-Wechsler Scale* is an adaptation, for use with French-speaking Canadians, of the Wechsler Bellevue Intelligence Scale. Since the Ottawa-Wechsler is the particular scale which we have most often used in our work with aphasics, it is the one which will be specifically discussed. With the exception of certain details of our test description which are not true of all adaptations or revisions† of the original Wechsler Bellevue Scale, the following discussion is generally applicable to the use of Wechsler Intelligence Scales in aphasiology.

The Ottawa-Wechsler scale provides a measure of intelligence, that is, an intelligence quotient. It is composed of ten subtests, five constituting a verbal scale and the other five constituting a performance (non-verbal) scale. Test performance is summarized by three figures, namely a Full Scale Intelligence Quotient (IQ), a Verbal IQ (summarizing results on the verbal subtests), and a Performance IQ (summarizing results on the non-verbal subtests).

The names of the five subtests comprising the *verbal scale* are, respectively: General Information, General Comprehension, Digit Span, Arithmetic and Similarities:

1. The *General Information* subtest consists of a series of 25 questions intended to explore the extent and availability of factual knowledge (acquired through formal education and personal pursuits). The expected responses range from quasi-definitions ('How many musicians in a trio?'‡) to academic knowledge ('Who was Alexander VI?')
2. The *General Comprehension* subtest consists of ten spoken stimuli (e.g., 'Why should a country have an army?') to which subjects must respond by stating their opinion or describing what their behaviour would be in hypothetical circumstances. The expected responses represent widespread social and moral precepts (e.g., the answer to the above question might be 'To defend the country!'). This subtest presumably explores the subjects' 'judgement', their ability to keep their thoughts within a precise frame of reference, and to maintain adequate contact with 'reality'. We are doubtful of its current validity, however, since many of the expected responses appear clearly outmoded. Furthermore, it is not self-evident that the degree of adherence to convention constitutes a measure of an individual's 'intelligence'.

* Maurice Chagnon. Editions de l'Université d'Ottawa (1953).

† A widely-used revision of the Wechsler Bellevue Intelligence Scale is the Wechsler Adult Intelligence Scale or WAIS (Psychological Corporation, 1955). The WAIS includes subtests very similar to those described here (with an increased number of items per subtest) and a vocabulary subtest in which the subject is asked to explain the meaning of increasingly difficult words.

‡ All examples are fictitious.

3. The *Digit Span* subtest examines the ability to repeat series of digits spoken by the examiner. The length of digit series is progressively increased and both forward repetition (i.e., in order of presentation) and backward repetition (reverse order) are examined. This subtest mainly measures immediate memory and provides information about the use of different reproduction strategies. The properly verbal aspects of this subtest are limited to the instrumentality involved in its administration (i.e., audiophonatory transposition).
4. The *Arithmetic* subtest examines the ability to solve 'concrete' arithmetical problems ('Yves has seven apples and Mary has two more than Yves. How many apples do they have both together?'). Ten progressively more difficult problems are thus presented, the first eight being spoken by the examiner and the last two presented in writing. This subtest involves language comprehension and logical reasoning; it requires that the subjects focus their attention, retain the information provided and carry out the four types of elementary arithmetical operations within specified time limits.
5. On the *Similarities* subtest, the subject must identify a common meaning shared by two words spoken by the examiner ('swallow' and 'crow'→'bird'). Ten pairs of words are presented: depending on the particular pair, the conceptual relationship between the two words is either 'concrete', 'functional' or 'abstract'. Successful completion of this subtest presupposes the ability to effect a comparative analysis of meaning and depends on the integrity of linguistic functioning to a greater extent than do the other subtests included in the verbal scale.

Each of the five subtests comprising the *performance* or *non-verbal scale* must be completed within a specified time limit. The names of these subtests are, respectively: Picture Arrangement, Picture Completion, Block Design, Object Assembly and Digit Symbol:

1. During the *Picture Arrangement* subtest, subjects are given between three and six separate pictures: their task is to arrange them in the appropriate sequential order to illustrate a story without words. A total of six picture series are presented. Successful performance requires the adequate perception of the forms shown in each picture, abstraction of their meaning and, for each series, deduction of the conceptual links permitting the pictures to be ordered in such a way that they constitute a congruent ('logical') whole. Although linguistic production is not requested, it is not prevented, and verbalization, even if only covert, usually enters into a normal subject's approach to this task.
2. The *Picture Completion* subtest is composed of 15 pictures. Each is a simple concrete figure which lacks an essential, and in some cases lateralized, detail (e.g., a picture of a cat with only one ear). The subject's task is to identify the part required to complete the picture: this requires visual exploration of the entire stimulus, its identification as an entity and explicit recognition of the omitted part (and thus of its essential nature). Although this subtest does not necessarily entail linguistic mediation, it is, again, common in normal subjects.
3. During the *Block Design* subtest, the subject must successively reproduce seven, two-colour, increasingly complex geometric designs. On each trial, a model is presented which does not clearly indicate the edges of the individual blocks. Subjects are then given from 4 to 16 cubes, each with a single colour on certain sides and two different colours on the other sides, for their reproduction. This subtest mainly entails visual-motor performance in two-dimensional space.
4. The *Object Assembly* subtest requires the successive completion of three puzzles forming pictures related to the human body. Each puzzle is composed of six or seven pieces. This subtest also assesses mainly visual-motor behaviour.
5. The *Digit Symbol* subtest requires that each of nine arbitrary symbols be rapidly associated with one of the Arabic numerals between 1 and 9. The test material, including a display of the digit-symbol relationships, is presented visually and the subject is asked to reproduce the corresponding symbol for each of the digits presented. Initially a test of fine motor coordination, it gradually becomes a learning task as the subject progresses. The score obtained depends on the number of correct associations—up to a maximum of 67—made within the specified time limit.

In clinical neuropsychology, the scores obtained on the Wechsler Scale are interpreted by comparisons with the expected scores, taking into account the patient's age, educational level and his or her premorbid social, cultural and occupational status, etc. In certain cases, cerebral disease may be reflected by a large decrease in the Full Scale IQ. Certain discrepancies in the results obtained on the different subtests are, however, the best indicators of organic pathology. A commonly cited example is a clear discrepancy between the Verbal IQ and Performance IQ: when the former is considerably higher than the latter, the existence of a right hemisphere lesion may be suspected (in a right-hander); the opposite relationship suggests the possible presence of a left hemisphere lesion. It should nevertheless be noted that many left hemisphere lesions may impair behaviours required on certain subtests of the performance scale as well as those required on the subtests of the verbal scale (Fig. 16-4)

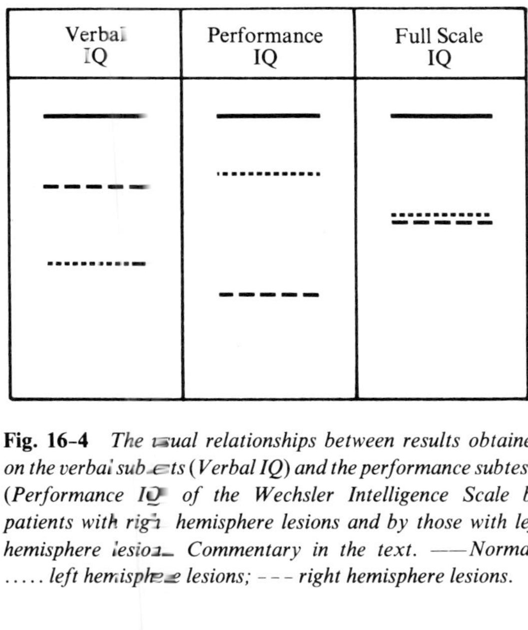

Fig. 16-4 *The usual relationships between results obtained on the verbal subtests (Verbal IQ) and the performance subtests (Performance IQ) of the Wechsler Intelligence Scale by patients with right hemisphere lesions and by those with left hemisphere lesions. Commentary in the text. ——Normal; ..... left hemisphere lesions; - - - right hemisphere lesions.*

The following points should be borne in mind when interpreting discrepancies in the results obtained by right-handed patients on the different subtests of the Ottawa-Wechsler or Wechsler Bellevue Scales:

1. Age-related involution might explain particularly marked impairment on the Digit Span subtest; on the other hand, results on the General Comprehension and the Picture Completion subtests are relatively less affected by normal senescence.
2. If they cannot be attributed to other evident causes (instrumental, involutional, educational, etc.), clear asymmetries in the profile established from results obtained on the ten different subtests (Barnett's psychograph) suggest the possibility of a cerebral lesion (and the need to confirm or refute this hypothesis by other examinations). It is generally taught that the Digit Span and the Digit Symbol subtests are particularly sensitive to the presence of cerebral damage, regardless of type and localization.
3. Different memory disturbances may be manifested on certain subtests, for example the General Information and Arithmetic subtests or, if immediate memory is impaired, on the Digit Span subtest.
4. An impairment of abstract attitude[32, 33], of the type often observed in aphasia (see Insertion 10.2), may affect results on the General Comprehension, Similarities, Digit Symbol, Object Assembly, Block Design and Picture Arrangement subtests.
5. Constructional apraxia or a disturbance of visual function—such as agnosia—may hinder performance on the Digit Symbol, Object Assembly, Block Design or Picture Arrangement subtests. Visual neglect may be the source of impaired performance on several of the tests comprising the non-verbal scale, for example the Picture Completion subtest.
6. The Wechsler Scale profiles of aphasics vary according to the patients' age, the localization and size of their lesions, the nature of associated neuropsychological disorders, the time since onset of their disease,* etc. The anomalies presented by aphasics are rarely, if ever, confined solely to the subtests of the Verbal Scale [this can be attributed as much to the content of certain so-called 'non-verbal' tests of the Wechsler Scale (cf. above) as to the nature of aphasia itself]. The Digit Symbol and, usually, the Picture Arrangement subtests are affected in proportion to the verbal scale subtests, whereas performance may be relatively intact on the Picture Completion, Block Design and Object Assembly subtests. When this is the case, and results on the

* Severe aphasia (and particularly a severe disturbance of comprehension) may preclude presentation of the Wechsler Scale. This is especially true early in the course of evolution.

Standard Progressive Matrices (cf. p. 380) are normal or nearly so, it can be assumed that there is no significant parietal lesion, either left or right[34].

WECHSLER MEMORY SCALE*

The Wechsler Memory Scale was developed to permit the quantitative measurement of an individual's mnemonic capacities. They are represented by a single score which is calculated on the basis of results obtained on the following seven subtests:

1. *Personal and Current Information*: the subject is questioned about personal information ('What is your date of birth?'†) and about presumably well-known facts ('Who is the President of China?').
2. *Immediate Orientation*: the subject is questioned about simple spatial-temporal facts ('What season is it now?').
3. *Mental Control*: different tasks are presented (e.g., reciting the alphabet backwards) to examine behaviours based on early learning. These tasks have time limits.
4. *Logical Memory*: after telling the subject about the test procedure, the examiner reads aloud a short text which includes various facts. The subject's task is (immediately) to recount the story in as much detail as possible. Two different texts are presented.
5. *Digit Span*: this subtest requires the immediate repetition, both forward and backwards, of increasingly longer series of digits.
6. *Visual Reproduction*: the stimuli are cards displaying one or two abstract designs. Each stimulus card is exposed for ten seconds and, after its removal, the subject must reproduce the drawings.
7. *Associate Learning*: the stimuli consist of ten word pairs, five considered 'easy' because there is an obvious conceptual relationship between the associated words and five considered 'hard' because of the absence of any obvious relationship. The examiner reads all the word pairs aloud and, after a five-second pause, successively reads the first member of each pair; the subject's task is to respond to each word by supplying the second (associated) member of the pair (within five seconds). This whole procedure is carried out three times with a ten-second pause between the end of each recall phase and the beginning of the next presentation of the word-pairs. The same ten word pairs are used throughout but their order of presentation is varied.

The figure which summarizes results on these seven subtests is called the memory quotient (MQ). Its significance can be fully appreciated only by comparison with the IQ value obtained on one of the Wechsler Intelligence Scales (preferably the WAIS). The MQ-IQ comparison provides a quantitative index: when it is strongly negative, that is, when the MQ is much less than would be expected from the IQ, it suggests a possible organic memory disorder (the opposite discrepancy and a comparable decrease in both scores are of less interest in aphasiology).

HALSTEAD-REITAN BATTERY‡

In our opinion, the particularly extensive normative research which has been carried out on the Halstead-Reitan Battery‡[15-25, 35-45] makes it a choice instrument for a neuropsychological assessment. The aims of this battery are to identify the presence of an organic brain lesion, to determine its lateralization and, finally, to specify its location. Although the first two goals are of secondary interest in aphasiology, the Halstead-Reitan Battery may nevertheless be valuable in the study of neuropsychological disturbances associated with aphasia or even in the interpretation of certain symptomatological elements of the aphasia itself.

The Halstead-Reitan Battery was developed in two phases, the first directed by Halstead from 1935 to 1947 and the second by Reitan from 1951 to 1959. Seven subtests were studied during the first phase. We shall collectively refer to them as the Halstead Battery. Presentation of these subtests yields ten different scores which are combined to obtain an *impairment index*. This index is of great value in the diagnosis of the presence or absence of a cerebral lesion. The subtests comprising the Halstead Battery are as follows:

---

* Wechsler, D. A standardized memory scale for clinical use. *Journal of Psychology*, **19**, 87-95, 1945.

† All examples are fictitious or have been paraphrased.

‡ Neuropsychology Laboratory, Indiana University Medical Center, Indianapolis, Indiana 46202, USA (1968).

1. During the *Category Test*, seven series of slides (a total of 208) are successively projected on a screen. In most of the series, each slide shows four designs: the expected response is the selection of one of them according to a principle which the subject must discover. Subjects indicate their choice by pushing one of four levers (numbered 1 to 4). Having been informed about the meaning of these consequences, the subjects receive feedback after each response with correct choices being followed by a 'pleasant' sound (bell) and incorrect ones being followed by an 'unpleasant' sound (buzz). Subjects are told when a new series is to begin and thus know that the principle guiding correct selections, which remains constant within a series, may now change. The principles involved in the earlier series are simpler than in the later ones: their discovery presupposes the ability to form more or less complex concepts through observation of the similarities and differences between the stimuli, to formulate hypotheses on the basis of these observations and then to test these hypotheses according to the feedback received after each response. Although the performance of certain subjects with small brain lesions may not differ from that of normal subjects on the Category Test, it is generally very sensitive to the presence of cerebral lesions.
2. The *Critical Flicker Frequency Test*, which is carried out using an electronic instrument (Strobotac), permits identification of the frequency at which intermittent light is perceived as continuous. The subject manipulates a button which controls the frequency of the visual stimulus and then stops as soon as the light appears to be continuous. The examiner notes the frequency of this stimulus (frequency threshold). This frequency is then used as a reference to calculate the mean of the deviations observed on five further trials (deviation threshold).
3. The *Tactual Performance Test* is an adaptation of the Séquin–Godard formboard. The test is completed in four steps with the first three requiring blind performance. The subject is given ten wooden geometric figures and a formboard with indentations, each of which corresponds in shape to one of these figures. During the first step, subjects use only their dominant hand. They must palpate each figure and then, by the same means, find the corresponding form on the formboard and fit the figure into it. The task is the same during the second step, in which subjects use their other hand, and during the third step, in which they use both hands. The examiner records the time required to complete each step: besides providing information on subjects' learning abilities, these measures alone may yield valuable clues about the site of possible cerebral lesions (particularly in certain cases of parietal or callosal lesions). The fourth step is carried out under visual control and requires graphic production. The stimuli are removed from the subjects' view and they are asked to draw from memory the ten figures which they had previously manipulated; they must reproduce them on a single page, arranging them in the same way as on the formboard. The behaviours observed during this stage may also provide clues to the localization of possible cerebral lesions (especially in the case of retrorolandic lesions).
4. The *Rhythm Test* corresponds to a part of the *Seashore Test of Musical Talent*. Thirty pairs of tape-recorded rhythmical sequences are presented: subjects must compare the members of each pair and say whether or not they are identical (15 pairs are the same and 15 are different). In aphasiology, this test may be useful in studying patients whose symptomatology includes a clear element of word deafness[27] (see Chapters 4 and 5).
5. In the *Speech Sound Perception Test*, the subject is asked to indicate which of four written syllables corresponds to a tape-recorded stimulus. The test comprises 60 nonsense syllables. Aphasic symptomatology including an element of word deafness[27] or alexia for syllables[28] (see Chapters 4 and 5) may be a source of abnormal performance on this subtest.
6. The *Finger Tapping Test* measures the speed of oscillation of the right and left index fingers by means of a counter which records the movements of a lever which is pushed with a finger. The subject is asked to carry out the task as rapidly as possible and a score is obtained, for each index finger, by calculating the mean number of oscillations over five periods of ten seconds each. Possible differences between the two index fingers and a comparison between the index finger of the dominant and that of the non-dominant hand are taken into account when interpreting the scores on this test.

7. The *Time Sense Test* is carried out using a special stop-watch which is controlled by the subject. The test is completed in several steps, certain ones being carried out under visual control and presumably resulting in learning (a total of 40 trials), and others involving blind performance and measuring the subject's ability to appreciate a predefined time period (a total of 20 trials). The subject's score is obtained by adding the deviations observed during the blind performance trials.

To obtain Halstead's *Impairment Index*[25], the figure (0.1) is assigned to each of the following results: 51 errors or more on the Categories Test; a frequency threshold of 20.9 or less on the Flicker Frequency Test; a deviation threshold of 15.7 or more on the Flicker Frequency Test; a total time of 15.7 minutes or more for the first three steps of the Tactile Performance Test; reproduction of five figures or less on the fourth step of the Tactile Performance Test; correct disposition of four figures or less on the Tactile Performance Test; six errors or more on the Rhythm Test; eight errors or more on the Speech Sound Perception Test; 50 oscillations or less for the most efficient index finger on the Finger Tapping Test; a cumulative deviation of 261 seconds or more on the Time Sense Test. The impairment index is then calculated simply by adding the assigned figures; thus it may range between 0 and 1, with a value of (0.5) being strongly suggestive of the presence of an organic brain lesion.

REITAN'S BATTERY

Reitan's battery of neuropsychological tests comprises: (a) *Halstead's battery*; (b) the *Wechsler-Bellevue Intelligence Scale* (Form 1, 1944); (c) the *Reitan-Indiana Aphasia Screening Test*; (d) the *Minnesota Multiphasic Personality Inventory* (*MMPI*); (e) the *Trail Making Test*; (f) the *Reitan-Klove Sensori-Perceptual Examination*; and (g) a *Lateral Dominance Examination*. We have already discussed the different subtests of Halstead's Battery as well as those of a French-Canadian adaptation of the Wechsler Scale (cf. pp. 381 and 385). We shall omit discussion of the Reitan Indiana Test since it is too abbreviated, given the aims of this text (see Chapter 15). Neither shall we discuss the MMPI, a test of marginal utility in clinical aphasiology. The remaining components of Reitan's battery are as follows:

1. The *Trail Making Test*[38–40] has two parts. In the first, the subject must join a series of numbered circles (from 1 to 25) scattered in random order over a sheet of paper. The task is similar on the second part of the test, except that the circles must be joined by alternating between numerical ordering (1 to 13) and alphabetical ordering (A to L). If errors are made, they are pointed out as they occur and the subject corrects them. The subject is instructed to work as quickly as possible and the time taken to complete each part of the test is recorded. A third score is obtained by transforming the total performance time into a weighted score. Different neuropsychological disorders (constructional apraxia, visual neglect, etc.) may impair performance during the Trail Making Test; in addition, and apart from these disturbances, aphasics generally have difficulty in doing the second part of this subtest.
2. The *Reitan–Klove Sensori-Perceptual Examination* represents a systematization of certain particular aspects of a routine neurological examination. The behaviours assessed were mainly selected for their localizing value, particularly in relation to the temporo-parieto-occipital regions. The test has several parts (in each one, the observed behaviours are numerically defined in terms of the number of errors).
   (a) The main goal of the first part is to test for the presence of tactile, visual or auditory *extinction* by means of bilateral simultaneous stimulation. For each sensory modality, a threshold of unilateral perception is first determined and then a fixed number of unilateral and bilateral stimuli are presented (48 tactile, 16 auditory and 48 visual).
   (b) The second part is especially intended to reveal the presence of *finger agnosia*. It begins by the preliminary learning of a code linking each finger, from the thumb to the little finger (for example), to the corresponding number (from 1 to 5). The rest of the subtest requires blind finger identification. The examiner stimulates (lightly touches) each finger four times in a predetermined random order for a total of 20 stimulations per hand. A separate score is recorded for each hand.
   (c) The third part is based on the presence of *agraphaesthesia* in certain patients with

cerebral lesions. In a preliminary step, the examiner demonstrates the nature of the task by successively tracing the numbers 3, 4, 5 and 6 on the palm of the patient's hand. The rest of the test requires blind, verbal identification of the same stimuli as they are traced by the examiner, in a predetermined random order, on the tips of the fingers. Four stimuli are thus traced on each finger for a total of 20 per hand. A separate score is recorded for each hand.

(d) The fifth part requires the identification of coins by blind palpation.

(e) The main goal of the sixth part is also to identify the presence of *astereognosia*, this time by the use of the *Reitan–Klove Tactile Form Recognition Test*. This test is based on the blind palpation of four simple geometric figures (plastic): an intentionally non-verbal, multiple-choice response is required; after having palpated the stimulus with one hand, the subject must use the contralateral hand to select its duplicate from a board containing duplicates of all four forms. Each of the four figures is presented four times to each hand in a predetermined random order. Each hand is scored separately in terms of the number of identification errors and total palpation time.

(f) Finally, the Reitan–Klove Test includes the identification of the limits of the visual field (cf. p. 378).

3. The *Lateral Dominance Examination* aims to identify the dominant eye, hand and foot. It consists of a questionnaire and observations of different requested behaviours. The latter include dynamometric measurement of hand grasp force and use of a test intended to determine ocular dominance (*Miles ABC Test of Ocular Dominance*).

THE TOKEN TEST (DE RENZI AND VIGNOLO)*

The Token Test is carried out using tokens which differ in size, shape and number. In the original version of this test[47], the tokens include five large circles, five small circles, five large rectangles, and five small rectangles: each of these series contains one red, one blue, one green, one yellow and one white token. The test is divided into five parts, with each of the first four consisting of ten commands and the fifth part consisting of 21 commands. The commands are spoken and become progressively more difficult from one part of the test to the next:

Part 1: each command requires the identification of a single token specified by shape and colour.

Part 2: each command requires the identification of a single token specified by size, shape and colour.

Part 3: each command requires the identification of two tokens, each one specified by shape and colour.

Part 4: each command requires the identification of two tokens, each one specified by size, shape and colour.

Part 5: the commands are more complex and include grammatical elements requiring, for example, that the tokens be manipulated in relation to each other ('Put the red circle on the green rectangle'), that exceptions ('Pick up all the rectangles except the yellow one') and conditions ('When I touch the green circle, you take the white rectangle') be understood, etc. In this part of the test, the tokens are specified only by shape and colour.

In our French-language adaptation of the original† Token Test, we have used squares rather than rectangles and added one further command to part 5. We have found that many normal subjects make up to seven errors during part 5 (and sometimes a few during part 4 as well).

Performance on the Token Test may be affected by several factors of which language comprehension is certainly among the most important[49–51]. This test is particularly useful for the study of comprehension disturbances in Broca's aphasics: the last part often permits demonstration of impaired comprehension of grammatical words. To permit a comparison of

* Token Test, Clinica Delle Malattie Nervrose et Mentale, Universita de Milano, Italy.

† After the original Token Test was published (without norms)[47], many investigators developed modified or shorter versions. De Renzi and Faglioni[48] have recently reported normative data on a shortened version and propose that it be adopted as the standard form of the Token Test. This version differs from the original (cf. above) by: a reduction in the number of commands to a total of 36; the introduction of an initial part containing easier items (identification by shape or colour only); the use of squares instead of rectangles; and the use of black, instead of blue, tokens.

oral comprehension and written language comprehension, the Token Test commands may also be presented in writing.

TESTS USED AT THE CENTRE DU LANGAGE DE L'HÔPITAL DE LA SALPÊTRIÈRE

One of us (F.L.) and Blanch Ducarne[52] recommend the use of following tests (or, in some cases, English language equivalents) for the neuropsychological assessment of aphasics:

1. *Intelligence tests*
   (a) Wechsler Adult Intelligence Scale (Verbal Scale; Performance Scale).
   (b) R.B. Cattel Intelligence Scale. Scale 2. Forms A and B.
   (c) Progressive Matrices (Fould and Raven) (PM-38).
   (d) Terman-Merrill Scale.
2. *Performance tests*
   (a) Kohs' Cubes (Grace Arthur).
   (b) Porteus Maze Test (Vineland revision).
   (c) Stick Test (Gelb, Goldstein).
   (d) Borelli-Oléron Performance Scale.
3. *Perceptual-motor tests*
   (a) L. Bender's perceptual-motor tests.
   (b) The Complex Figure of Rey.
   (c) Benton Visual Retention Test (Forms C and D).
4. *Perceptual tests*
   (a) Experimental Scale of Visual Acuity (Rossano).
   (b) Thurstone's Identical Forms Test.
   (c) Polak's Colour-test.
   (d) Farnsworth's Dichotomous Test for Colour Blindness.
5. *Head's tests*
   (a) Hand-Eye-Ear Test.
   (b) Time Test.
   (c) Colour Test.
6. *Academic achievement and verbal tests* (*paper and pencil*)
   (a) Achievement tests to determine grade level.
   (b) Forms F and C of the National Institute for Professional Orientation.
   (c) General Classification Test.
7. *Memory tests*
   (a) Wechsler Memory Scale.
   (b) Benton Visual Retention Test—Form F.
8. *Verbal tests*
   (a) Vocabulary test (Binois-Pichot).
   (b) Spelling test (P. Rennes).
   (c) Test of Textual Comprehension (P. Rennes).*

ILLUSTRATIVE CASES

A neuropsychological disturbance, aphasic or other, may sometimes be so mild that its presence remains questionable after a routine neurological examination. The results of a neuropsychological battery are then of greatest value since they may permit a definitive answer. Such cases are nevertheless rare in clinical aphasiology, where the patient's aphasia is generally obvious and often associated with other localizing signs such as hemiparesis or hemianopsia: a psychometric battery would then lose its justification if its only goal was to identify the presence of a cerebral lesion or to determine its lateralization. Consequently, the aim is usually to reveal the presence of associated disturbances, that is, to objectify features which permit better understanding of certain aspects of the aphasic symptomatology itself. We shall close the present chapter by presenting psychometric results for four illustrative cases. While not discussing all possible cases, the four which are presented represent prototypes and, as such, include elements drawn from several files.

Case 1

The patient was a 57-year-old right-handed school teacher with no familial history of left-handedness or ambidexterity. Myocardial infarction had occurred at the age of 55 and been followed by periods of auricular fibrillation. Following the sudden onset of a neurological disorder, he presented a suppression of language and right hemiplegia without loss of consciousness or obvious disturbance of comprehension; after five or six days, rapid recovery took place over about a week and then became much slower. At the time of the psychometric assessment (five weeks after the onset of the neurological dis-

* Lhermitte, F. and Ducarne, B., Plan de l'examen clinique des aphasiques: *Revue pratique*, 15, 2365–2374, 1965.

order) he presented a relatively mild Broca's aphasia with a predominant articulatory disturbance (phonetic disintegration in the dystonic phase); a buccofacial apraxia of moderate severity; and a mild, mainly brachiofacial, right hemiparesis (he could manipulate a pencil with his right hand although with some difficulty): no sensory deficits were detected during a routine neurological examination; visual acuity, perimetry and audiometry were normal. His general state was good; arrythmia was controlled by medication. The diagnosis was left, prerolandic cortical–subcortical softening of probable embolic origin; results of paraclinical examinations were consistent with this diagnosis. The lesion was thought to be centred, at the cortical level, on the caudalmost part of the left, third frontal convolution and on the precentral gyrus. It was suggested that it also might spread to the caudalmost part of the second frontal convolution and to the anterior third of the insula[53] (see Chapter 8-3 and 8-4). Results of the psychometric assessment were as follows:

Colour vision: normal. The few hesitations observed during *colour naming* and *colour evocation* tests can reasonably be attributed to word-finding difficulty.

Bender Visual Motor Gestalt Test: nearly normal with the exception of graphic awkwardness related to the mild, right hemiparesis.

Complex Figure of Rey: copy: type IV; 50th percentile; four minutes. These results are compatible with the presence of a cerebral lesion but have no localizing value. Reproduction from memory: type IV; 10th percentile; four minutes, 30 seconds (same comments as above). No constructional apraxia. The graphic awkwardness is related to the mild right hemiparesis; it might also explain the long performance time.

Standard Progressive Matrices (*PM-38*): Slow performance (45 minutes) with a score corresponding to the 75th percentile. Although within the range of normal, the patient's score is presumably lower than that which he would have obtained before onset of neurological disease; impaired inner language (i.e., difficulty in nonvocal self-verbalization) may have hindered reasoning during certain portions of the PM-38.

Ottawa-Wechsler Intelligence Scale (Fig. 16-5)

(a) *General Information*: Weighted Score = 13; normal.
(b) *General Comprehension*: weighted Score = 10; points were lost as a result of the patient's lack of verbal incentive.
(c) *Digit span*: weighted Score = 7; the patient was handicapped by his articulatory disturbance (recall appeared to be hindered by the slow speaking rate) and probably also by impaired inner language.
(d) *Arithmetic*: weighted score = 9; the subject was probably handicapped by impaired inner language; failures on the last two problems can be attributed to inaccurate reading.
(e) *Similarities*: weighted score = 13; normal.
(f) *Picture Arrangement*: weighted score = 10; the subject was probably handicapped by impaired inner language.
(g) *Picture Completion*: weighted score = 14; normal.
(h) *Block Design*: weighted score = 8; time penalties partially related to the hemiparesis; performance suggests the possibility of mild, upper limb apraxia; as in the case of the Figure of Rey, this finding may be an effect—which becomes clearer as the stimuli become more complex—which is related, without localizing value, to the presence of a cerebral lesion.
(i) *Object Assembly*: weighted score = 10; the three puzzles were correctly assembled but the patient worked rather slowly and obtained only one bonus point for time.
(j) *Digit Symbol*: weighted score = 5; performance was hindered by the hemiparesis; some impairment of visual-motor coordination is suspected.

Verbal IQ = 105; Performance IQ = 105; Full Scale IQ = 107. No discrepancy between Verbal IQ and Performance IQ. The Verbal, Performance, and Full Scale IQs are all within the normal range and the Performance IQ is consistent with results obtained on the Progressive Matrices (PM-38). The scores obtained on several subtests nevertheless suggest that the premorbid IQ was higher; in certain respects the decrease is specifically related to the presence of an aphasiogenic lesion; in other respects it appears related, without localizing specificity, to cerebral dysfunction.

Wechsler Memory Scale: MQ = 101. No discrepancy between MQ and IQ. The same factors can explain the decrease in both; there is no evidence of a specific memory disturbance.

Halstead's Tests

(a) *Category Test*: 69 errors; this result is consissistent with the presence of a cerebral lesion.

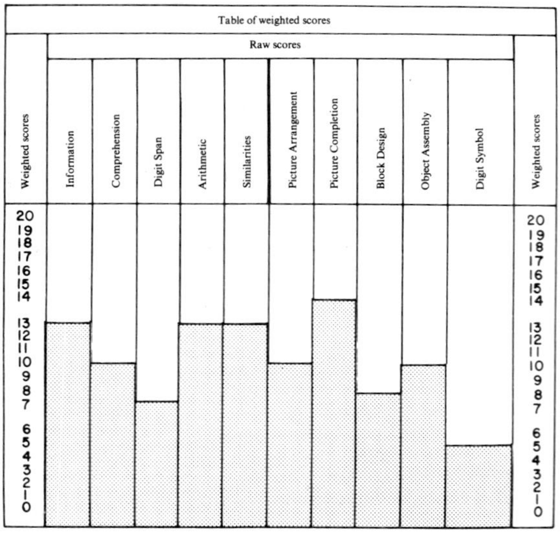

Fig. 16-5 *Wechsler Scale: profile of Case 1 (schoolteacher). Commentary in the text.*

(b) *Tactual Performance Test*: right hand: eight minutes; left hand: three minutes; both hands: three minutes. Five figures were drawn correctly, of which four were correctly situated. The paretic impairment certainly enters into the explanation of right-hand performance; results on the last part of the test may be evidence of disturbed inner language and/or of a 'general' factor (without localizing value).

(c) *Rhythm Test*: results within the normal range.

(d) *Finger Tapping Test*: right hand: 28; left hand: 45. The right-hand performance is related to the residual hemiparesis.

Reitan's Tests

(a) *Trail Making Test:* the score was 9 on the first part (Trail Making A) and 3 on the second (Trail Making B). The total performance time was abnormally long; this can be partially attributed to the hemiparesis and probably also to some impairment of visual-motor coordination. Results on the second part also indicate disturbed letter identification and a (non-specific) difficulty in systematically alternating between numbers and letters.

(b) *Reitan–Klove Test*: the results confirm the integrity of the retrorolandic regions. Only one anomaly was observed, namely increased palpation time for the right hand during the sixth part of the subtest; this is explained by the hemiparesis.

Token Test: there were four errors on the fourth part of the test and 13 on the fifth part. There is a mild disturbance of oral comprehension; understanding of grammatical words is particularly affected.

Case 2

The patient was a 42-year-old, bilingual (French and English) right-handed architect with no familial history of left-handedness or ambidexterity. His medical history was uneventful prior to a highway accident which was followed by a coma lasting six days. After the comatose period, it was observed that the patient had great difficulty understanding what was said to him and that his language, while fluent and normally articulated, could hardly be understood. His general state having improved, a detailed neuropsychological assessment was carried out five weeks after the accident. He then presented a Wernicke's aphasia with the main symptomatological elements being as follows: fluent discourse but including many hesitations and all types of paraphasias (the patient was relatively aware of this disturbance); severely impaired repetition with relatively better oral reading; writing to dictation relatively more impaired than other aspects of written expression; relatively good oral language comprehension at an elementary level (which represented an improvement) but frequent failures on more complex tests (the patient often requests that spoken directions be repeated); impaired comprehension of written language, although clearly less affected than comprehension of oral language. With the exception of a right superior quadranopsia, the remainder of the neurological examination was normal. The diagnosis was cerebral contusion with damage mainly in the left temporal region; results from paraclinical examinations were consistent with this diagnosis. The lesion was thought especially to involve the first temporal convolution (including the *planum*) and perhaps the second as well; questions were raised concerning its possible extension to Heschl's zone and to the posterior part of the insula (see Chapters 8–3 and 8–4). Results of the psychometric assessment were as follows:

Colour vision: normal results on the *Polak*, *Ishihara* and *Hardy–Rand–Ritter* tests as well as on colour-matching tests. No abnormalities in colouring pictured objects. Since the patient did not appear to understand the instructions, the *Holmgren* and *Farnsworth* tests were not presented. Despite this and some errors, attributable to the aphasia, during tests of *colour identification*, *naming*, *recognition* and *evocation*, colour vision is presumed to be normal.

Bender Visual Motor Gestalt Test: very nearly normal.

Benton Visual Retention Test (*form C*, *procedure A*) the main anomalies (omission of a small figure placed to the right and quite removed from the central part of the stimulus) can be attributed to the quadranopsia.

Complex Figure of Rey: copy: type IV; 70th percentile; three minutes. These results are compatible with the presence of a cerebral lesion. No constructional apraxia. The visual deficit in the upper right quadrant explains the omission of some details. Reproduction from memory: no meaningful production.

Standard Progressive Matrices (*PM-38*): although the score was normal (75th percentile) it can be assumed that this patient would have obtained a higher score before onset of his neurological disease. Reasoning during certain parts of the PM-38 may have been hindered by impaired inner language.

Ottawa–Wechsler Intelligence Scale (Fig. 16–6)

(a) *General Information*: weighted score = 5; abnormally low.

(b) *General Comprehension*: weighted score = 7; lower limit of the normal range; less than the expected score (given this patient's background).

(c) *Digit Span*: weighted score = 4; abnormally low.

(d) *Arithmetic*: weighted score = 4; abnormally low.

(e) *Similarities*: weighted score = 7; lower limit of the normal range; less than the expected score.

(f) *Picture Arrangement*: weighted score = 9; handicap related to impaired inner language.

(g) *Picture Completion*: weighted score = 12; almost normal.

(h) *Block Design*: weighted score = 8; increasingly inadequate behaviour with increased stimulus complexity (compatible with the presence of a cerebral lesion but without localizing value).

(i) *Object Assembly*: weighted score = 10; the three puzzles were correctly assembled but points were lost because of slow performance.

(j) *Digit Symbol*: weighted score = 7; lower limit of the normal range; less than the expected score.

Verbal IQ = 78; Performance IQ = 93; Full Scale IQ = 75. The Verbal IQ is relatively more affected than Performance IQ, a discrepancy compatible with a left hemisphere lesion. The relatively better performance on the *Standard Progressive Matrices* (PM-38), than on the *Wechsler Scale* suggests the relative intactness of the left inferior parietal lesion.

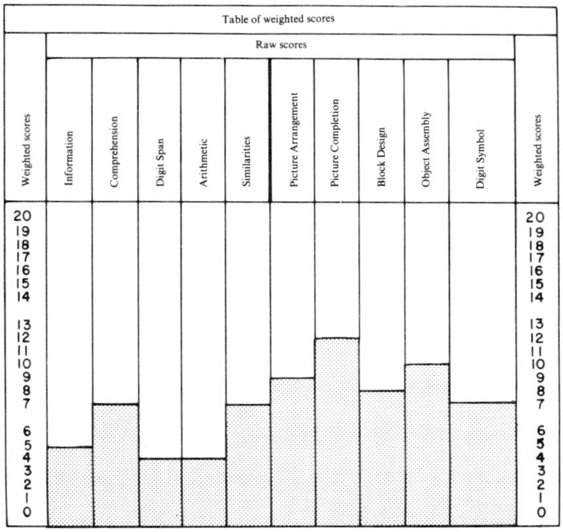

Fig. 16–6 *Wechsler Scale: profile of Case 2 (architect). Commentary in the text.*

Wechsler Memory Scale: results near zero and thus a large discrepancy between MQ and IQ. The syndrome presumably includes a significant amnesic element.

Halstead's Tests

(a) *Category Test*: more than 100 errors before the test was discontinued. At certain times, the patient did not appear to distinguish between the two types of auditory feedback; suspected presence of agnosia for (non-verbal and non-musical) sounds.

(b) *Tactual Performance Test*: right hand: six minutes; left hand: five minutes; both hands: four minutes. Four figures were correctly drawn, of which two were correctly situated. Results on the last part of the test may be evidence of disturbed inner language, an associated amnesic disturbance and/or a 'general' factor (without localizing value).

(c) *Rhythm Test*: score indicative of severe impairment.

(d) *Speech Sound Perception Test* (English version): score indicative of severe impairment. An obvious element of word deafness; temporal localization.

(e) *Finger Tapping Test*: right hand: 37; left hand: 36. Compatible with the presence of a cerebral lesion (without localizing value).

Reitan's Tests

(a) *Trail Making Test*: the score was 8 on the first part and 2 on the second. Total performance time was abnormally long; at certain moments the quadranopsia clearly entered into account. The results on the second part were particularly affected by literal alexia (which, in this patient, is much more severe than verbal alexia[46]).

(b) *Reitan-Klove Test*: the subtests requiring verbal responses were not presented. Besides the quadranopsia, no other visual field deficits were observed; on the other hand, the results suggested the possibility of right auditory extinction.

Token Test: impaired comprehension of oral language was evident even on the first part of the test; during the last part; the patient appeared to respond at random. When the Token Test was presented in written form, the results were normal for the first two parts and below normal for the next two: 13 errors were made on the fifth part.

Case 3

The patient was a 61-year-old, right-handed journalist having a left-handed father and an ambidexterous brother. He had suffered occasional periods of vertigo during the past year. More severe and prolonged than previously, the last of these episodes had been followed by temporary dimming of vision and a period of obnubilation. Some hours later, the patient felt that he had completely recovered but it was then that he discovered, when looking at a newspaper, that he could no longer read. An aphasia assessment carried out on the following day revealed the presence of very mild word-finding difficulty and of word blindness: written language was not understood and oral reading was impossible; copying was servile; on the other hand, writing to dictation and spontaneous writing were normal, as were results on all other parts of the aphasia assessment. During a routine neurological examination, the presence of a right homonymous hemianopsia was noted; perimetry indicated that the hemianopsia did not spare macular vision. The diagnosis was vertebrobasilary insufficiency with softening in the area of the left posterior cerebral artery; results from paraclinical examinations were consistent with this diagnosis. Although there was agreement about the territory affected, there was some dispute about the exact localization of the lesions (see Chapter 5 and Fig. 8-21). Results of the psychometric assessment were as follows:

Colour Vision: normal results on the *Polak* and *Ishihara Tests* as well as on *Head's Test* (matching of coloured bands) and *Holmgreen's Test*. On the other hand, errors were made on the *Hardy-Rand-Ritter Test*, and the *Farnsworth Test (100-Hue)* revealed the presence of pseudo-dyschromatopsia (Fig. 16-7). Performance was abnormal on tests of *colour naming* and *evocation* but less impaired on tests of colour *identification* and *recognition*. Some peculiar colour selections were noted during the *colouring test*. In summary, this patient presents the most frequent symptomatological constellation currently designated by the name of colour agnosia[28].

Bender Visual Motor Gestalt Test: normal.

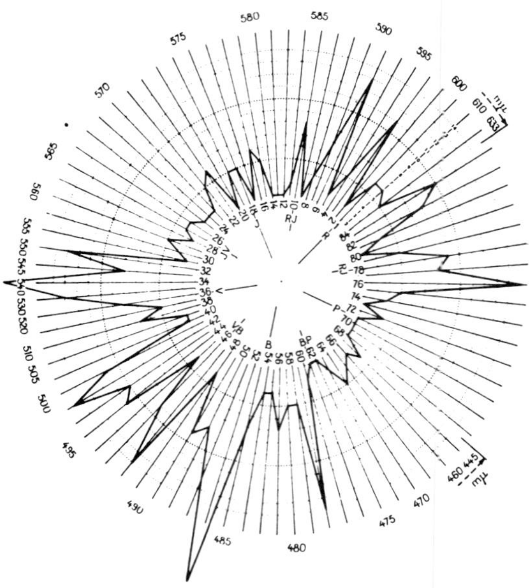

Fig. 16-7 *Farnsworth Test (100-Hue): pseudo-dyschromatopsia. From Lhermitte et al*[28].

Benton Visual Retention Test (*form C, procedure A*) certain anomalies attributable to the hemianopsia.

Complex Figure of Rey: copy: type I; 50th percentile four minutes. Omission of certain details on the right side of the stimulus. Reproduction from memory: type I; 10th percentile; four minutes. The framework was reproduced as well as the most noticeable structures; numerous details were nevertheless omitted, especially those on the right side of the stimulus. The results suggest a possible memory dysfunction.

Standard Progressive Matrices (*PM-38*): the patient's score is in the 90th percentile; one hour was required to complete the test. The patient was very aware that exploration of all the visual material was needed before selecting his response.

Ottawa–Wechsler Intelligence Scale (Fig. 16–8)

(a) *General Information*: weighted score = 17; this score is above average.
(b) *General Comprehension*: weighted score = 16; although critical, the patient completely grasped the type of expected replies; his score is above average.
(c) *Digit Span*: weighted score = 13; the patient could repeat eight digits forward and five backwards.
(d) *Arithmetic*: weighted score = 11; being unable to read them, the patient lost the points associated with the last two problems.
(e) *Similarities*: weighted score = 17; this score is above average.
(f) *Picture Arrangement*: weighted score = 11; certain visual details, both literal and other, appeared not to have been noticed.
(g) *Picture Completion*: weighted score = 13; this score is at the upper limit of the average range.
(h) *Block Design*: weighted score = 7; the patient lost points for having three times used yellow, rather than white, elements; performance was abnormally slow but the stimuli were adequately reproduced in terms of the designs.
(i) *Object Assembly*: weighted score = 13; the three puzzles were correctly assembled but the time bonuses were relatively small.
(j) *Digit Symbol*: weighted score = 7; alexia for numbers, although less severe than the literal alexia partially explains this relatively low score; an element of amnesia may also enter into account.

Verbal IQ = 123; Performance IQ = 109; Full Scale IQ = 121. The discrepancies observed between different subtests, as well as the score on the Standard Progressive Matrices (PM-38), suggests that the premorbid IQ was higher than the present IQ. The abnormally low scores are mainly related to the alexia, colour agnosia and hemianopsia.

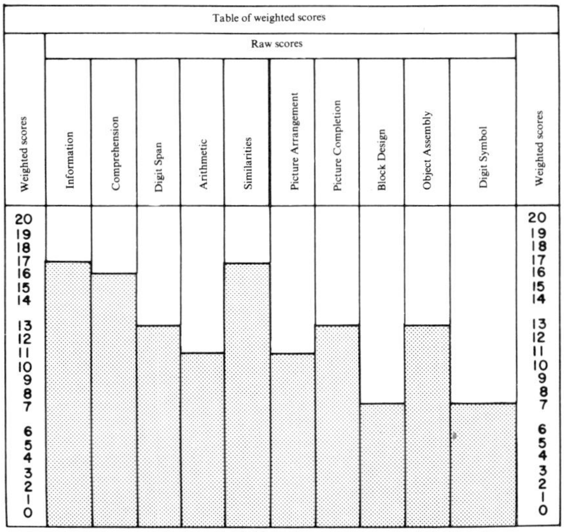

Fig. 16-8 *Wechsler Scale: profile of Case 3 (journalist). Commentary in the text.*

Wechsler Memory Scale: MQ = 110; QM – QI = – 11. The discrepancy suggests an associated memory disturbance. Performance was poorest on the *Visual Reproduction* and *Associate Learning* subtests.

Halstead's Tests

(a) *Category Test*: the number of errors is abnormally high. Many can be explained as a result of impaired recognition of colours, numbers and letters; memory dysfunction also appears possible.
(b) *Tactual Performance Test*: right hand: five minutes; left hand: four minutes; both hands: three minutes. Six figures were correctly drawn, of which five were correctly situated. Being at the limit of the normal range, the last result may be evidence of a mild memory disturbance.
(c) *Rhythm Test*: normal results.
(d) *Finger Tapping Test*: right hand: 46; left hand: 46. Normal scores; the identical

performance of each hand is noteworthy (cf. family history of handedness).

Reitan's Tests

(a) *Trail Making Test*: the score was 9 on the first part of the test; the second was not presented because of the patient's difficulty in identifying literal symbols.

(b) *Reitan–Klove Test*: the only abnormal results are related to the hemianopsia.

Token Test: errors were made on each of the five parts of the test; all can be attributed to the colour agnosia.

Case 4

The patient was a 64-year-old, right-handed Jesuit without any familial history of left-handedness or ambidexterity or any personal or familial history of developmental dyslexia–dysorthographia. Other than mumps at the age of 22, his medical history was uneventful. He complained of disturbed 'concentration' and 'memory loss' which resulted in, among other things, difficulty in 'finding words'. He was unable to specify when these troubles began; a colleague, however, reported that he had found the patient somewhat 'strange' at least a year ago, and particularly mentioned that his Sunday sermons were a little 'disconnected' and redundant. An aphasiological assessment revealed the presence of mild dysorthographia and moderately severe word-finding difficulty. The latter was little aided by facilitating cues and was manifested in spontaneous language and during word evocation tests to the same extent as during naming tests (amnesic aphasia). A consultant suggested the possibility of a mild tendency towards echolalia and of paraphasic production slightly beyond the limits of normal language (see Chapter 14). Repetition and oral reading were nevertheless normal. With the exception of a certain slowness in responding, results on the usual comprehension tests were nearly normal for both oral and written language. With the exception of the inability to copy the drawing of a cube, results on the remainder of the neurological examination were normal. A degenerative disease, such as Alzheimer's, for example, or the presence of a slowly growing left hemisphere tumour (see Chapter 9) was suspected. Results of the psychometric assessment were as follows:

Colour vision: reading of the pseudo-isochromatic plates was almost normal and colours were matched without error. Similarly, no errors were made during the *Holmgreen Test*. The *Farnsworth Test* (*100-Hue*) was discontinued because the patient appeared to be responding at random. The patient completed the tests of *colour identification* and *colour recognition* without error but certain anomalies, mostly related to word-finding difficulty, were observed during the tests requiring the *naming* and *evocation* of colours.

Bender Visual Motor Gestalt Test: signs of organicity without localizing value (rotations, displacements, simplifications, dots replaced by dashes, etc.)

Complex Figure of Rey: type IV; 10th percentile; six minutes. Displacements, omissions, duplication of details etc. Obvious constructional apraxia[30]; the results suggest a possible element of left visual neglect. Reproduction from memory: no production.

Standard Progressive Matrices (*PM-38*): The patient scored in the 25th percentile. Errors were made within the first part of the test; by the third series of problems, the patient often appeared to respond at random.

Ottawa–Wechsler Intelligence Scale (Fig. 16–9)

(a) *General Information*: weighted score = 8; aphasic and memory impairments obvious.

(b) *General Comprehension*: weighted score = 12; the patient appeared more at ease with this type of material and obtained a score within the normal range.

(c) *Digit Span*: weighted score = 6; memory impairment obvious.

(d) *Arithmetic*: weighted score = 6; dyscalculia; faulty reasoning.

(e) *Similarities*: weighted score = 9; this score is within the normal range: some bizarre, dissociated and paraphasic responses (e.g., the similarity between 'airplane' and 'falcon': by the movement and position of his arms, the patient conveyed the idea of flying; verbally, he said they were both 'birds').

(f) *Picture Arrangement*: weighted score = 6; the patient neglected pertinent features and did not adequately apprehend the logical links in sequences containing more than three pictures.

(g) *Picture Completion*: weighted score = 9; this score is within the normal range but below that which could be expected given the patient's background and the usual imperviousness of this subtest to the presence of a cerebral lesion.

(h) *Block Design*: weighted score = 5; obvious disturbance (praxic and/or agnosic) of visuo-spatial organization. Colour selections were correct.
(i) *Object Assembly*: weighted score = 3; obvious praxic disturbance and faulty identification of certain parts of the puzzle.
(j) *Digit Symbol*: weighted score = 3; obvious praxic factor; some instances of perseveration; almost no learning.

Verbal IQ = 96; Performance IQ = 82; Full Scale IQ = 88. Global deterioration, slightly more marked on the Performance Scale; most of the scores are clearly pathological. These results, together with those on the *Standard Progressive Matrices* (PM-38) suggest the presence of degenerative disease rather than a tumour.

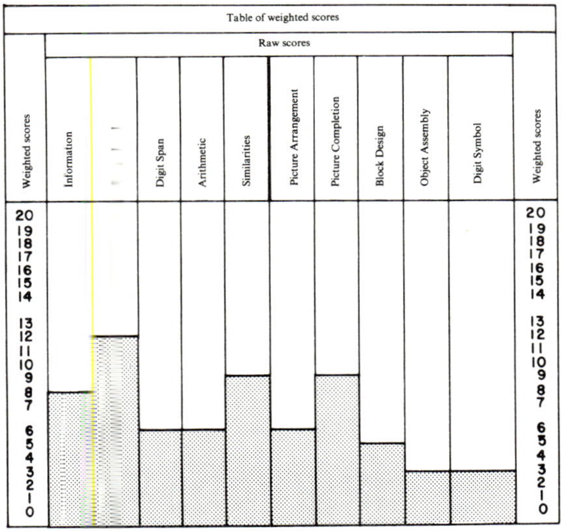

Fig. 16-9 *Wechsler Scale: profile of Case 4 (Jesuit). Commentary in the text.*

Wechsler Memory Scale: MQ = 75; MQ − IQ = −13. The overall picture undoubtedly reflects a memory disturbance as much as aphasic, agnosic and praxic impairments.

Halstead's Tests

(a) *Category Test*: a large number of errors; the patient appeared to respond at random and testing was discontinued after the third series of stimuli.
(b) *Tactual Performance Test*: right hand: 10 minutes; left hand: 11 minutes; both hands: 10 minutes. Test time clearly pathological; no learning. Only two figures were drawn from memory and only one was correctly situated.
(c) *Finger Tapping Test*: right hand: 27, left hand: 25. Variable rhythm; the index finger was not continuously in contact with the lever. The scores are pathological but without localizing value.

Reitan's Tests

(a) *Trail Making Test*: the score was 7 on the first part and 1 on the second part. During the latter, systematic alternation between letters and numbers was impossible. The scores are pathological but without localizing value.
(b) *Reitan–Klove Test*: mild extinction phenomena, equal on the left and on the right, were observed in all modalities (visual, auditory, tactile). Mild finger agnosia may be present.

Token Test: an increasing number of errors beginning on the third part of the test (16 errors during the fifth part). No improvement when the commands were presented in writing.

The presence of acquired aphasia constitutes clear evidence of a cerebral lesion, one which is generally irreversible. Thus, as we have already pointed out, the major goal of a psychometric assessment of an aphasic is neither the identification of the presence of such a lesion nor of its lateralization. Disregarding certain exceptional cases, a psychometric assessment is of value for other reasons: (a) it sometimes contributes to an aetiological diagnosis (see Case 4 above); (b) it may permit the systematic description, particularly within the context of a research programme, of disturbances which often accompany aphasia and perhaps even lead to hypotheses regarding certain aspects of the aphasic dysfunctions themselves; (c) it may sometimes permit the identification of mild deficits which escaped notice during a routine neurological examination and, as a result, lead to greater precision in the diagnosis of localization (see Cases 3 and 4 above); (d) when repeated on successive occasions, it may provide objective measures of a favourable or worsening course of evolution; (e) finally, it may be of great significance when decisions are to be taken regarding the patient's possible reintegration into the work force (see Chapter 17).

REFERENCES

1. Hécaen, H. (1972) *Introduction à la neuropsychologie.* Paris: Larousse.
2. Marie, P. (1926) *Travaux et mémoires*. Vol. I. Paris: Masson.
3. Klippel, M.M. (sous la présidence de) (1908) Compte rendu de la réunion de la société neurologique de Paris du 11 juin 1908: discussion sur l'aphasie. *Revue neurologique*, **16,** 611.
4. Klippel, M.M. (sous la présidence de) (1908) Compte rendu de la réunion de la société neurologique de Paris du 9 juillet 1908: discussion sur l'aphasie (suite). *Revue neurologique*, **16,** 974.
5. Klippel, M.M. (sous la présidence de) (1908) Compte rendu de la réunion de la société neurologique de Paris du 23 juillet 1908: discussion sur l'aphasie (fin). *Revue neurologique*, **16,** 1025.
6. Lhermitte, F., Chain, F., Escourolle, R., Ducarne, B. & Pillon, B. (1972) Etude anatomoclinique d'un cas de prosopagnosie. *Revue neurologique*, **126,** 329.
7. Lhermitte, F., Lecours, A.R., Ducarne, B. & Escourolle, R. (1973) Unexpected anatomical findings in a case of fluent jargon aphasia. *Cortex*, **9,** 433.
8. Lecours, A.R. & Lhermitte, F. (1976) The 'pure form' of the phonetic disintegration syndrome ('pure anarthria'); anatomo-clinical report of a historical case. *Brain and Language*, **3,** 88.
9. Tissot, R., Lhermitte, F. & Ducarne, B. (1963) Etat intellectuel des aphasiques. Essai d'une nouvelle approche à travers des épreuves perceptives et opératoires. *Encéphale*, **52,** 285.
10. Alajouanine, Th. (1965) Sur l'état intellectuel des aphasiques. *Revue pratique* (Paris), **5,** 2325.
11. Lhermitte, F. (1976) Peut-on penser sans langage? *Réalités*, **363,** 40.
12. Bay, E. (1957) Untersuchungen zum Aphasie Problem. *Nervenartz*, **28,** 450.
13. Bay, E. (1964) Aphasia and intelligence. *International Journal of Neurology*, **4,** 252.
14. Jackson, J.H. (1958) *Selected Writings of John Hughlings Jackson*. New York: Basic Books.
15. Reitan, R.M. (1956) Investigation of relationships between 'psychometric' and 'biological' intelligence. *Journal of Nervous and Mental Diseases*, **123,** 536.
16. Reitan, R.M. (1958) Qualitative versus quantitative mental changes following brain damage. *Journal of Psychology*, **46,** 339.
17. Reitan, R.M. (1959) Impairment of abstraction ability in brain damage: quantitative versus qualitative changes. *Journal of Psychology*, **48,** 97.
18. Reitan, R.M. (1960) The significance of dysphasia for intelligence and adaptive abilities. *Journal of Psychology*, **50,** 355.
19. Reitan, R.M. (1962) Psychological deficit. *Annual Review of Psychology*, **13,** 415.
20. Reitan, R.M. (1962) Psychological deficits resulting from cerebral lesions in man. In *The Frontal Granular Cortex and Behavior* (Ed.) Warren, J.M. & Akert, K. p. 295. New York: McGraw-Hill.
21. Reitan, R.M. (1966) Diagnostic inferences of brain lesions based on psychological test results. *Canadian Psychologist*, **7a,** 368.
22. Reitan, R.M. (1966) Problems and prospects in studying the psychological correlates of brain lesions. *Cortex*, **2,** 127.
23. Reitan, R.M. (1966) A research program on the psychological effects of brain lesions in human beings. *International Review of Research in Mental Retardation*, **1,** 153.
24. Reitan, R.M. (1970) Sensorimotor functions, intelligence and cognition, and emotional status in subjects with cerebral lesions. *Perceptual and Motor Skills*, **31,** 275.
25. Halstead, W.C. (1947) *Brain and Intelligence*. Chicago, IL: University of Chicago Press.
26. Lordat, J. (1843) Analyse de la parole pour servir à la théorie de divers cas d'alalie et de paralalie (de mutisme et d'imperfection de parler) que les neurologistes ont mal connus. *Journal de la Société pratique de Montpellier*, **7, 8;** 333 and 417; 1.
27. Lhermitte, F., Chain, F., Escourolle, R., Ducarne, B., Pillon, B. & Chedru, F. (1971) Etude des troubles perceptifs auditifs dans les lésions temporales bilatérales. A propos de trois observations dont deux anatomocliniques. *Revue neurologique*, **124,** 329.
28. Lhermitte, F., Chain, F., Aron, D., Leblanc, M. & Souty, O. (1959) Les troubles de la vision des couleurs dans les lésions postérieures du cerveau, à propos de 42 observations. *Revue neurologique*, **121,** 5.
29. Bender, L. (1933) Disturbances in visuomotor Gestalt function in organic brain disease associated with sensory aphasia. *Archives of Neurology and Psychiatry* (Chicago), **30,** 514.
30. Ducarne, B. & Pillon, B. (1974) La copie de la figure complexe de Rey dans les troubles visuo-constructifs. *Journal de Psychologie normale et pathologique*, **4,** 449.
31. Benton, A.L. (1962) The visual retention test as a constructional praxis task. *Confinia Neurologica* (Basel), **22,** 141.
32. Goldstein, K. (1933) L'analyse de l'aphasie et l'étude de l'essence du langage. *Journal of Psychology*, **30,** 430.
33. Goldstein, K. & Sheerer, M. (1941) Abstract and concrete behavior—an experimental study with special tests. *Psychological Monographs*, **329,** 1.
34. Lhermitte, F. & Signoret, J.L. (1969) Analyse d'un apprentissage associatif: résultats obtenus chez 42 aphasiques. *Cortex*, **5,** 415.
35. Reitan, R.M. (1953) Intellectual functions in aphasic and non-aphasic brain-injured subjects. *Neurology*, **3,** 202.
36. Reitan, R.M. (1954) Intelligence and language functions in dysphasic patients. *Diseases of the Nervous System*, **15,** 131.
37. Reitan, R.M. (1955) Certain differential effects of left and right cerebral lesions in human adults. *Journal of Comparative and Physiological Psychology*, **48,** 474.

38. Reitan, R.M. (1955) The relation of the trail making test to organic brain damage. *Journal of Consulting Psychology*, **19,** 393.
39. Reitan, R.M. (1958) Validity of the trail making test as an indicator of organic brain damage. *Perceptual and Motor Skills*, **8,** 271.
40. Reitan, R.M. (1959) Correlations between the trail making test and the Wechsler-Bellevue scale. *Perceptual and Motor Skills*, **9,** 127.
41. Reitan, R.M. (1959) Effects of brain damage on a psychomotor problem solving task. *Perceptual and Motor Skills*, **9,** 211.
42. Reitan, R.M. (1972) Verbal problem solving as related to cerebral damage. *Perceptual and Motor Skills*, **34,** 515.
43. Reitan, R.M. & Reed, H.B.C. (1962) Consistencies in Wechsler-Bellevue mean values in brain-damaged groups. *Perceptual and Motor Skills*, **15,** 119.
44. Reitan, R.M. & Fitzhugh, K.B. (1971) Behavioral deficits in groups with cerebral vascular lesions. *Journal of Consulting and Clinical Psychology*, **37,** 215.
45. Reitan, R.M. & Tarshes, E.L. (1959) Differential effects of lateralized brain lesions on the trail making test. *Journal of Nervous and Mental Diseases*, **129,** 257.
46. Alajouanine, Th. (Ed.) (1960) *Les grandes activités du lobe occipital*. Paris: Masson.
47. Renzi, E. (de) & Vignolo, L.A. (1962) The token test: a sensitive test to detect receptive disturbances in aphasics. *Brain*, **85,** 665.
48. Renzi, E. (de) & Faglioni, P. (1978) Normative data and screening power of a shortened version of the Token Test. *Cortex*, **14,** 41.
49. Albert, M.L. (1972) Certains aspects des troubles de la compréhension auditive du langage. *Langages*, **7,** 37.
50. Poeck, K., Kerschensteiner, M. & Hartje, W.A. (1972) A quantitative study on language understanding in fluent and nonfluent aphasia. *Cortex*, **8,** 299.
51. Poeck, K., Orgass, B., Kerschensteiner, M. & Hartje, W. (1974) A qualitative study on token test performance in aphasic and non-aphasic brain damaged patients. *Neuropsychologia*, **12,** 49.
52. Lhermitte, F. & Ducarne, B. (1965) Plan de l'examen clinique des aphasiques. *Revue pratique* (Paris), **17,** 2365.
53. Dejerine, J. (1926) *Séméiologie des affections du système nerveux*. Paris: Masson.
54. Weisenburg, T.H. & McBride, K.E. (1933) *Aphasia*. New York: Commonwealth Fund.
55. Bastron, J.A. (1957) *Clinical Examination in Neurology*, p. 3. Philadelphia and London: W.B. Saunders.

BIBLIOGRAPHY

Ajuriaguerra, J. (de) & Hécaen, H. (1949) *Le cortex cérébral*. Paris: Masson.

Albert, M.L. (1976) Short-term memory and aphasia. *Brain and Language*, **3,** 28.

Alberoni, F. (1956) Il metodo delle funzioni discriminati alla diagnosi di deterioramento mentale. *Archivio di Psicologia, Neurologia e Psichiatria*, **17,** 1.

Alford, L.B. (1937) Defects of intelligence from focal lesions within the central part of the left cerebral hemisphere. *American Journal of Psychiatry*, **94,** 615.

Andersen, A.L. (1951) The effect of laterality localization of focal brain lesions on the Wechsler-Bellevue subtests. *Journal of Consulting and Clinical Psychologist*, **7,** 149.

Archibald, Y.M., Wepman, J.M. & Jones, L.V. (1967) Nonverbal cognitive performance in aphasic and nonaphasic brain-damaged patients. *Cortex*, **3,** 275.

Archibald, Y.M., Wepman, J.M. & Jones, L.V. (1967) Performance on nonverbal cognitive tests following unilateral cortical injury to the right and left hemisphere. *Journal of Nervous and Mental Diseases*, **45,** 25.

Arrigoni, G. & Renzi, E. (de) (1964) Constructional apraxia and hemispheric locus of lesion. *Cortex*, **1,** 170.

Assal, G., Eisert, H.-G. & Hécaen, H. (1969) Analyse des résultats du test de Farnsworth D15 chez 155 malades atteints de lésions hémisphériques droites ou gauches. *Acta Neurologica Belgica*, **69,** 705.

Balthazar, E.E. (1963) Cerebral unilateralization in chronic epileptic cases: Wechsler object assembly subtest. *Journal of Clinical Psychology*, **19,** 169.

Barbizet, J. & Duizabo, Ph. (1977) *Abrégé de neuropsychologie*. Paris: Masson.

Barnes, G.W. & Lucas, G.J. (1974) Cerebral dysfunction vs psychogenesis in Halstead-Reitan tests. *Journal of Nervous and Mental Diseases*, **158,** 50.

Beauvois, M.F. & Lhermitte, F. (1975) Répétition immédiate et apprentissage d'une série de mots chez 30 sujets aphasiques. *Neuropsychologia*, **13,** 247.

Bender, L. (1938) *A Visual Motor Gestalt Test and Its Clinical Use*. New York: American Orthopsychiatry Association.

Bender, M.B. & Teuber, H.L. (1946) Phenomena of fluctuation, extinction and completion in visual perception. *Archives of Neurology and Psychiatry* (Chicago), **55,** 627.

Benson, D.F. & Denckla, M.B. (1969) Verbal paraphasia as source of calculation disturbance. *Archives of Neurology* (Chicago), **21,** 96.

Benton, A.L. (1967) Problems of test construction in the field of aphasia. *Cortex*, **3,** 32.

Benton, A.L., Elithorn, A., Fogel, M.L. & Kerr, M. (1963) A perceptual maze test sensitive to brain damage. *Journal of Neurosurgery and Psychiatry*, **26,** 540.

Benton, A.L. & Fogel, M.L. (1962) Three-dimensional constructional praxis. *Archives of Neurology* (Chicago), **7,** 347.

Benton, A.L. & Joynt, R.J. (1959) Reaction time in unilateral cerebral disease. *Confinia Neurologica*, **19,** 247.

Berko, J. (1951) Mental evaluation of the aphasic child. *American Journal of Occupational Therapy*, **5,** 241.

Birch, H.G. (1957) Experimental investigations in expressive aphasia. *New York State Journal of Medicine*, **24,** 3849.

Boller, F. (1968) Latent aphasia: right and left 'non aphasic' brain-damaged patients compared. *Cortex*, **14,** 245.

Boller, F. & Vignolo, L.A. (1966) Latent sensory aphasia in hemisphere-damaged patients: an experimental study with the token test. *Brain*, **89,** 815.

Botez, M.I. (1951) Mild forms of aphasia, apraxia and agnosia. *Acta Psychiatrica Scandinavica*, **37,** 111.

Boyd, H.F. (1949) A provisional quantitative scoring with preliminary norms for the Goldstein-Scheerer cube test. *Journal of Clinical Psychology*, **5,** 148.

Brown, I. (1955) Abstract and concrete behavior of dysphasic patients and normal subjects. *Journal of Speech Disorders*, **20,** 35.

Bruell, J.H. & Albee, G.W. (1962) Higher intellectual functions in a patient with hemispherectomy for tumors. *Journal of Consulting and Clinical Psychology*, **26,** 90.

Caramazza, A., Gordon, J., Zurif, E.B. & DeLuca, D. (1976) Right-hemispheric damage and verbal problem solving behavior. *Brain and Language*, **3,** 41.

Chansky, N.M. (1967) Validity of the Benton visual retention test. *Perceptual and Motor Skills*, **24,** 1126.

Costa, L.D. & Vaughan, H.G. (1962) Performance of patients with lateralized cerebral lesions: I. Verbal and perceptual tests. *Journal of Nervous and Mental Diseases*, **134,** 162.

Delacato, C.H. (1957) Hemiplegia and concomitant psychological phenomena. *American Journal of Occupational Therapy*, **10,** 157.

Delay, J., Pichot, P., Dursap, R. & Perse, J. (1950) L'aphasie latente. Son diagnostic dans l'artériosclérose cérébrale au moyen d'un test de vocabulaire. *Revue neurologique*, **83,** 180.

Denny-Brown, D. (1958) The nature of apraxia. *Journal of Nervous and Mental Diseases*, **126,** 9.

Denny-Brown, D. & Banker, B.Q. (1954) Amorphosynthesis from left parietal lesion. *Archives of Neurology, Neurosurgery and Psychiatry* (Chicago), **71,** 302.

Denny-Brown, D., Meyer, J.S. & Horenstein, S. (1952) Significance of perceptual rivalry resulting from parietal lesion. *Brain*, **75,** 433.

Dissez, C., Crouigneau, C., Fenelon, J. & Arne, L. (1970) Examen psychologique d'un aphasique; discussion d'une observation: aphasie de Broca post-traumatique chez l'enfant. *Journal français d' Oto-rhino-laryngologie*, **19,** 195.

Doehring, D.G. & Reitan, R.M. (1960) MMPI performance of aphasic and nonaphasic brain-damaged patients. *Journal of Clinical Psychology*, **16,** 307.

Doehring, D.G. & Reitan, R.M. (1961) Language disorders in brain-damaged patients. *Archives of Neurology* (Chicago), **5,** 294.

Drewe, E.A. (1974) The effect of type and area of brain lesion on Wisconsin card sorting test performance. *Cortex*, **10,** 159.

Ducarne, B. & Pillon, B. (1974) La copie de la figure complexe de Rey dans les troubles visuo-constructifs. *Journal de Psychologie normale et pathologique*, **4,** 449.

Edwards, A.E. & Auger, R. (1965) The effect of aphasia on the perception of precedence. *Proceedings of the 73rd Annual Convention of the American Psychological Association*, 207.

Ferguson, G. (1966) *Statistical Analysis in Psychology and Education*. New York: McGraw-Hill.

Fillenbaum, S. & Jones, L.V. (1962) An application of 'cloze' technique to the study of aphasic speech. *Journal of Abnormal and Social Psychology*, **65,** 183.

Fitzhugh, K.B. & Fitzhugh, L.C. (1964) WAIS results for subjects with longstanding, chronic, lateralized and diffuse cerebral dysfunction. *Perceptual and Motor Skills*, **19,** 735.

Fitzhugh, K.B. & Fitzhugh, L.C. (1965) Effects of early and later onset of cerebral dysfunction upon psychological test performance. *Perceptual and Motor Skills*, **20,** 1099.

Fitzhugh, L.C. & Fitzhugh, K.B. (1964) Relationships between Wechsler-Bellevue from I and WAIS performances of subjects with long-standing cerebral dysfunction. *Perceptual and Motor Skills*, **19,** 539.

Fitzhugh, K.B., Fitzhugh, L.C. & Reitan, R.M. (1956) Effects of 'chronic' and 'current' lateralized and nonlateralized cerebral lesions upon trail making test performances. *Journal of Nervous and Mental Diseases*, **137,** 82.

Fitzhugh, K.B., Fitzhugh, L.C. & Reitan, R.M. (1961) Psychological deficits in relation to acuteness of brain dysfunction. *Journal of Consulting Psychology*, **25,** 61.

Fitzhugh, K.B., Fitzhugh, L.C. & Reitan, R.M. (1962) Wechsler-Bellevue comparisons in groups with 'chronic' and 'current' lateralized and diffuse brain lesions. *Journal of Consulting Psychology*, **26,** 306.

Flowers, C.R. (1975) Proactive interference in short-term recall by aphasic, brain-damaged non aphasic and normal subjects. *Neuropsychologia*, **13,** 59.

Fogel, M.L. (1964) The intelligence quotient as an index of brain damage. *American Journal of Orthopsychiatry*, **34,** 555.

Frances, R., Lhermitte, F. & Verdy, M.F. (1973) Le déficit musical des aphasiques. *Revue internationale de Psychologie appliquée*, **22,** 117.

Giroire, J.M., Fenelon, J. & Arne, L. (1972) Etude de la mémoire chez les aphasiques par l'échelle P.R.M de Rey. *Annales médico-psychologiques*, **1,** 424.

Giroire, J.M., Fenelon, J. & Arne, L. (1972) Etude de la mémoire chez les aphasiques par l'échelle P.R.M. de Rey. *Bordeaux Médicale*, **5,** 103.

Goldstein, H. & Cameron, H. (1959) A new mental mensuration method for the motor and sensory aphasic. *Pennsylvania Medical Journal*, **62,** 1513.

Goldstein, K. & Sheerer, M. (1941) Abstract and concrete behavior—an experimental study with special tests. *Psychological Monographs*, **329,** 1.

Hain, J.D. (1964) The Bender-gestalt test; a scoring method for identifying brain damage. *Journal of Consulting Psychology*, **28,** 34.

Halstead, W.C. *Manual for the Halstead-Wepman Screening Test for Aphasia*. Chicago, IL: University of Chicago Clinics.

Halstead, W.C. (1939) Behavioral effects of lesions of the frontal lobe in man. *Archives of Neurology and Psychiatry* (Chicago), **42,** 780.

Halstead, W.C. (1940) Preliminary analysis of grouping behavior in patients with cerebral injury by the method of equivalent and non equivalent stimuli. *American Journal of Psychiatry*, **96,** 1263.

Hartje, W., Kerschensteiner, M., Poeck, K. & Orgass, B. (1973) A cross-validation study on the token test. *Neuropsychologia*, **11,** 119.

Hartlage, L. (1966) Common psychological tests applied to the assessment of brain damage, *Journal of Projective Techniques*, **30,** 319.

Hays, W.L. (1963) *Statistics for Psychologists*. New York: Holt, Rinehart and Winston.

Hécaen, H. (1960) Les apraxies. *Revue neurologique*, **102,** 541.

Hécaen, H. (1972) *Introduction à la neuropsychologie*. Paris: Larousse.

Hécaen, H. & Assal, G. (1970) A comparison of constructive deficits following right and left hemisphere lesions. *Neuropsychologia*, **8,** 289.

Hécaen, H. & Gimeno Alava, A. (1960) L'apraxie idéomotrice unilaterale gauche. *Revue neurologique*, **102,** 648.

Heilman, J.H. (1975) A tapping test of apraxia. *Cortex*, **11,** 259.

Heilman, K.M., Scholes, R. & Watson, T.R. (1976) Defects of immediate memory in Broca's and conduction aphasia. *Brain and Language*, **3,** 201.

Heimburger, R.F. & Reitan, R.M. (1961) Easily administered written test for lateralizing brain lesions. *Journal of Neurosurgery*, **18,** 301.

Hirschenfang, S. (1960) A comparison of WAIS scores of hemiplegic patients with and without aphasia. *Journal of Clinical Psychology*, **16,** 351.

Hirschenfang, S., Berman, D. & Benton, J.G. (1967) Follow-up study of Bender-Gestalt reproductions by right and left hemiplegic patients. *Perceptual and Motor Skills*, **25,** 339.

Janota, O. (1938) Sur l'apraxie constructive et sur les troubles apparents de l'aperception et de l'expression des rapports spatiaux. *Encéphale*, **2,** 173.

Kinsbourne, M. & Warrington, E.K. (1962) A study of finger agnosia. *Brain*, **85,** 47.

Kinsbourne, M. & Warrington, E.K. (1964) Observations on color agnosia. *Journal of Neurology, Neurosurgery and Psychiatry*, **27,** 296.

Klebanoff, S.G., Singer, J.L. & Welensky, H. (1954) Psychological consequences of brain lesions and ablations. *Psychological Bulletin*, **51,** 1.

Klein, R. (1949) Dynamic factors in aphasia. *Journal of Mental Sciences*, **95,** 874.

Klein, R. & Mayer-Gross, W. (1957) *The Clinical Examination of Patients with Organic Cerebral Disease*. London: Cassel.

Lansdell, H. (1961) The effect of neurosurgery on a test of proverbs. *American Psychology*, **16,** 448.

Leicester, J., Sidman, M., Stoddard, L.T. & Mohr, J.P. (1971) The nature of aphasic responses. *Neuropsychologia*, **9,** 141.

Létourneau, P. (1976) Le rendement au Ottawa-Wechsler dans le cas d'hémiplégie non-traumatique. *Bulletin de l'Institut de Réadaptation de Montréal*, **22,** 4.

Lhermitte, J. (1939) *L'image de notre corps*. Paris: Editions de la nouvelle revue critique.

Luria, A.R. (1964) Neuropsychology in the local diagnosis of brain damage. *Cortex*, **1,** 3.

Marie, P., Bouttier, H. & Bailey, P. (1922) A propos des faits décrits sous le nom d'apraxie idéomotrice. *Revue neurologique*, **29,** 973.

Matthews, C.G., Guertin, W.H. & Reitan, R.M. (1962) Wechsler-Bellevue subtest mean rank orders in diverse diagnostic groups. *Psychological Reports*, **11,** 3.

Matthews, C.G. & Reitan, R.M. (1964) Correlations of Wechsler-Bellevue rank orders of subtest means in lateralized and non-lateralized brain-damaged groups. *Perceptual and Motor Skills*, **19,** 391.

McFie, J. & Zangwill, O.L. (1960) Visual-constructive disabilities associated with lesions of the left cerebral hemisphere. *Brain*, **83,** 243.

Mencher, G.T. (1967) The reliability of electrodermal audiometry with aphasic adults. *Journal of Speech Research*, **10,** 328.

Miller, G.A. (1975) *The Psychology of Communication*. New York: Basic Books.

Miller, M.H. (1960) Audiologic evaluation of aphasic patients. *Journal of Speech Disorders*, **25,** 333.

Orgass, B. & Poeck, K. (1968) Rechts-links-störung oder Aphasie? Eine experimentelle Untersuchung zur diagnostischen Gültigkeit der rechtslinks-Prüfung. *Deutsche Zeitschrift für Nervenheilkunde*, **194,** 261.

Orgass, B. & Poeck, K. (1969) Assessment of aphasia by psychometric methods. *Cortex*, **5,** 317.

Orgass, B., Poeck, K., Hartje, W. & Kerschensteiner, M. (1973) Zum Vorschlag einer Kurzform des Token Tests zur Auslese von Aphasikern. *Nervenarzt*, **44,** 93.

Piercy, M. (1964) The effects of cerebral lesions on intellectual function; a review of current research trends. *British Journal of Psychiatry*, **110,** 310.

Piercy, M.F., Hécaen, H. & Ajuriaguerra, J. (de) (1960) Constructional apraxia associated with unilateral cerebral left and right sided cases compared. *Brain*, **83,** 225.

Poeck, K., Kerschensteiner, M. & Hartje, W.A. (1972) A quantitative study on language understanding in fluent and nonfluent aphasia. *Cortex*, **8,** 299.

Poeck, K. & Orgass, B. (1966) Gerstmann's syndrome and aphasia. *Cortex*, **2,** 421.

Poeck, K., Orgass, B., Kerschensteiner, M. & Hartje, W. (1974) A qualitative study on token test performance in aphasic and non-aphasic brain damaged patients. *Neuropsychologia*, **12,** 49.

Poeck, K. & Stachowiak, F.J. (1975) Farbbenennungsstörungen bei aphasischen und nicht aphasischen Hirnkranken. *International Journal of Neurology*, **209,** 95.

Pommez, J. (1970) Présentation du test logométrique V.V.V.A. (données préliminaires). *Journal français d' Oto-rhino-laryngologia*, **19,** 197.

Porch, B.E. (1966) *Multidimensional Quantification of Ges-*

tural, Verbal and Graphic Responses of Patients with Cerebral Pathology. PhD dissertation, Stanford University.

Prick, J.J.G. & Colon, P.J.A. (1950) Aphasieprobleem na 125 jaren. *Nederlands Tijdschrift voor de Psychologie*, **5,** 369.

Provins, K.A. & Cunliff, P. (1972) The reliability of some performance tests of handedness. *Neuropsychologia*, **10,** 199.

Reed, H.B.C. & Reitan, R.M. (1963) Intelligence test performances of brain damaged subjects with lateralized motor deficits. *Journal of Consulting Psychology*, **27,** 102.

Reitan, R.M. (1974) *Clinical Neuropsychology: Current Status and Application*. New York: Wiley.

Renzi, E. (de) & Faglioni, P. (1965) The comparative efficiency of intelligence and vigilance tests in detecting hemispheric cerebral damage. *Cortex*, **1,** 410.

Renzi, E. (de), Faglioni, P., Scotti, G. & Spinnler, H. (1972) Impairment in associating colour to form, concomitant with aphasia. *Brain*, **95,** 293.

Renzi, E. (de), Pieczuro, A. & Vignolo, L.A. (1968) Ideational apraxia: a quantitative study. *Neuropsychologia*, **6,** 41.

Renzi, E. (de) & Spinnler, H. (1967) Impaired performance on color tasks in patients with hemispheric damage. *Cortex*, **3,** 194.

Rogers, E.J. (1957) Hemiplegia—its incidence and association with aphasia and fractures in a chronic disease hospital. *New York State Journal of Medicine*, **57,** 2220.

Rosenberg, B. (1965) The performance of aphasics on automated visuo-perceptual discrimination, training and transfer tasks. *Journal of Speech Research*, **8,** 165.

Rosenberg, B. & Edwards, A.E. (1964) The performance of aphasics on three automated perceptual discrimination programs. *Journal of Speech Research*, **7,** 295.

Sall, M. & Wepman, J.M. (1945) A screening survey of organic impairment. *Journal of Speech Disorders*, **10,** 283.

Satz, P., Richard, W. & Daniels, A. (1967) The alteration of intellectual performance after lateralized brain-injury in man. *Psychonomic Science*, **7,** 369.

Sauguet, J., Benton, A.L. & Hécaen, H. (1971) Disturbances of the body schema in relation to language impairment and hemispheric locus of lesion. *Journal of Neurology, Neurosurgery and Psychiatry*, **34,** 496.

Schuell, H. (1965) *Differential Diagnosis of Aphasia with the Minnesota Test*. Minneapolis: University of Minnesota Press.

Schuell, H. & Benson, L. (1973) *Card Materials for the Minnesota Test for Differential Diagnosis of Aphasia*. Minneapolis: University of Minnesota Press.

Schuell, H., Jenkins, J.J. & Carroll, J.B. (1963) A factor analysis of the Minnesota test for differential diagnosis of aphasia. *Journal of Speech Disorders*, **5,** 349.

Shapiro, D.Y., Sadowsky, D.A., Henderson, W.G. & Buren, J.M. (van) (1973) An assessment of cognitive function in post-thalamotomy Parkinson patients. *Confinia Neurologica* (Basel), **35,** 144.

Sidman, M. (1971) The behavioral analysis of aphasia. *Journal of Psychiatric Research*, **8,** 413.

Sidman, M., Stoddard, L.T., Mohr, J.P. & Leicester, J. (1971) Behavioral studies of aphasia: methods of investigation and analysis. *Neuropsychologia*, **9,** 119.

Signoret, J.L. (1966) *Etude d'un apprentissage associatif chez 28 sujets présentant une aphasie par lésion cérébrale localisée*. Medical thesis, Paris.

Singer, H.D. & Low, A.A. (1933) Acalculia. *Archives of Neurology and Psychiatry*, **29,** 467.

Smith, A. (1966) Verbal and nonverbal test performances of patients with 'acute' lateralized brain lesions (tumors). *Journal of Nervous and Mental Diseases*, **141,** 517.

Smith, A. (1971) Objective indices of severity of chronic aphasia in stroke patients. *Journal of Speech Disorders*, **36,** 167.

Société Française de Neurologie (1960) Les apraxies—rapports, sous la direction de M.H. Hécaen. In *Revue neurologique*, tome 102, p. 1, XXIVe Réunion neurologique internationale. Paris: Masson.

Speigel, D.K., Jones, L.V. & Wepman, J.M. (1965) Test responses as predictors of free speech characteristics in aphasia patients. *Journal of Speech Research*, **4,** 349.

Stam, C. (1953) The significance of aphasia in otology. *Laryngoscope*, **1,** 44.

Stengel, E. (1944) Loss of spatial orientation, constructional apraxia and Gertsmann's syndrome. *Journal of Mental Sciences*, **90,** 753.

Swisher, L.P. & Sarno, M.T. (1969) Token test scores of three matched patients groups: left brain-damaged with aphasia, right brain-damaged without aphasia, non brain-damaged. *Cortex*, **5,** 264.

Tyler, H.R. (1969) Defective stimulus exploration in aphasic patients. *Neurology*, **19,** 105.

Weigl, E. (1966) On the construction of standard psychological tests in case of brain damage. *Journal of the Neurological Sciences*, **3,** 123.

Weisenburg, T.H. (1934) A study of aphasia. *Archives of Neurology and Psychiatry* (Chicago) **31,** 1.

Weinstein, S. (1964) Deficits concomitant with aphasia or lesions of either hemisphere. *Cortex*, **1,** 154.

Wepman, J.M. (1961) *A Selected Bibliography on Brain Impairment Aphasia and Organic Psychodiagnosis*. Chicago, IL: Language Research Association.

Wepman, J.M. & Jones, L.V. (1961) *Studies in Aphasia: an Approach to Testing*. Chicago, IL: Education-Industry Service.

Wertheim, N. & Botez, M.I. (1961) Receptive amusia: a clinical analysis. *Brain*, **84,** 19.

Wheeler, L. (1963) Predictions of brain damage from an aphasia screening test: an application of discriminant functions and a comparison with a non-linear method of analysis. *Perceptual and Motor Skills*, **17,** 63.

Wheeler, L. (1964) Complex behavioral indices weighted by linear discriminant functions for the prediction of cerebral damage. *Perceptual and Motor Skills*, **19,** 907.

Wheeler, L. & Reitan, R.M. (1962) Presence and laterality of brain damage predicted from responses to a short aphasia screening test. *Perceptual and Motor Skills*, **15,** 783.

Whitaker, H.A. & Noll, J.D. (1972) Some linguistic parameters of the Token Test. *Neuropsychologia*, **10,** 395.

Wiener, G. (1965) Review: differential diagnosis of aphasia with the Minnesota test, by H. Schuell. Minneapolis, MN: University of Minnesota Press. (*Journal of Nervous and Mental Diseases*, **144,** 334, 1967).

Wilson, S.A.K. (1908) A contribution to the study of apraxia with a review of the literature. *Brain*, **31,** 164.

Yates, A.J. (1954) Validity of some psychological tests for brain damage. *Psychological Bulletin*, **51,** 359.

17. Aphasia Therapy*

'Well, then, two years ago I was wounded and I need to continue my work to accustom myself to the French language. I'm getting better and, in the year since I've been working, I've made a lot of progress. So, I work a little in all directions. We have two young ladies who know the French language very well and who give me difficult work. I work once each week and I cotol of this ... of this ... of this work, I write, I talk and I talk to the young ladies who always talk to me. Besides, I don't have any men. I never see any men. I only see women who are very nice, who are very well, who are older or younger but who are very nice to me.'

(*Conversation with Mr Co.; November 1969*)

An overview of aphasiological research carried out during a century or more immediately reveals striking differences in the progress achieved: certain aspects of aphasia have been at least partially clarified while others, which cannot be considered inaccessible, have scarcely been explored. Knowledge has accumulated about the forms of aphasia (see Chapters 3 to 7), the nature and localization of aphasia-producing lesions (see Chapters 8 and 9) and the linguistic characteristics of aphasics' language (see Chapters 2 to 4, and 12), but very little research attention has been focused on aphasia therapy. Indeed, if the advances achieved in medical management have been such that the aetiological treatment of certain diseases which may cause aphasia is now possible, only fragmentary progress has occurred in disciplines which could eventually lead to a theory of aphasia therapy, that is, the psychophysiology of language and the psychophysiopathology of aphasia and its evolution in the presence of a stabilized cerebral lesion. Unexplained or poorly understood phenomena remain so numerous in these areas that students of speech and language pathology generally feel ill at ease when confronted with the uncertain, or even arbitrary, principles governing one of their future professional activities, that of providing therapy to adults with acquired aphasia. The feelings of uneasiness are almost always reinforced by a few years of professional experience which serve to illustrate the seemingly insoluble theoretical problems raised by aphasia and its rehabilitation and to convince beginning therapists of the irreversibility of the aphasic deficits in many patients. On the other hand, experience will also permit therapists to observe the usefulness of their work, as well as its limitations. The demoralizing effects of absolute failures will be balanced by spectacular successes and therapists will become increasingly aware that language recovery, even if quite limited in numerous cases, is seen as a priceless gain by aphasic individuals. The attitudes and comments of patients and their families will demonstrate the great value which they place on aphasia therapy (Insertion 17.1), even in cases where it provides only a linguistic crutch. Thus, for example, patients with softening in the area of the anterior sylvian artery will show that they attach as much importance to the recovery of relative autonomy in speech, which allows partial compensation for the effects of their aphasia, as to the recovery of relative autonomy in movement, which allows partial compensation for their hemiplegia.

Although interest in aphasia therapy dates from the end of the last century[1-3], the provision of therapy to aphasic patients did not become common practice until the last world war[4, 5] and has not yet yielded universally accepted guiding

* Through their contribution to this text, Louise Coderre, Michèle Bergeron and Denise Lafond wish to pay tribute to Mme Blanche de Ribaucourt-Ducarne and to acknowledge the influence of her teaching.

Insertion 17.1

'Et puis alors depuis euh, dix jours à peu près, les↓ les cours de↓ de /ʀee/↓ *de* /ʀee/↓ /ʀe/↓ *oui* /dyka/↓/ʀedydy/↓ /ʀedykas/↓ /ʀedykasjɔ̃/ *ont commencé. Et↓ et voilà. Ca se passe euh, ou↓ pour essayer de↓ Ca dépend de ce qu'on a. Ca dépend si on ne* /susjɛ̃/ *pas↓ si on ne se* /susjɛ̃/ *pas de ce qu'on entend ou de ce qu'on ne dit pas↓ de ce qu'on dit, de ce qu'on ne dit pas plutôt ou de↓ Ca depend si l'on se DIT↓ si l'on se rappelle de↓ de ce que l'on écrit. Et on se sert de↓ de magnétos pour savoir comment les↓ les↓ les mots s'écrivent—en ce qui me concerne du moins, c'est le cas—et puis ensuite pour↓ euh pour se↓ se↓ pour se rappeler euh, comment on↓ on les prononce↓ on les prononce. Et puis euh, ben il faut essayer de↓ de↓ de↓ pas↓ pas de↓ pas de se rappeler le nombre de↓ le plus grand nombre de mots, mais il faut que ça revienne, enfin. Il faut↓ il faut↓ Je pense que c'est un moyen* /kɔ/↓ /kɔ/↓ *commode, utile, pratique, efficace, c'est ça surtout pour mettre, non seulement les mots mais le↓ le mécanisme, le remettre en↓ en* /ʒ/↓ *en↓ en* /mumɑ̃/↓ *en mouvement. Et puis alors il faut* /li/↓ *LIVRE aussi des↓ des textes en essayant de↓ de dire les syllabes et puis aussi quelque-fois se↓ finir↓ euh, au début surtout se↓ se demander ce que ça veut dire, le PROBLÈME↓ le text. C'est pas tellement évident; pour essayer de↓ pour faire un↓ une* /sɛ̃sɛ/↓ *une synthèse de ce qui a été↓ de ce qui est dit, c'est quelquefois difficile, pour se↓ pour se↓ pour euh↓ Une↓ une phrase, c'est déjà pas mal, et quand il y en a plusieurs, quelquefois ça↓ ça fait un tout qui ne veut pas dire grand-chose, surtout au DÉPART↓ au↓ au début. Six heures par jour au moins. C'est une bonne chose parce que, comme ça, on ne se↓ on ne s'ennuie pas mais enfin! Sur le* /mɔ/↓ *pour le moral, c'est une bonne chose, c'est une↓ main enfin c'est↓ Non puis oui, c'est quand même↓ c'est↓ c'est quand même extrêmement intéressant, je dois en le dire. Ah! puis en plus de ça c'est↓ c'est necessaire. Mais enfin c'est↓ c'est passionnant.'*

'And so then about uh, ten days ago, the↓ programme of↓ of /ʀee/↓ of /ʀee/↓ /ʀe/↓ yes /dyka/↓ /ʀedydy/↓ /ʀedykas/↓ /ʀedykasjɔ̃/ began. And↓ there you are. That takes place uh, or↓ in order to try to↓ That depends on what one has. That depends if one doesn't /susjɛ̃/↓ if one doesn't /susjɛ̃/ what one hears or what one doesn't say↓ what one says, what one doesn't say rather or on↓ That depends if one SAYS↓ if one remembers what↓ what one writes. And one uses some↓ some tape recorders to know how the↓ the↓ the words are written—in what concerns me at least, that's the case—and then after in order to↓ uh in order to↓ to↓ in order to remember uh, how one↓ one↓ pronounces them↓ one pronounces them. And then uh, well you must try to↓ to↓ to↓ not↓ not to↓ not to remember the number of↓ the largest number of words, but it's necessary that that returns, finally. It must↓ it must↓ I think that it's a /kɔ/↓ /kɔ/↓ convenient, useful, practical, effective way, it's that especially to put, not only the words but the↓ the mechanism, to put it back in↓ in↓ /ʒ/↓ in↓ in /mumɑ̃/↓ in movement. And so then you must /li/↓ BOOK also some↓ some texts in trying to↓ to say the syllables and then also sometimes to finish↓ oneself↓ uh, at the beginning especially↓ to ask oneself what that means, the PROBLEM↓ the text. It's not very obvious; to try to↓ to make an↓ a /sɛ̃sɛ/ a synthesis of what was↓ of what is said, it's sometimes difficult, to↓ to↓ to uh↓ A↓ a sentence, it's not bad already, and when there are several of them, sometimes that↓ that makes a whole which doesn't mean very much, especially at the DEPART↓ at the↓ at the start. Six hours a day at least. It's a good thing because, like that, one isn't↓ one isn't bored but still! For the /mɔ/↓ for the morale, it's a good thing, it's a↓ but finally it's↓ No then if, all the same it's↓ it's↓ it's extremely interesting all the same, I must certainly say. Ah! then in addition to that it's↓ it's necessary. But finally, it's↓ it's fascinating.'

(*Conversation with Mr Spo.; March 1969*)

principles. In some centres, the approach is essentially psychotherapeutic, while in others it is a global form of language stimulation which excludes or de-emphasizes remedial methods aimed at specific aphasic behaviours. In still others, therapists follow our own approach (which will be subsequently described) in using procedures derived from empirical observations of aphasic symptomatology and the structures of normal language. Despite differing approaches to therapy, there is general agreement that constant attention must be given to patients' global personality as determined by their genetic, cultural, and social background and as modified by their state of health. In this regard, supportive psychotherapy may be useful in many cases, particularly when patients' reactions to their linguistic handicap are so negative that it constitutes a significant obstacle to speech and language therapy.

The present chapter is primarily based on empirical considerations. Lacking the direction of a clearly formulated theory of aphasia therapy, our approach can be only pragmatic. We shall first discuss certain general aspects of therapy and indicate the benefits which can be derived from appropriate modifications of audiovisual methods of foreign-language teaching and of teaching programmes which were not originally intended for aphasics. We shall next introduce the concept of pre-language therapy involving procedures which precede formal language retraining and are appropriate in some cases. We shall then consider different aspects of aphasia therapy under different symptomatological headings. Finally, we shall conclude with a brief outline of problems associated with the termination of therapy and the patient's social and professional reintegration.

GENERAL ASPECTS OF APHASIA THERAPY

A limited number of studies on the effects of aphasia therapy have been published during the last 20 years. With only a few exceptions, they were carried out on poorly defined populations and were much too limited by the criteria for subject selection (it is extremely difficult to find 'comparable' aphasic subjects). In some cases, the nature of the training exercises was so limited that they are hardly representative of aphasia therapy (a finding that three intensively trained global aphasics name six common objects more accurately than untrained controls contributes to the physiopathology of aphasia but scarcely demonstrates the utility of aphasia therapy[6]). However, the recent studies of the Milan group[7-9] provide what may represent the closest possible approximation to a scientific demonstration of partial, but functional, language recovery as a result of therapy given to adult aphasics. If one hesitates, for methodological reasons, to accept the results of previous studies completely, the utility of aphasia therapy can be evaluated according to criteria other than the scientific method. Excluding those who approach the question with rigid and negative preconceptions, clinicians who provide aphasia therapy or observe it being carried out are usually convinced by their observations, in spite of their anecdotal nature, of the benefits which many patients derive from aphasia therapy. This being recognized, either with or without major reservations, it remains to determine which modes of language (or psychological) therapy appear to be the most useful, considering what is known about linguistic functioning in normal speakers and in aphasics.

THE FOUNDATIONS OF APHASIA THERAPY

Aphasia therapy is founded, at least in our view, on a complete study of the patient and of his or her disease. Such a study obviously involves a multidisciplinary approach:

1. Before beginning therapy, the patient is examined by various specialists, including a neurologist, a psychologist, a speech pathologist and, possibly, a linguist. Their assessment procedures were described in other chapters of this text (3 to 7, 12, 15 and 16) and will not be discussed here.
2. The role of the social worker varies in different countries. For example, in Quebec it is the social worker who, in the larger and more organized centres, obtains and records information on the aphasic's personal, family and social background. It is often the social worker who can best interact with the patient's family and provide necessary information about aphasia therapy, the results which may be expected, the role which the family may play and the attitude which they should adopt towards the aphasic member of their family. When well conducted, this intervention will frequently reduce anxiety, lead to easier acceptance of the behavioural changes associated with aphasia and prevent the creation of unfavourable therapy context. Since they lead to an awareness of premorbid socio-familial dynamics, the results of this inquiry will also help the therapist to understand the reaction of patients and their family to the

Insertion 17.2

'Practical use defines language which functions to facilitate ongoing action, above all action carried out in collective conditions of collaboration or of rivalry ... What essentially characterizes the practical use of language, what fundamentally distinguishes it from representational use is the importance of what is given by the situation, the importance of what is supposedly known by all. It is not a question here of narrating, of exposing or of explaining, but a question of quickly adapting the action of each one to the circumstances which are perceived by all ... Practical language is eminently elliptical and, in this elliptical language, one sees imperatives without specification of the object ... indications of objects without specification of what should be done with them ... circumstantial indications without mention of the objects, the subjects and the actions ... The meaning is ensured by the situation.' [From Ombredane[41].]

aphasic handicap and facilitate the selection of long-term therapy goals. A family interview will also permit judgement about the possible participation of family members in language retraining (cf. p. 409) and provide information on the ideomatic characteristics of the patient's social environment (predominant type of verbal interaction; structural variations; usual topics of conversation) which must be considered when planning a therapy programme (which will initially focus on recovery of the most common premorbid linguistic behaviours).

3. The occupational and physical therapists can often be led to assume a useful role in increasing a patient's readiness for language therapy, especially in the case of certain motor aphasics (cf. p. 412).
4. Although aphasia therapy is influenced by a certain empiricism, which generally increases with the therapist's experience, it is also strongly guided by theoretical and clinical findings from several disciplines:
   (a) The psychology of language: the speech pathologist must recognize and elicit the major uses of language (*affective use, pragmatic or practical use, referential or representational use*). The context in which the clinician works may lead to an over-emphasis on referential language. If this becomes an obstacle to progress, the therapist must rely on imagination to create situations which elicit linguistic expressions of affect or, even better, pragmatic linguistic behaviours (Insertion 17.2). In some cases, the latter best lend themselves to facilitating techniques and particularly favour the generalization of acquired behaviours.
   (b) The psychology of learning helps the therapist to identify ways to establish an effective working relationship with the patient and also provides guiding principles for the organization of relearning experiences.
   (c) Linguistics and neurolinguistics guide the therapist in the choice and progressive sequencing of linguistic materials used in therapy activities (cf. pp. 408 and 420).
   (d) Pedagogical methodology includes various approaches to foreign-language teaching which may be useful to the therapist when preparing therapy exercises (cf. p. 411).

SELECTING CANDIDATES FOR THERAPY

No matter how great the therapist's enthusiasm and desire to help as many patients as possible, he/she* must confront the issue of selecting suitable candidates for aphasia therapy. This question is partially related to the patient's medical prognosis, which, if good, is a favourable indicator for therapy. This prognosis is established on the basis of aetiological, clinical and anatomical considerations focused on the identification

* For purposes of clarity, the clinician will henceforth in this chapter be designated only by the pronoun 'she', in contrast to the patient who will be referred to using the masculine pronoun.

of the nature and extent of the lesions causing aphasia and, when appropriate, the disturbances associated with it (see Chapters 4, 8 and 9). Thus a patient whose aphasia is related to the presence of an inoperable glioblastoma would obviously be a poor therapy candidate while another, whose aphasia results from focalized softening, may, especially if he is young, benefit greatly from therapy. Other variables, which are more difficult to appreciate, must also be considered. The time since onset of the cerebral lesion is important when considering whether the aphasic deficits are probably transitory or permanent. Their severity, not at onset but after the acute stage, must also be considered, for severity is of even greater importance than the clinical form of aphasia when establishing a prognosis. The patient's age[10, 11] (Fig. 11-2), his handedness and that of his relations[11, 12], his personality, language background, interests and employment history influence language recovery to various degrees. The patient's ability to adapt to his handicap, his motivation to provide the effort required during language therapy, and the support he receives to this end from his entourage are all extremely important. The patient's premorbid intellectual level and whether or not the aphasia is accompanied by 'intellectual deterioration' must obviously be considered (see Chapter 16).

As a general rule, global aphasics derive few benefits from aphasia therapy. The gains observed with training—increased comprehension of spoken language, improvement of copying and sometimes of repetition—may also occur, to a similar degree, in patients who do not receive therapy. In Wernicke's aphasia proper, a significant component of auditory agnosia or the presence of repetitive, undifferentiated jargon are unfavourable indicators for recovery. On the other hand, partial, spontaneous improvement in auditory comprehension and reduction of anosognosia are favourable signs. Wernicke's aphasia with predominant impairment of written language almost always merits an early attempt at therapy, especially when the aphasia is of vascular origin and the patient is relatively well educated. The same is true for cases of pure word blindness. Even in patients whose clinical picture is unrelated to degenerative aetiology, a Wernicke's aphasia with preserved repetition has, in our experience, a rather poor prognosis for recovery when comprehension is severely disturbed. On the other hand, patients presenting nearly pure conduction aphasia are usually good therapy candidates. This is also true for those presenting the phonetic disintegration syndrome, even when severe, provided that the other signs of aphasia are relatively mild (see Chapters 3 and 4).

With the exception of those cases where therapy is clearly indicated or clearly contra-indicated, it is usually advisable to provide therapy on a trial basis. An assessment is then carried out in the initial session, with consideration, when indicated, for the tension which may be generated by the patient's first encounter with the therapist and the effect this may have on his performance. A second assessment is generally carried out after one or two months of intensive therapy. Comparison of results obtained from the two evaluations will indicate whether improvement has occurred and permit the team responsible for the patient to reach a decision to continue or to terminate therapy. In the latter case, a further assessment may be recommended for some months later in order to monitor evolution in the absence of therapy. Should indications of some spontaneous recovery be later observed, therapy may be resumed.

Opinions differ concerning the best moment to begin therapy, mostly because it is frequently impossible to distinguish between its effects and those of spontaneous recovery. We believe that the effects of one usually add to those of the other and that the questions surrounding this issue do not prevent the formulation of some guiding principles about beginning therapy. It is almost never advisable to begin during the acute stage of disease: the patient's general state and need for medical treatment generally preclude therapy in any case. Moreover, during the acute stage, certain Wernicke's aphasics are in a state of excitation which is incompatible with the start of systematic therapy. The therapist can nevertheless visit her future patient and establish initial contact through attempts at dialogue but this involves only global language stimulation revolving around points of immediate personal interest to the patient. In our opinion, it is not worth while to prolong this type of intervention beyond the time when the pathology is under medical control and the patient's general state will permit a detailed assessment of his aphasia and the beginning of a therapy programme. This moment may arrive some days, weeks, or even months after the onset of aphasia.

We consider the frequency of therapy sessions

to be of prime importance. Our observations suggest that progress is greater and more durable when successive therapy sessions are separated by only short intervals. With the exception of those patients who would be overly fatigued by such a schedule, we therefore recommend daily or twice-daily sessions during the initial stage of therapy. These sessions, which are carried out by the therapist and involve her active participation, should ideally be supplemented by exercises which the patient may work on alone or with the help of a family member or an acquaintance. The therapist's role includes judgement of the appropriate time to reduce the frequency of therapy sessions, something which will generally be carried out in a gradual fashion.

The termination of therapy often creates a dilemma. Theoretically, this decision is taken when the patient's language performance has reached a plateau. However, it is difficult to affirm, solely on the basis of a formal language assessment, that a given patient has, or has not, reached such a plateau. Opinions on the patient's progress expressed by family members or others with whom he has contact can provide information which should be suitably weighed. Taylor-Sarno[13] recommends the use of a systematic questionnaire to elicit judgements on the patient's progress from family members. It may also be useful to have the language assessment carried out by someone other than the patient's therapist. Whenever possible, the patient's case should be discussed with his physician, the psychologist and the social worker. They may contribute new perspectives, which although not directly related to language performance, may nevertheless provide guidance when reaching a decision concerning the possible termination of therapy. In this regard, a programme of aphasia therapy will rarely need to be prolonged over a period of more than two to three years.

LEARNING CHARACTERISTICS OF APHASIC ADULTS

Although the question of the relationships between aphasia and intelligence will not be considered here (see Chapters 16 and 19), we shall nevertheless discuss certain learning characteristics of aphasic adults which are relevant to therapy programming. It has been shown[14, 15], generally in regard to both verbal and non-verbal activities, that the majority of aphasics are slow to learn and require more practice than normal to reach predetermined criteria; that their learning curves are often irregular (variability of performance); and that they typically make more errors than normal subjects—errors which usually reflect a greater or lesser tendency to perseverate. However, aphasic patients frequently show improvements with practice and, on certain tasks, demonstrate transfer of learning and generalization of acquired knowledge. Learning by aphasic subjects is not limited to simple memorization but often involves the use of facilitating strategies. They tend, however, to be less diversified and less effective than those of normal subjects in the same learning situations. In a study of operant conditioning, Brookshire[16] showed that the majority of aphasic subjects were sensitive to short delays introduced between responses and consequent events. Other findings suggest that learning of relatively easy items may be hindered when preceded by failures on more difficult items[17].

The learning characteristics of aphasic patients may vary with the site of their cerebral lesions and, therefore, with the clinical form of aphasia which they present (see Chapters 4 and 8-3). Using a simple non-verbal learning task, one of us (F.L.) and Signoret[18, 19] showed that certain learning approaches of aphasics with purely frontal or purely temporal lesions were similar to those of normal subjects. However, organizational activities which subtend learning processes were grossly disturbed when the lesion involved the left parietal region in addition to frontal or temporal structures.

PROCEDURAL ASPECTS OF APHASIA THERAPY

Before presenting details of various therapy procedures, we shall discuss some general principles guiding their development and application. These principles are concerned with the therapy environment, the selection of therapy materials and the ways in which they are presented during therapy[20]. These principles are all related to the fact that aphasia therapy, even when viewed as a learning situation, is aimed at the resurgence of past knowledge and not at the acquisition of new knowledge.

The therapy context

Our personal experience has repeatedly illustrated the need for attention to the therapy context in order to avoid the inadvertent establishment of a schoolroom atmosphere characterized by a teacher–student type of relationship, rigidity, formalism and neutral linguistic exchanges. Such a context is not conducive to the patient's progress, especially at the start of therapy. Consequently, the therapist should strive to create a context aimed as far as possible towards the reproduction of natural language situations. This can be partially accomplished by ensuring that the therapy room does not have the sterile appearance of a laboratory and also by adopting an accepting, supporting, and dynamic attitude towards the patient. Even though the patient's aphasia may render verbal communication very difficult, the therapist will often find it beneficial to devote some time to the establishment of a mutually comfortable linguistic relationship. Aphasic patients generally appreciate discussion of topics related to their personal interests such as family, work, etc. Although they usually respond poorly to irony, patients are frequently grateful to the therapist who does not avoid the appropriate use of humour.

Aphasic individuals are generally very susceptible to the effects of fatigue (functional exhaustion of the neuro-axonal networks underlying the varied aspects of linguistic functioning); its presence can usually be detected by the appearance of perseverative behaviours. The insertion of an appropriate number of pauses into each therapy session is generally effective in avoiding fatigue and, furthermore, can prevent the occurrence of catastrophic reactions. Such reactions must be avoided at all costs because they may have a very negative effect on therapy, sometimes even including a total inhibition of learning. The therapy should be carried out in a manner such that the patient produces the greatest number of adequate responses: the use of positive verbal reinforcement can be very useful in this regard. Although some failures are inevitable during therapy, each session should usually conclude on a positive note, that is, with a task which the patient can complete successfully[21]. Even when the therapist knows that successful performance does not represent genuine progress, it can prevent feelings of self-disparagement resulting from repeated failures.

Selection of materials

The selection of linguistic materials to be used in therapy is based on criteria derived from knowledge of descriptive linguistics and psycholinguistics. Several variables are considered, including the length and phonological and syntactical complexity of the linguistic units, their frequency of usage in the linguistic community and the level of language which they would normally elicit. The stimuli presented in therapy generally follow a progression from shorter to longer, from simpler to more complex, from higher to lower frequency of usage, and from affective and pragmatic use to referential use.

The linguistic units used in therapy must also be selected with regard to their picturability[22] and, for certain exercises, it may be necessary to choose linguistic materials which are particularly concrete. However, the therapist should exercise caution in regard to an exaggeration of this dimension. While a certain concreteness, or what Goldstein[23] described as the loss of the categorical attitude (see Insertion 10.2), is spontaneously shown in the behaviour of most aphasics, it is also possible that certain therapy practices may contribute to its increase[20].

Aphasia therapy typically involves the use of a wide array of objects, drawings, pictures and photographs which provide support for the language exercises. Control of the visual quality of the stimuli is important, especially since aphasic patients may frequently have an associated right hemianopsia or quadranopsia. Control of physical stimulus properties is also essential in the case of written passages or lists of words, expressions or sentences which are to be used in therapy. In addition to being highly legible, the content of the written stimuli should be adapted to the patient's needs. When selecting stimuli for written language exercises, the therapist may find useful ideas in certain school books; they must, however, be used with care. Aphasics frequently experience feelings of reduced self-worth, feelings which should not be reinforced through the use of materials which are obviously intended for children.

Stimulus presentation

The therapist may use various procedures in attempts to elicit predetermined linguistic behaviours. For example, to facilitate the production of words which cannot be evoked during a naming exercise, the therapist may resort to the provision of the initial sound (phonemic cueing) (see Chapter 4), a sentence completion cue, or presentation of the response in written form, etc. During other types of exercises, stimulus repetition, prosodic modification of the stimulus or other facilitating procedures may be employed. The observation that a particular mode of facilitation is usually effective for a particular patient (i.e., it generally permits adequate stimulation) can provide direction for the first stages of his therapy programme, since the most intact mode of stimulation will be the first one used in therapy[21]. However, the therapist must gradually reduce the use of facilitating techniques and attempt to foster the patient's use of increasingly voluntary language.

The stimuli for a therapy session should be selected in advance and, as a general rule, be relatively numerous and diversified. Attempting to achieve extremely stable responses to a small number of stimuli is often a valid procedure in teaching situations but is not recommended during aphasia therapy as it may often be too discouraging for the patient. It is better to work on exercises involving several items from the same inventory and, when the patient's performance is too unstable, to review some or all of the items in a later session. The rate of stimulus presentation should be studied for each patient and be accelerated as progress occurs. The study of stimulus presentation rate is guided, like the insertion of pauses into the therapy session (cf. above) and for the same reasons, by the observation of perseverative phenomena. In many aphasics, perseverative behaviours increase in frequency with increasing similarity among the stimuli (in terms of their form and meaning). Thus we recommend the initial use of stimuli which are dissimilar in both form and meaning and a later, gradual, transition to stimuli drawn from the same field of forms or of meanings (see Chapter 2).

THE ROLE OF THE FAMILY

We shall here discuss the direct role in therapy which may be assumed by the aphasic's family, a role involving supervision of exercises to be carried out by the patient. Participation of a family member is often necessary because the limited availability of speech pathology services in many centres (at least in certain countries) does not permit therapy sessions to be provided with adequate frequency. When properly guided, the participation of a family member can compensate for the inadequate number of sessions which can be provided by professional therapists. An additional, and perhaps major, advantage is the enhanced opportunity for the transfer of acquired gains into more natural language situations. It is nevertheless essential that the relative or friend who will assist the therapist meet two requirements. First, he must have a very clear idea of the exercise procedures, something which he may gain through observation of sessions carried out by the therapist and explanations which she will provide concerning the nature and goal of each exercise. Second, the relationship between the family member or friend and the aphasic patient must be devoid of significant tensions. If the exercises to be carried out at home become a source of excessive pressure on the patient, they will have no beneficial effects and may even compromise the benefits derived from sessions carried out by the therapist. In cases where these two essential requirements cannot be met, it is probably best to forgo family participation in therapy or to reduce their direct intervention to a minimum and, whenever possible, to rely on the help of an outside tutor.

PROGRAMMED INSTRUCTION IN APHASIA THERAPY

Work in psychology by Skinner[24-26] and later Holland[27] led to the identification of the principles of *operant conditioning*. The subsequent application of these principles to various educational programmes gave birth to *sequential* or *programmed instruction*. During the last 20 years, the adaptation of this form of teaching to aphasia therapy has been the subject of experimental investigation[16, 28, 29] and the results of certain studies appear quite promising.

Beginning with the principle that behaviour is the result of the interaction between an organism and its environment, and knowledge that it is possible to analyse behaviour (responses), its consequences (reinforcement or punishment) and its antecedents (discriminative stimuli), investigators developed a teaching method in which the behaviours to be acquired are organized in a hierarchical sequence involving numerous stages and substeps. The subject's responses are continually controlled by the presentation of appropriate stimuli and reinforcement so that he is gradually led, through successive approximations, to the acquisition of preselected terminal behaviours. Use of programmed instruction, as outlined above, requires (1) the specification of all responses to be elicited from the subject and of all behavioural elements considered to represent sub-stages in the acquisition of the terminal behaviours, that is, a detailed analysis of terminal behaviours and of their prerequisites; (2) the specification of all stimuli and their order of presentation in small, graduated steps, from the simplest to the most complex, so that each step provides the basis for further learning; and (3) the specification of reinforcement contingencies and their mode of application. Most instructional programmes rely on modelling and imitation to guide the subject and some include stages specifically intended to increase response generalization and the eventual transfer of acquired responses into the subject's usual environment.

The importance of selecting appropriate reinforcers has received much emphasis in programmed instruction. While not denying that this choice may significantly influence the course of learning, especially in children, we believe that it seldom constitutes a major problem in therapy for adult aphasics. Knowledge of correct responses conveyed by verbal approval, a nod or smile from the therapist or, even better, by marked improvement in the patient's performance, often constitutes adequate positive reinforcement. On the other hand, the specification and ordering of the stimuli raises greater difficulties, since there are various descriptive models of language, each of which could provide a basis for the selection and hierarchical ordering of stimuli at each of the different levels: phonetic, phonological, morphological, syntactical and semantic.

Previous research on the use of programmed instruction with aphasic subjects, including that of Doehring, Dudley and Coderre[30, 31], has shown that it may permit global aphasics to acquire certain elementary behaviours related to visual perception. In addition, it may result in notable improvement in several types of linguistic performance (however, it has not yet been demonstrated, particularly in cases of severe aphasia, that the results of programmed instruction are generally superior to those obtained through the application of more traditional methods). Finally, the most impressive results of programmed instruction obtained to date appear to be those which resulted from the development of rigorous instructional programmes specifically tailored to the needs of individual patients.

Programmed instruction, whether or not dispensed with the help of a *teaching machine* (instruments which are sometimes convenient but frequently too rigid or cumbersome) has thus provided some proof of its merits in the domain of aphasia therapy. The rigour required in the development of instructional programmes appears especially propitious for individualized therapy. On the other hand, the rigour required in its development is also a particular source of difficulty in the objective evaluation of its effects on a population as unstable and heterogeneous as that of aphasics.

The information presented above on programmed instruction and its application to aphasia therapy suggests two major conclusions. On the one hand, research findings have not yet demonstrated that the application of methods other than programmed instruction is unjustified. Even if this point was eventually reached and widespread generalization of programmed instruction would be desirable, there are obvious reasons why this could only take place gradually. On the other hand, therapists who at present use more traditional methods already have information on programmed instruction for aphasics at their disposal, information which can lead to particularly useful reflection concerning the orientation of their work. Most speech pathologists are now aware of the great importance of the hierarchical ordering, in terms of complexity, of the behaviours to be recovered and of the stimuli which will be employed to this end. They are also aware—although sometimes in a confused fashion—that their conveyed attitudes or their smallest gestures may constitute a form of reinforcement or punishment and must, therefore, be judiciously controlled and, especially, predefined. With regard to this last point, it should be noted that marked inconsistency in the therapist's attitude towards her patient's successes and failures may constitute an unrecognized hindrance to his progress in therapy.

USE OF AUDIOVISUAL METHODS IN APHASIA THERAPY

Aphasia therapy should not focus on recovery, achieved through intensive cramming, of a lexicon almost devoid of relational terms. By itself, a restricted ability (i.e., non-generalized) to name a certain number of pictures is of no particular advantage in daily conversational exchanges. Although recovery of words designating objects and actions, and later of the ability to use these words in natural verbal exchanges, is of major importance, recovery of other linguistic units which are frequently used in the linguistic community is also essential. Aphasia therapy should be aimed, whenever possible, towards the production of habitually-well-structured syntagms and not towards agrammatical listings. Consequently, the use of pictured contexts illustrating the commonest syntactic structures of the patient's language is of major importance in aphasia therapy. When selecting appropriate visual illustrations, the therapist will find several advantages in the use of audiovisual methods originally intended for foreign language teaching. Having clinically studied certain of the numerous and varied programmes currently available for French-language teaching, we shall briefly describe those programmes which we have found particularly useful with aphasic populations. (We do so on the assumption that similar types of English-language programmes could be beneficially employed with English-speaking aphasics.)

The three French-language programmes which we consider the most functional are called *Voix et Images de France*[32], *De Vive Voix*[33] and *Dialogue Canada*[34-36]. They were developed by teams composed of linguists, phoneticians, psychologists and educators and are intended to promote the acquisition of the vocabulary of daily life as well as the manipulation of the most commonly-used grammatical structures. Language is developed through situations which are clearly illustrated by pictures, and the audiovisual materials are presented chiefly as instruments for dialogue. The teaching materials consist of picture sequences, presented in a book or on film strips, which can be paired with tape-recorded linguistic stimuli. These varied, lively and ordered pedagogic kits also include other materials (texts, slides, etc.).

Methods of foreign-language teaching intended for strangers wishing to acquire another language obviously require some procedural modifications for use with aphasics, modifications which will be dictated by a systematic evaluation of each patient's symptomatology and cultural background. The foreign-language teaching programmes move too rapidly for many aphasics but their usual progression can be slowed, within a given lesson, by inserting a greater number of sentences illustrating the same structure and/or by increasing the number of lexical variations. We have found that these measures are usually effective in increasing generalization of acquired gains. Although some difficulties with form or content may be encountered with regard to the regional linguistic particularities of individual aphasics, we have not found them to be a major obstacle. Our experience in using audiovisual methods from France (*Voix et Images de France*, *De Vive Voix*) with Francophone aphasics in Quebec has shown that any needed modifications can usually be easily introduced. If particular difficulties are encountered in this regard, the therapist may elect to use a method (e.g., *Le Français International*[37]) which specifically focuses on the linguistic features common to the various communities which share the same language.

Finally, our experience has frequently illustrated the utility of the successive use of different audiovisual methods. With certain patients, we begin therapy using the *Méthod Audiovisuelle de Français*[38]. Although its basis is similar to that of *Voix et Images de France*, the former begins with illustrations of more global situations which are more easily perceived and verbally described. After improvement has occurred with use of this somewhat simpler programme, the therapist will usually find it advantageous to progress to other methods (e.g., *Dialogue Canada*, *Voix et Images de France* or *De Vive Voix*).

Other audiovisual equipment or materials are valuable aids in aphasia therapy. Useful items include tape-recorders, particularly the easy-to-handle cassette models, which permit recording and playback of the patient's responses; collections of photographs, slides, film strips and certain film loops such as those prepared by the National Film Board of Canada to illustrate particular nominal inventories and the corresponding categories of action verbs; the *Language Master* (Bell and Howell, Chicago), which permits the combined presentation of spoken and written language stimuli and their corresponding pictures, as well as the recording and playback of the patient's responses; and finally, certain types of programmable equipment. With the help of these accessories, the therapist can plan a therapy programme which is focused as closely as possible on the individual problems of each patient and also includes a supplement to the therapy sessions which she personally conducts.

PRE-LANGUAGE THERAPY

Pre-language therapy[21] consists of series of empirically selected exercises which are presented with the aim of minimizing the clinical manifestations of various neuropsychological disturbances which are frequently associated with aphasia (see Chapters 4 and 16). Pre-language therapy is thus intended to prepare the patient to derive the maximum possible benefit from subsequent language retraining. As indicated by its name, pre-language therapy generally begins before language retraining, although the later stages of the former may sometimes be carried out concurrently with the initial stages of the latter. Pre-language therapy is primarily focused on the remediation of attentional disturbances, problems of spatial and temporal orientation, of memory, or of calculation, as well as on paretic and/or dyspraxic deficits which may constitute obstacles to the retraining of spoken or written language.

In ideal situations, responsibility for the provision of pre-language therapy is shared between the occupational therapist and the speech pathologist, but when this is not possible the latter must assume full responsibility. In some cases, the therapist must begin with repeated instructions, conveyed both linguistically and through gestured demonstrations, in order to focus and maintain the patient's attention to a particular activity; in so doing, she will progressively encourage the patient's attention to her spoken interventions. In this regard, we have found various activities, including dominoes, card games, chequers, chess, classification tasks, picture completion tasks, etc., to be useful for many patients, and particularly for certain Wernicke's aphasics (see Chapter 4) whose logorrhoea should be stemmed and attention focused on the external world before beginning language therapy proper. Different methods, whose effectiveness varies with particular patients, can be used in therapy for associated disturbances affecting memory, orientation and calculation. The speech pathologist will usually integrate exercises aimed at the remediation of these deficits into the earlier stages of language retraining. Several types of occupational therapy activities are useful in pre-language therapy for cases in which aphasia is associated with constructional apraxia or an element of visual agnosia, for example, form board games, two- and three-dimensional puzzles and copying exercises (simple drawings and geometric figures). Miming exercises, first requiring imitation and then responses to verbal commands, may lessen the effects of an ideomotor or ideational apraxia. Colouring exercises or the matching of objects with appropriate colours may be used with patients presenting an associated disturbance of colour recognition. Clearly, the results obtained from the use of these different exercises will vary among patients.

In cases of pure (or nearly pure) anarthria or Broca's aphasia (see Chapters 3 and 4), it is generally the speech pathologist who assumes responsibility for the development of a pre-language therapy programme for buccofacial apraxia, i.e., a programme of preparatory exercises for phonetic-level therapy. Such exercises are aimed at control of respiratory amplitude and steadiness, control of intra-oral pressure and imitation, then performance, on command, of various movements of the speech organs[21]. In many patients, generally those with a Broca's aphasia, preparatory exercises for written language therapy are also indicated and are intended to counter the effects of a residual hemiplegia affecting the dominant hand or to increase control of the non-dominant hand when it is the one which must be used for writing. Useful exercises include the copying of progressively smaller, simple forms and of forms corresponding to graphic features (see Chapter 2), as well as the copying of numbers, letters and words from a model or on a dotted outline. Since these types of activities are typically carried out by patients whose aphasia is of recent onset, the words to be copied should usually represent basic concrete concepts which can be easily associated with pictures or with simple actions. We shall further discuss these preparatory exercises for therapy centred on articulatory and graphic disturbances in subsequent sections of this chapter.

THERAPY FOR LINGUISTIC REDUCTION AND FOR JARGON

The common forms of Broca's aphasia and of Wernicke's aphasia were described in a preceding section of this text (see Chapter 4). In Broca's aphasia, linguistic production is typically poor and very meagre: there is a *reduction* of language which is sometimes accompanied by a *lack of verbal incentive*. In Wernicke's aphasia, linguistic production is typically copious but, to use Baillarger's[39] expression, perverted: there is *jargon* and, in prototypical cases during the initial stages of evolution, *logorrhoea*. It is mainly through contrasting these two types of symptomatology that the two major classes of aphasia can be clinically identified[40]. Under the present heading, we shall discuss aspects of aphasia therapy which are directly related to the reduction and/or aspontaneity of the frontal aphasics on the one hand and, on the other, aspects of therapy related to the logorrhoea of certain temporoparietal aphasics. Other aspects of therapy for these patients, concerning, for example, the articulatory disturbances of Broca's aphasics or the comprehension disturbances of Wernicke's aphasics, will be discussed later. In other sections of this chapter we shall also describe therapy methods for both the more and the less common forms of aphasia. Thus we shall describe therapy for phonemic disturbances, as most characteristically manifested in conduction aphasia, therapy for lexical disturbances observed within the context of complex symptomatology or as a nearly isolated impairment as in the case of amnesic aphasia etc.

LINGUISTIC REDUCTION IN BROCA'S APHASIA

Management of the linguistic reduction presented by Broca's aphasics (and by certain patients with mixed aphasia) is divided into two major stages, the first called *demutization* and the second called *spontaneous production*[21]. During the first stage, therapy is aimed at the recovery of the most automatic uses of language or, in Ombredane's[41] terminology, at the recovery of emotional and practical language (see Insertion 17.1). In general, the patient's inhibition can be overcome (or partially overcome) only by the use of various facilitating procedures: phonemic cues, contextual cues in the form of sentences to be completed by an appropriate word, complete sentences requiring a brief, more or less stereotyped reply, etc. The efficacy of such cues will usually be enhanced if they are paired with gestures, mime and prosodic exaggerations which the therapist has found useful through experience, and if the patient's responses are positively reinforced. Thus, through a dynamic and energetic approach including multiple cues, the therapist gradually leads certain patients to produce meaningful linguistic units in unison with her. These productions typically include concrete substantives, frequently used expressions and other fixed syntagms, imperative predicates, short expressions of emotions, etc. Further attempts at therapy will generally be terminated (cf. p. 407) if it becomes clear that the patient cannot progress beyond this stage of automatic production almost devoid of propositional value. On the other hand, when further therapy appears warranted, the reliance on facilitating cues is quickly de-emphasized since their prolonged use is non-productive and may actually impede further progress. Thus the use of facilitating cues is gradually faded in order to move towards the controlled repetition of spoken linguistic stimuli, that is, towards repetition which is voluntary even if it is often defective in terms of articulatory production. When voluntary repetition is possible, the patient is ready to advance to the stage of spontaneous production (Insertion 17.3).

The transition between these therapy stages is carried out gradually, and occasional recourse to facilitating cues or to short repetition exercises is not excluded in the spontaneous production stage, especially in the beginning. However, this stage is essentially based on use of audiovisual methods developed for foreign-language teaching and adapted to the particular needs of aphasic patients (cf. p. 411). In the context of conversational exchanges incorporating progressively more complex linguistic structures and supported by the simultaneous presentation of the corresponding written material and pictures, the therapist guides the patient's participation in dialogues which include increasingly more propositional questions, replies and comments. Unless the severity of the articulatory disturbance is such that an analytical method (cf. p. 414) must be temporarily employed, the use of isolated words is avoided in the spontaneous production stage. This measure is taken in an attempt (which frequently proves inadequate) to counter the tendency of many Broca's aphasics to evolve towards agrammatism during the course of therapy. The use of audiovisual methods in therapy must generally be supplemented, either concurrently or subsequently, by sessions devoted to the enrichment of available vocabulary and to the remediation of syntactical deficits (cf. p. 52 and 420–453).

LOGORRHOEA IN WERNICKE'S APHASIA

The goal of aphasia therapy for the linguistic reduction associated with Broca's aphasia is to elicit as much language as possible from the patient. Exactly the opposite is true during the preliminary stage of therapy for Wernicke's aphasics presenting logorrhoeic jargon (cf. p. 412 under the heading 'Pre-Language Therapy') in which the goal is to silence the patient and to focus his attention on various tasks which include mostly non-linguistic stimuli and require gestural rather than spoken production. Once this goal has been attained, that is, attending behaviour has been established[21], language retraining is begun using exercises based on the analysis of complex linguistic units into their phonological constituents. These exercises entail various types of transposition, namely, audiophonatory (repetition), visuophonatory (oral reading), audiographic (writing to dictation) and visuographic (copying) beginning, for each patient, with the least impaired transposition mode (or modes). When later attempting to transfer acquired responses into dialogue situations, careful control and possible slowing of the speech flow may be required in order to prevent the reappearance of jargon.

THERAPY FOR PHONETIC AND PHONEMIC DISTURBANCES

In the language of aphasics, it is (in general) easy to recognize two types of transformations which affect correctly selected words. In the first case, articulation is laboured, numerous individual speech sounds are distorted and sometimes difficult to identify, and their syllabic enchaining is disturbed. The patient is then said to present the syndrome of phonetic disintegration[42] [which may occur in an isolated or nearly isolated form, as in pure anarthria, or in a more complex symptomatological context, as in Broca's aphasia (see Chapters 3 and 4)]. In the second case, the individual phonemic units are normally produced, are easily identified by the listener, and their syllabic enchaining appears undisturbed.* However, words are altered by phoneme omissions, additions, substitutions and transpositions: the patient is then said to produce phonemic paraphasias, a fact which is especially characteristic of certain forms of Wernicke's aphasia and, in particular, of conduction aphasia[43, 44] (see Chapter 4). Speaking very schematically, phonetic disintegration can generally be considered as a disorganization of the third linguistic phase and phonemic paraphasias as a disorganization of the second phase[50] (see Chapter 2). Nevertheless, while it is not uncommon to see patients without articulatory difficulty who produce numerous phonemic paraphasias, it is frequent, if not typical, to observe that patients with an evident articulatory disturbance also produce a greater or lesser number of phonemic paraphasias[51]. Evidence of the latter, which can be considered as a particular instance of Pierre Marie's law[52] (see Chapter 1-1), is particularly clear after a certain period of evolution, that is, with a decrease in the severity of the reduction and the articulatory disturbance. Although therapy procedures for phonetic and for phonemic deviations will be discussed separately, the above considerations imply that therapy for a given patient, and particularly in the case of a Broca's aphasic, must be based on a careful analysis of the patient's linguistic productions and, when indicated, include exercises for the disturbance of the second linguistic phase as well as for that of the third phase.

PHONETIC DISTURBANCES IN BROCA'S APHASICS

Therapy for impaired articulation

In the early post-onset period, the presence of severe apraxia often prevents the voluntary execution of buccofacial movements including those involved in phoneme production, namely features. Pre-language therapy is therefore required if other demutization procedures (cf. p. 413) prove ineffective. The patient is given exercises requiring imitation, and then production on verbal command, of movements inherent in the articulation of features into phonemes:

* This assertion excludes consideration of the phonemic approaches which may be demonstrated by these patients and the fact that during recovery, and generally as an effect of therapy, they often develop an intermittent and temporary tendency towards slowed, syllabic speech.

Insertion 17.3

Albert, Sparks and Helm[45], from Boston University, briefly described (1973) a therapy method intended to facilitate recovery in patients showing severe reduction of oral expression (see Chapter 4). The novelty of this method, now known as *Melodic Intonation Therapy* (MIT), resides in an initial emphasis on singing; patients first attempt to intone linguistic targets rather than to produce them with normal speech prosody.* Sparks, Helm and Albert[46] studied the effects of this form of therapy in a group of patients who had shown no improvement during an earlier period of more traditional therapy. Their results clearly indicated that MIT may result in a significant recovery of oral expression, although the positive effects appeared dependent on careful selection of patients. While further research is necessary to confirm the characteristics of appropriate therapy candidates, it presently appears that MIT is particularly suited to patients with very little oral expression who show impaired repetition (even for monosyllabic stimuli) as well as relatively good comprehension of spoken language. (Patients who made the greatest gains during MIT were those with a z-score of 0 to +0.5 on the auditory comprehension tests of the *Boston Diagnostic Aphasia Examination*[47]†.) If these criteria are met, production of stereotypes—contrary to what first might be thought—constitutes a favourable indicator (especially if the stereotypes are produced without evident articulatory difficulty). In contrast, MIT did not lead to improvement in the presence of a relatively severe comprehension disturbance nor—and perhaps more significantly—when repetition was relatively good (it should be noted that the small number of subjects to date does not permit definitive conclusions in this regard).

As in more traditional therapy for reduced oral expression (cf. p. 413), the stimuli for MIT must be carefully selected. The therapist assembles a group of highly functional linguistic phrases and then composes a melody for each one, with the tonal sequence, accents and rhythm of the melody reflecting an intonation pattern which would normally be associated with the spoken stimulus. Thus the therapy materials consist of groups of written phrases, each one accompanied by its musical notation. The use of familiar melodies is strictly avoided as their effects have been observed to be detrimental[46, 47].

1. As most recently described[47], MIT involves four progressive levels of difficulty. In the first, which has no linguistic component, the patient and the therapist hum the stimulus melodies‡ and handtap their rhythms in unison. In this regard, it is useful to have the therapist and patient facing each other while seated at a table large enough so that both may rest their forearms on it. The patient usually taps with his left hand which may initially be guided by the therapist, who usually uses her right hand. During this first level, a gestural code may be established to indicate to the patient when he should passively observe the therapist and when he should attempt to respond.
2. In Level II, the linguistic targets are added to the melody and the patient is helped to achieve independent repetition of the stimulus through a sequence of increasingly difficult steps: (a) the therapist and patient handtap and intone the melodic linguistic stimulus in unison; (b) the therapist gradually reduces her participation to encourage solo repetition by the patient; (c) the therapist presents the sung linguistic stimulus for immediate unaided repetition by the patient; (d) the therapist presents a sung request for immediate (intoned) production of the target phrase. A similar sequence is followed in Level III but the difficulty of the last steps is increased by (a) imposing a delay between the therapist's presentation of the stimulus and the patient's intoned response and by (b) encouraging the patient to use only some element of the stimulus phrase in response to an appropriate question from the therapist.
3. The goal of the fourth and final level of MIT is a return to normal prosody during

* This procedure appears clearly related to one, previously described in this chapter, which entails the use of exaggerated prosody and mimicry during the first steps of demutization.

† In certain respects, this clinical picture is reminiscent of that of Goldstein's[23] central motor aphasia (see Chapter 10).

‡ Humming the melody from visual notation may be difficult for therapists with poor sight-reading skills. One of us (B.B.) has found it useful first to play the melody on a small, portable instrument (xylophone) before attempting to hum it.

propositional use of some element of the stimulus phrase. This transition is facilitated by the presentation of the stimulus phrases in speech-song to encourage production, in an exaggerated form, of the principal prosodic features of the stimulus phrase. Again, this level is composed of carefully sequenced steps in which the patient responds to each stimulus by (a) delayed, intoned repetition; (b) immediate repetition in speech song; (c) delayed repetition in speech song; (d) delayed repetition with normal speech prosody and (e) normal prosody and the production of elements of the linguistic stimulus in response to a question.

4. When the patient fails to respond adequately to a particular stimulus, work with that stimulus is either discontinued immediately or, for some steps, when failure still occurs after a backup procedure. Another stimulus is then presented and the sequence of steps is begun again. During all but the first level, the patient's responses are scored during each session of MIT. Progression from one level to a higher one is contingent on 90 per cent response accuracy based on a mean of ten consecutive sessions.

In cases where MIT has led to recovery of a certain degree of functional oral expression, the patient's productions were usually of an agrammatic type with defective articulation. It thus appears that MIT must eventually be followed by other types of therapy. The time at which this shift should occur must be determined through consideration of individual cases since research on this question is presently limited. Sparks et al[46] suggest that MIT should be provided on an intensive (i.e., daily) basis during three months, with other methods excluded, before considering the introduction of other procedures. Although this position might seem dogmatic, it could also be the result of a sound empirical approach.

The number of aphasics who have received systematic melodic intonation therapy remains quite limited. However, the observations reported to date are consistent with others found in the aphasiological literature on:

1. *Motor aphasia*: 'Singing is, quite often, more intact than speech. When singing, the patient not only retains the melody of the song but very often clearly articulates words which he cannot produce when speaking' (Dejerine[48]).
2. Therapy for the *phonetic disintegration syndrome*: 'The rhythmical repetition of the same phonatory movement, at different speeds, the rhythmical succession of starts, stops and repetitions, the repeated and rhythmical passage from one to another of two phonemes, then of three and of four phonemes, [when continued] at length with the same phonemes, always appeared to us as eminently effective training procedures'... 'The patient engages in veritable psalmody, first at the same time as the therapist, then alone' (Alajouanine et al[42]).
3. Articulation therapy in *efferent motor aphasia*: 'In devising methods for overcoming the inertia of articulatory patterns, we began with the observation that even though a patient was unable to carry out a single complex movement smoothly, he had no difficulty in carrying out two successive acts if they were sufficiently different from one another. On the basis of this we tried to find a means of transforming a two-phoneme syllable into two distinct articulatory movements'... 'One technique was to have him pronounce the two syllables at different pitches' (Luria[49]).

The above observations raise questions of obvious theoretical interest, especially concerning the reasons for the facilitating effect of melody. Personal observations (B.B.) suggest that this facilitation occurs at the level of articulatory actualization and, more specifically, at the level of phoneme sequencing; and that it may be related to the differentiation of articulatory sequences by different musical characteristics (rhythms, pitch, changes, rests, accents). The occurrence of such facilitation at the level of motor encoding in no way excludes the possibility that other effects occur earlier during the process of word evocation. In other words, these suggestions do not conflict with the hypothesis of Sparks et al[46] that melodic stimulation acts to increase the role of the right cerebral hemisphere in the interhemispheric control of oral expression.

exhalation, elevation of the tongue tip, labial-dental contact, lip protrusion, etc. Whenever possible, the exercises follow a gradual progression from movements executed in concrete situations to movements performed on verbal command and in the absence of a contextual support[21]. For example, voluntary control of exhalation may be increased by training the patient to blow out a lighted candle, then to repeat the same movement in the presence of an unlighted candle and, finally, in the absence of a candle.

Once elementary movements can generally be executed in a voluntary fashion, therapy is aimed at the concomitant production of certain groups of features, that is, at the production of phonemes. On the basis of indicators drawn from linguistic theory and knowledge of the order of phoneme acquisition during language development[53, 54], the following progression in therapy exercises is frequently recommended: vowels before consonants, stops before fricatives, anterior consonants (with visible place of articulation) before posterior consonants, etc. While this progression is generally valid, it should not preclude some flexibility during the course of therapy. Patients attempting to articulate a particular phoneme may succeed in producing another and the therapist will often find it advantageous to capitalize on these 'errors' by temporarily reorienting the remainder of the therapy session. In the very early stages of phonetic therapy, sounds are produced nearly simultaneously by the patient and therapist and the therapist provides much assistance in the form of exaggerated articulatory gestures and accompanying hand movements, each of which is associated with a specific phoneme[21, 55]. Use of these supports is gradually faded as soon as possible in order to advance to the stage where the patient repeats the sound only after it has been produced by the therapist without exaggerated articulation or hand movements.

At the start of therapy, an emphasis on perfect articulation of isolated phonemes is generally inadvisable. As soon as the patient's approximations are sufficient to permit accurate identification of a certain number of phonemes, the exercises should include phonemic sequences forming, in order of increasing complexity, words, phrases and sentences. At the beginning of this stage of *syllabic enchaining*, the stimulus sequences should require minimal muscular synergy. In other words, they should follow the principle of coarticulation as outlined by Ohman[56] and McDonald[57]. Thus the initial stimuli consist of syllables in which the consonant and vowel share the maximum possible number of common features (/si→sɛ→sæ/; /ʃu→ʃo/→ʃə) and, as the exercises gradually progress, the number of common features is gradually reduced (/sɔ→su/; /ʃɛ→ʃi/). The juxtaposition of syllables requiring rapid shifts of the articulatory organs and maximal muscular synergy is avoided until a later stage of phonetic-level therapy, especially in cases of severely disturbed articulation.

Although the principles outlined above constitute general guidelines for the planning of phonetic therapy, they must be adapted to particular cases. When planning a therapy programme for a given individual, attention must also be given to associated disturbances (reduced output, phonemic deviations, etc.), i.e., to factors which are not all directly related to the properly phonetic disturbance. An analysis of the patient's productions in terms of acoustic and motor parameters and comparisons of his misarticulations during different types of activities (conversation, repetition, etc.) are extremely important. The study of contamination effects resulting from the juxtaposition and proximity of certain phonemes, the identification of the most effective facilitating mechanisms, etc. must also be taken into account. This type of investigation will allow the therapist to distinguish the properly phonetic aspect of the deficit and to recognize its paretic and/or dystonic components (see Chapter 3).

No matter what particular problem has been selected as a target for one or more sessions of phonetic therapy, the linguistic stimuli should be presented to the patient in order of increasing articulatory difficulty. For example, the following progression could be used to promote voicing by an aphasic who tends to devoice voiced consonants:

1. HAMMER A NAIL /hæmɚənel/: all the phonemic constituents are voiced and none has an unvoiced cognate in English. Consequently, when the patient places his hand over his larynx, he will feel the continuous vibration of his vocal folds.
2. IS-OF-OTHER /ɪs-ɑv-ʌðɚ/: the vowel facilitates voicing of the following voiced fricative.
3. THERE IS THE ZOO /ðɚɪzðəzu/: here again, all the elements are voiced. The consonants are fricatives which, because they can be prolonged, are more easily voiced than plosives. Although voicing is often partial and discontinuous at the start of therapy, it progressively becomes more reliable and stable.
4. HAVE FUN /hævfʌn/: there is both a voiced and an unvoiced fricative within the same sentence.
5. MAID-ROBE-LEG-A BIG BOWL /med-rob-lɛg-əbɪgbol/: only voiced plosives are included.

6. IT'S COLD TODAY /ɪtskoldtəde/: two words within the same sentence include both a voiced and an unvoiced plosive.

At each stage of therapy, the work is planned so that learning exercises are followed by drills and exercises to promote stabilization, generalization, and transfer to oral reading, conversation, etc. Several methods intended for foreign-language teaching (cf. p. 410) include phonetic exercises on contrasting phonemes. These exercises are generally arranged in order of increasing difficulty and the speech pathologist will find them extremely useful in work with aphasic individuals.

Therapy for impaired prosody

Certain suprasegmental features of discourse are generally disturbed in the phonetic disintegration syndrome (see Chapters 3 and 4). The rhythm of speech is disturbed by syllabic scanning, faulty transition from one word to the next, the excessive prolongation of certain phonemic sequences and the shortening of others[43, 58]. Depending on the patient, certain aspects of intonation may be monotonous or exaggerated, leading to a loss or disturbance of normal speech melody.

Although complete recovery of normal prosody cannot generally be expected in Broca's aphasia, the therapist can try to attenuate those dysprosodic aspects which interfere with the modulation of speech and reduce the intelligibility of discourse. Thus the patient may be given exercises centred on vocalic chaining, transitions between words, stress and melodic line. In this last case, the exercises are aimed at recovery of the intonation patterns of interrogatives, exclamations, negatives, etc. Similarly, it may be useful to carry out exercises involving the repetition of emotional expressions or utterances in which different emotions—joy, doubt, surprise, irony, impatience, indignation, fear—are expressed mainly through variations in intonation. Dialogues excerpted from narratives and plays may provide useful materials for such exercises. We have found that methods combining the use of books and tape-recordings and originally intended for improvement of pronunciation in adults learning a foreign language[59–61] can also be easily adapted to the needs of aphasic patients.

As phonetic therapy draws to an end, the therapist must usually devote some sessions to the establishment of simultaneous control over both articulation and prosody. Having achieved approximate control of each one separately, it is not unusual for patients to encounter difficulty in monitoring both at once. For example, a patient may be able to achieve adequate voicing and control of word transitions only when speaking in a monotone voice. The voluntary nature of the control which is finally achieved, and thus its fragility, is often seen when conscious control is lessened by the patient's absorption in a conversational exchange. Nevertheless, a certain degree of articulatory and prosodic automaticity can generally be re-acquired through prolonged retraining.

PHONEMIC DISTURBANCES IN WERNICKE'S APHASIA

The production of numerous phonemic transformations (see Chapter 2) is characteristic of both conduction aphasia and of Wernicke's aphasia proper. It dominates the picture of conduction aphasia but is only one element of a more complex symptomatological group in Wernicke's aphasia (see Chapter 4). As already mentioned, the clinical picture of Broca's aphasia may include the production of phonemic paraphasias in addition to the characteristic articulatory disturbance. In conduction aphasia, the disorganization of phonemic encoding may be quite selective and the patient is aware of his impairment (see Fig. 14-1) so that therapy is usually begun immediately. Despite the usual presence of word-finding difficulty, therapy is usually facilitated by the facts that the patient's lexical choices are usually adequate and the phonemic transformations which characteristically pepper his conversation do not usually prevent recognition of the underlying linguistic segments. In the more frequent case of Wernicke's aphasia proper, attempts to remediate the phonemic disturbance can be undertaken only after a course of pre-language therapy (cf. p. 412) aimed at the establishment of attending behaviours and the patient's recognition of his impairment. Such recognition is indicated by the appearance of successive approximations (*conduites d'approche phonémique*), that is, attempted corrections at the beginning of words [(17.1) /aktivite/→tak - tak - ta - tati - ativite - aktivite/]. These successive approximations quite often appear when many of the neologistic productions lose their seemingly aberrant aspect, that is, when their structure is such that they can be identified, with reasonable certainty, as being phonemic paraphasias (see Chapter 2).

The variability of phonemic transformations and their unpredictable nature prevent planning of a therapy programme rigorously based on an analysis of the linear structure of each patient's errors. However, certain characteristics can be noted[62] which provide some direction for therapy. In this regard it is useful to determine whether the patient shows a clear trend towards *anticipation* errors [(17.2) /aktivite→taktivite/, (2.20) /malabil→amababil/] or, on the contrary, a clear tendency towards errors by *reiteration* [(2.15) /inaktif/→/inaktik/, (17.3) /malabil/→ /malababim/]. In the latter case, is there consistent evidence of phonemic *contamination* from one stimulus to another, that is, do the responses suggest that the patient *perseverates* [(17.4) /flœʀ→flœʀ/, /laʀm→flam/, /ʀamo→flaʀmo/, /ʀɛgl→frɛg/]?* Additional guidelines to planning the progression of a therapy programme are provided by knowledge of the stimulus characteristics which are most likely to elicit the production of phonemic transformations. In general, more transformations will be elicited by longer than by shorter words and by words with a more complex phonemic structure than by words with a simpler structure. Thus words containing groups of consonants or vowels, pairs of identical or similar phonemes, and ending with a consonant etc. [fast /fæst/ and calisthenics /kæləsθɛnɪks/] elicit more transformations than words which are simpler in structure, for example, those composed of successive consonants and vowels [day /ce/ and happiness /hæpɪnɛs/]. In addition, words which are members of a large paradigm [/bæt; kæt, fæt, hæt, mæt, næt, pæt, ræt, sæt, væt/] are more difficult than those from a more restricted paradigm [/bʌd, dʌd, mʌd/] and phrases containing a large number of grammatical morphemes [no matter how the weather will be] elicit more transformations than those containing only a few [a big bowl of hot soup], etc.

Since relatively few errors are usually made on monosyllables, the stimuli used in the earliest exercises are usually bi-syllables. The initial series are composed of words which are simple in structure, are very different from each other, and whose constituent phonemes share few common features [hammer /hæmɚ/, pillow /pɪlo/, bacon /beʀən/]. Later, stimuli are presented in more homogeneous groups with each stimulus including identical or similar phonemes [saucer /sɔsɚ/, seaside /sisaɪd/, seashore /siʃor/, satin /sætɪn/, session /sɛʃən/]. The subsequent groups meet the same criterion but each word also includes consonant clusters [concrete /konkrit/, construct /kənstrʌkt/, structure /strʌktʃɚ/, staircase /stɛrkes/]. Once control of bi-syllables has been established, the stimuli generally consist of short, structurally simple syntagms. They are often more accurately produced than structurally complex, multisyllabic words, which are reserved for a later stage of therapy. For each of these successive stages, the therapy exercises are planned to follow an order of increasing difficulty. The insertion, within the same sentence, of words containing identical or similar units and differing only in the position of these units [conservation – conversation /kənsɚveʃən – kɑnvɚseʃən/, fine-knife /faɪn-naɪf/, leading-dealing /lidiŋ – dilɪŋ/] is usually reserved for an advanced stage of therapy: such sentences are particularly difficult for aphasics with disturbances of phonemic encoding.

Since oral reading is usually less impaired than repetition in these patients[43], visual support, namely the written word, is often paired with the presentation of the auditory model. In the rarer cases where writing to dictation is the most intact transposition mode, the therapist will train the patient to write each stimulus word before repeating it, and then to write and repeat simultaneously. The combined use of three transposition modes (generally repetition, oral reading, writing to dictation) is often feasible. Use of the Language Master (cf. p. 411) is then convenient, as this device allows the patient to record his reading of a written stimulus, to compare his production with that recorded by the therapist on another channel of the tape, to erase his production if inadequate, and to start over, keeping in mind what he has heard and what he sees. When needed, he can also copy the printed word which he sees or write the one which is dictated.

The final stages of therapy are characterized by the gradual removal of facilitating patterns

* At the start of therapy, a marked tendency towards anticipation errors can be countermanded, in oral reading, by use of a covering card so that the stimuli are exposed syllable by syllable and, in repetition, by presenting the stimuli in segments. Effects of a tendency to perseverate generally become more marked as the therapy session progresses and can be partially controlled by lengthening the interval between successive stimuli.

and by concentrated work in the most impaired transposition mode (which is usually repetition). Once phonemic encoding has been generally re-established and the successive approximations have been internalized, sometimes at the expense of a relative slowing in rate of speech, the therapy sessions will consist of exercises to increase generalization and transfer of adequate encoding to narration, conversation, etc.

An attempt at therapy can sometimes be undertaken with certain particularly 'intelligent' Wernicke's aphasics whose disorder affects all modes of transposition, leaving no clearly favoured pathway for language therapy. In such cases, the therapist may follow the *method of codes* described by de Ribaucourt-Ducarne[21]. In this method, the therapist more or less intuitively attempts to facilitate recovery by providing various associations of sound and meaning to certain of the patient's spontaneous oral or written productions. For example, if he spontaneously said /kɑr/ (car), the therapist would immediately try, by associating repetition, the written word, a gesture or a rapid sketch, etc., to elicit the production of /kɑrbɑn/ (carbon), /kɑrpɪt/ (carpet), /pɪt/ (pit), /pɪtɪ/ (pity), etc. Certain patients clearly grasp the principle of this approach and, after some time, they themselves direct its application. The therapist then assumes the role of an informed interlocutor.

THERAPY FOR AGRAMMATISM AND DYSSYNTAXIA

The concepts of agrammatism and dyssyntaxia (or paragrammatism) were previously defined (see Chapter 2). The frequent occurrence of agrammatism in the symptomatological context of an evolving Broca's aphasia and of dyssyntaxia in the symptomatological context of Wernicke's aphasia were also discussed (see Chapter 4). When therapy for morphological and syntactical deficits appears necessary, and this is more frequent in the case of Broca's aphasics or certain conduction aphasics than in the common forms of Wernicke's aphasia, the development of an appropriate therapy programme is a complex endeavour and the results are seldom spectacular, especially in the case of agrammatism. They are, nevertheless, sufficient to justify attempts at intervention for longer or shorter periods. Having empirically observed their (relative) value, we rely on the use of exercises whose progression is based on knowledge accumulated from research in several disciplines.

Linguistics. Syntactical structures differ in complexity; for example, the production of two juxtaposed affirmatives is simpler than the production of a negative main clause followed by a subordinate clause. Some syntactical structures are used frequently and others rarely; for example, statements indicating actions carried out by the subject are far more frequent than statements describing actions affecting the subject.

Neurolinguistics (see Chapter 12). Several investigators[63-69] have carried out exhaustive synchronic analyses of aphasic language which have permitted descriptions of agrammatism in linguistic terms.* Others have carried out diachronic studies of recovery from agrammatism (spontaneous recovery[70] or recovery subsequent to a systematic therapy programme[71]). The results of such studies permit a hierarchical ordering or grammatical complexity and thus provide a basis for the development of progressively more complex exercises for use in therapy with agrammatic patients. Furthermore, a study by Holland and Levy[71] suggests that certain tasks have a positive influence on the relearning of agrammatic subjects; for example, certain structures are more effectively recovered through repetition and comprehension tasks than through other means.

---

* Certain syntactical structures are more intact than others in Broca's aphasia. For example, VS + NS is immediately more available than NS + VS or NS + VS + NS[63]. Few Broca's aphasics demonstrate regular or appropriate use of the copula (segment relating the subject to the predicate), expansion of nominal syntagms, use of the passive form, etc.[63] Morphological rules, especially those governing morphological markers of verbs and particularly those which indicate tense, constitute a major difficulty for Broca's aphasics. They have somewhat less difficulty with gender and number agreements for certain determiners, adjectives, and nouns. Use of function words is also a source of difficulty, with their omission being an important characteristic of agrammatism and their paraphasic usage being characteristic of dyssyntaxia (this is particularly true for prepositions indicating spatial-temporal relations)[66].

Psycholinguistics. Knowledge of the chronological order in which various syntactical structures are acquired during language development can also provide guidelines to the hierarchical ordering of exercises to be used in therapy for morphosyntactical disturbances. For example, it is known that many syntactical rules are acquired before morphological rules, early syntactical groupings extend beyond simple syntagms, and the relations subject–object, subject–verb, and verb–object are among those most frequently used by young children[72].

Our reference to developmental data in this discussion of aphasia therapy does not imply that we consider aphasia to involve a regression to an earlier developmental stage. Such an assertion cannot be easily supported given its unlikely implications concerning brain structure and functioning. However, this does not preclude certain resemblances between some aphasic language behaviours and those of children, nor that the linguistic behaviours which are acquired later in the course of normal development are generally those which are most disturbed and the last to be recovered in aphasia[43, 73]. Thus we consider it justified, in the absence of a firm theory of aphasia, to base certain stages of aphasia therapy on this type of data.

AGRAMMATISM IN BROCA'S APHASIA

More or less complete recovery from Broca's aphasia or mixed aphasia may occur in the absence of any tendency towards agrammatism. Nevertheless, it often happens, even in patients whose therapy was carefully centred on the use of global methods during the spontaneous production phase, that progressive recovery and the use of a propositional lexicon are accompanied by more or less severe agrammatism. In this case, the therapy programme should include exercises intended to increase the availability of the commonest morphosyntactic rules.

In developing such exercises, we have tried to adhere to the following principles as closely as possible:

1. Lexical elements (nouns, adjectives and verbs) are selected according to their frequency of usage in the language. Common words are selected rather than less frequent words but the inventories, especially of verbs, are not limited to concrete words. Words whose phonological structure is particularly complex are initially excluded.
2. When questions are asked, at least during the early stages of therapy, they are formulated in such a manner that the syntactical structure of the (correct) response is predetermined.
3. Most of the exercises are presented with visual support in the form of illustrations: drawings and series of drawings; materials from audiovisual language teaching methods (Fig. 17.1) are usually employed.
4. When necessary, exercises to ensure comprehension of the semantic meaning of common syntactical structures should precede exercises involving the production of these structures. Procedures used in comprehension exercises include pointing to pictures in response to spoken commands and the matching of written sentences to their corresponding pictures.
5. In the production exercises proper, transposition tasks—repetition and copying, reading and copying—precede oral evocation (i.e., exercises in which the aphasic must formulate a sentence using given lexical elements) and oral evocation generally precedes written evocation. Depending on the case, the most intact expressive modalities will be emphasized (or used exclusively).
6. The exercises are presented in order of increasing linguistic difficulty, and the transition from one stage to another is accomplished through small variations, at least during the initial stages of therapy.
7. Imperative and assertive forms precede negative, interrogative and other transformations. For each one, the exercises aimed at recovery of the syntactical convention (relationships between words and simple syntagms in the context of sentences) precede exercises aimed at recovery of the morphological convention (relationships between lexical monemes and morphological markers in the context of words) (see Chapter 2).
8. For each series of exercises aimed at recovery of the syntactical convention, the relationships between simple syntagms (syntagms-I) in the context of sentences (syntagms-III) are treated before the relationships between words within the context of syntagms-I (see Chapter 2).
9. Exercises in narration, carried out with progressively decreasing assistance, are included

with the aim of increasing the transfer and generalization of acquired gains.

To our knowledge, there is presently no available therapy programme for the syntactical deficits of aphasics which is based on an explicit theory of aphasia and has been demonstrated to be effective through experimental evaluation. We must also emphasize that the practical suggestions to be discussed in the following paragraphs are not presented as a proven method of aphasia therapy. We say only that they were based on a consideration of research findings (some of which were previously cited), that they are generally consistent with the principles enumerated above and that they describe those procedures which we have found, up till now, to be the most effective in our own attempts at therapy for the syntactical disturbances of aphasics. In our opinion, a therapy programme for agrammatism must be based on several types of exercises, be carried out in several successive (but not mutually exclusive) stages, and follow a re-acquisition order of increasing difficulty with respect to morphosyntactic structures. The provision of facilitating cues, universally used in therapy with Broca's aphasics, remains an essential complement which we shall discuss later.

Finally, the therapy should be as dynamic and natural as possible. Thus it should be based on familiar language, that is, the language of everyday conversational exchanges, and the types of tasks usually done in school should generally be avoided. Since the primary objective is the recovery of oral expression, the usual structures of spoken language should be emphasized. Exercises involving non-conversational behaviours (e.g., repetition, oral reading, etc.) may sometimes be required but their only goal is the eventual facilitation of syntactical spontaneous production.

Exercises

The following sequence of exercises is suggested for each stage of therapy.

Comprehension. Exercises in (oral and written) comprehension of syntactical structures are used only when the results of the aphasia assessment (see Chapter 15) indicate faulty comprehension of grammatical features.

Repetition. Repetition exercises permit systematic prosodic variation. In numerous agrammatic patients, this greatly facilitates normal or near normal morphosyntactic production.

Oral reading. Even within the context of an oral reading task, a dialogue approach is possible and is usually advisable (for example, a question or comment from the therapist can facilitate the reading of a complete sentence containing the target structure).

Oral production (in response to a situation or question). In this type of exercise the patient comments verbally on an action mimed by the therapist, illustrated by a picture or a picture sequence, or demonstrated by the manipulation of one or more objects (object manipulation often involves natural actions which favour corresponding verbal commentary). When a target utterance is to be elicited by a question, the therapist must formulate it in such a way that the answer must be the target utterance or a very close approximation.

Written production. The written production exercises are usually a form of homework (completed between the sessions personally conducted by the therapist) and are intended to reinforce the most recent gains in oral production.

Besides introducing variety into the therapy exercises, which may help attract and maintain the patient's interest, the inclusion of these different forms of language behaviour permits repetition of the same target structures, this practice often being necessary for their stabilization and generalization. The presentation order proposed above is not invariable. Depending on the patient's most intact modality, the therapist might, for example, find it advantageous to reverse the order of the repetition and oral reading exercises.

Stages in therapy for agrammatism

When all goes well, therapy for agrammatism usually consists of three successive stages involving: (1) the teaching of thematically unrelated sentences (this initial stage is intended to focus the patient's attention on structural aspects, i.e., on the syntactical features of the stimulus utterances); (2) the teaching of thematically related sentences (this intermediate stage focuses on the simultaneous control of semantic and syntactic constraints; the patient must attend to both the syntactical structure of the target sentences and the messages conveyed); and (3) expressive discourse (this final stage aims at the transfer of gains into narration).

Teaching thematically unrelated sentences

Following a procedure developed by Goodglass[63] in the Story Completion Test (see Chapter 12), the therapist promotes sentence formulation through the help of a short 'story' consisting of two to four utterances presented in a manner which will elicit a grammatically structured sentence. To overcome difficulty in lexical retrieval, which is common in agrammatic patients as in almost all other aphasics, the lexical elements of the target responses are included in the therapist's preliminary remarks. The following examples illustrate this approach:

[1] (NS − VS)*	'I want to go out. So I open the door and ... What do I do?' |I GO OUT.|†
[2] (NS − VS + NS)	'I want to buy a hat. So I go to the store and ... What do I do?' |I BUY A HAT.|
[3] (NS − VS + PS)	'The little boy wants to play in the snow. He puts on his snowsuit and goes outside. Then ... what does the little boy do?' |HE PLAYS IN THE SNOW.|
[4] (NS + Cop + PS)	'The man is fixing his car in the garage. Where is he? I could say that ...' |THE MAN IS IN THE GARAGE.|

This type of exercise is preceded by repetition and oral reading exercises, one of their purposes being to accentuate the unequivocal nature of expected responses. This is particularly important in the case of target sentences which include a prepositional phrase, a unit which is frequently optional (see the third example above where the response could have been |HE PLAYS|). Furthermore, each type of sentence is presented in several variations of the basic pattern. Initially, these substitutions are carried out in one paradigm at a time, beginning with that of the NS object, then that of the VS, and finally that of the NS subject.

[1] Substitutions in the NS object paradigm:
|THE BOY WASHES THE CAR.|
|THE BOY WASHES THE WINDOW.|
|THE BOY WASHES THE DISHES.|
etc.

[2] Substitutions in the VS paradigm:
|THE BOY WASHES THE CAR.|
|THE BOY FIXES THE CAR.|
|THE BOY DRIVES THE CAR.|
etc.

[3] Substitutions in the NS subject paradigm:
|THE BOY WASHES THE CAR.|
|THE GIRL WASHES THE CAR.|
|PETER WASHES THE CAR.|
etc.

For patients who are progressing well, it may also be useful to include exercises requiring the substitution of pNS‡ for nNS‡ subject (see Chapter 2).

[1] |THE BOY REPAIRS THE WINDOW.|
[2] |HE REPAIRS THE WINDOW.|
etc.

Through these paradigmatic exercises, the therapist provides each patient with the practice needed to stabilize the target structures. We are unable to provide experimental data on the optimal number of practice sentences to ensure recovery of a particular structure. It seems unlikely that such figure could ever be established since it would probably vary widely as a function of the subject's age, educational level, nature and extent of lesions, etc.

The use of different types of facilitation is generally necessary during the first, and sometimes the second, stage of therapy for agrammatism. The main types of facilitation which are used are as follows.

* NS = nominal syntagm; VS = predicate; Cop = Copula; Adv = adverb; Adj = adjective; PS = prepositional syntagm (see Chapter 2).

† In the beginning, the therapist may facilitate production by providing the pronoun (or first word) of the target response.

‡ pNS = pronominal nominal syntagm; nNS = nominal nominal syntagm (see Chapter 2).

Phonemic cues (see Chapter 4). Phonemic cues may be vocalized or silent. In the latter case, only visual information is provided.

Verbal context cues (see Chapter 4). The efficacy of this type of facilitation can be enhanced by prosodic exaggeration (intonation and accentuation).

Gestures and mime. These types of cues include symbolic gestures intended to elicit particular elements of the target sentence (pronouns, verbs, prepositions, adverbs). We have found that evocation of (action) verbs may be especially difficult in agrammatism and is often facilitated by this type of cue. Coded gestures, a bit like those used by orchestra conductors, may also be useful as their temporal-spatial progression may evoke that of the target sentence.

Visual code. Although the presentation of corresponding written messages as a supplement to spoken stimuli is a type of facilitation which may be used during therapy for agrammatism, we are referring here to the use of tokens. Through preliminary learning, tokens of different sizes and shapes may be associated with a specific syntactic unit of the target sentence ['red square' = (subject), 'blue triangle' = (verb), etc.]. Manipulation of these tokens, that is, their selection and sequential arrangement, facilitates retrieval of the constituents of the target sentence and is especially effective in eliciting production of syntactically complete utterances.

Phonemic code. Experience shows that certain formal auditory associations may permit the production of certain utterances which are otherwise unavailable. The cueing usually involves a transition from a lexical unit to a grammatical homophone. For example, the patient unable to retrieve the interrogative form 'what' may be able to do so after numerous exercises in reading, repeating and identifying the word (watt) on lightbulbs, electrical appliances, etc. Similarly, difficulty with the form 'which' may be overcome through reading, repeating and identifying the stimulus (witch).

When beginning therapy, the clinician generally uses these different types of facilitation in combination. However, in keeping with the final goal of syntactic production which is as normal and as autonomous as possible, the facilitating cues are faded as soon as their removal does not hinder the patient's progress.

Teaching thematically related sentences

The second stage of therapy for agrammatism is generally begun as soon as there is relatively consistent production of the constituents of *simple affirmative declaratives* [SAD: e.g., (nNS + VS): |THE BOY WALKS|, (nNS + VS = nNS): |THE BOY WASHES THE CAR|, etc.]. In other words, the first and second stages of therapy are then carried out concurrently [the first stage continued for structures other than the imperative (cf. p. 426), and the second stage for structures of the SAD type]. The first and second stages are related in terms of the progression of exercises (repetition, reading, evocation) but they are distinguished by the nature of the material included in the therapy exercises. It is during the second stage that materials from certain audiovisual foreign language teaching methods are particularly useful (cf. p. 411). The method *De Vive Voix* was adapted for use with French speaking agrammatic patients by Coderre[74]. This adaptation will be illustrated by examples of the first five items from an early lesson in this programme. The target sentences, each of which corresponds to a picture (Fig. 17-1), are composed of elementary structures (NS + VS), (NS + VS + NS), or (NS + VS + PS) and are as follows:

[1] |A LADY IS WALKING ON THE SIDEWALK.|
[2] |SHE TRIPS AND FALLS.|
[3] |A MAN HELPS HER.|
[4] |THE LADY HURT HER KNEE.|
[5] |SHE CALLS A TAXI.|
etc.

Since dialogue is the essence of most audiovisual programmes for foreign-language teaching, this approach should be retained when they are used with aphasics: furthermore, such an approach is consistent with the aims of therapy for agrammatism (cf. above). It does, however, require attention to the therapist's participation in each dialogue since the questions which she will ask must be carefully formulated. These questions must be both vague enough (lexically) that they cannot be answered by a single element of the target sentence and precise enough that the target sentence is unequivocally the required response. The following questions, for example, could be asked to elicit the target sentences [1 to 5] listed above:

[1] *What's going on?*
[2] *What happens to the lady?*

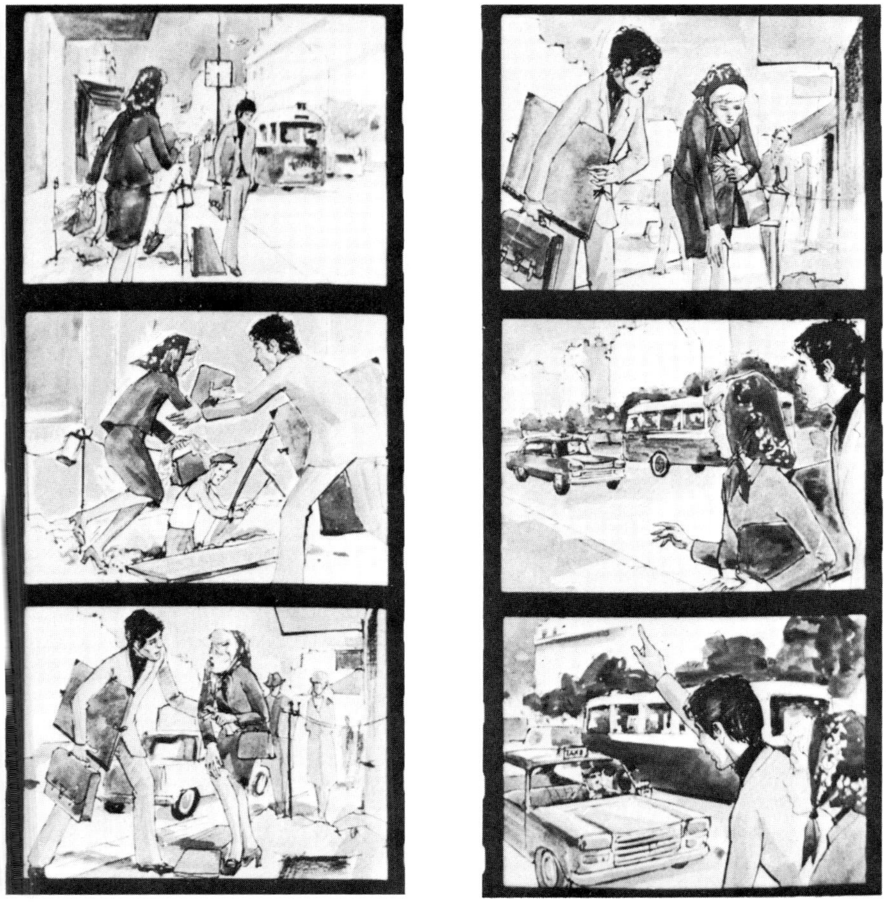

Fig. 17-1 *Example of sequenced illustrations from a film strip used in certain exercises during therapy for agrammatism. Commentary in the text. From Mauget*[33].

[3] *What is the man doing?*
[4] *What did the lady do to herself?*
[5] *What does she do because walking is too painful?*

Consider the fourth target sentence, [4], for example. If the therapist asked, *'Where did the lady hurt herself?'* the natural reply, *'on the knee'*, would include only one element of the target structure. On the other hand, if the question is *'What is going on?'* (as for the first item), the number of possible replies is too great and the expected structure is too imprecisely specified. By asking *'What did the lady do to herself?'*, the patient is almost obliged to answer, *'She hurt her knee'* [this is true provided that the patient's attention is focused on the corresponding picture and, when needed, on a relevant detail in the picture (Fig. 17-1)]. As indicated by this brief discussion of the fourth example, it is through constant reference to the illustrations that the target response for each picture is pre-determined in terms of its syntactical structure. In addition, the unequivocal responses expected during the oral production exercises have been carefully coached. First, the therapist produced the target sentence for each picture in the lesson while the patient listened passively, and then these target sentences were practised in repetition and/or oral reading exercises.

Narration

During the final stage, the patient is asked to narrate stories of increasing length and complexity which are based, at least in the beginning, on pictured stimuli (projections, picture sequences, etc.). Certain themes or stories from the second stage can often be usefully reviewed during this final stage but the therapist's interventions are then reduced to a minimum (consisting of non-specific remarks intended to encourage the patient to continue if he stops, or to signal an omission, etc.). When the patient reaches the stage of syntactically adequate narration in the presence of visual support, this assistance is removed and the patient attempts narration based only on a suggested theme or topic. When moving into this last step, it is sometimes useful to begin with the recounting of well-known stories (e.g., *Little Red Riding Hood*, *Cinderella*, etc.) and then to progress to more personal narratives which are not dependent on such formalized learning ('A day at work', 'My last holiday', etc.).

Notes on the sequencing of exercises with respect to syntactical structure

In each of the three stages which we have discussed, it is important that the required productions follow an order of increasing difficulty with respect to syntactic structure (this is more crucial during the first stage than during the second and more important during the second stage than during the third). The exercises are restricted to basic structures, that is, to those which are characteristic of language centred on the facts, ideas and needs of daily life. Although we have not determined its validity through systematic experimentation, we nevertheless suggest the following (largely empirically derived) progression.

Imperative sentences. Presenting imperatives at the start of the progression may be contrary to certain linguistic hypothesis concerning the hierarchy of grammatical difficulty[74] but experience has shown that this structure is particularly easy for agrammatic patients. Nevertheless, the therapist may sometimes find it useful to replace it by affirmative declaratives of the (NS + VS) type. In this case, the therapist supplies the subject of the target sentence (cf. [1], [2], p. 421) and the segment elicited is an artefact in the sense that its surface aspect does not correspond to its underlying meaning. This facilitating technique often proves to be an excellent way of initiating therapy for agrammatism.

Simple or extended declarative affirmative sentences. These sentences can include various elements which we suggest be introduced in the following order:

[1] (NS + VS)	|PETER WALKS.|
[2] (NS + VS + NS)	|PETER OPENS THE WINDOW.|
[3] (NS + VS + PS)	|PETER WALKS IN THE GARDEN.|
[4] (NS + VS + NS + PS)	|PETER THROWS THE BALL ON THE ROAD.|
[5] (NS + VS + PS + PS)	|PETER JUMPS OVER THE FENCE IN THE YARD.|

Within this first group, the VSs are action verbs. It is usually advisable to form a second group intended to re-establish use of the copula. Use of the verbs 'to be' and 'to have' (and 'to do' in English) is more complicated, since they can function as either main or auxiliary verbs. Their appropriate use must usually be the target of several varied exercises. The polysemic nature of the verb 'to be'* makes it particularly difficult, and each of its principal meanings, for example the expression of state ('He is sick') and of place ('He is in Marseilles'), must usually be treated separately:

[1] (NS + Cop + Adv)	|THE BOY IS FAR.|
[2] (NS + Cop + Adj)	|THE BOY IS BIG.|
[3] (NS + Cop + NS)	|PETER IS A MECHANIC.|
[4] (NS + Cop + PS)	|PETER IS IN THE ATTIC.|
etc.	

Exercises in expansion by coordination are then introduced, initially following an affirmative model of the type (NS + VS + NS):

[1] [nNS + VS + (nNS and nNS)]	|THE BOY OPENS THE WINDOW AND THE DOOR.|
[2] [nNS + (VS and VS) + nNS]	|THE BOY WASHES AND FIXES THE CAR.|

* In our work with French-speaking patients, the first stages of therapy involve almost exclusive emphasis on the present indicative. For English-speaking patients, we think that the continuous present (aux$^+$ing) tense should also be reviewed and could be appropriately introduced at this point. In exercises on the continuous present, the habitual use of contracted forms in spoken language should be respected when evaluating the patient's responses. (See Section on Negative Sentences.)

[3] [(nNS and nNS) +VS+nNS] |THE BOY AND THE MAN FIX THE CAR.|

[4] [nNS+(VS+nNS) and (VS+nNS)] |THE BOY OPENS THE DOOR AND WASHES THE WINDOW.|

etc.

It is not uncommon that structures of the last type must be approached through successive steps:

[1] |THE BOY OPENS THE DOOR.|
[2] |THE BOY WASHES THE WINDOW.|
[3] |THE BOY OPENS THE DOOR AND WASHES THE WINDOW.|
etc.

Negative sentences. Once affirmative declaratives have been re-acquired or almost mastered, a series of exercises on negative transformations is begun. The sequencing of these exercises is analogous to that described for affirmatives. The clinician should then respect certain dialectical features of spoken language, particularly the omission of *'ne'* (in French). However this remark applies only to the patient's responses: in effect, even if the complete form does not appear in the surface structure, it is nevertheless part of the speaker's competence (see Chapter 12). We have found that omission of the particle *'ne'* in the material presented by the clinician does not facilitate the patient's production but rather hinders it because the stimuli appear unnatural. In other words, the clinician should use the uncontracted negative form in the material presented to the patient (in repetition or in reading for example) but should not require it in the patient's productions.

Interrogative sentences. Exercises on the use of the interrogative generally follow those intended to facilitate production of negative transformations. Prosodic expression of interrogation, by a rising inflection at the end of the sentence, is the first to appear during language development[75] and remains frequent in adult language. Thus it is the focus of initial exercises on the interrogative for patients in whom the prosodic form is not preserved. Subsequent exercises are ordered with respect to data obtained from analyses of aphasic language[64–69, 74]: the easiest interrogatives are those introduced by interrogative words, that is, *quel* (what), *qui* (who), *où* (where), *quand* (when), *pourquoi* (why), *comment* (how), followed by those introduced by interrogative locutions, that is, *est-ce que* (is it that), *qu'est-ce que* (what is it that). Interrogatives requiring inversion of the respective functions of the subject and the verb are introduced last and only to those whose progress allows it.*

Sentences with a subordinate object clause (introduced by 'that' or 'what'). Inclusion of this structure at this stage in the progression was suggested to us only by the relative ease with which it is spontaneously produced by some agrammatics. This is perhaps related to the fact that the clause functions as the object of the sentence, a constituent which may be particularly well preserved in agrammatism.

Sentences with adverbial or relative clauses. The sequence of exercises ends with these complex structures. It should be emphasized that very few agrammatics achieve functional mastery in this regard. If it is considered worth while to present exercises on these structures, the stimuli should be in the form of a main clause followed by a subordinate clause.†

Notes on the sequencing of exercises with respect to different sentence constituents

The following statements provide general guidelines to the sequencing of the different functional elements of the target sentences.

Subject. Animate subjects precede inanimate ones and, within the animate group, (determiner + noun) and (proper nouns) precede (pronouns). To introduce the propositional use of personal pronouns, the therapist will often find it advantageous to resort to particularly evocative contextual situations and to the use of a simple, previously established code (speaker's finger pointing to own chest = 'I', circular movement of

* In English, the stress on the initial word of a WH-question appears to facilitate their production[65] so that they may generally be easier than yes–no questions which begin with an unstressed auxiliary.

† The passive transformation usually remains almost unavailable to agrammatic patients. In very favourable cases, the therapist may attempt to promote production through exercises in which the patient must transpose, into the passive voice, sentence stimuli which are presented, orally and in writing, in the active voice.

both hands = 'we', etc.). Third-person pronouns (he, she, it, they) can be readily introduced in a NS subject paradigm illustrated by pictures (e.g., Fig. 17-1). Particular attention is given to 'I' because of its very high frequency of usage in normal language and the usual tendency of agrammatic patients to omit it or to substitute the pronoun 'me'[66, 69].

Object. To avoid the additional difficulty associated with reversibility[76], it is better to begin with the inanimate object and to introduce the animate object later. In regard to subjects and objects, the therapist may find it useful to devote some exercises to certain syntagmatic expansions (which may be particularly difficult); for example, the use of attributive adjectives and predicative adjectives, the addition of a noun complement, etc. It is usually best to proceed in two stages, the exercises first being aimed at the syntagmatic expansion and then at its insertion into a sentence.

[1]	[(nNS + PS)]	|A PIECE OF CAKE.|
[2]	[nNS + VS + (nNS + PN)]	|THE BOY EATS A PIECE OF CAKE.|
	etc.	

Determiners. The definite article precedes the indefinite article which in turn precedes possessive adjectives and other determiners. Morphological variations are presented in the following order: number, person, and then gender.

Prepositions. The first prepositions introduced are those which (in French) are most directly dependent on the verb or the noun, namely *à* (to), *de* (of, from), *en* (in, to, at). They are followed by prepositions marking place, spatial relationships, time, goal and destination, instrument and agent, manner, etc. In the case of prepositions, it is particularly important to respect their frequency of use and their frequency of association with particular words. Prepositions can often be introduced through the use of facilitating contexts, that is, through ready-made expressions which include the target preposition. For example, the locution *une voiture de course* (racing car) would be introduced before *la voiture de Paul* (Paul's car) (or, in English, 'out of order' would be introduced before 'out of the box').

Verb inflections. In the first stages of therapy for agrammatism, the target syntactical structures are presented only in the present indicative. Expression of the future (immediate and simple future) and of the past is then taught, but review of all possible tenses and moods is generally worth while only in exceptional cases. Classical conjugation exercises may sometimes be a useful supplement to re-establish the association between verb inflections and the corresponding personal pronouns.* In therapy for morphological disturbances, it may be useful to present exercises in which the patient must construct sentences by arranging word cards and in which the selection of some words depends on that of morphological markers (e.g., personal pronouns, substantive subjects, adverbs of time).

Exercises centred on the use of derived and compound words (see Chapter 1, concept of a syntheme[77]) will be discussed later in the section on therapy for lexical disturbances. Use of these words, whose realization does not fall within the realm of morphology strictly defined, does not represent a problem which is particular to agrammatism. Although the disturbance involves both morphology and features which may be part of the clinical picture of agrammatism proper, therapy for disturbances affecting the use of monemes marking the gender (in French) and number of certain nouns and adjectives is incorporated (for empirical reasons) into exercises for the remediation of lexical disturbances. The problems of gender and number of certain grammatical words have already been mentioned.

In severe cases of agrammatism, the agrammatic character of discourse rarely disappears completely. Nevertheless, therapy helps to decrease it in many cases and it is not unusual to see patients who demonstrate continued improvement over a period of several years. Neither is it unusual to observe the relative fragility of the gains achieved. The evocation of relational words and appropriate grammatical structures remains slow and, in urgent situations, the most extensively re-educated patients will spontaneously revert to agrammatic forms of discourse. Once word-finding difficulty has been more or less overcome, the high information value of the

* Verbs are more highly inflected in French than in English.

agrammatic style makes it clearly more effective in urgent situations than language whose syntactical appropriateness is obtained only at the price of a considerable loss of time (see examples 2.88, 2.89 and 4.1).

PARAGRAMMATISM IN WERNICKE'S APHASIA

It is the clinical characteristics of agrammatism which determine the approach to its remediation (cf. pp. 52 and 86). The patient produces little speech and, during the first stages of evolution, his utterances are generally reduced to the juxtaposition of lexical words. There is an obvious disturbance specifically affecting syntax: in this regard, almost everything must be reviewed and experience demonstrates the soundness of a systematic therapy programme which is sequenced in order of increasing linguistic difficulty. It is also the clinical characteristics of dyssyntaxia, or paragrammatism, which determine the need for therapy and the approach to therapy. In the most typical cases, the patient speaks freely and his discourse includes both grammatical and lexical words in what appear to be almost normal proportions if repetitions indicative of word-finding difficulty (see Chapters 2 and 4) are ignored. However both grammatical and lexical words give rise to paraphasic substitutions which are more or less frequent, depending on the case and the stage of evolution of the patient's disease. Some of these substitutions, especially among those affecting grammatical words, result in dyssyntactic sentences[50, 78]. Nevertheless, the great majority of sentences are normal in terms of morphology and syntax, regardless of whether or not they contain paraphasic transformations. Furthermore, the ability to generate sentences following all types of syntactical patterns is well preserved (in spontaneous utterances), in contrast to what is observed in agrammatism. This is true even for such syntactically complex structures as subordinate, relative, and object clauses (see examples 2.83, 2.90, 4.20 and 4.28). Thus, in cases where it appears useful to attempt 'syntactical' therapy, it is clear that a therapy programme can be planned only after a detailed study of each patient's productions. In this regard, the most useful productions are obtained by asking the patient to tell a familiar story and to describe different pictures or scenes (see Chapter 15). Such samples can be analysed, at least to a certain point, by reference to a norm.

In certain cases of conduction aphasia, this analysis will permit the identification of a clear disturbance of syntax and, especially, of morphology (see Chapter 4). In our opinion, these patients are the only aphasics who produce a more or less major number of morphological errors in conversation, narration, and especially, in written compositions [(17.5) *'J'ai pris'*→*'J'ai prendu'* ('I took'→'I taken'), *'Je vais manger'*→*'Je vais mangerai'* ('I'm going to eat'→'I'm going to will eat')]. Although we cannot provide a definitive answer, it nevertheless seems worth while to question whether this clinical picture, which is relatively rare, might not suggest the possibility of a specific morphosyntactic disturbance which differs from agrammatism. However this may be, morphosyntactic therapy for these cases will be intuitively guided following those principles of therapy for agrammatism which appear most appropriate. Although this will generally involve the last stages of the programme for agrammatism outlined above, some flexibility is required because the nature of the therapy programme will be partially determined by an inventory of the various morphological and syntactical errors made by the patient. The sentence stimuli used in the therapy exercises will include correct examples of the syntactical structures erroneously produced by the patient. He will be asked to read the stimuli, to repeat them (if possible) and to reproduce them from memory in speech and in writing. Finally, the therapist will attempt to elicit the stimulus sentences and other structurally similar sentences during directed dialogue. Other useful procedures include written multiple-choice exercises in which the patient must select the matching card which shows the grammatical element needed to complete a grammatically incomplete stimulus sentence. Also useful are error scanning and/or correction exercises, exercises requiring the joining of sentence fragments written on different cards, and exercises requiring the selection of morphological markers with reference to other sentence constituents [e.g., choice of the morphological marker *'erons'* in the presence of the personal pronoun *'nous'* (we) and the adverb of time *'demain'* (tomorrow) (or, in English, choice of the marker ('s) given the words 'children' and 'shoes')]. When preparing these different exercises, the therapist attempts to follow an order of increasing linguistic complexity.

In the common forms of Wernicke's aphasia (see Chapter 4), an analysis of linguistic productions, at least of oral productions, almost always leads to the conclusion that, in these cases, there is not a specific disturbance of syntax. The utterances typically include paragrammatic transformations which vary in frequency among different cases. However, these transformations are not essentially different from the much more common paraphasic transformations which do not lead to a disorganization of the morphosyntactic dimension of discourse (see Chapter 2, concept of dyssyntaxia). Furthermore, in these patients, certain types of syntactical errors disappear when lexical retrieval improves. This may be the case, for example, for obviously wrong choices and for the repetition of articles and determiners whose frequency gradually decreases as word-finding difficulty lessens. Nevertheless, the clinician often considers it useful to devote some therapy sessions to the use of grammatical morphemes. Such sessions will usually be focused on the use of prepositions or of personal pronouns, since they are often erroneously selected in jargonaphasia, and less frequently on the use of coordinating and subordinating conjunctions and relative pronouns. The therapy procedures will reflect the fact that the common forms of Wernicke's aphasia are characterized by difficulty in word selection proper, rather than by difficulty in production, and that this is also true for verb inflections. If use of these markers is to be specifically treated in the therapy programme, the exercises will be focused on their selection and, especially, on their agreement in tense. It is probably advisable to follow an order of increasing linguistic difficulty in each aspect of morphosyntactical therapy but the importance of a sequential progression is much less crucial than in the case of agrammatism. While the general direction of therapy should always remain clear, the clinician must nevertheless be flexible in temporarily reorienting individual sessions according to the successes and failures of her patient. It is not uncommon for paragrammatism to be more marked in written than in oral expression so that the therapy exercises may emphasize the production of written language, depending on the patient's educational and cultural background. The materials used in the therapy exercises are very similar to those used in the last stages of therapy for agrammatism and in therapy for dyssyntaxia appearing in the clinical context of conduction aphasia (cf. p. 429). The differences between therapy for morphosyntactical disturbances in Broca's aphasics and in Wernicke's aphasics are far less evident in the linguistic materials of the exercises themselves than in the manner in which they are employed.

THERAPY FOR LEXICAL DISTURBANCES

Therapy for all 'true aphasias'—an expression of C. Foix[79] which excludes pure anarthria, pure agraphia (if it exists), pure word deafness and pure word blindness (see Chapters 3, 5 and 10)—includes a phase specifically aimed at the remediation of lexical impairment. In other words, a greater or lesser degree of word-finding difficulty (see Chapter 4) is observed in all 'true aphasias' and its modification must constitute the specific goal of a certain number of exercises as soon as it appears advisable to begin a therapy programme.

The physiopathology of word-finding difficulty is not well known but observations of aphasics suggest that it is not the same in all forms of aphasia[80]. On the one hand, patients with Broca's aphasia or conduction aphasia typically apprehend the links uniting corresponding meanings (*signifiés*) and forms (*signifiants*) but they experience difficulty in the evocation and production of the latter. In our experience, phonemic cueing with exaggerated visual information is often an effective type of facilitation for these patients. On the other hand, patients presenting a common form of Wernicke's aphasia or Pitres' aphasia typically have little difficulty in emitting words but do have difficulty in apprehending certain links between meanings and forms[21]. In the common forms of Wernicke's aphasia, this results in disturbed comprehension and paraphasic word usage. In Pitres' aphasia, the semantic disturbance is more subtle but nevertheless demonstrable (and moreover, may be only quantitatively different from that of the common forms). It is perhaps because of the absence of anosognosia in Pitres' aphasia that word-finding difficulty is manifested by circumlocutory productions rather than by paraphasic productions. Facilitation by phonemic cueing is generally less effective for these patients than for

Broca's aphasics. Although they suggest physiopathological differences, these behavioural distinctions, which are not always very clear-cut, do not provide a basis for an explicit dichotomy in the development of remedial exercises for lexical impairment in the various clinical forms of aphasia. Here again, those features of therapy which are specifically related to the clinical form of aphasia are less evident in the content of the therapy exercises than in the manner of their use and in the exchanges which are established between the clinician and the patient. The nature of these differences will become increasingly clear to each clinician during the course of accumulated experience in aphasia therapy.

Although the exercises to be discussed here are primarily intended to increase the vocabulary available for propositional use, it is clear that they are not exclusively focused on the lexical disturbance. As we have indicated in the previous paragraph, this term encompasses a varied group of behaviours and it should not be assumed that it designates a precise pathological entity. Word retrieval exercises may be preceded by ones in which the patient must identify (by pointing or matching responses) words spoken by the clinician so that lexical therapy is related to therapy for disturbed comprehension (cf. p. 434). Similarly, when working on lexical exercises, the therapist soon requires that the elicited words be used in appropriate linguistic contexts so that therapy for word-finding difficulty is related to morphosyntactic therapy (cf. p. 427). The headings used in the present chapter reflect divisions necessary for didactic purposes and should not be thought to imply that aphasia therapy can be fragmented into unrelated units.

The preparation of word-finding exercises is influenced by findings from linguistics and related domains in psycholinguistics and neurolinguistics (see Chapter 12): distributional analyses; studies of the frequency of word usage, such as those* by Gougenheim[81] in Europe or by Vikis-Freibergs in Quebec[82]; studies on the organization of semantic fields (work by Mounin[85], Fodor[86], and Greimas[87] appears particularly relevant), studies on the most effective types of facilitation in the different forms of aphasia (see Chapter 4); Jakobson's research[88] leading to a distinction, with regard to aphasic disorganizations of the first linguistic phase, between disorders of word selection and those of the integration of words into sentences; qualitative studies of semantic paraphasias in aphasia and investigations of aphasic difficulties in apprehending the existence and in recognizing the extent of meaningful relationships which may exist between words[89]. Lexical therapy always includes exercises in oral and written word finding but, depending on particular cases, these exercises may or may not be preceded by oral reading and copying exercises or exercises requiring word identification or matching, multiple-choice selection of target words from a list enumerated by the therapist or presented on separate cards, or word classification. Such facilitating procedures are frequently used at the start of therapy but are progressively discarded as the focus of therapy gradually shifts from an emphasis on word retrieval exercises to the use of re-acquired vocabulary in the context of directed dialogue. When appropriate, lexical therapy progresses to a point where it merges with syntactical therapy.

When lexical reduction is clearly evident, the first stage of lexical therapy almost always consists of naming exercises: this early stage is intended to promote recovery of a basic vocabulary. The initial series of exercises should be based on words which have been carefully selected so that they are semantically diverse and have a high frequency of usage. Refinements are introduced into later series: on the one hand, the patient is asked to name not only each stimulus but also its different parts (e.g., first 'watch' and then its 'hands' and 'bracelet'; first 'leaf' and then its 'stem' and 'veins'; 'lighter' then 'flame' and 'flint'); on the other hand, the words included within each exercise have lower frequencies of usage and are increasing related in terms of conceptual association (e.g., chicken - table - book - etc., then chicken - dog - fish - etc., then chicken - owl - parrot - etc., then chicken - turkey - duck - etc.). During this first stage of therapy, the use of drawings and pictures is generally necessary and simultaneous presentation of the written words corresponding to the pictures is frequently advantageous. Because of their rich illustrations and attention to the structure of the lexicon, various teaching publications (for example, *l'Imagier de Père Castor*[90]) can provide appropriate materials for many therapy sessions. Once a stage has been reached where the help of

* Or, in English, those by Thorndike and Lorge[83] or Howes[84].

facilitating cues is no longer required for the retrieval of basic vocabulary items, it is often useful to reinforce their availability by devoting some time to exercises in *rotated naming* (*dénominations alternées*), a procedure described by Ombredane[41]. The patient is presented with a pictured object which he is asked to name at his own speed and in the absence of facilitating cues. After correct naming, a second picture is presented in the same way. Correct naming is then followed by another presentation of the first stimulus to verify the continued availability of the appropriate response. The second picture is then presented again and, when both the first and second have been successfully named, a third picture is introduced. Evocation of the third word is followed by the presentation of the first two stimuli, etc. This method is one which we have found to be particularly useful in therapy for patients with amnesic aphasia.

For Broca's aphasics who show a tendency towards agrammatism, it is important that the lexical exercises are regularly followed by others aimed at the use of recovered vocabulary within the context of short sentences. This is the case if it means that the series of lexical exercises must be completed more slowly, and is true not only for the early exercises which we have outlined above but also for other exercises which we shall now describe. These exercises are somewhat more linguistically orientated (although they cannot be reconciled with rigorous linguistic purism) and are intended for use in the second stage of lexical therapy, that is, in the stage which follows recovery of a certain basic vocabulary. These exercises are all aimed towards the associated production of words which are defined in relation to others by different types of semantic associations. We have not included an exhaustive listing of all possible types of such exercises. Rather we have described basic therapy procedures, intended for therapists who have not yet developed their own batteries, and limited discussion to comments on those exercises which we have found useful in our own work with aphasics.

Antonyms. A stimulus word is presented orally or in writing and the patient's task is to find a word of opposite meaning or, during preliminary exercises, to select the antonym from a list of words spoken by the therapist or written on separate cards. This type of exercise is particularly suited to adjectives (pretty↔ugly; thick↔thin; useful↔useless) but may also involve pairs of substantives which are antonyms or are generally opposed in everyday usage (summer↔winter; day↔night; sugar↔salt), as well as verbs involving opposite actions (pull↔push; empty↔fill; buy↔sell). By providing contextual elements in the case of words having multiple meanings, the therapist can attempt to elicit several antonyms ('hard' referring to a physical-attribute→soft; 'hard' referring to difficulty→easy). Two types of exercises should be distinguished, the first requiring the production of *morphological opposites* (*bound opposition*: useful→useless; patient→impatient; logical→illogical) and the second requiring production of *lexical opposites* (*free opposition*: pretty→ugly; good→bad; true→false)[91]. Production of the former may be relatively more difficult than that of the latter in cases of Broca's aphasia with agrammatism or conduction aphasia with dyssyntaxia while the opposite dissociation may sometimes be observed in the common forms of Wernicke's aphasia and, even more clearly, in amnesic aphasia[66] (see Chapter 4). Where evident, these differences in relative difficulty will be taken into consideration when planning word-retrieval exercises for particular patients.

Synonyms. Analogous exercises can be carried out with synonyms. In this case, the patient's task is to retrieve as many synonyms or near-synonyms as possible in response to a stimulus word presented orally or in writing (dirty→soiled, stained, filthy, muddy; silly→foolish, senseless; stupid, simple).

Derived words. The therapist presents a spoken or written stimulus word and, if necessary, supporting information in the form of incomplete linguistic contexts or short definitions. The patient's task is to supply some derived forms of the stimulus word (front→affront, frontier, forefront; form→inform, formation, formal, format, reform). Certain classes of words which are easily paired, for example, names of work sites and occupations, (bank→banker; pharmacy→pharmacist; bakery→baker)* can pro-

* Additional exercises may be presented in parallel. They are analogous but involve words which are paired on a purely conceptual basis (hospital↔doctor; school↔teacher; garage↔mechanic).

vide material for exercises in derivation. It is relatively unimportant whether or not this type of exercise is considered to be part of morphological therapy rather than of lexical therapy. What is important is that the exercises be selected as a function of the facts observed during the aphasiological assessment of the patient (cf. p. 428).

Compound words. Similar exercises can be done using stimulus lexemes which constitute the first element of a compound word (key→keyhole, keyboard, keynote, keypunch, keystone; sun→sunrise, sunset, sunflower, sunburn, sunshine, sunlight, sunbeam, sunspot). The patient's educational and cultural background must be carefully considered when selecting stimulus words and those whose usage is to be promoted by these exercises.

Categories. The stimulus is a word designating a category of similar items and the patient's task is to retrieve the name of some category members (tools→hammer, screwdriver, saw, etc.; clothes→dress, coat, socks, etc.). In this type of exercise, the extent of the stimulus category can be gradually narrowed (animals, then four-legged animals, then four-legged domestic animals, four-legged animals in a zoo, etc.).* The therapist will initially provide information and assistance but the patient's productions must become increasingly autonomous. In this regard, it is often useful to present these exercises after some preliminary tasks in which the patient selects appropriate exemplars of a specified category from a group of words written on separate cards.

Other conceptual associations. Other analogous exercises may be used. The patient may be asked to name the parts of a whole specified by the stimulus name (car→engine, wheels, steering wheel, windshield, hood, headlights, etc.; tree→roots, trunk, branches, leaves, bark, fruit, etc.), or to retrieve, in a relatively unstructured manner, words which bear some conceptual relation to a specified stimulus heading† (winter→snow, cold, skiing, Christmas, mitts, season, etc.; geography→travel, school, country, ocean, globe, Africa, etc.). It may be useful to first carry out this type of exercise in the presence of iconographic support. The most useful illustrations have two advantages. First, they permit the introduction of more abstract and/or relatively low frequency words into the word finding exercises. Second, in the more advanced stages of therapy, the patient's productions may provide material which is particularly well suited to exercises involving the integration of recovered vocabulary into progressively more complex sentences (cf. pp. 420–429).

Paradigms.‡ The stimulus consists of an incomplete sentence with the omitted element being a lexical word. The sentence is presented orally and in writing and the therapist provides explanations and any needed examples. The patient must evoke different words which would each be appropriate to fill the blank in the stimulus sentence ('Peter buys a ______ in the department store'→comb, sweater, screwdriver, pencil, corkscrew, etc.; 'Peter lives in a ______ house'→big, small, old, new, beautiful, magnificent, etc.). As illustrated by the second example, this type of exercise can be particularly useful in promoting the recovery of lexical elements other than substantives.

Homonyms. The stimulus word has multiple meanings and the patient's task is to produce different words which are each related to one of the possible meanings. In the case of *homographs*, the stimulus word may be presented orally and in writing (mean→dog, temperature, well; tap→water, dance, telephone). In the case of *homophones*, that is, homonyms whose different meanings are associated with different spelling patterns, the therapist tries to proceed using stimuli which are only presented orally (/si/→view, waves, letter; /pɛr/→gloves, fruit, cut). In cases where the patient is unable to respond, the therapist facilitates correct production by presentation of written cues (/si/—see, sea, c; /pɛr/—pair, pear, pare). Other types of exercises may also be centred on homonyms: thus the patient may be asked to write the stimulus word

* At this point, lexical therapy merges with therapy for disturbed comprehension.

† For certain patients, it may be advantageous to begin with exercises in which the clinician enumerates lists of words and asks the patient to respond to each stimulus as quickly as possible by uttering the first word which comes to mind. In these exercises, the 'best' words produced in response to previous stimuli may then be presented as stimuli on subsequent trials.

‡ See definition of this term in Chapter 2 (p. 36).

in short syntagms, each of which illustrates one of the possible contextual meanings (turn→turn down an offer, turn back in time, turn over a page, turn to a friend, turn off the lights, a turn of a screw, do a good turn, take your turn, to turn a phrase, a turn for the worse; /saɪt/→out of sight, a sight for sore eyes, sightseers, to cite a verse, site of the explosion).

Semantic analysis and synthesis. In synthesis exercises, certain features of a word are listed by the therapist or provided in a short definition. The patient's task is then to produce the appropriate word ('part of a car which controls its direction'→steering wheel; 'the shortest line between two points'→straight; 'a count of all people who live in a country'→census). The procedure is reversed in analysis exercises, where the stimulus is a single word and the patient attempts to list semantic features or provide a short definition (the stimulus 'horse'→animal, domestic, etc.). It is often advisable to present these exercises after preliminary ones in which the patient can select elements of his response from words which are written on separate cards.

THERAPY FOR DISTURBANCES OF ORAL LANGUAGE COMPREHENSION

Although comprehension of spoken language is generally not completely intact in Broca's aphasia or in conduction aphasia, the observed impairment is relatively mild (see Chapters 4 and 15) and may often show spontaneous improvement. In cases where it is considered worth while to integrate exercises specifically aimed at linguistic decoding into the patient's therapy programme, they will usually be centred on the comprehension of grammatical words and of the general meaning of discourse (i.e., the comprehension of wholes). On the other hand, the therapy programme will be much more comprehensive for Wernicke's aphasics and, if therapy appears useful, for global aphasics. In both cases, partial spontaneous improvement of spoken language comprehension is quite often observed (when the aphasia is not a result of progressive disease) and recovery is probably accelerated, or even accentuated, by the early and intensive use of various exercises.

In cases of Wernicke's aphasia, a therapy programme can generally be started as soon as the anosognosia and logorrhoea have decreased (cf. p. 412, pre-language therapy). We shall here discuss the main characteristics of two therapy approaches. The first is intended for aphasics whose difficulties in oral comprehension are especially related to failures in the recognition of the auditory features of spoken language [agnosic disturbance of oral comprehension; auditory aspect; word deafness (see Chapters 4 and 5)]. The second approach is intended for aphasics who demonstrate normal discrimination of auditory features but nevertheless present impaired comprehension resulting from a rupture of the links between linguistic forms and meanings, that is, from difficulty in associating linguistic stimuli with traces of past experience which impart meaning to the stimuli [phasic—psycholinguistic—disturbance of oral comprehension (see Chapter 4)]. Here again, it is as much for didactic purposes as in recognition of actual symptomatological configurations that we clearly distinguish between these two types of disturbances. Nevertheless, the clinical picture is very often mixed so that, for many patients, the therapy programme should involve a combination of the two suggested approaches.

AGNOSIC DISTURBANCES OF ORAL COMPREHENSION

The auditory basis of an oral comprehension disturbance can be easily recognized only when the comprehension of written language is normal, or at least much less disturbed, than the comprehension of spoken language (see Insertion 8.2). The severity of the oral comprehension disturbance is of prime importance in regard to the prognosis for recovery and consequently, in regard to decisions about the advisability of an intensive therapy programme. When word deafness is severe, the prognosis for recovery of oral comprehension may be very poor regardless of the efforts extended during language therapy. On the other hand, there is hope for some improvement, which is probably at least partially related to therapy, when word deafness is of moderate severity at onset. As a complement, the prognosis is relatively better if the underlying lesions, which are usually the result of a cerebral vascular accident, are left temporal rather than bi-temporal (see Chapters 8 and 9).

In general, the exercises centred on an agnosic disturbance of oral comprehension attempt to improve the discrimination of linguistic forms (i.e., sounds)[92, 93]. To ensure that the exercises are appropriate, the therapist first determines the level of segmental complexity at which the patient shows difficulty in discriminating phonemic contrasts. This can be examined using multiple-choice procedures in which the patient points to written stimuli corresponding to those presented orally by the therapist. Is difficulty apparent at the level of isolated monosyllables? If so, does the disturbance even affect phonemes belonging to the same paradigm but sharing few constituent features [/bi↔si/ (see Chapter 2)], or does it affect only contrasts between structurally related phonemes (/bi↔pi/)? Or again, does the discrimination difficulty only become evident in the context of longer and more complex segments (baby↔body /bebɪ↔bɑdɪ/; rocket↔pocket /rɑkɪt↔pɑkɪt/; filling↔fishing /fɪlɪŋ↔fɪʃɪŋ/; cattle↔camel /kætl↔kæml/; bowling↔boating /bolɪŋ↔botɪŋ/; button↔mutton /bʌtn↔mʌtn/; medal↔metal /mɛdl↔mɛtl/; thread↔shred /θrɛd↔ʃrɛd/; prices↔prizes /praɪsɪz↔praɪzɪz/; knife↔fine /naɪf↔faɪn/; potato↔tomato /pəteto↔təmeto/; magazine↔mezzanine /mægəzin↔mɛzənin/); etc. Once the effects of factors related to stimuli, especially to their length and phonological complexity, have been explored, the therapist will determine whether the rate at which the stimuli are spoken,* stimulus repetition and the emphasis of contrasting phonemes have a facilitating or an adversive effect.

Having identified the threshold of segmental complexity above which oral comprehension is impaired, the therapist then considers different details of the therapy programme. On the basis of our empirically defined approach, we suggest that therapy be composed of three stages[21]† with materials selected according to the principles of increasing similarity and complexity.

The first stage of therapy is based on exercises involving maximal facilitation of auditory analysis, that is on exercises combining oral and written stimulus presentation. The sessions carried out by the therapist can be supplemented as needed by periods in which the patient works alone using a tape recorder or a *Language Master*. Because it permits the simultaneous presentation of auditory and visual stimuli, as well as any needed recording and playback of the patient's own productions, the *Language Master* proves to be a valuable accessory in certain cases. As therapy progresses, presentation of written stimuli is gradually faded, thus marking the end of the first stage of therapy.

In the next stage, exercises are ordered to include progressively more complex linguistic stimuli (words, sentences) which are spoken by the clinician and matched to their corresponding picture by the patient. In the first exercises, the patient must select the appropriate picture from a group which illustrate words having no formal relationship to each other ('hat' among 'sheep', 'hat', 'train'; 'pillow' among 'donkey', 'pillow', 'cup'; 'fly' among 'bolt', 'house', 'fly'). Subsequent exercises require a choice among pictures illustrating words from the same field of forms ('hat' among 'hat', 'cat', 'mat'; 'pillow' among 'window', 'pillow', 'willow'; 'fly' among 'pie', 'fly', 'tie'). In this type of exercise, patients whose disturbed comprehension is due to an agnosic disorder will often make spontaneous attempts at speech reading (lip reading). If this visual facilitation no longer appears to be required after a certain period of therapy, the therapist will gradually remove it by using a card to cover the lower part of her face when speaking. On the other hand, if it becomes clear that the patient can progress only by improving his speech reading skills, the therapist will attempt to facilitate such learning by initially exaggerating her buccophonatory movements. At times it may even be useful to have the patient mimic these movements in the hope that the visual message will be paired with proprioceptive feedback.

In the final stage, for those who progress to this point, therapy consists mainly of exercises in audiophonatory and audiographic transposition (lists of words and syntagms are repeated and written to dictation). In the beginning, the patient prepares for these exercises by reading the stimuli, first orally and then silently. This

* Slowness of decoding is the main problem in certain patients (see Chapter 1; Lordat's self-observation[94]).

† When possible, regular reading exercises are also recommended, even in cases of severe word deafness (where significant improvement in oral language comprehension is not expected): they are then intended to reduce the tendency, generally observed in these cases, towards a progressive decrease in vocabulary and a progressive increase in the production of phonemic paraphasias (see Chapter 5).

written facilitation is later removed. As in other stages of therapy, the stimuli are initially short and include large contrasts and subsequently become longer and include minimal contrasts (/bi↔si/ then /bi↔mi/ before /bɪt↔kɪt/ then /bɪt↔pɪt/, with these last two contrasts preceding billow↔willow /bɪlo↔wɪlo/ then billow↔pillow /bɪlo↔pɪlo/ etc.). Generally speaking, we find it useful to work first on initial contrasts, then on final contrasts, and lastly, on contrasts between medial sounds (/bæt↔kæt and bæt↔pæt/, then /bæt↔bæk and bæt↔bæd/ and then /bæt↔bɪt and bæt↔bʌt/). Stimuli consisting of longer words or sentences are also arranged in order of increasing length and increasing similarity of phonemic contrasts. The exercises are presented in an increasing order of difficulty and, whenever possible, involve a progression from a single contrast to multiple contrasts.

PHASIC (PSYCHOLINGUISTIC) COMPREHENSION DISTURBANCES

In certain aphasics, the recognition and elementary discrimination of the constituent features of language remains nearly normal but a rupture of the links between forms and meanings (*signifiants-signifiés*) results in impaired comprehension of both oral and written language. One speaks of a phasic, or psycholinguistic, disorder proper. The disturbance may be mild or severe, depending on the case and the time elapsed since onset (see Chapters 4 and 8). In cases where the aphasia is not associated with a massive lesion or progressive disease, it is our opinion that therapy will often accelerate and complement a tendency towards partial spontaneous improvement (see Chapter 11). When planning and instituting a therapy programme, it should be borne in mind that in the case of a phasic disturbance of comprehension, short sentences are generally better understood than are isolated words (see Chapter 4). The therapist will also take into account the fact that increased stimulation may sometimes enable patients to grasp the meaning of a stimulus which was not previously understood. A common way of increasing stimulation is by pairing the auditory stimulus with the corresponding written message. When such visual facilitation is used, it must be gradually withdrawn as soon as possible.

Here again, the therapy is carried out in stages and progresses from simple to more complex exercises.

During the initial stage, which is only necessary in cases of a severe phasic disturbance of comprehension, therapy is initially aimed at the production of short replies to concrete linguistic stimuli. Propositioned usage, particularly of 'yes' and 'no', is fostered in the context of questions about the patient's family and work and, especially, about people and objects in the patient's immediate environment, that is, in the therapy setting. The therapist will frequently find it necessary, especially at the beginning, to increase available stimulation by repeating questions, rephrasing them in different words, pairing them with visual and auditory support, etc.: these forms of facilitation should be removed as soon as possible. Even if very simple responses are required, the therapist must take the possible occurrence of paraphasias into account when evaluating the patient's level of comprehension. Paraphasic transformations, which do not necessarily indicate failures in comprehension, may occur in the context of very simple productions and involve the mutual substitution of 'yes' and 'no'. They can sometimes be detected by a dissociation between the patient's utterance and facial expression or gestures or by the spontaneous correction of the initial utterance.

In subsequent exercises, the patient successively identifies spoken stimuli by pointing to the appropriate illustration in a group of matching pictures. When beginning these exercises, it is often necessary to use gestures, to repeat directions, etc., in order to focus the patient's attention on the multiple-choice stimuli. Because of possible attentional deficits, the visual stimuli should be composed of clear, high-quality drawings or reproductions. We suggest the following progression for the first matching exercises:*

1. Identification by pointing to pictures of objects successively named by the therapist (the target name is presented in the context of a

* The next section of the text has three headings with a separate progression described for each one. There is also an implied progression from one heading to the other: first, identification of names by pointing to a picture in a group of unrelated pictures, then identification from description by pointing to a picture in a group of unrelated pictures, then identification of names by pointing to a picture among a group of semantically related ones, etc.

short sentence in which it is the only important semantic element). The group of matching pictures is initially composed of unrelated items (the patient must point to 'apple' among pictures of a tie, apple and chicken; 'scarf' among pictures of a pear, scarf and turkey; 'duck' among lemon, belt and duck). Later, the matching pictures represent items from the same semantic field (the patient must point to 'apple' among pictures of a pear, apple and lemon; 'scarf' among pictures of a tie, scarf and belt; 'duck' among chicken, turkey and duck). In many cases, it is useful to do some exercises of this type on the names of colours, geometric forms, and body parts (the patient must point to 'red' among illustrations of red, pipe, and table and then 'red' among yellow, red and green; 'square' among illustrations of a bottle, a tyre, and a square and then 'square' among a square, triangle and rectangle; 'nose' among pictures of a lighter, nose and pencil and then 'nose' among ear, chin and nose). In addition, for certain lexical paradigms, a single complex picture may be presented and the patient asked to point out different parts (the wheels, bumper and headlights of a car; a cow's muzzle, horns and tail; a man's knee, elbow and neck). These early comprehension exercises can often be usefully paired with picture and/or written word categorization tasks in which the stimuli are grouped according to different conceptual headings (hammer, screwdriver, plane, etc. under 'tools'; radish, turnip, beet, etc. under 'vegetables'). These are tasks which some patients can carry out on their own after a preparatory period supervised by the therapist.

2. The patient then progresses to identification-by-pointing exercises in which the therapist does not name the stimulus but rather defines or briefly describes it. If the patient has word-finding difficulty, as is usually the case, a lexical dimension is added to these exercises by asking for the name in response to the double stimulation provided by the therapist's description and the correctly selected picture. The therapy materials may be almost the same as those used in the preceding exercises and are presented in an analogous sequence (the patient identifies 'a tool used to pound nails' among pictures of an apple, hammer and rabbit and then among pictures of a hammer, screwdriver and plane; 'a geometric form with four equal sides' among pictures of an ashtray, glove and square and then among a triangle, square and rectangle).
3. The final series of identification exercises requires the matching of pictures to action words which are spoken by the therapist. Here again, the matching pictures are presented in an order of increasing conceptual similarity (the patient must identify 'The girl is drinking water' among pictures illustrating a girl drinking water, a dog biting a thief and a man smoking a cigarette; and then the stimulus 'The boy is pushing the car' among pictures showing a boy washing a car, a boy pushing a car, and a boy driving a car; 'The man smokes a cigarette' among pictures of a man holding a lighter, a man filling his pipe, and a man smoking a cigarette; and 'The girl reads a letter' among pictures of a girl writing a letter, a girl reading a letter, and a girl reading a book).

In the above exercises, the patient identifies a spoken stimulus by selecting the corresponding picture from a group of matching pictures. It may be useful to present other exercises in which picture matching is determined by the corresponding written stimuli, each one being presented on a separate card. When therapy materials are organized so that the written stimuli review those previously presented in spoken form, the patient may sometimes be able to complete these exercises on his own.

In some cases, the above exercises, based on picture matching, can be profitably followed by others in which the patient identifies spoken stimuli by selecting the corresponding written one from a group of written stimuli. These exercises follow the same principles outlined above (selection among written stimuli which are at first unrelated and later among written stimuli from the same semantic field) but when appropriate, the use of written materials permits an increase in the level of linguistic difficulty beyond that which can be achieved using picture matching tasks. Relatively abstract substantives and verbs, attributive adjectives etc. cannot be easily pictured but can be readily introduced in the context of multiple choice tasks involving selection from a group of written stimuli.

After mastery or near mastery of the identification by matching exercises, the patient advances to exercises centred on the execution of increasingly complex spoken commands. The materials for these exercises consist of progressively larger and less disparate groups of objects. Increasing complexity of the commands is ensured by controlling the number of objects, their nature, and the natural and imposed relations between them. It is also controlled by the nature of the commands: from usual to arbitrary ('Put the cup on the saucer'→'Put the fork in the cup'); from explicit to implicit ('Give me the pencil and paper'→'Give me what I need to write'); from general to more specific ('Give me a cup'→'Give me a green cup'); and from simple to multiple ('Give me the yellow pencil'→'Give me the yellow pencil and put the blue one in your pocket').

At this stage, a certain period of therapy must often be specifically focused on the comprehension of morphological markers and grammatical words and structures. For some categories, this can be approached using exercises in which spoken stimuli are identified by pointing to pictures ('Show me the cat *on*, *under*, *in front of*, *behind* the chair'); ('Show me *the horse*, *the horses; the book, the books*'; 'Show me *your*, *my*, *his* shoes'; etc.). Subsequent exercises involve the execution of arbitrary commands requiring comprehension of object–object relations ('Put the pencil *in*, *under* the box) or object–person relations ('Give the apple to *me*, *him*'; 'Give it to *me*, *him*'). Mime and gestures may be useful supports when these exercises are first introduced but their use should be as limited as possible and soon discontinued. At the end of this stage of therapy, it may be convenient to use tokens and increasingly difficult commands from the Token Test[95] (see Chapter 16) or equivalent exercises.

The final stages of therapy for a phasic disturbance of comprehension merge with the final stage of therapy for word-finding difficulty (cf. p. 430). They are based on stories tape-recorded by the therapist, texts read by the patient, picture sequences, or films whose plots become increasingly more complicated and less obvious. The patient's task is to provide a suitable title, summarize the story and answer questions about the meaning of different grammatical and lexical units in the particular contexts in which they occur. At an advanced stage, the texts used in these exercises are based on multiple word meanings, homophones and homographs, implicit communication, puns and other humorous forms and, finally, absurdities.

THERAPY FOR DISTURBANCES OF WRITTEN EXPRESSION

Two factors are of prime importance in relation to disturbances of written language, namely the patient's educational level and habitual use of written language since completing his formal education. Quite often, a third factor, which is partially related to the first two, must also be considered, that is, the premorbid existence of dysorthographia (cultural or developmental). In certain cases, the disturbance of written language can be adequately appreciated only by inspecting samples produced before the onset of aphasia. In any event, information on these factors must be as complete as possible in order to permit appropriate planning of an eventual therapy programme.

Nowadays, clinicians working with aphasic populations usually encounter patients who present one of two main cultural profiles with respect to written linguistic expression.

In the first case, the patients have usually received an elementary education (often interrupted) and have sometimes even completed higher grades. However, their subsequent employment required little writing and their acquired skills were seldom practised. They continued to sign their names on various papers (and often remain able to do so despite their aphasia) and occasionally wrote short letters and grocery lists. Reading remained laborious or gradually became so through lack of practice and, in some cases, was almost totally limited to the headlines and eye-catching announcements of a weekend paper. Given these conditions, it is scarcely reasonable to focus an entire section of the therapy programme on the disturbance of written expression (which in these cases, more than in others and despite the clinical form of aphasia, is readily manifested by a suppression or severe reduction). On the other hand, if written language is at least partially spared, and the patient's symptomatology suggests its feasibility or advisability, it may be advantageous to use written language as a support during exercises which are primarily intended to promote recovery of spoken language.

In the second case, the patients' education was sufficient to ensure firm mastery of written language and, more importantly, reading and writing were integrated into their usual activities after their education was completed. Therapy specifically aimed at the recovery of written expression should usually be attempted with patients in this group unless ruled out by the clinical form of aphasia, the nature of associated neurological disorders or the aetiology of the causal disease.

A disturbance of written expression is, by definition, absent in the clinical picture of pure anarthria.* On the other hand, it is present in an isolated state, and limited to the properly graphic aspects of writing, in pure agraphia (see Chapters 3 and 6). In pure word deafness, written expression is impaired only when writing to dictation. In pure word blindness, anomalies of written expression are confined to servile copying and to occasional errors attesting to a lack of self-monitoring which is normally ensured, as production progresses, by continuous feedback (see Chapter 5). In all the other forms of aphasia, the clinical picture may include, among other aphasic impairments, a significant disturbance of written expression (see Chapter 4). It may affect all three phases of written expression (see Chapter 2), as is often the case in Broca's aphasia, or may spare graphic execution and be evident only at the second and first linguistic phases. The disturbance may sometimes be clearly predominant at one or the other of these two phases. In therapy for written expression, disturbances of graphic execution (third phase) and of orthography (second phase) are treated separately from oral expressive disturbances. On the other hand, therapy for the lexical and morphosyntactical aspects of written expression is paired with that for oral expression when written exercises are primarily intended to reinforce recently recovered aspects of oral expression. In the few cases where lexical and morphosyntactical therapy focused specifically on written language appears worth while, it will be deferred until the final stage of the patient's therapy programme.

THERAPY FOR IMPAIRED WRITING (GRAPHIC EXECUTION)

Broca's aphasia is typically associated with a right-sided motor deficit which often precludes use of the dominant hand for writing. When this situation appears permanent, attempts will be made to improve left hand control of writing movements. Pretraining in occupational therapy, intended to increase fine motor control of the left hand, is then indicated.

When a right-handed aphasic must use his left hand for writing, the therapy exercises are primarily aimed at the acquisition of the movements involved in writing, a goal which obviously will be more easily attained in the absence of an associated left-side apraxia (see Chapter 4). Experience also demonstrates that left-handed writing is more quickly mastered by certain 'right-handers' whose hemispheric dominance for handedness was not absolute[12] (see Chapter 11). When the right upper limb is spared or sufficiently intact to permit continued use of the right hand for written expression, the observed impairment may reflect, as in the case of an articulatory disturbance (see Chapter 3), paretic, dystonic or dyspraxic components. Either at onset or during evolution, one of these components may clearly be the predominant source of the graphic impairment. One speaks of apraxic agraphia, whether the lesion is frontal or parietal, in cases where muscular force and tone do not appear to explain, or no longer explain, the observed impairment.

In therapy for graphic execution proper, the exercises are generally the same regardless of which hand is used for writing and whether the impairment is related to paretic, dystonic or dyspraxic factors.

The first stage entails the graphic reproduction of forms corresponding to different segments of letters (see Chapter 2, concept of graphic features). When beginning the exercises, the therapist uses her hand to guide that of the patient, which initially remains a passive tool. If all goes well, the patient soon takes the initiative, something the therapist easily perceives through the pressure exerted by the patient's hand against her own. On this signal, when the patient's initiatives appear adequate, the therapist gradually decreases her participation and allows the patient to work alone.

When the patient has achieved satisfactory unaided control of the production of graphic features, the next exercises entail the production of letters by using a pencil to follow their con-

* Ignoring the natural awkwardness of left-handed writing in cases where an associated hemiplegia precludes writing with the right hand.

tours on dotted outlines. The patient first traces letters which involve continuous movements and the fewest directional changes and later progresses to those requiring discrete movements and more directional changes[21]. Appropriately sequenced exercises for this stage of therapy can be found in certain workbooks used in elementary schools.

Subsequent exercises are centred on the servile copying of letters, and then of progressively longer words, and may be more or less extended depending on the case.

Simple copying is then followed by transposed copying (from print to cursives or vice versa). Although the use of cursives is more conventional, printed letters may be more legible, especially in the presence of motor deficits affecting the hand used for writing. The transcription exercises will emphasize production in whichever mode (print or cursives) appears to be most appropriate for habitual use by each patient.

The final stage of therapy for graphic impairment is based on writing to dictation exercises. Their complexity and the frequency and duration of therapy will be determined by the needs of individual patients.

THERAPY FOR DYSORTHOGRAPHIA

In certain languages, including French and English, the rules governing the transition from the oral to the written code are needlessly complex, frequently arbitrary and sometimes so restrictively applied that they are confined to exceptions (Insertion 17.4). These factors favour the emergence of dysorthographia of either cultural or biological origin. Like word-finding difficulty, dysorthographia may belong, and usually does belong, to the clinical picture of most forms of aphasia (see Insertion 19.1) and, again like word-finding difficulty, it may be the precursor or the residual of a symptomatological constellation which includes many other elements. Two principles relative to therapy for an aphasic dysorthographia emerge from these preliminary considerations. First, in cases where therapy appears advisable, the goals should not exceed the patient's premorbid performance and often must remain below this level. Second, even though the therapist may occasionally correct spelling during various therapy exercises, it is generally better to delay exercises specifically aimed at the dysorthographia until later stages of the therapy programme. They are often introduced only in the stage of *residual dysorthographia*[21], a stage which is common when the patient's premorbid cultural background, as well as the nature, site and extent of the aphasia producing cerebral lesion, permit a favourable evolution of his aphasia.

Many school books can be used as sources of material when planning therapy to improve spelling. However, the exercises must be carefully selected so that they progress from the simple to the more complex. In the earlier stages of therapy, it may be useful, when this is not ruled out by the clinical form of aphasia, to combine copying with oral spelling and then oral spelling with writing to dictation. In therapy with French-speaking patients, a series of exercises on the spelling of words containing graphemic homophones (see Chapter 2) cannot be avoided.* In addition, exercises emphasizing the orthographic aspects or morphosyntactical agreements (*les accords*) are usually necessary. Here again, school books provide useful material for the preparation of different exercises.

Type III Wernicke's aphasia is characterized by a predominant, or even nearly exclusive, impairment of written language which is presumably related to a lesion of the angular gyrus (see Chapters 4 and 8). For patients presenting this form of aphasia, it is often advisable to reject a global approach in favour of more analytical methods similar to those commonly used in the remediation of developmental reading and spelling disabilities[96]. These methods are primarily aimed at mastery, initially at the level of the second linguistic phase (see Chapter 2), of phoneme–grapheme correspondences. In the initial stage of therapy, the exercises require phonemic differentiation and the association of a distinctive gesture (facial and manual) to each phoneme. When the gestural associations have been acquired, the exercises progress to the identification and production of graphemes in response to auditory stimuli and, finally, to the recognition and evocation of these graphemes in the context of syllables, words and sentences. The

* English-speaking patients would probably also benefit from exercises reviewing graphemic homophones and the spelling of morphological markers.

Insertion 17.4

Consider, for example, possible graphemic representations of the vowel

/ɑ̃/ in French		or	/u/ in English	
" (*AN*)	as in *RUBAN*		" (O)	as in TO
" (*ANS*)	as in *DEDANS*		" (OO)	as in TOO
" (*ANC*)	as in *BANC*		" (WO)	as in TWO
" (*ANCS*)	as in *BANCS*		" (EW)	as in THREW
" (*AND*)	as in *QUAND*		" (OUGH)	as in THROUGH
" (*ANDS*)	as in *GLANDS*		" (UE)	as in BLUE
" (*ANG*)	as in *ÉTANG*		" (EU)	as in MANEUVER
" (*ANGS*)	as in *ÉTANGS*		" (OU)	as in GROUP
" (*ANT*)	as in *POURTANT*		" (U)	as in RUDE
" (*ANTS*)	as in *CHANTS*		" (UI)	as in JUICE
" (*EN*)	as in *EN*			
" (*ENS*)	as in *GENS*			
" (*END*)	as in *RÉVÉREND*			
" (*ENDS*)	as in *RÉVÉRENDS*			
" (*ENG*)	as in *HARENG*			
" (*ENGS*)	as in *HARENGS*			
" (*ENT*)	as in *SOUVENT*			
" (*ENTS*)	as in *PARENTS*			
" (*AM*)	as in *AMBRE*			
" (*AMP*)	as in *CHAMP*			
" (*AMPS*)	as in *CHAMPS*			
" (*EM*)	as in *EMBOLIE*			
" (*EMPS*)	as in *TEMPS*			
" (*AON*)	as in *PAON*			
" (*AONS*)	as in *PAONS*			
" (*EAN*)	as in *JEAN*			
" (*AEN*)	as in *CAEN*			
" (*EMPT*)	as in *EXEMPT*			
" (*EMPTS*)	as in *EXEMPTS*			

progression of the exercises is based on several factors:

1. Single-letter graphemes precede multi-letter graphemes [(F)=/f/ before (PH)=/f/, for example, (FILTER) before (PHOTO)].
2. Graphemes with a single or few phonemic correspondents precede graphemes with multiple phonemic correspondents [(B)=/b/ before (G)=/g/ or /dʒ/, for example, (BALL) before (GAS) or (GIN)].
3. Letters corresponding to one grapheme precede letters corresponding to several graphemes [(C)=/k/ or /s/ before (X)=/ks/ or /gz/), for example, (CAR) and (CENT) before (EXTRA) and (EXAMPLE)].
4. Graphemes having few possible forms precede those having many possible forms [(G), (GG), (GU), (GUE)=/g/ before (O), (OH), (OE), (EW), (OW), (OA), (OUGH), etc.=/O/, for example, (BIG), (EGG), (GUARD), (VOGUE) before (AGO), (OH), (TOE), (SEW), (FLOW), (BOAT), (THOUGH), etc.].
5. Segments with a CV structure precede those with a CSV or CCV structure [for example, (DIP) and (RIP) before (DRIP)].
6. Shorter units precede longer ones with syllables introduced before words and words before sentences.

LEXICAL AND MORPHOSYNTACTICAL THERAPY

Although there are rare cases in which recovery is less probable for oral than for written expression, therapy for the latter can almost always be paired, in a supportive fashion, with therapy for oral expression related to all aspects of the first phase of language (cf. p. 34). Moreover, as a general rule, written production is to a certain degree dependent on oral production (as is the case when writing is formally taught to children). Thus, when aphasia therapy is aimed at those aspects of written symptomatology which concern linguistic reduction, syntax, and different verbal and syntagmic transformations (see Chapter 2), it generally follows the principles and progressions outlined in the preceding discussion of therapy for oral expression (cf. p. 420). However, if the therapist opts for a relatively comprehensive programme of therapy for written expression (realizing that the results will often be limited), she will then include certain exercises in which the written aspect has priority over the oral aspect. These exercises concern features specific to written language, especially those related to its manner of acquisition, as well as to its particular automatisms and specific forms. For example:

1. When necessary, preliminary exercises will be focused on presumably automatized written productions (name, address, letter headings, days of the week, etc.).
2. Different exercises are then presented to elicit written production of single lexical words: copying words presented in conjunction with their corresponding pictures; copying from memory; writing words to dictation; and written naming. The approach is generally global and orthography is not a primary consideration at this stage of therapy. The exercises can nevertheless be prepared using elementary spelling books: they contain lists of words which are grouped according to level of difficulty and their use facilitates global recovery of the most common spelling patterns.
3. Subsequent tasks require the writing of simple sentences: exact copying; copying with the selection of a particular item ('When I'm sick, I call the plumber—the doctor—the baker', 'When I'm thirsty, I drink—I eat—I walk'); copying incomplete sentences with written evocation of the missing word ('You cut wood with a ______'); writing to dictation, at first of complete stimuli, then of stimuli requiring recall and production of a particular segment, and finally of partially dictated sentences which must be appropriately completed. All exercises including incomplete sentences progress from highly restricted contexts ('A rolling stone gathers no ______'; 'You cut wood with a ______') to less restricted contexts ('Mary ate ______'; 'Mary bought ______'). Moreover, in the initial exercises, the missing element is always at the end of the sentence (and is usually the object or complement) but is later an initial word (subject) and then an intrasyntagmic word. Finally, the sentences are also arranged so that missing substantives precede missing verbs which in turn precede missing attributive adjectives. When appropriate, incomplete sentences can also be used as stimuli to elicit written evocation of grammatical words.
4. At this stage, therapy for written expression is less and less separable from other aspects of aphasia therapy. When further progress appears possible, the following types of complex activities can be introduced:
   (a) Written questions are presented about a written text which remains in the patient's view. The text may be one which is used for the first time, one which has been copied, or one which was written to dictation. Written questions may also be based on a picture, a sequence of pictures or a film.
   (b) The lexical exercises described for oral expression may be done in written form (cf. pp. 430–434);
   (c) The syntactical exercises described for oral expression may be done in written form (cf. pp. 420–430).
5. Therapy for written expression may terminate with compositions which the patient prepares on his own. They should become progressively longer, be written on progressively more abstract topics, and include increasingly complex syntactical constructions.

THERAPY FOR DISTURBANCES OF WRITTEN LANGUAGE COMPREHENSION

As in the case of oral language comprehension (cf. p. 434), the disturbances of written language comprehension observed in aphasia may reflect an agnosic impairment (visual aspect; word blindness) or a psycholinguistic impairment (see Chapters 4 and 5). The former is frequently called *agnosic alexia* and the latter *aphasic alexia*[97]. Since a dissociation between these two types of disturbances is generally not obvious, their coexistence must usually be presumed when planning an eventual therapy programme. For purposes of discussion, we shall nevertheless separate therapy exercises into those especially aimed at agnosic alexia and those especially aimed at aphasic alexia.

AGNOSIC ALEXIA

The techniques discussed under this heading are useful in therapy for pure word blindness. They may also be beneficial for certain Wernicke's aphasics, particularly in cases where there is clearly predominant disturbance, both in reception and production, of written language.*

In total agnosic alexia, even the recognition of isolated letters is impaired, that is, there is a literal alexia (see Chapter 5). In these cases, the goal of the initial stage of therapy is to palliate the visual agnosic deficit (which is specific to linguistic features) by increasing the role of proprioceptive feedback associated with writing movements[21]. The patient is gradually led to recognize letters solely on the basis of their constituent movements. In the first step, the therapist executes the movements corresponding to a pre-selected target letter as if she were writing the greatly-enlarged letter in space with her finger. The patient is then asked to imitate the therapist's movements. This active imitation usually leads to improvement—which is frequently quite spectacular—in the recognition of letters which could not be identified from conventional (static) visual stimuli. This initial stage is immediately paired with other exercises requiring the blind identification of letters from movements passively traced with the patient's hand (the therapist manipulates the patient's index finger as if it were a pencil). Next, the patient is required to trace letters actively, using the end of his index (or another) finger. In some cases, the goal of accurate identification of target letters can be attained more rapidly if the stimuli to be traced consist of enlarged letters cut out of sandpaper. In the following stage, the stimulus letters are static and increasingly conventional in size and visual characteristics. Although letter recognition is still to be achieved through finger tracing, it must now be done at some distance from the letter. The tracing gradually becomes more and more subtle and is soon merely a sketch which is barely visible to an observer. Finally, even this is no longer necessary or is only required occasionally.

When the agnosic disturbance is limited to visual verbal stimuli or includes only an additional difficulty with colours (see Chapters 5 and 16), the method outlined above typically leads to improvement of the literal alexia. Such improvement is more easily achieved if the stimuli are sequenced so that the immediate succession of letters which are similar in form [(*u*) and (*n*), (*m*) and (*n*), (*d*) and (*b*), etc.] is avoided at the start of therapy and only introduced during later stages.

Most speech pathologists work at present in social contexts where their clients have had more previous experience with printed letters in reading and more experience with cursives in writing. This situation has two implications for therapy: on the one hand, therapy for literal alexia should often begin with the recognition of cursive letters and, on the other hand, the gains achieved in recognition must subsequently be generalized to printed letters. The transition from one code to the other can be facilitated by beginning with letters having a similar form in both codes [(*o*) and (o), (*i*) and (i), (*u*) and (u), (*c*) and (c), etc.] and reserving, for the final stage, those which are less similar in form [(*a*) and (a), (*f*) and (f), (*l*) and (l), (*s*) and (s), etc.]. Since progress is generally rapid during this type of exercise, the therapist will not hesitate to add others, when necessary, on certain contrasts between capital and small letters. Such exercises will follow the same principles as those outlined above.

If the therapist judges that progress in letter recognition is not sufficiently rapid, she may attempt to accelerate improvement by placing a card displaying the alphabet (in cursives and in print) within the patient's view. This is done because, in agnosic alexia, the ability to read letters is usually preserved if letters are presented in alphabetical order. Thus the comparison of an unidentified stimulus letter with the alphabetical list may contribute to its identification. If this strategy is employed, the therapist will abandon this form of facilitation as soon as possible.

* It should be noted that Dejerine[48, 98–100] made no qualitative distinction between word blindness occurring in isolation and word blindness associated (in certain lesions of the angular gyrus) with agraphia.

Once the problem of literal alexia has been entirely or almost overcome, therapy is oriented towards recovery of reading which is as global, accurate and rapid as in the patient's premorbid state. As a general rule, this point can be approached but will seldom be attained. The reading exercises include progressively longer and more complex segments—syllables, increasingly longer words, sentences, and passages of text—and should be sequenced so that they progress from the more to the less familiar. The intermediate stages of therapy may be particularly laborious. If paralexias are frequently observed, a formal study of their characteristics (in terms of omissions, substitutions, anticipations, etc.) may be useful. If certain types of deviations appear to predominate, appropriate remedial exercises can then be introduced.

If visual deficits are associated with the alexia, for example unilateral visual neglect, coloured marks can be placed at the beginning and the end of each line to encourage complete visual scanning. Similarly, for certain patients with abnormal eye movements, the temporary use of a screening card can often facilitate perception of letter and word sequences and prevent inappropriate shifts from one line to another.*

APHASIC ALEXIA

When a word or a sentence is accurately read by an agnosic alexic, its meaning is as fully understood as it was premorbidly. In contrast, an aphasic alexic may be unable to grasp the meaning of a word which he has just read aloud without error. This shows that his (psycholinguistic) disturbance is analogous to the one which impairs his comprehension of spoken language (see Chapter 4). This is why, as we have previously implied, therapy procedures for a psycholinguistic disturbance of comprehension are similar in many respects for both auditory and visual information. In other words, the nature of many remedial exercises for the improvement of aphasic alexia can be deduced, when the tasks are not in fact identical, from the exercises already described for a psycholinguistic disturbance of oral comprehension (cf. p. 436). They include:

1. Increasingly difficult exercises in the matching of written words (especially nouns and verbs) to their corresponding pictures. These exercises may or may not be preceded by, or paired with, others which require the identification of words spoken by the therapist by pointing to written words in lists which are graded in difficulty (lists of semantically unrelated words before lists of semantically related words, etc.). Depending on the case, the therapist will decide whether these exercises, and all therapy for aphasic alexia, will include correction of the patient's oral productions or whether this aspect will be ignored and attention focused on comprehension only.
2. Increasingly difficult exercises in the matching of written sentences to pictures and then in matching each of a series of written sentences to the appropriate picture in a picture sequence.
3. Execution of written commands which are progressively more complex, more arbitrary and less explicit.
4. Reconstruction of written sentences from constituents displayed on separate cards (with or without multiple choices); completion of sentences with a missing element (with or without multiple choices); definition of a paradigm from sentences with a missing element and from word lists; classification of written words under various written conceptual headings; reconstitution of written texts from constituent sentences displayed on separate cards, etc.
5. Exercises centred on the comprehension of written discourse (i.e., the comprehension of wholes). These exercises are based on textual passages which are graded in terms of their content and formulation. In this respect, it is often convenient to adapt texts selected from school books. The therapist asks a predetermined series of questions intended to guide the patient's understanding of the most important meaningful elements of the text, their reciprocal relationships, and then the main idea emerging from the entire passage. Depending on the case, it may or may not be advisable, in the context of these exercises, to comment in passing on the meaning of various grammatical structures which are particularly difficult for aphasic patients.

* The following training task is sometimes useful in this regard: the patient interrupts his reading, looks away from the text and then attempts to redirect his view to the exact spot where he stopped reading.

GROUP THERAPY

Throughout this chapter, we have emphasized that the nature and progression of a therapy programme must be planned and carried out with as much regard for aphasic individuals as for the clinical forms of aphasia, which are themselves very variable in many respects. For certain aphasic individuals, the therapy programme proves to be more stimulating and effective when it is partially provided in the context of group therapy. Such therapy is carried out in one of two ways, the first called *closed group* and the other *open group*[101, 102]. In the first case, as in individual therapy, the primary goal is recovery from the linguistic disturbance. In contrast, in the second case, group therapy is aimed at promoting maximal use of residual (and recovered) language during social interactions between group members (both aphasic and non-aphasic). It is, of course, possible for the same patient to participate first in a closed group and then join an open group.

CLOSED GROUPS

Closed group therapy is usually directed by a speech pathologist, although joint direction by a speech pathologist and an occupational therapist is sometimes desirable. The ideal group consists of three aphasics. They may differ, to a certain extent, in the clinical picture which they present or even in their stage of recovery. The group sessions are conducted more informally than the individual therapy sessions. In the group sessions, the therapist's main concern is to structure situations which, while eliciting all language functions (cf. p. 404), will particularly stimulate the participants' propositional use of progressively more varied and complex utterances. Because this requires a certain amount of improvisation, the group leaders' previous experience is extremely important. They follow only a single fundamental rule but one which is initially difficult to apply, namely that the situations created must not only promote the participation of the most impaired patient (who would otherwise be exposed to constant failure) but must also be stimulating to the least impaired patient (who would otherwise lose the motivation necessary for further progress).

OPEN GROUPS

In open groups, the speech pathologist's interventions give way to those of the psychologist and the social worker. Open group therapy sessions may benefit from the participation of normal speakers, for example, the patients' friends or family members. The aphasics included in open groups are those whose therapy programme is approaching completion and who will soon reach their maximal level of linguistic performance. Within an open group, the severity of the linguistic handicap will therefore vary among the participants. The group sessions have two primary goals: on the one hand, to permit each aphasic member to express his feelings about his handicap and, on the other, to foster the habitual use of his residual abilities in the context of social exchanges.

In open groups, the clinicians' attitude is relatively non-directive. Even more than in closed groups, the course of exchanges (both linguistic and other) in open groups is gradually allowed to depend on the aphasic participants' particular interests and concerns at the time of each meeting. Once this type of therapy is well underway, it is the patients themselves who decide on the frequency of future sessions. As implied by this description, open group therapy is appropriate only for those aphasics who have recovered at least some ability to communicate verbally, who are aware of their handicap, and whose personality characteristics—including those which may depend on their medical condition—are such that social relationships remain possible.

SOCIAL AND PROFESSIONAL REINTEGRATION OF APHASIC PATIENTS

Whether or not such hopes are realistic, most aphasic patients long to return to their premorbid social environment. In concrete terms, the most usual case is that of the patient who wishes to return to both his family and friends and to his work and earnings. While resumption of employment might first appear of lesser importance, this is often not the case, at least in contemporary

Western countries. Such value is often placed on work, and sometimes on its associated remuneration, that the inability to work may generate feelings ranging from shame to marked depression. Without work, it may thus be difficult for the patient to maintain a sense of psychological well-being.

THE RETURN TO THE FAMILY

Whenever possible, an aphasic patient should return to his family, or to his circle of friends, as soon as there are no medical or socio-economic contra-indications. For many aphasics, this return constitutes an important step in their therapy programme, a step in which the social worker and psychologist will (ideally) participate as fully as the speech pathologist and the physician.

An aphasic's return home, particularly in the case of a patient with Wernicke's aphasia, is sometimes the cause of conflicts which rapidly become unbearable. Besides the linguistic impairment which impedes communication, the cerebral lesions responsible for the aphasia may also be the source of physical and intellectual disturbances (see Chapters 4 and 16) and even, in either a direct or reactional manner, of behavioural disturbances. Those close to the aphasic may find his return extremely disconcerting and their inappropriate attitudes towards him may not only hamper his reintegration into the home, but may also affect the gains—which are often unstable—which have been achieved through language therapy. The patient's family and friends often have little knowledge of aphasia and, in the absence of significant premorbid family conflicts, this ignorance, especially on the part of the aphasic's spouse, often constitutes the greatest obstacle to the successful reintegration of an aphasic into the family environment. The family's understanding of aphasia can be increased through counselling which may be provided on either an individual basis (particularly with a family member or a friend who has assumed the role of tutor during the patient's therapy programme) or in group sessions organized for people who are closely involved in the daily life of aphasic individuals[103]. The advantages of group sessions include the more economic use of available personnel and the opportunity to present more complete information in a systematic manner.

In cases where resumption of even part-time work is impossible, it sometimes becomes necessary to resort to a programme of recreational activities. This is best managed by an occupational therapist. Whether or not the family members participate in the planned activities, the programme will provide them with some relief and reduce the isolation which is sometimes imposed by the responsibilities which they have assumed in regard to their aphasic relative. The latter will also benefit, since a well-planned programme may eventually come to be viewed as an acceptable alternative to conventional employment. In addition, when the recreational activities take place in a suitably oriented context, they may help conserve the gains made during language therapy and possibly even stimulate further language recovery.

THE RETURN TO WORK

Once his handicap has stabilized, the victim of a cerebral vascular accident (see Chapter 9) may sometimes be able to return to paid employment. However, those whose aphasia was caused by cerebral softening are generally disadvantaged in this regard. At *l'Hôpital de la Salpêtrière*, it was estimated that about 35 per cent of aphasic patients (considered without regard to aetiology) were eventually able to return to some form of employment[104]. This figure merits reflection, as follows.

Although it perhaps suggests an order of magnitude, hasty generalizations may be faulty. The figure came from an aphasia therapy centre and was therefore based primarily, if not solely, on the consideration of patients whose medical condition was sufficiently good to envisage a long term therapy programme. In addition, it came from a very well-known centre whose clientele included a high proportion of patients in particularly favourable socio-economic circumstances.

The figure is a function of several factors, many of which will vary among different countries such as: the average educational level; the availability of aphasia therapy and the usual approach to therapy; union and management policies concerning the employment of handicapped persons; national policies regarding social assistance programmes; the local unemployment rate; etc.

The figure includes all patients who resumed

employment and does not distinguish between full and part-time work, employment of workers (who must meet predefined quotas) and of proprietors (whose deficiencies can be palliated through tightened controls), employment at the premorbid level (with respect to functions and salary) and employment—as is often the case—at an inferior level.

Following Rothschild's formulation[105], we shall list the variables related to professional re-adaptation under five headings:

1. *Medical variables*: nature of the disease; clinical characteristics; severity and duration of the handicap; associated pathologies; residual potential for professional activity (level of recovery).
2. *Psychological variables*: 'intelligence' (see Chapter 16): capacity for self-evaluation and adaptation to the changes related to cerebral pathology.
3. *Professional variables*: premorbid employment history; professional status.
4. *Psychosociological variables*: nature of the patient's premorbid relationships with his milieu; reaction in this milieu to the patient's handicap and the degree of the patient's dependence on his milieu; the predominant scale of values in the surrounding society.
5. *Demographic variables*: age groups; family situations; educational levels, number of dependents, sexes, salary (and/or benefit) scales.

A combination of circumstances may sometimes exist which is particularly auspicious for the resumption of work by an aphasic with a stabilized cerebral lesion. It includes a professional background resulting in well-anchored knowledge, a certain degree of flexibility in regard to hours of work and production, the support of informed and caring people and, especially, a relatively mild residual handicap. A return to work can then be expected to cause no problems other than those related to increased fatigue during convalescence and those resulting from discouragement generated by the realization of reduced capability, problems which can usually be circumvented with adequate support. In less favourable cases, which are also commoner, the therapist frequently hesitates to raise the question—and the hope—of a return to work. Certain tests intended to determine the potential for employment may occasionally be useful but we do not consider them sufficiently valuable to recommend their general use. As soon as the chances of relative success in a working situation appear sufficiently high, and a possible failure could be tolerated, the preferred solution may well be a trial period of employment. Analysis of the aphasic's performance during this period will often provide a clearer answer than the use of available tests.

The following considerations are generally relevant when planning the return to work:

1. The optimal setting for a trial period of employment might be within a sheltered workshop. It must nevertheless be recognized that governments usually support workshops designed to ease the problems of the mentally retarded, the emotionally disturbed or workers with motor handicaps, rather than the very different problems of aphasic persons.
2. In certain countries, consultation with an employment counsellor is often useful. His/her familiarity with government programmes, the functioning of community agencies and the hiring practices of different employers will allow the counsellor to act as an intermediary between those agencies and the handicapped worker.
3. If the selected employment will involve regular contact with other people, it is important that they be informed about aphasia and the limits which it imposes on the aphasic person. It is often the speech pathologist or the physician who assumes the responsibility of providing suitable information to those in the setting where the aphasic, after having completed his therapy programme, will attempt to return to work.

REFERENCES

1. Féré, Ch. (1886) La rééducation des aphasiques. *Revue générale de Clinique et de Thérapeutique*, **785.**
2. Thomas, A. and Roux, E. (1895) Essai sur la psychologie des associations verbales et sur la rééducation de la parole dans l'aphasie motrice. *Bulletin de la Société de Biologie*, 16 November.
3. Froment, I. (1921) *La rééducation des aphasiques moteurs.* Medical thesis, Paris.
4. Eldridge, M. (1968) *A History of the Treatment of Speech Disorders.* Edinburgh and London: Livingstone.
5. Travis, L.E. (1957) *Speech Pathology.* New York: Appleton-Century Crofts.

6. Sarno, M.T., Silverman, M. & Sands, E. (1970) Speech therapy and language recovery in severe aphasia. *Journal of Speech Research*, **13,** 607.
7. Vignolo, L.A. (1964) Evolution of aphasia and language rehabilitation: a retrospective exploratory study. *Cortex*, **1,** 344.
8. Basso, A. (1977) Aphasia rehabilitation. Communication to the *International Symposium on Aphasia* (*World Federation of Neurology*), Göteborg, September.
9. Basso, A., Capitani, E. & Vignolo, L.A. (1979) Influence of rehabilitation on language skills in aphasic patients: a controlled study. *Archives of Neurology*, **36,** 190.
10. Brown, J.W. (1976) The neural organization of language: aphasia and lateralization. *Brain and Language*, **3,** 482.
11. Brown, J.W. & Hécaen, H. (1976) Lateralization and language representation. *Neurology*, **26,** 183.
12. Subirana, A. (1969) Handedness and cerebral dominance. In *Handbook of Clinical Neurology* (Ed.) Vinken, P.J. & Bruyns, G.W. Vol. 4, p. 248. Amsterdam: North-Holland.
13. Taylor-Sarno, M. (1965) A measurement of functional communication in aphasia. *Archives of Physical Medicine*, **46,** 101.
14. Tikofsky, R.S. & Reynolds, G.L. (1962) Preliminary study: nonverbal learning and aphasia. *Journal of Speech Research*, **5,** 133.
15. Tikofsky, R.S. & Reynolds, G.L. (1963) Further studies of nonverbal learning and aphasia. *Journal of Speech Research*, **6,** 329.
16. Brookshire, R.H. (1969) Probability learning by aphasic subjects. *Journal of Speech and Hearing Research*, **12,** 857.
17. Brookshire, R.H. (1972) Effects of task difficulty on naming performance of aphasic subjects. *Journal of Speech and Hearing Research*, **15,** 551.
18. Signoret, J.L. (1966) *Etude d'un apprentissage associatif chez 28 sujets présentant une aphasie par lésion cérébrale localisée*. Medical thesis, Paris.
19. Lhermitte, F. & Signoret, J.L. (1969) Analyse d'un apprentissage associatif: résultats obtenus chez 42 aphasiques. *Cortex*, **5,** 415.
20. Eisenson, J. (1957) Aphasia in adults. In *Handbook of Speech Pathology* (Ed.) Travis, L.E. p. 436. New York: Appleton-Century Crofts.
21. Lhermitte, F. & Ducarne, B. (1965) La rééducation des aphasiques. *Revue pratique* (Paris), **15,** 2345
22. Goodglass, H., Hyde, M.R. & Blumstein, S. (1969) Frequency, picturability and availability of nouns in aphasia. *Cortex*, **5,** 104.
23. Goldstein, K. (1948) *Language and Language Disturbances*. New York: Grune and Stratton.
24. Skinner, B.F. (1968) *La révolution scientifique de l'enseignement*. Brussels: Dessart.
25. Skinner, B.F. (1971) *L'analyse expérimentale du comportement*. Brussels: Dessart.
26. Skinner, B.F. (1972) *Cumulative Record: a Selection of Papers*. New York: Appleton-Century Crofts.
27. Holland, J.G. (1960) Teaching machines: an application of principles from the laboratory. In *Teaching Machines and Programmed Learning* (Ed.) Lumsdaine, A.A. & Glaser, R. Washington: National Education Association.
28. Brookshire, R.H. (1973) *An Introduction to Aphasia*. Minnesota: BRK Publishers.
29. Brookshire, R.H. (1971) Effects of delay of reinforcement on probability learning by aphasic subjects. *Journal of Speech Research*, **14,** 92.
30. Doehring, D.G., Dudley, J.G. & Coderre, L. (1967) Programmed instruction in picture-sound association for the aphasic. *Folia phoniatrica* (Basel), **19,** 414.
31. Dudley, J.G., Doehring, D.G. & Coderre, L. (1968) Speed of visual perception in aphasic and non-aphasic patients with hemiplegia. *Cortex*, **4,** 389.
32. Guberina, P. & Rivenc, P. (1971) *Voix et images de France*. Paris: Didier.
33. Mauget, M.I. (1972) *De vive voix*. Paris: Didier.
34. Commission de la Fonction Publique du Canada (1974) *Dialogue Canada, I*. Ottawa: Approvisionnements et Services Canada.
35. Commission de la Fonction Publique du Canada (1974–1975) *Dialogue Canada, II*. Ottawa: Approvisionnements et Services Canada.
36. Commission de la Fonction Publique du Canada (1975) *Dialogue Canada (programmé)*. Ottawa: Approvisionnements et Services Canada.
37. Rondeau, G., Vinay, J.P., Calvé, P., Germain, C., Le Blanc, R. & Rondeau, F. (1972) *Le français international*. Montreal: Centre Éducatif et Culturel.
38. Gauvenet, H., Guberina, P., Neveu, P., Rivenc, P. & Valtier, R. (1969) *Méthode audiovisuelle du français*. Paris: Didier.
39. Baillarger, J. (1890) De l'aphasie au point de vue psychologique. Aphasie simple. Aphasie avec perversion de la faculté du langage. In *Recherches sur les maladies mentales* (Ed.) Baillarger, J. p. 584. Paris: Masson (first edition in 1865).
40. Goodglass, H., Quadfasel, F.A. & Timberlake, W.H. (1964) Phrase length and the type and severity of aphasia. *Cortex*, **1,** 133.
41. Ombredane, A. (1951) *L'aphasie et l'élaboration de la pensée explicite*. Paris: Presses Universitaires de France.
42. Alajouanine, Th., Ombredane, A. & Durand, M. (1939) *Le syndrome de désintegration phonétique dans l'aphasie*. Paris: Masson.
43. Alajouanine, Th., Lhermitte, F., Ledoux, Renaud, D. & Vignolo, L.A. (1964) Les composantes phonemiques et semantiques de la jargonaphasie. *Revue neurologique*, **110,** 5.
44. Lecours, A.R. (1975) Aphasie. *Encyclopédie médico-chirurgie, 17019 A^{10}*, 7.
45. Albert, M.L., Sparks, R.W. & Helm, N.A. (1973) Melodic intonation therapy for aphasia. *Archives of Neurology* (Chicago), **29,** 130.
46. Sparks, R., Helm, N. & Albert, M. (1974) Aphasia rehabilitation resulting from melodic intonation therapy. *Cortex*, **10,** 303.

47. Sparks, R.W. & Holland, A.L. (1976) Method: melodic intonation therapy for aphasia. *Journal of Speech and Hearing Disorders*, **41,** 287.

48. Dejerine, J. (1914) *Séméiologie des affections du système nerveux*. Paris: Masson.

49. Luria, A.R. (1970) *Traumatic Aphasia*. The Hague: Mouton.

50. Lecours, A.R. & Rouillon, F. (1976) Neurolinguistic analysis of jargonaphasia and jargonagraphia. In *Studies in Neuro-linguistics* (Ed.) Avakian-Whitaker, H. & Whitaker, H. Vol. II, p. 95. New York: Academic Press.

51. Poncet, M., Degos, C., Deloche, G. & Lecours, A.R. (1972) Phonetic and phonemic transformations in aphasia. *International Journal of Mental Health*, **1,** 46.

52. Marie, P. (1906) Révision de la question de l'aphasie: la troisième circonvolution frontale ne joue aucun rôle spécial dans la fonction du langage. *Semaine médicale* (Paris), **26,** 241.

53. Jakobson, R. (1962) *Selected Writings—I: Phonological Studies*. The Hague: Mouton.

54. Ingram, D. (1976) *Phonological Disability in Children. Studies in Language Disability and Remediation*. London: Edward Arnold.

55. Borel-Maisonny, S. (1966) *Langage oral et écrit*. Tome 1: pédagogie des notions de base. Paris: Delachaux-Niestlé.

56. Ohman, S.E.G. (1965) Coarticulation in VCV utterance: spectrographic measurement. *Journal of the American Society of Acoustics*, **39,** 151.

57. McDonald, E.T. (1964) *Articulation Testing and Treatment—a Sensory-motor Approach*. Pittsburgh, PA: Stanivix House.

58. Alajouanine, Th., Pichot, P. & Durand, M. (1947) Dissociation des altérations phonétiques avec conservation relative de la langue la plus ancienne dans un cas d'anarthrie pure chez un sujet français bilingue. *Encéphale*, **28,** 245.

59. Barrel, L. (1968) *Méthode de prononciation du français*. Paris: Didier.

60. Calacue-Andron, E. (1971) *Trente-deux exercises de phonétique française*. Paris: Didier.

61. Léon, M. (1970) *Exercices systématiques de prononciation française*. fasc. I. Paris: Hachette-Larousse.

62. Lecours, A.R. & Lhermitte, F. (1969) Phonemic paraphasias: linguistic structures and tentative hypotheses. *Cortex*, **5,** 193.

63. Goodglass, H., Berko-Gleason, J., Bernholz, N.A. & Hyde, M.R. (1972) Some linguistic structures in the speech of a Broca's aphasic. *Cortex*, **8,** 191.

64. Myerson, R. & Goodglass, H. (1972) Transformational grammars of three agrammatic patients. *Language and Speech*, **15,** 40.

65. Gleason, J.B., Goodglass, H., Green, E., Ackerman, N. & Hyde, M.R. (1975) The retrieval of syntax in Broca's aphasia. *Brain and Language*, **2,** 451.

66. Dordain, G. (1968) *Contribution à l'étude neurolinguistique de l'aphasie. Analyse comparative des performances grammaticales de 28 aphasiques dont 14 agrammatiques*. Medical thesis, Paris.

67. Nespoulous, J.L. (1973) *Approche linguistique de divers phénomènes d'agrammatisme*. Thesis, Departement de linguistique, Université de Toulouse-le-Mirail, Toulouse.

68. Rouillon, F. (1971) *A propos de quelques observations d'agrammatiques et de dyssyntaxiques; essai d'analyse comparative de certaines de leurs performances grammaticales*. Medical thesis, Paris.

69. Tissot, R., Mounin, G. & Lhermitte, F. (1973) *L'agrammatisme. Etude neuropsycholinguistique*. Brussels: Dessart.

70. Ludlow, C. (1973) *The Recovery of Syntax in Aphasia: an Analysis of Syntactic Structures Used in Connected Speech during the Initial Recovery Period*. Phd Dissertation, New York University, New York.

71. Holland, A.L. & Levy, C.B. (1971) Syntactic generalization in aphasics as a function of relearning an active sentence. *Acta Symbolica*, **2,** 34.

72. Bloom, L. (1970) *Language Development, Form and Function in Emerging Grammars*. Cambridge, MA: MIT Press.

73. Jakobson, R. (1971) *Studies on Child Language and Aphasia*. The Hague: Mouton.

74. Coderre, L. *Le discours agrammatique*. Ecole de Réadaptation, Faculté de Médecine, University of Montreal (unpublished manuscript).

75. Dale, P.S. (1976) *Language Development*. Montreal: Holt, Rinehart and Winston.

76. Forster, K.I. & Olbrei, I. (1973) *Semantic heuristics and syntactic analysis. Cognition*. The Hague and Paris: Mouton.

77. Martinet, A. (1967) *Eléments de linguistique générale*. Paris: Colin.

78. Cyr-Stafford, C. & Boisclair-Papillon, R. (1974) *La dyssyntaxie: essai de définition*. Medical thesis, University of Montreal.

79. Marie, P. & Foix, C. (1917) Les aphasies de guerre. *Revue neurologique*, **1,** 53.

80. Lhermitte, F. (1965) Sémiologie de l'aphasie. *Revue pratique* (Paris), **15,** 1.

81. Gougenheim, G. (1958) *Dictionnaire fondamental de la langue française*. Paris: Didier.

82. Vikis-Freibergs, V. (1974) *Fréquence d'usage des mots au Québec*. Montreal: Presses de l'Université de Montréal.

83. Thorndike, E.L. & Lorge, I. (1944) *The Teacher's Word Book of 30 000 Words*. New York: Teacher's College, Columbia University.

84. Howes, D. (1966) A word count of spoken English. *Journal of Verbal Learning and Verbal Behavior*, **5,** 572.

85. Mounin, G. (1972) *Clefs pour la sémantique*. Paris: Seghers.

86. Fodor, J.A. & Katz, J.J. (Ed.) (1964) *The Structure of Language*. Englewood Cliffs, NJ: Prentice Hall.

87. Greimas, A.J. (1966) *Sémantique structurale*. Paris: Larousse.

88. Jakobson, R. (1964) Towards a linguistic typology of aphasic impairments. In *Disorders of Language* (Ed.) de

Reuck, A.V.S. & O'Connor, M. p. 21. London: Churchill.

89. Lhermitte, F., Derouesné, J. & Lecours, A.R. (1971) Contribution à l'étude des troubles sémantiques dans l'aphasie. *Revue neurologique*, **125,** 81.
90. In Collaboration (1957) *Imagier du Père Castor*. Paris: Flammarion.
91. Hécaen, H. & Angelergues, R. (1965) *Pathologie du langage*. Paris: Larousse.
92. Schuell, H. (1953) Auditory impairment in aphasia: significance and retraining technique. *Journal of Speech Disorders*, **18,** 14.
93. Schuell, H. (1953) Aphasic difficulties understanding spoken language. *Neurology*, **3,** 176.
94. Lordat, J. (1969) Analyse de la parole pour servir à la théorie de divers cas d'alalie et de paralalie (de mutisme et d'imperfection de parler) que les neurologistes ont mal connus. In *La naissance de la neuropsychologie du langage* (Ed.) Hécaen, H. & Dubois, J. p. 130. Paris: Flammarion.
95. Renzi, E. (de) & Vignolo, L.A. (1962) The token test: a sensitive test to detect receptive disturbances in aphasics. *Brain*, **85,** 665.
96. Maistre, M. (de) (1968) *Dyslexie Dysorthographie*. Paris: Editions Universitaires.
97. Alajouanine, Th., Lhermitte, F. & Ribaucourt-Ducarne, B. (de) (1960) Les alexies agnosiques et aphasiques. In *Les grandes activitiés du lobe occipital* (Ed.) Alajouanine, Th. p. 235. Paris: Masson.
98. Dejerine, J. (1891) Sur un cas de cécité verbale avec agraphie, suivi d'autopsie. *Mémoires de la Société de Biologie*, **3,** 197.
99. Dejerine, J. (1892) Des différentes variétés de cécité verbale. *Mémoires de la Société de Biologie*, **4,** 1.
100. Dejerine, J. (1892) Contribution à l'étude anatomo-pathologique et clinique des différentes variétés de cécité verbale. *Mémoires de la Société de Biologie*, **4,** 61.
101. Bloom, L.M. (1962) A rationale for group treatment of aphasic patients. *Journal of Speech and Hearing Disorders*, **27,** 11.
102. Malone, R.L. (1969) Expressed attitudes of families of aphasics. *Journal of Speech and Hearing Disorders*, **34,** 146.
103. Turnblom, M.L. & Myers, J.S. (1952) A group discussion program with families of aphasic patients. *Journal of Speech Disorders*, **17,** 393.
104. Ducarne, B. (1967) La rééducation des troubles du langage d'origine cérébrale. *Acta Neurologica Belgica*, **67,** 1059.
105. Safilios-Rothschild, C. (1970) *The Sociology and Social Psychology of Disability and Rehabilitation*. New York: Random House.

BIBLIOGRAPHY

Adams, G.F. & Hurwitz, L.J. (1963) Mental barriers to recovery from strokes. *Lancet*, **2,** 533.

Agranowitz, A. (1954) Group therapy as a method of retraining aphasics. *Quarterly Journal of Speech*, **40,** 170.

Agranowitz, A. & McKeown, M.R. (1964) *Aphasia Handbook for Adults and Children*. Springfield, IL: Thomas.

Albertson, E.T. (1947) A glimpse into an aphasic's world. *American Journal of Occupational Therapy*, **1,** 361.

Albrecht, M.A. (1962) A suggested neurological theory that justifies speech therapy for the adult aphasic. *Journal of Rehabilitation*, **28,** 20.

Albright, J.S. & Albright, R.W. (1959) The role of linguistics in speech and hearing therapy. *Language Learning*, **9,** 51.

Anderson, J.O. (1945) Eighteen cases of aphasia studied from the view-point of a speech pathologist. *Journal of Speech Disorders*, **10,** 9.

Anderson, J.O. (1948) Aphasia and its treatment. In *Twentieth Century Speech and Voice Correction* (Ed.) Froeschels, E. p. 39. New York: Philosophical Library.

Aronson, M., Shatin, L. & Cook, J.C. (1956) Socio-psychotherapeutic approach to the treatment of aphasic patients. *Journal of Speech Disorders*, **21,** 352.

Backus, O.L. (1945) The rehabilitation of aphasic veterans. *Journal of Speech Disorders*, **10,** 149.

Backus, O.L. & Dunn, H.M. (1947) Intensive group therapy in speech rehabilitation. *Journal of Speech Disorders*, **12,** 39.

Backus, O.L. & Henry, I.D. (1947) *Aphasia in Adults*. Ann Arbor, MI: University of Michigan Press.

Barbizet, J. & Métellus, J. (1973) Que peut-on attendre de la rééducation de l'aphasique? *Gazette Médicale Française*, **80,** 1035.

Barger, W.C. (1953) Experimental approach to aphasic and to nonreading children. *American Journal of Orthopsychiatry*, **23,** 158.

Benson, D.F. (1973) Psychiatric aspects of aphasia. *British Journal of Psychiatry*, **123,** 555.

Berko, J. (1958) The child's learning of English morphology. *Word*, **14,** 150.

Berko, J. & Palmer, M.F. (1952) The education of the aphasic child. *American Journal of Occupational Therapy*, **6,** 241.

Berman, M. & Peele, L.M. (1967) Self-generated cues: a method for aiding aphasic and apractic patients. *Journal of Speech and Hearing Disorders*, **32,** 372.

Bertin, Dissez, C. & Arne, L. (1971) Observations de quelques dysarthries neurologiques post-traumatiques rééduquées. *Revue de Laryngologie* (Bordeaux), **92,** 562.

Beyn, E.S. & Shokhor-Trotskaya, M.K. (1966) The preventive method of speech rehabilitation in aphasia. *Cortex*, **2,** 96.

Biorn-Hansen, V. (1957) Social and emotional aspects of aphasia. *Journal of Speech Disorders*, **22,** 53.

Birch, H.G. & Bitterman, M.E. (1949) Reinforcement of learning: the process of sensory integration. *Psychological Review*, **56,** 292.

Birdwhistell, R.L. (1970) *Kinesics and Context: Essays in Body Motion Communication*. Philadelphia, PA: University of Pennsylvania Press.

Black, J.W. & Jancosek, C.G. (Ed.) (1968) *Proceedings of the Conference on Language Retraining for Aphasics*. Washington: USA Department of Health, Education and Welfare.

Blackman, N. (1950) Group psychotherapy with aphasics. *Journal of Nervous and Mental Diseases*, **111,** 154.

Blackman, N. & Tureen, L.L. (1948) Aphasia—a psychosomatic approach in rehabilitation. *Transactions of the American Neurological Association*, **73,** 193.

Boone, D.R. (1961) Relationship of progress in speech therapy to progress in physical therapy. *Archives of Physical Medicine*, **42,** 30.

Brisay, A.N. (de) & Stuart, C.K. (1964) Restoration of communication in the elderly, with special reference to hemiplegic patients: interim report on program. *Journal of the American Geriatric Society*, **12,** 687.

Britton, D. (1951) Rehabilitation of aphasics. *Physical Therapy*, **3,** 477.

Broida, H. (1979) *Coping with Stroke: Communication Breakdown of Brain Injured Adults*. Houston, TX: College Hill.

Brookshire, R.H. & Lommel, L. (1974) Perception of sequences of visual temporal and auditory-spatial stimuli by aphasics, right hemisphere damaged and non brain damaged subjects. *Journal of Communication Disorders*, **7,** 155.

Bryans, B. & Poncet, M. (1979) La rééducation d'une aphasie dynamique. *Folia Phoniatrica*, **31,** 259.

Buck, M. (Ed.) (1968) *Dysphasia: Professional Guidance for Family and Patient*. Englewood Cliffs, NJ: Prentice Hall.

Burr, H.G. (1964) *The Aphasic Adult: Evaluation and Rehabilitation*. Charlottesville, VA: Wayside Press.

Butfield, E. (1960) Acquired receptive dysphasia. *Speech Pathology and Therapy*, **3,** 8.

Butfield, E. & Zangwill, O.L. (1946) Re-education in aphasia; a review of 70 cases. *Journal of Neurology, Neurosurgery and Psychiatry*, **9,** 75.

Caceres, V. (1971) Readaptation et rééducation dans le syndrome aphasique. *Revue de Neuro-psiquiatrie*, **34,** 309.

Carson, D.H., Carson, F.E. & Tikofsky, R.S. (1968) On learning characteristics of the adult aphasic. *Cortex*, **4,** 92.

Castner, B. (1940) Language development. In *The First Five Years of Life* (Ed.) Gesell, A. p. 189. New York: Harper and Row.

Chapey, R. (Ed.) (1981) *Language Intervention Strategies in Adult Aphasia*. Baltimore, MD: Williams and Wilkins.

Clarke, E. (1972) On the child's acquisition of antonyms in two semantic fields. *Journal of Verbal Learning and Verbal Behavior*, **11,** 750.

Cole, E.M. (1950) Work of the aphasia unit at Cushing V.A. hospital. *Journal of Nervous and Mental Diseases*, **112,** 75.

Copland, J. (1883) A case of aphasia; recovery. *Lancet*, **2,** 896.

Corbin, M.L. (1951) Group speech therapy for motor aphasia and dysarthria. *Journal of Speech Disorders*, **16,** 21.

Delacato, C.H. (1963) *The Diagnosis and Treatment of Speech and Reading Problems*. Springfield, IL: Thomas.

Darley, F.L. (1982) *Aphasia*. Philadelphia: W.B. Saunders.

Darley, F.L. (1972) The efficacy of language rehabilitation in aphasia. *Journal of Speech and Hearing Disorders*, **37,** 3.

Delay, J. & Lhermitte, F. (1963) Aphasie: problèmes neuropsychologiques; rééducation. *Encyclopédie médico-chirurgie, 17019 A^{50}*, 4.

Dissez, C. (1971) Etude de la méthode audio-visuelle dans le rééducation des aphasiques. *Revue de Laryngologie* (Bordeaux), **92,** 555.

Douglass, E. (1953) Diagnostic, classification and reeducation in aphasia. *Canadian Medical Association Journal*, **69,** 376.

Ducarne, B. (1976) Troubles neuropsychologiques des traumatisés crâniens ayant subi un coma plus ou moins prolongé. *Psychologie Française*, **21,** 59.

Edwards, A.E. (1965) Automated training for matching-to-sample task in aphasia. *Journal of Speech and Hearing Research*, **8,** 39.

Eimas, P.D., Siqueland, E.R., Jusczyk, P. & Vigorito, J.M. (1971) Speech perception in infants. *Science*, **171,** 303.

Eisenson, J. (1947) Aphasics: observations and tentative conclusions. *Journal of Speech Disorders*, **12,** 290.

Eisenson, J. (1949) Prognostic factors related to language rehabilitation in aphasic patients. *Journal of Speech Disorders*, **14,** 262.

Eisenson, J. (1960) When and what in aphasia. *Monographs of the Society for Research in Child Development*, **25,** 90.

Eisenson, J. (1964) Aphasia: a point of view as to the nature of the disorder and factors that determine prognosis for recovery. *International Journal of Neurology*, **4,** 287.

Eliasberg, W.G. (1947) Social implications of dysphasia. *Journal of Nervous and Mental Diseases*, **105,** 469.

Eliasberg, W.G. (1963) Wills in stroke and aphasia. *Disorders of the Nervous System*, **24,** 105.

Elvin, M.B. & Olfield, R.C. (1951) Disabilities and progress in a dysphasic university student. *Journal of Neurology, Neurosurgery and Psychiatry*, **14,** 118.

Ettlinger, G. & Moffett, A.M. (1970) Learning in dysphasia. *Neuropsychologia*, **8,** 465.

Fabian, A. (1955) Reading disability; index of pathology. *American Journal of Orthopsychiatry*, **24,** 319.

Filby, Y. & Edwards, A.E. (1963) An application for automated teaching methods to test and teach form discrimination to aphasics. *Journal of Programmed Instruction*, **2,** 25.

Fink, S.L. (1961) The clinical psychologist evaluates aphasia rehabilitation. *Journal of the American Speech Association*, **3,** 177.

Froment, J. (1921) La rééducation des aphasiques moteurs: principes, procédés et résultats. *Paris médicale*, **41,** 267.

Froment, J. & Monod, O. (1914) La rééducation des aphasiques moteurs. *Lyon médicale*, **122,** 157, 213 and 283.

Gainotti, G. (1972) Emotional behavior and hemispheric side of lesion. *Cortex*, **8,** 41.

Galkowski, T. (1964) Phoniatric rehabilitation in cases of speech disorders of central origin. *Zdrowie Psychiczne*, **5,** 2.

Gardner, R.A. & Gardner, B.T. (1969) Teaching sign-language to a chimpanzee. *Science*, **165,** 664.

Gens, G.A. (1949) Let's be realistic about aphasia. *Training School Bulletin*, **46,** 49.

Giden, F.M., Eno, M.L. & Bosley, E.C. (1950) The occupational therapist discusses aphasia. *American Journal of Occupational Therapy*, **4,** 160.

Gloning, K. & Quatember, R. (1964) Some classification of aphasic disturbances with special reference to rehabilitation. *International Journal of Neurology*, **4,** 296.

Goldstein, H. & Cameron, H. (1952) New method of communication for the aphasic patient, *Arizona Medicine*, **9,** 17.

Granich, L. (1947) *Aphasia: a Guide to Retraining*. New York: Grune and Stratton.

Hackworth, H.B. & Best, J. (1965) Practical therapy for aphasics. *Rehabilitation Record*, **5,** 19.

Hassard, G.H. & Brien, L. (1962) Referral of aphasic patients. *Texas State Journal of Medicine*, **58,** 75.

Held, J.P. (1977) Rééducation de l'hémiplégique. *Concours médicale*, **99,** 80.

Helm, A. & Benson, D.F. (1978) *Visual Action Therapy for Global Aphasia*. Paper presented at the Academy of Aphasia Annual Meeting, Chicago.

Henske, A.A. (1880) Case of hemiplegia and aphasia ending in recovery. *Alienist and Neurologist*, **1,** 193.

Hillbon, E. (1965) Rehabilitation of brain-injured war veterans. *Suomen Hammaslaakariseuran Toimituksia*, **15,** 1104.

Holland, A.L. (1970) Case studies in aphasia rehabilitation using programmed instruction. *Journal of Speech and Hearing Disorders*, **35,** 377.

Holland, A.L. (1971) *Psycholinguistic and Behavioral Variables Underlying Recovery from Aphasia*. Washington: USA Department of Health, Education and Welfare.

Holland, A.L. (1978) Some practical considerations in aphasia therapy. In *Communication Disorders: an Audio Journal for Continuing Education* (Ed.) Bradford, L.J. Vol. 3. New York: Grune and Stratton.

Holland, A.L. & Harris, A.B. (1968) Aphasia rehabilitation using programmed instruction. In *Operant Processes in Remedial Speech and Language Training* (Ed.) Sloane, H. & MacAulay, B.D. Boston, MA: Houghton Mifflin.

Holland, A.L. & Levy, C.B. (1971) Syntactic generalization in aphasics as function of relearning an active sentence. *Acta Symbolica*, **2,** 2.

Holland, A.L. & Sonderman, J.C. (1974) Effects of a program based on the token test for teaching comprehension skills to aphasics. *Journal of Speech Research*, **17,** 589.

Horwitz, B. (1962) An open letter to the family of an adult patient with aphasia. *Rehabilitation Literature*, **23,** 141.

Houchin, T.D. & Delano, P.J. (1964) *How to Help Adults with Aphasia*. Washington: Public Affairs Press.

Howes, D. (1966) Comments on the so-called acquiescence set in aphasia. *Journal of Abnormal Psychology*, **71,** 151.

Huber, M. (1942) Re-education of aphasics. *Journal of Speech Disorders*, **1,** 112.

Hughes, T.M. (1961) Guidelines for aphasia. *American Archives of Rehabilitation Therapy*, **9,** 4.

Hurwitz, L.J. (1971) A neurologist's view on aphasia. *Gerontologia Clinica* (Basel), **13,** 307.

Ince, L.P. (1968) Desensitization with an aphasic patient. *Behavioral Research Therapy*, **6,** 235.

Jenkins, J.J. & Schuell, H. (1961) Changing concepts of aphasia. *Perceptual and Motor Skills*, **13,** 270.

Jenkins, J.J. & Schuell, H. (1964) Further work on language deficit in aphasia. *Psychological Review*, **71,** 87.

Jenkins, J.J. & Schuell, H. (1965) Acquiescence response set in aphasics. *Journal of Abnormal Psychology*, **70,** 111.

Johns, D.F. (Ed.) (1978) *Clinical Management of Neurogenic Communicative Disorders*. Boston, MA: Little, Brown and Company.

Jones, M.V. (1956) Rebuilding language in stroke patients. *Journal of Rehabilitation*, **22,** 9.

Jones, M.V. (1965) Programs for dyslexics. *Rehabilitation Literature*, **26,** 236.

Jong, P.C. (1962) Research into the possibilities of rehabilitation of patients with aphasia. *Gerontologia Clinica* (Basel), **4,** 134.

Keenan, J.S. (1966) A method for eliciting naming behavior from aphasic patients. *Journal of Speech and Hearing Disorders*, **31,** 261.

Keith, R.L. & Aronson, A.E. (1975) Singing as therapy for apraxia of speech and aphasia: report of a case. *Brain and Language*, **2,** 483.

Keith, R.L. & Darley, F.L. (1967) The use of a specific electric board in rehabilitation of the aphasic patient. *Journal of Speech and Hearing Disorders*, **32,** 148.

Kendrick, D.C. (1965) Speed and learning in the diagnosis of diffuse brain damage in elderly subjects: a Bayesian statistical approach. *British Journal of Social and Clinical Psychology*, **4,** 141.

Kennedy, L. (1947) Remedial procedures for handling aphasic patients. *Archives of Neurology and Psychiatry* (Chicago), **57,** 646.

Kiml, J. (1967) Re-education of speech in total aphasia. *Folia phoniatrica* (Basel), **19,** 34.

Kimmel, H.D. (1966) Inhibition of the unconditioned response in classical conditioning. *Psychological Review*, **3,** 232.

Klima, E.S. & Bellugi, U. (1974) Language in another mode. *Neurosciences Research Program Bulletin*, **12,** 539.

Klingbeil, G.M. (1939) The historical background of the modern speech clinic; part 2: aphasia. *Journal of Speech and Hearing Disorders*, **4,** 267.

Kushner, H., Hubbard, D.J. & Knox, A.W. (1973) Effects of punishment on learning by aphasic subjects. *Perceptual and Motor Skills*, **36,** 283.

Lapoint, L.L. (1977) Base-10 programmed stimulation: task specification, scoring and plotting performance in aphasia therapy. *Journal of Speech and Hearing Disorders*, **42,** 90.

Lashley, K.S. (1938) Factors limiting recovery after central nervous lesions. *Journal of Nervous and Mental Disorders*, **88,** 733.

Lee, L.L. (1961) Some semantic goals for aphasia therapy. *ETC: a Review of General Semantics*, **43,** 261.

Leischner, A. (1974) Le fonctionnement et les méthodes d'une clinique d'aphasiologie. *Le Langage et l'Homme*, **24,** 17.

Levy, C.B. & Holland, A.L. (1971) *Influence of Grammatical Complexity and Sentence Length on Comprehension in Adult Aphasics*. Washington: USA Department of Health, Education and Welfare.

Lhermitte, F. & Ducarne, B. (1968) Problèmes psychologiques, sociaux et professionnels des aphasiques: l'aphasique dans la société. *Evolution médicale*, **12,** 547.

Linn, L. (1967) Sodium Amytal in treatment of Aphasia. *Archives of Neurology and Psychiatry*, **58,** 357.

Linn, L. & Stein, M. (1946) Sodium amytal in treatment of aphasia: preliminary report. *Bulletin of US Army Medical Department*, **5,** 705.

Longerich, M. (1958) *Manual for the Aphasic Patient*. New York: McMillan.

Longerich, M. & Bordeaux, J. (1958) *Aphasia Therapeutics*. New York: McMillan.

Lowman, E.W. & Rusk, H.A. (1962) Self-help devices: aphasia therapy. *Postgraduate Medicine*, **32,** 79 and 182.

Luria, A.R. & Tzetkova, L.S. (1967) The re-education of victims of cerebral lesions and its psychopedagological implications. *Bulletin of Psychology*, **20,** 880.

Malone, R.L. (1969) Expressed attitudes of families of aphasics. *Journal of Speech and Hearing Disorders*, **34,** 146.

Marks, M.M., Taylor, M.L. & Rusk, H.A. (1957) Rehabilitation of the aphasic patient: a survey of three years experience in a rehabilitation setting. *Archives of Physical Medicine*, **38,** 219.

Martin, B.R. (1962) *Communicative Aids for the Adult Aphasic*. Springfield, IL: Thomas.

Mason, C.F. (1961–1962) Hypnotic motivation of aphasics. *Journal of Clinical and Experimental Hypnosis*, **9,** 297.

McArthur, J.A. (1972) Speech and language disorders in the adult. *Rehabilitation*, **7.**

McLeod, J. (1964) Aphasia and dysarthria. *New Zealand Speech Therapy Journal*, **2,** 4.

McLeod, J. (1965) Dyslexia and speech defects. *Journal of the Australian College of Speech Therapy*, **15,** 46.

Medico-legal section (Ed.) (1950) Testamentary capacity: aphasia. Lewin v. Lewin. *South African Medical Journal*, **38,** 815, 834.

Mehrabian, A. (1972) *Nonverbal Communication*. Chicago, IL: Aldine Atherton.

Meyers, R. (1937) Aphasia: a problem in differential diagnosis and re-education. *Quarterly Journal of Speech*, **23,** 357.

Mills, C. (1904) Treatment of aphasia by training. *Journal of the American Medical Association*, **43,** 1940.

Mills, C.K. & Weisenburg, T.H. (1905) Word-blindness with a record of a case due to a lesion in the right cerebral hemisphere in a right-handed man; with some discussion of the treatment of visual aphasia. *Medicine*, **11,** 822.

Modgins, E. (1964) *Episode*. New York: Atheneum.

Modgins, E. (196[illegible]) *Having a Stroke and Getting Over It*. New York: Atheneum.

Montague, U. (1962) *Behavioral Changes in Patients Following Strokes*. Springfield, IL: Thomas.

Morley, J.H. (196[illegible]) Applying linguistics to speech and language therapy for aphasics. *Language Learning*, **10,** 135.

Moser, D. (1961) An understanding approach to the aphasic patient. *American Journal of Nursing*, **61,** 52.

Moss, C.S. (1972) *Recovery from Aphasia: the Aftermath of My Stroke*. Springfield, IL: University of Illinois Press.

Mowrer, O.H. (1960) *Learning Theory and the Symbolic Processes*. New York: Wiley.

Nedelec, Y. (1970) Rythme et évolution de la rééducation chez l'aphasique. *Journal française d'Oto-rhino-laryngologie*, **19,** 199.

Nielsen, J.M. (1963) Speech defects in middle life. *Geriatrics*, **18,** 827.

Nielsen, J.M. & Schultz, D.A. (1948) Treatment of traumatic aphasics of World War II at Birmingham General VA Hospital, Van Nuys, California. *Military Surgeon*, **102,** 351.

Palmer, M.F. (1950) Aphasia and occupational therapy. *American Journal of Occupational Therapy*, **4,** 95.

Pause, B.E. & McCroskey, R.L. (1962) Treatment of the adult hemiplegic patient with aphasia. *Journal of the American Physical Therapy Association*, **2,** 111.

Peacher, W.G. & Peacher, G.M. (1948) Management of speech disorders in a hospital clinic. *Diseases of the Nervous System*, **9,** 3.

Peuser, G. (1974) Le rôle du linguiste dans une clinique d'aphasiologie. *Le Langage et l'Homme*, **24,** 24.

Pfaff, P.L. (1940) The moto-kinaesthetic method applied to aphasia. *Journal of Speech Disorders*, **5,** 271.

Pialoux, P., Valtat, M., Freyss, G. & Legent, F. (1975) *Précis d'orthophonie*. Paris: Masson.

Pizzamiglio, L. & Roberts, M. (1967) Writing in aphasia: a learning study. *Cortex*, **3,** 250.

Reeves, E.W. (1963) The aphasic patient. *Nursing Outlook*, **11,** 522.

Reynolds, G.L. & Tikofsky, R.S. (1961) Further investigation of nonverbal learning with adult aphasics. *Journal of the American Speech Association*, **3,** 343.

Ritchie, D. (1961) *Stroke: a Study of Recovery*. Garden City, New York: Doubleday.

Robbins, S.D. (1939) Examination and re-education of aphasics. *Journal of Speech and Hearing Disorders*, **4,** 15.

Rosenberg, B. & Edwards, A.E. (1965) An automated multiple response alternative training program for use with aphasics. *Journal of Speech Research*, **8,** 415.

Sadek-Khalil, D. (1971) Essai de présentation de deux cas d' 'aphasie'. *Revue de Laryngologie* (Bordeaux), **92,** 546.

Sahs, A.L., Martman, E.C. & Aronson, S.M. (1976) *Guidelines for Stroke Care*. Washington: USA Department of Health, Education and Welfare.

Sarno, M.T. (1972) *Aphasia*. New York: Appleton-Century-Crofts.

Sarno, M.T. & Levita, E. (1971) Natural course of recovery in severe aphasia. *Archives of Physical Medicine*, **52,** 175.

Sarno, M.T. & Silverman, M. (1970) Psychological factors and recovery in geriatric patients with severe aphasia. *Journal of the American Geriatric Society*, **18,** 405.

Scargill, H.M. (1954) Modern linguistics and recovery from aphasia. *Journal of Speech Disorders*, **19,** 504.

Schafer, J.A., Mumber, R.S. & Psaki, R.C. (1954) Understanding aphasia. *Archives of Physical Medicine*, **35,** 228.

Schuell, H. (1955) Diagnosis and prognosis in aphasia. *Archives of Neurology and Psychiatry* (Chicago), **74,** 308.

Schuell, H. (1960) Review of the month: speech and brain mechanisms. *Rehabilitation Literature*, **21,** 181.

Schuell, H. (1975) *Aphasia: Theory and Therapy*. Baltimore, MD: University Park Press.

Schuell, H., Carroll, V.A. & Street, B.S. (1955) Clinical treatment of aphasia. *Journal of Speech Disorders*, **20,** 43.

Schuell, H., Jenkins, J.J. & Jimenez-Pabon, E. (1964) *Aphasia in Adults: Diagnosis, Prognosis and Treatment*. New York: Harper and Row.

Seron, X., Lambert, J.-L. & der Linden (van), M. (1977) *La Modification du Comportement*. Brussels: Dessart and Margada.

Shankweiler, D.P. (1959) Effects of success and failure instructions on reaction time in patients. *Journal of Comparative and Physiological Psychology*, **52,** 546.

Sheehan, V.M. (1946) Rehabilitation of aphasics in an army hospital. *Journal of Speech Disorders*, **11,** 149.

Sheehan, V.M. (1948) Techniques in the management of aphasics. *Journal of Speech Disorders*, **13,** 241.

Smith, M. (1948) Teaching an aphasic how to write again. *Journal of Clinical Psychology*, **4,** 419.

Smith, S. & Turton, E.C. (1951) Restoration of speech in severe aphasia by intravenous and oral priscol. *British Medical Journal*, **2,** 891.

Stoicheff, M.L. (1960) Motivating instructions and language performance of dysphasic subjects. *Journal of Speech Research*, **3,** 75.

Subirana, A. (1956) Vision neurologique des troubles du langage d'intérêt phoniatrique: le pronostic des aphasies de l'adulte. *Folia Phoniatrica* (Basel), **8,** 147.

Swezey, R.L., Friedman, R.E. & Gales, M.R. (1970) A communication device for severely dysarthric persons with agraphia. *Archives of Physical Medicine*, **51,** 501.

Taylor, M.L. (1958) *Understanding Aphasia: a Guide for Families and Friends*. New York: Institute of Physical Medicine and Rehabilitation.

Taylor, M.L. (1964) Linguistic considerations of the verbal behavior of the brain-damaged adult. *Linguistic Reporter*, **6,** 1.

Taylor, M.L. & Marks, M. (1955) *Aphasia Rehabilitation: Manual and Workbook*. New York: Institute of Physical Medicine and Rehabilitation.

Taylor, M.L. & Marks, M. (1959) *Aphasia Rehabilitation: Manual and Therapy Kit*. New York: McGraw-Hill.

Taylor, M.L. & Rusk, H.A. (1957) Speech problems of hemiplegics. *Public Health Reports* (Washington), **72,** 832.

Teitelbaum, H.A. (1950) Communication for the paralyzed. *Nursing World*, **124,** 351.

Tissot, A. (1972) Ré-éducation des aphasies de Broca. *Médecine et Hygiène* (Geneva), **30,** 1820.

Tobis, J.S. (1959) Physical medicine and rehabilitation management in aphasia. *Journal of the American Medical Association*, **169,** 393.

Tobis, J.S., Lowenthall, M. & Simon, M. (1957) Evaluation and management of the brain-damaged patient. *Journal of the American Medical Association*, **165,** 2035.

Travis, L.E. (1971) *Handbook of Speech Pathology and Audiology*. New York: Appleton-Century Crofts.

Turnblom, M. & Myers, J.S. (1952) A group discussion program with the families of aphasic patients. *Journal of Speech Disorders*, **17,** 393.

Tyrer, J.H. (1965) The re-education of aphasics. Experiences in the language re-education centre of the Salpêtrière hospital. *Journal of the Australian College of Speech Therapy*, **15,** 43.

Ulatowska, H.K. & Richardson, S.M. (1974) A longitudinal study of an adult with aphasia: considerations for research and therapy. *Brain and Language*, **1,** 151.

Valladares, C.M. (1959) Classification et nomenclature des syndromes aphasiques: thérapies orthophoniques suggérées. *Acta Audiologica y Foniatrica Hispano-americana*, **1,** 143. (In Spanish.)

Velletri-Glass, A., Gazzaniga, M.S. & Premack, D. (1973) Artificial language training in global aphasics. *Neuropsychologia*, **11,** 95.

Voinescu, I., Dobrota, I. & Gheorghita, N. (1972) Aspects psychothérapiques de la rééducation de l'aphasie. *Revue roumaine de Neurologie*, **9,** 387.

Wartenberg, R. (1961) Testamentary capacity in aphasia. *Neurology*, **2,** 749.

Watzlawick, P., Beavin, J.H. & Jackson, D.D. (1967) *Pragmatics Human Communication: a Study of Interactional Patterns, Pathologies and Paradoxes*. New York: Norton.

Weidner, W. & Lasky, E. (1976) The interaction of rate and complexity of stimulus on the performance of adult aphasic subjects. *Brain and Language*, **3,** 34.

Weinstein, S. (1959) Experimental analysis of an attempt to improve speech in cases of expressive aphasia. *Neurology*, **9,** 632.

Wepman, J.M. (1947) The organization of therapy for aphasia: 1. The in-patient treatment center. *Journal of Speech Disorders*, **12,** 405.

Wepman, J.M. (1951) *Recovery from Aphasia*. New York: Ronald Press.

Wepman, J.M. (1953) A conceptual model for the process involved in recovery from aphasia. *Journal of Speech Disorders*, **18,** 4.

Wepman, J.M. (1958) The relationship between self-correction and recovery from aphasia. *Journal of Speech Disorders*, **23,** 302.

Wepman, J.M. (1958) Aphasia and the 'whole-person' concept. *American Archives of Rehabilitation Therapy*, **1,** 1.

Wepman, J.M. (1962) New frontiers of aphasia therapy. *Hearing News*, **5,** 11.

Wepman, J.M. & Morency, A. (1963) Filmstrips as an adjunct to language therapy for aphasia. *Journal of Speech Disorders*, **28,** 191.

Wepman, J.M. & Pelt, D. (van) (1955) A theory of cerebral language disorders based on therapy. *Folia Phoniatrica* (Basel), **7,** 223.

West, J.A. (1973) Auditory comprehension in aphasic adults: improvement through training. *Archives of Physical Medicine*, **54,** 78.

West, R. & Stockel, S. (1965) The effect of meprobamate on recovery from aphasia. *Journal of Speech Research*, **8,** 57.

Wulf, H.H. (1973) *Aphasia: My World Alone*. Wayne, MI: Wayne State University Press.

18. Aphasia in Bilinguals and Polyglots

[Did you see the doctor again?]* Euh oui. Oui. [When did you see him?] Euh, lundi passé. [What did he say?] Euh, il m'a dit . . . Ah! je . . . Ha! I don't know what you say. [Do you still happen to speak English?] Oui, euh, to mes enfants . . . to everybody . . . [Did your mother or your father speak English?] N . . Mon père. [Was your father English-speaking? Was he of English origin?] Non, Non, à la maison, c'était tout français. A la maison, my . . . my house, c'est tout français. C'est tout français everywhere . . . [What sort of difficulty do you have?] Euh, when . . . Quand je veux parler à mes amis—n'importquoi—je parle anglais. Je parle, euh anglais. You know. [When you speak English, do you also have difficulty in finding words? Or is it only in French?] J'ai de la difficulté aussi, mais . . . not much though.

(Conversation with Mrs Son.; February 1977)

The study of language pathology in bilinguals and polyglots can provide important information about the organizational principles underlying language comprehension and production and thus can suggest directions for the development of explanatory models in theoretical linguistics, supply material for a theory of bilingualism, and possibly contribute to the diagnosis and prognosis of aphasic syndromes in patients who have mastered two or more languages.

RECOVERY OF DIFFERENT LANGUAGES

Little progress has been made since Pitres' famous study of aphasia in polyglots, a study which has been referred to since its publication in 1895[1-4]. Pitres briefly cited 16 cases gleaned from the medical literature of the past 40 years and added seven more detailed case studies of his own. He noted that polyglots who become aphasic generally lose, to the same extent, the use of all languages with which they are familiar and simultaneously recover the ability to use all languages as their condition improves. Nevertheless, this is not always the case; certain languages are sometimes more affected or, if all are equally impaired, certain ones may be less fully recovered than others, or not be recovered at all, during the course of evolution. Pitres raised questions about the explanation of these differences and the laws governing the pattern of language recovery.

The different languages of polyglot aphasics may indeed be recovered in numerous and varied ways: at least six different patterns have been identified in the cases which have been described during the last century[5]:

1. Recovery is said to be *parallel* when all the languages known by the patient are similarly impaired and are restored at the same rate. This recovery pattern appears to be by far the most common.
2. Recovery is said to be *differential* when the patient does not recover all previously spoken languages to the same extent or when one or more languages are recovered more slowly than another one or others.
3. Recovery is described as *successive* when restoration of one language does not begin before another one has been recovered (at least partially).

* In this sample, only the questions have been translated into English. The answers remain untranslated in order to show the switches between French and English.

4. Recovery is called *selective* when one or more of the patient's languages is not restored. Among reported cases of this recovery pattern, certain patients have been described as having lost both comprehension and expression. In contrast, others who did not recover the expressive use of one or more languages nevertheless retained or recovered comprehension.
5. Recovery is said to be *antagonistic* when one language regresses as recovery of another one progresses during evolution.
6. Finally, recovery is said to be *mixed* when bilinguals systematically mix their two languages. This intermingling has been reported at all levels: intrusion of words of the other language within sentences, endings from one language added to words of the other, telescoping at the level of morphemes, thus forming hybrid words [e.g., *jahno* from the German word *ja* and the Czechoslovakian word *ahno* (yes)][6], or formation of words using morphemes of two languages [e.g., *heftag* from the German word *Montag* and the Hungarian word *hefto* (Monday)][7]. The substitution of Cyrillic for Latin letters and vice versa has also been reported.

These different modes of recovery are not necessarily mutually exclusive either with respect to time or several different languages. Thus, for example, antagonistic recovery may occur after a period of successive recovery, and parallel recovery of two languages may occur while a third language remains selectively unavailable.

FACTORS RELATED TO DIFFERENTIAL RECOVERY

The search for an explanation of non-parallel recovery of different languages began with Ribot. Formulated in 1881, his *law of regression* predicts preferential recovery of the mother tongue in polyglot aphasics: according to this law, the most recent memory formations are the first to be destroyed while the oldest are the most stable and, consequently, the most resistant to morbid dissolution[8]. Several other factors have since been evoked, always with the aim of explaining the exceptions to the rules which had been previously formulated.

Primacy

Linguistic habits acquired in childhood are more resistant to aphasia than those acquired later, regardless of the respective degree of familiarity at the time of insult. Consequently, the mother tongue will be the least impaired and thus the first to reappear in cases of successive recovery, the most fully restored in differential recovery and the only one restored in selective recovery in bilinguals: such are the teachings of what is called *Ribot's rule*[8]. It should be noted that this explanation, like those which follow, cannot account for either the mixed or antagonistic modes of recovery.

Automaticity

What is acquired later to a high degree of automaticity may supplant earlier acquisitions of the same type. The order of recovery is thus from the language which was most automatic to the language which was least automatic at the time of insult. The determining factor is the degree of practice. It is thus the subject's most commonly used language (which is usually but not always the mother tongue) which first reappears, because it is based on the most solidly established associations: such is the content of *Pitres' rule*.

Affect

Links of affection between the patient and a particular speaker, or a group of speakers, of one of his languages; strong occupational motivation, such as the desire to regain the language of the work place, or the desire to improve social standing by regaining the most prestigious language, may result in recovery of a language which is neither the patient's most commonly used one nor his mother tongue. Psychosexual and psychosocial components of the patient's emotional life are able to play, through a powerful psychoneurobiological force, a decisive role in the selection of a particular language for recovery: such is the content of *Minkowski's rule*.

Visualization

The recovery of a standard language (which can be written), instead of a dialect which is only spoken, might possibly be due to the potential for mental visualization of written words in the former case. Particularly in cases where there is no damage to areas of the brain involved in reading and writing, the visual element of a language may facilitate the recovery of other elements[9]. A classical (i.e., dead) language, acquired through reading and writing, may then be less affected than the mother tongue acquired through listening and speaking[10].

Nature of the written code

Recovery of a phonetically written language (in which there is a high degree of correspondence between graphemes and phonemes, as in Russian, or between written characters and syllables, as in kana representations in Japanese) may be better or poorer, depending on the site of lesion, than that of an ideographically written language (such as Chinese in which there is no correspondence between written characters and pronunciation)[11, 12]. Languages usually written without vowels, such as Hebrew, would be somewhere in between but closer to ideograms since they are difficult to read out of context, that is, without prior knowledge about meaning[13–15].

Orientation of writing

In cases of right or left hemianopsia, reading of one language may be favoured over another, depending on whether the language is written from left to right, such as English and French, or from right to left, such as Arabic and Hebrew[14].

Severity

Parallel recovery of all known languages may occur in certain patients after a first aphasic episode while only one language is recovered after a second, more severe stroke[16, 17]. This observation led to the hypothesis that there probably exists in the brain 'a functional substratum common to all languages' [8] and that, in conditions of global weakening, the polyglot aphasic can accomplish only a limited number of linguistic functions. If the language zone is severely damaged, polyglots would thus be limited, at least temporarily, to the use of one language. Moreover, the choice of a particular language would be increasingly restricted with increased impairment of brain functioning[19]. It may be that, in severe cases, the patient concentrates on one language in order to economize his/her resources while this psychological defence mechanism against the catastrophic impairment of an important faculty is not needed in cases of mild impairment[20].

Appropriateness

Certain patients do not recover either their mother tongue or most commonly used language but rather the one used in the hospital environment during their convalescence. This fact led to the hypothesis that the language which is preferentially recovered is the one which is most useful to the patient[21] and most adapted to his/her purposes[22]. The language available may also depend on the subject to be discussed[23], on the interlocutor[24], or on the habitual use of a particular language in a given situation[25].

Context of acquisition

The patient's different languages are likely to be more or less interdependent, depending on whether they were learned in the same context (e.g., the parents sometimes used one language and sometimes the other) or in separate contexts (e.g., the mother tongue was used in the family setting and another language was later acquired in a foreign country). It can be expected that languages acquired in the same context would be more likely to be recovered in a parallel fashion after the onset of aphasia, while languages acquired in different contexts would be more susceptible to differential recovery[26].

When considered individually, none of the above factors appears to be responsible for a particular mode of recovery. While certain patients regained the language of the hospital setting although it was neither their mother tongue nor most familiar language, other patients did not regain the language used in their environment even though it was both their mother tongue and most commonly used language. In other cases, the language recovered was neither the patient's mother tongue, nor his most familiar language, nor that of the environment in which he regained consciousness. It is clear that other factors enter into play besides acquisition order and the degree of familiarity or utility in the circumstances of convalescence. The patient may sometimes be completely unable to use the language to which he is emotionally most attached (for political–religious reasons and because it is the only language allowing communication with his children)[27]. The patient's proficiency in a particular language does not appear to provide a better explanation of preferential recovery. Gelb[28] has even maintained that preferential recovery of a foreign language, or especially of a classical language, may occur precisely because it is less automatized and requires greater effort of reflection. Such mental effort may stimulate the damaged mechanism where the mother tongue appears insufficient.

Similarly, increasing severity of aphasia does not necessarily lead to the use of only one language, as shown by Zierer's description[29] of a five-year-old child who was fluent in German and Spanish. Twelve days after the surgical ablation of a cerebral tumour, symptoms of aphasia began to appear, first of a motor aphasia and then of a receptive aphasia which gradually became total. As the patient's state deteriorated and the aphasia became progressively more severe, increasing but always parallel impairment of both languages was observed until there was a total absence of both comprehension and production.

It should not be forgotten that, as first implied by Pitres[1], cases of non-parallel recovery are the exception rather than the rule[30]. Despite this, they are as interesting and as instructive as cases of 'pure' aphasia which are equally rare, if not even rarer, in unilingual aphasics (see Chapter 4). It is nevertheless true that, regardless of whether their languages were acquired in identical or very different contexts, most aphasics recover them in proportion to their degree of mastery before the onset of aphasia.

There does not appear to be any correlation between the pattern of recovery of different languages and the type of aphasia[5]. Neither this nor any of the other factors discussed can be considered to be the only cause of a given pattern of evolution. It is far more likely that a polyglot's particular mode of recovery of different languages depends on multiple and interacting factors, including the order in which the languages were acquired, the respective degrees of proficiency attained in each language, the emotional attachment to each of the languages used, the size and the site of lesion, patients' age at the onset of aphasia, their intellectual level, their degree of literacy and particularly the extent to which reading and writing are part of their daily activities, the ways and the context in which each language is used, as well as the way each language is organized at the phonological, morphological, syntactical and semantic levels[31].

FUNCTIONAL AND ANATOMICAL ORGANIZATION IN BILINGUALS AND POLYGLOTS

Regardless of the particular characteristics of the language preferentially recovered (i.e., whether it be the mother tongue, the most familiar language, the most useful one, the one preferred emotionally, etc.), an important question remains: how can one language be almost completely recovered to the exclusion of all others? This question has given rise to three hypotheses: (1) each language is stored in a different location in the brain; (2) the unrecovered language is not lost but inhibited; (3) there is a locus in the brain which functions as a switch mechanism and allows the patient to shift from one language to another.

The first hypothesis has not found many supporters but did attract a large number of critics[7, 9, 18, 32–36]. The second hypothesis, which is in accord with the general laws of excitation, interference and inhibition between all types of neural phenomena[36], is more widely accepted. Differential recovery does not appear attributable to organic destruction of physiologically specialized centres but seems to reflect functional disturbances. A selective deficit is not caused by the destruction of the language stored in a certain part of the cortex, but by the inability to retrieve the stored information. Several facts provide support for this hypothesis: (a) in many cases, the patient is unable to utter a word of a given language but nevertheless understands it; thus the selective aphasia cannot be caused by the destruction of the traces or engrams[16]; (b) the loss of a language (sometimes of both comprehension and expression), is often only temporary; in certain cases, the subsequent recovery from the linguistic disturbance is too rapid to be explained by (re)learning[1, 4]; (c) neurotic patients without evident focal cerebral lesions exhibit the same types of reactions as polyglots[37–39]; (d) the unavailable languages do return during particular cerebral states[40], such as delirium[41], epileptic attacks or under hypnosis[37].

The hypothesis that one language is inhibited while another is used and that, in certain pathological states, this inhibition is permanent, is compatible with (although independent of) the hypothesis of a localized mechanism which permits switching from one language to another. The latter hypothesis has given rise to two interpretations, one localizationist and the other functional.

THE SWITCH MECHANISM

Several observations suggested a close relationship between a lesion of the supramarginal gyrus and selective language recovery. Thus this cortical region was thought to function as a shunting device, or switch mechanism, permitting the shift from one language to another[17, 42–45]. A lesion in this zone would cause the patient either to speak only one language or to shift involuntarily from one language to another.

Two types of contradictory evidence were nevertheless reported: on the one hand, cases were observed in which there were difficulties in shifting from one language to another, or again, utterances consisting of a mixture of several languages, despite the anatomical intactness of the left temporoparietal region[7, 9, 46, 47]; on the other hand, there were cases in which a left temporoparietal lesion did not cause difficulty in switching between languages[7, 47, 48]. However, it is not necessary to postulate that if a switching mechanism is a fact of cerebral functioning, it must then have a specific anatomical localization.

In fact, the ability to switch need not be a particular faculty of bilinguals and polyglots. It may be conceived as a more general function put to a particular use, one which does not involve a mechanism specific to these groups. The decision to speak Russian or English is perhaps of the same order as the decision to speak or to remain silent. The decision to switch from one language to another, just like the decision initially to speak in a particular language, is more economically explained by the functioning of a general neural mechanism than by a specialized mechanism serving only that particular purpose. There is no need to postulate a specific functional organization other than that possessed by each unilingual speaker and which permits him or her, among other things, to switch registers, changing from colloquial to formal language, using different vocabulary and more standard syntax. Goldstein[40] pointed out that any alteration of cerebral functioning impairs the ability to make sudden changes in mental processing (*attitude mentale*) and that shifts from one language to another can occur only if the faculty of abstraction is preserved. Along the same line, Jakobson[49] assumed that aphasics with *similarity disorders*, being unable to recognize equivalences, have great difficulty in translating or in switching from one language to another.

LATERALIZATION OF LANGUAGE FUNCTIONS

The study of bilingual aphasics and results from dichotic listening tests and tachistoscopic tests in normal bilingual subjects has led to various conclusions: (1) both languages are subserved by the dominant hemisphere for language (almost always the left)[50, 51]; (2) one language is represented in the left hemisphere and the other in the right hemisphere[52]; (3) one language is lateralized to the left hemisphere and the other is bilaterally represented[52–55]; (4) in bilinguals, the non-dominant hemisphere participates in linguistic functioning to a greater extent than in unilinguals and does so for both languages[7]; (5) both languages are represented in the two hemispheres, the organization of linguistic functioning being less lateralized in bilinguals[56].

At first sight, these conclusions may appear contradictory. However, it must be considered that they were based on particular cases. This might indicate that different bilinguals may have their languages represented differently, depending on what Charcot called one's *psychic type* (see Chapter 1) and today is generally known as *cognitive style*, their tendency to use gestaltist strategies involving mainly the right hemisphere, or analytical and sequential strategies especially involving the left hemisphere, the age at which the languages were acquired, the age at the time of insult (or testing), sex, the degree of sinistrality, and several other factors.

Left hemisphere lateralization of one of a bilingual's languages has been attributed by two authors to the forced use of the right hand in a non-right hander. In the first case, a left-hander had been forced to write with his right hand, thus facilitating the participation of the left hemisphere in the acquisition of a second language learned during this period[27]. In the second case, an ambidexterous individual had learned to handle weapons with his right hand at the same time as learning a second language. The investigator presumed that the mother tongue was equally represented in both hemispheres in this illiterate woodcutter but that his second language was lateralized to the left hemisphere[53]. Such transfer has been reported to occur following cranial trauma during childhood[57]. Similarly, during convalescence, the non-dominant hemisphere may assume new functions benefiting the language in which the patient is given therapy[58].

Some studies have focused on cerebral dominance in non-aphasic bilinguals. Although results from certain tachistoscopic or dichotic listening tests have indicated dominant hemisphere lateralization for both languages[50] and even stronger lateralization in bilinguals than in unilinguals[51], a few subjects showed greater facility with one language on the right and with the other language on the left, while some others showed a substantial left–right difference in the processing of one language and almost no difference in the other[52]. Certain authors have thus suggested that, while the first language is lateralized in the left hemisphere, the learning of a second language during adulthood requires significant right hemisphere participation[55].

THE ASSESSMENT OF APHASIA IN BILINGUALS

If different descriptions of aphasia in bilinguals are to be usefully compared, it is important that certain aspects are not overlooked during the aphasia assessment, something which has occurred too often in the past and precluded all attempts at meaningful comparisons. Confirmation of the neuropsychological reality of certain aspects of bilingualism will require the accumulation of systematic and quantitatively sufficient data. Certain difficulties are inherent in the nature of aphasia itself. Moreover, it is seldom possible to obtain an adequate estimate of the patient's type or even degree of bilingualism before the onset of aphasia. The family can be of only limited help because their judgements are often very subjective and lacking in precision

Insertion 18.1

A. *Neurological examination*
1. Anamnesis
2. Orientation in time and space
3. Memory
4. Praxis
5. Gnosis
6. Neurological examination

B. *Aphasia assessment in each language*
1. Spontaneous language
2. Comprehension: identification by pointing; orders; semantic fields; matching pictures and sentences
3. Repetition
4. Naming
5. Automatic series
6. Sentence construction
7. Verbal fluency
8. Acceptability judgements; synonyms; semantic incongruities
9. Description of sequential pictures
10. Auditory verbal discrimination
11. Reading: letters, words, sentences
12. Writing: copying, writing to dictation, spontaneous writing
13. Mental calculation

C. *Specific assessment of a given pair of languages*
1. Translation (to be done orally except in the case of impaired articulation) words from L_1 to L_2; words from L_2 to L_1; sentences from L_1 to L_2; sentences from L_2 to L_1.
2. Acceptability judgements of sentences incorporating syntactic structures from the other language.

(Excerpt from M. C. Goldblum and M. Paradis, *The Assessment of Aphasia in Bilinguals*, in preparation.)

about the various elements of the patient's language such as syntax, phonology and vocabulary. The judgements of family members are usually made in terms of the extent of expressive fluency and it is sometimes impossible to obtain more precise information from either the patient or anyone else.

In order to permit comparisons, the case description should nevertheless include as much of the information specified above (Insertion 18.1) as can possibly be obtained. A complete assessment of aphasia in a bilingual should consist of three parts: a section concerned with the case history and the neurological examination; a detailed assessment of each language; and a specific evaluation of a given pair of languages indicating possible interferences. The assessment of the two languages should be carried out within a relatively short time period (i.e., 72 hours or less) in order to minimize possible recovery between the two testing sessions. The case history should include at least the information listed below (Insertion 18.2).

Insertion 18.2

Anamnesis
Name:
Date of birth:
Father's mother tongue:
Father's currently spoken language(s):
Mother's mother tongue:
Mother's currently spoken language(s):
Language(s) spoken at home by father:
Language(s) spoken at home by mother:
Language(s) spoken at home by the patient during childhood:
Language(s) spoken at home by the patient before onset of aphasia:
Language(s) spoken at work by the patient before onset of aphasia:
Age of language learning: L_1 spoken; L_2 spoken:
Language(s) of educational instruction (specify dates in cases of changes):
Methods of learning: L_1; L_2:
Age of learning to read: L_1; L_2:
to write: L_1; L_2:
Handedness:
Present linguistic milieu:
Periods spent in other linguistic surroundings
(location, dates, circumstances):
Educational level:
Occupation:
Reason and date of hospitalization:
Medical history:
Assessment carried out between

________________ and ________________
(day) (month) (year)   (day) (month) (year)

REFERENCES

1. Pitres, A. (1895) Etude sur l'aphasie chez les polyglottes. *Revue médicale*, **15,** 8[illegible]
2. Glass, L. (1976) Performance of bilingual Cuban-American aphasic patients on a task of body part identification. *Human Communication*, **1,** 29.
3. Obler, L.K. & Albert, M.L. (1977) Influence of aging on recovery from aphasia in polyglots. *Brain and Language*, **4,** 460.
4. Galloway, L. (1978) Language impairment and recovery in polyglot aphasia: a case of a heptaglot. In *Aspects of Bilingualism* (Ed.) Paradis, M. p. 139. Columbia: Hornbeam Press.

5. Paradis, M. (1977) Bilingualism and aphasia. In *Studies in Neurolinguistics* (Ed.) Whitaker, H. & Whitaker, A. Vol. 3, p. 65. New York: Academic Press.
6. Leischner, A. (1943) Die 'Aphasie der Taubstummen'. Beitrag zur Lehre von der Asymbolie. *Archives of Psychiatry*, **115,** 469.
7. Gloning, I. & Gloning, K. (1965) Aphasien bei polyglotten. Beitrag zur Dynamik der Sphrachabbaus sowe zur Lokalisationsfrage dieser Störungen. *Wiener Zeitschrift für Nervenheilkunde*, **22,** 362.
8. Ribot, Th. (1881) *Les maladies de la mémoire*. Paris: Baillière.
9. Minkowski, M. (1927) Klinischer Beitrag zur Aphasie bei Polyglotten, speziell im Hinblick auf das Schweizerdeutsche. *Schweizer Archiv für Neurologie und Psychiatrie*, **21,** 43.
10. Hinshelwood, J. (1902) Four cases of word blindness. *Lancet*, **1,** 358.
11. Lyman, R., Kwan, S.T. & Chao, W.H. (1938) Left occipito-parietal brain tumor with observations on alexia and agraphia in Chinese and English. *Chinese Medical Journal*, **54,** 491.
12. April, R.S. & Tse, P.C. (1977) Crossed aphasia in a Chinese bilingual. *Archives of Neurology* (Chicago), **34,** 766.
13. Luria, A.R. (1956) K voprosu o narushenii pis'ma i chteniia u poliglotov. *Fiziologicheskii Zhurnal* (Moscow), **2,** 127.
14. Halpern, L. (1941) Beitrag zur Restitution der Aphasie bei Polyglotten in Hinblick auf das Hebräische. *Schweizer Archiv für Neurologie und Psychiatrie*, **47,** 150.
15. Halpern, L. (1949) La langue hébraïque dans la restitution de l'aphasie sensorielle chez les polyglottes. *Semaine des Hôpitaux de Paris*, **58,** 2473.
16. Pick, A. (1921) Zur Erklarung gewisser Ausnahmen von der sogenannten Ribotschen Regel. *Abhandlungen aus der Neurologie, Psychiatrie, Psychologie und ihren Grenzgebieter, Beiheft 13 zur Monatschrift für Psychiatrie und Neurologie*, 151.
17. Pötzl, O. (1925) Uber die parietal bedingte Aphasie und ihren Einfluss auf das Sprachen mehrerer Sprachen. *Zentralblatt für die gesamte Neurologie und Psychiatrie*, **96,** 100.
18. Minkowski, M. (1936) Sur des variétés particulières d'aphasie chez les polyglottes. *Schweizerische Medizin Wochenschrift*, **66,** 697.
19. Krapf, E.E. (1957) A propos des aphasies chez les polyglottes. *Encéphale*, **46,** 623.
20. Charlton, M. (1964) Aphasia in bilingual and polyglot patients: a neurological and psychological study. *Journal of Speech Disorders*, **29,** 307.
21. Bay, E. (1964) General discussion. In *Disorders of Language* (Ed.) de Reuck, A.V.S. & O'Connor, M. p. 115. London: Churchill.
22. Goldstein, K. (1948) Disturbances of language in polyglot individuals with aphasia. In *Language and Language Disturbances* (Ed.) Goldstein, K. p. 138. New York: Grune and Stratton.
23. Bálint, A. (1923) Bemerkungen zu einem Falle von polyglotter Aphasie. *Zentralblatt für die gesamte Neurologie und Psychiatrie*, **83,** 277.
24. Herschmann, H. & Pötzl, O. (1920) Bemerkungen über Aphasie der Polyglotten. *Neurologisches Zentralblatt*, **39,** 114.
25. Krapf, E. E. (1955) Über das Sprachverhalten hirngeschädigter Polyglotten. *Wiener Zeitschift für Nervenheilkunde*, **12,** 121.
26. Lambert, W.E. & Fillenbaum, S. (1959) A pilot study of aphasia among bilinguals. *Canadian Journal of Psychology*, **13,** 28.
27. Halpern, L. (1950) Observations on sensory aphasia and its restitution in a Hebrew polyglot. *Monatschrift für Psychiatrie und Neurologie*, **119,** 156.
28. Gelb, A. (1937) Zur medizinischen Psychologie und philosophischen Anthropologie. *Acta Psychologica*, **3,** 193 (see especially pp. 247 and 250).
29. Zierer, E. (1974) Psycho-linguistic and pedagogical aspects in the bilingual education of a child of pre-school age. *Lenguaje y Ciencias*, **14,** 47.
30. Nair, K.R. & Virmani, V. (1973) Speech and language disturbances in hemiplegics. *Indian Journal of Medical Research*, **61,** 1395.
31. Paradis, M. (1977) The stratification of bilingualism. In *The Third LACUS Forum* (Ed.) di Pietro, R.J. & Blansitt, E.L. Jr. p. 237. Columbia, OH: Hornbeam Press.
32. Veyrac, G.-J. (1931) *Etude de l'aphasie chez les sujets polyglottes*. Medical thesis, Paris.
33. Ombredane, A. (1951) *L'aphasie et l'élaboration de la pensée explicite*. Paris: Presses Universitaires de France.
34. Penfield, W. (1953) A consideration of the neurophysiological mechanisms of speech and some educational consequences. *Proceedings of the American Academy of Arts and Sciences*, **82,** 199.
35. Penfield, W. & Roberts, L. (1959) *Speech and Brain Mechanisms*. Princeton, NJ: Princeton University Press.
36. Minkowski, M. (1963) On aphasia in polyglots. In *Problems of Dynamic Neurology* (Ed.) Halpern, L. p. 119. Jerusalem: Hebrew University.
37. Ghilarducci, F. (1892) Contribution au diagnostic différentiel entre l'hystérie et les maladies organiques du cerveau. *Achives neurologiques* (Paris), **24,** 287.
38. Krapf, E.E. (1955) The choice of language in polyglot psychoanalysis. *Psychoanalytic Quarterly*, **24,** 343.
39. Gerstenbrand, F. & Stepan, H. (1956) Polyglotte Reaktion nach Hirnschädigung; ein kasuistischer Beitrag. *Wiener Zeitschrift für Nervenheilkunde*, **13,** 167.
40. Goldstein, K. (1933) L'analyse de l'aphasie et l'étude de l'essence du langage. *Journal de Psychologie normale et pathologique*, **30,** 430.
41. Eskridge, J.T. (1896) Mind and word deafness after depressed fracture of the skull with subcortical hemorrhage-operation; complete recovery. *Medical News* (New York), **68,** 698.
42. Kaunders, O. (1929) Über polyglotte Reaktionen bei einer sensorischen Aphasie. *Zentralblatt für die gesamte Neurologie und Psychiatrie*, **122,** 651.
43. Pötzl, O. (1930) Aphasie und Mehrsprachigkeit. *Zentralblatt für die gesamte Neurologie und Psychiatrie*, **124,** 145.

44. Hoff, H. & Pötzl, O. (19[illegible]) Schiefe Körperhaltung und schiefer Gang bei Kleinhirnerkrankung. *Jb. Psychiat. Neurol.*, **48,** 217.
45. Leischner, A. (1948) Über die Aphasie der Mehrsprachigen. *Archiv für Psychiatrie und Nervenkrankheiten*, **180,** 731.
46. Stengel, E. & Zelmanowicz, J. (1933) Über polyglotte motorische Aphasie. *Zentralblatt für die gesamte Neurologie und Psychiatrie*, **149,** 292.
47. Lhermitte, R., Hécaen, H., Dubois, J., Culioli, A. & Tabouret-Keller, A. (196[illegible]) Le problème de l'aphasie des polyglottes: remarques sur quelques observations. *Neuropsychologia*, **4,** 515.
48. Schulze, H.A.F. (1968) Unterschiedliche Rückbildung einer sensorischer und einer ideokinetischen motorischen Aphasie bei einem Polyglotten. *Psychiatrie, Neurologie und medizinische Psychologie*, **20,** 441.
49. Jakobson, R. (1955) Aphasia as a linguistic problem. In *On Expressive Language* (Ed.) Werner, H. p. 69. Worcester, MA: Clark University Press.
50. Kershner, J.R. & Jeng, A.G.-R. (1972) Dual functional hemispheric asymmetry in visual perception: effects of ocular dominance and postexposural processes. *Neuropsychologia*, **10,** 437.
51. Stark, R., Genesee, F., Lambert, W.E. & Seitz, M. (1974) Multiple language experience and cerebral dominance. (Personal communication to M. Paradis.)
52. Hamers, J.F. & Lambert, W.E. (1974) Visual field and cerebral hemisphere preferences in bilinguals. (Personal communication to M. Paradis.)
53. Gorlitzer von Mundy, V. (1959) Ein 94 Jähriger mit einem deutschen Sprachzentrum und mit warscheinlich 2 slowenischen Sprachzentren. *Wiener Medizinische Wochenschrift*, **109,** 358.
54. Vildomec, V. (1963) *Multilingualism*. Leyden: Sythoff (see especially pp. 58 to 65).
55. Obler, L.K., Albert, M.L. & Gordon, H. (1975) Asymmetry of cerebral dominance in Hebrew–English bilinguals. Communication presented to the *Thirteenth Annual Meeting of the Academy of Aphasia*, Victoria, British Columbia.
56. Ovcharova, P., Raichev, R. & Gelava, T. (1968) Afaziia u Poligloti. *Neurologiia, Psikhiatriia i Neurokhirurgiia*, **7,** 183.
57. Anastasopoulos, G.K. (1959) Linkseitige Hemiplegie mit Alexie, Agraphie und Aphasie bei einem polyglotten Rechtshänder. *Deutsche Zeitschrift für Nervenheilkunde*, **179,** 120.
58. Bychowski, Z. (1919) Über die Restitution der nach einem Schädelschuss verlorenen Umgangssprache bei einem Polyglotten. *Monatschrift für Psychologie und Neurologie*, **45,** 183.

BIBLIOGRAPHY

Alajouanine, Th., Cathala, H.P. & Métellus, J. (1973) La problématique de l'aphasie dans les langues à écriture non alphabétique: à propos d'un cas chez un Chinois. *Revue neurologique*, **128,** 229.

Alajouanine, Th., Cathala, H.P., Métellus, J., Siksou, M., Alleton, V., Cheng, F., Turckheim, C. (de) & Chang, C. (1973) *Etude analytique d'un cas d'aphasie avec alexie et agraphie chez un malade chinois*. Hôpital Albert-Chenevier (Service H.P. Cathala), Créteil.

Alajouanine, Th., Pichot, P & Durand, M. (1949) Dissociation des altérations phonétiques avec conservation relative de la langue la plus ancienne dans un cas d'anarthrie pure chez un sujet français bilingue. *Encéphale*, **28,** 245.

Albert, M.L. & Obler, L.K. (1978) *The Bilingual Brain*. New York: Academic Press.

Critchley, M. (1974) Aphasia in polyglots and bilinguals. *Brain and Language*, **1,** 15.

Gloning, I. & Gloning, K. (1965) Aphasien bei Polyglotten. Beitrag zur Dynamik der Sprachabbaus sowie zur Lokalisationsfrage dieser Störungen. *Wiener Zeitschrift für Nervenheilkunde*, **22,** 3[illegible]2.

Hécaen, H., Mazars, G., Ramier, A.M., Goldblum, M.C. & Merienne, L. (1971) Aphasie croisée chez un sujet droitier bilingue (vietnamien-français). *Revue neurologique*, **124,** 319.

Hécaen, H., Mazars, G., Ramier, A.M., Goldblum, M.C. & Mérienne, L. (1971) Aphasie croisée chez un sujet droitier bilingue (vietnamien-français). *Annales médico-psychologiques*, **2,** 611.

Lambert, W.E. & Fillenbaum, S. (1959) A pilot study of aphasia among bilinguals. *Canadian Journal of Psychology*, **13,** 28.

Lambert, W.E. & Fillenbaum, S. (1961) A pilot study of aphasia among bilinguals. In *Psycholinguistics: a Book of Readings* (Ed.) Saporta, S. p. 455. New York: Holt, Rinehart and Winston.

Lambert, W.E. & Fillenbaum, S. (1972) A pilot study of aphasia among bilinguals. In *Language, Psychology and Culture* (Ed.) Lambert, W.E. p. 79. Stanford, CA: Stanford University Press.

Lebrun, Y. (1971) The neurology of bilingualism. *Word*, **27,** 179.

Lebrun, Y. (1975) Early bilingualism. In *The Context of Foreign Language Learning* (Ed.) Henting, J.M. & van Essen, A.J. p. 61.

Lebrun, Y. (1976) Recovery in polyglot aphasics. In *Recovery in Aphasics* (Ed.) Lebrun, Y. & Hoops, R. p. 96. Amsterdam: Swets and Zeitlinger.

Lebrun, Y. & Hasquin, J. (1971) Bilinguisme précoce et troubles du langage. In *Aspects sociologiques du plurilinguisme*. p. 60. Bruxelles, AIMAV, and Paris: Didier.

Lecours, A.R. & Lhermitte, F. (1976) The 'pure form' of the phonetic disintegration syndrome (pure anarthria):

anatomo-clinical report of a historical case. *Brain and Language*, **3**, 88.

Leischner, A. (1948) Über die Aphasie der Mehrsprachigen. *Archiv für Psychiatrie und Nervenkrankheiten*, **180**, 731.

Luria, A.R. (1960) Differences between disturbance of speech and writing in Russian and French. *International Journal of Slavic Linguistics and Poetics*, **3**, 13.

Minkowski, M. (1928) Sur un cas d'aphasie chez un polyglotte. *Revue neurologique*, **1**, 36.

Minkowski, M. (1963) On aphasia in polyglots. In *Problems of Dynamic Neurology* (Ed.) Halpern, L. p. 119. Jerusalem: Jerusalem Post Press.

Paradis, M. (1977) Bilingualism and aphasia. In *Studies in Neurolinguistics* (Ed.) Whitaker, H. & Whitaker, H.A. Vol. 3, p. 65. New York: Academic Press.

Paradis, M. (1982) *Readings on Aphasia in Bilinguals and Polyglots*. Montreal: Didier.

Silverberg, R. & Gordon, H. (1979) Differential aphasia in two bilinguals. *Neurology*, **29**, 51.

19. Thought and Language
Thought without Language

About this winter ago, I found myself in compny with my friend, Marie, Mathé and Helene, and we became engaged in a discution in speech and thought. They all said that it is (nessarssary) necessary to speak in order to think but I'm sceptical of that idea. Cause I say that there are several ranks in thought, that is to say that there is a (glogal) global sense more or les indefinite and a definite sense, more or less precise. It's degreed that thought depeloups more with speech but it's a question of family, school, (and) life education, even of manners. Men are not all equal in their thought and in their words but he thinks just the same, even if it's trifles. As for me, I lost speech two week, but I (imagination) imagined awl the same, I searched words, it's like a (morm) memory blank but I had the idea roughly, then the more I went along that returned to its place. It's true that I had a mentality completely anchored in myself.

(*Written essay; Miss Pie.; May 1971*)

Can one think without language[1, 2]? The question may at first appear surprising (at least to the layman) and most often elicits the answer 'No'.

This response is certainly understandable. Language and thought are so intimately linked in our mental activities that they might seem indissociable especially since, if we take an introspective approach, we are unable to analyse our reasoning and sentiments without resorting to language. Moreover, man's language is not only a means of communication but also an instrument which advances his thinking and without which he could not attain the very high levels of abstract and conceptual thought which are particular to humans. No one would think of minimizing the influence of language on thought, and it is undoubtedly more legitimate to magnify it in the manner of Paul Valéry[3]: *'honneur des hommes, saint langage'* (honour of men, sacred language).

Thought without language is indeed possible. There are very complex activities which may be carried out without involving language; moreover, language is probably a limiting constraint on some of them. Our intentions are to provide examples, to distinguish the types of mental activities in question, and to consider the cerebral mechanisms which then enter into play.

'Language' and 'thought' are words whose semantic vibrations are widespread and penetrating. Some go so far as to say that computers, and even flowers, have language and that computers possess intelligence! We must therefore define the meanings of these terms as they shall be used here in order to establish a common basis for the following discussion.

The definition of language is fairly simple. It here refers to human language which can be distinguished from all other languages by at least three characteristics: first, it consists of semantic signs and logical relationships which are totally arbitrary to the young brain which receives them and accepts all languages in the same way as a function of the linguistic environment; this is quite different from so-called animal languages which consist of universal signs transmitted by the genetic code. Second, human language is creative in the sense that with 30 to 40 phonemes and some thousands of words, man can express an infinite number of ideas through syntagmatic combinations which are often original: this was discussed elsewhere in this book (see Chapter 2) in recognizing that it is this multi-phased (and thus economical) nature which is specific to human language[4]. Finally, language serves a personal intent, that of communicating an idea to others, be it what one thinks or often even what one does not think. Such motivation does not exist in communication systems established through conditioning and experience between animals of the same or different species and it certainly does not exist in electronic machines.

Thought is more difficult to define. We shall here use the term in its largest sense to include all psychic activities: focusing attention, remembering, imagining, comparing, judging, thinking about thought processes. Times no longer require that it be viewed as double-sided with an objective and subjective aspect: thought includes dreams and the unconscious. Similarly, thought is no longer conceived as being an exclusive attribute of humans: it exists in higher animals, although no one is able to fix the limit above which mental processing begins. Our reflections on this topic will be based on animal psychology, on the ontogeny of intelligence and on cerebral pathology.

In the phylogenetic order, innate behaviours gradually give way to learning and to approaches based on reasoning. Since all learned behaviours are built on past experiences, experimental learning situations are useful in showing the progressively more complex behaviours which may be mastered by animals, that is, in providing information on the birth of intelligence and the development of processes which constitute the first stages of thought. We can list here only some of the abilities of animal brains such as: the mental representation of the task to be carried out; the establishment of relationships between different environmental elements, which are themselves variable and determine the adaptive action to be programmed by the animal; the development of strategies as a function of probability, as when a monkey must push one of two keys to obtain a reward, something which is easy when pushing one key is followed by positive reinforcement 100 per cent of the time but much more difficult when the probability of a reward is 70 per cent for one key and 30 per cent for the other; the monkey's ability to grasp an abstraction such as similarity or difference, as in learning to select an object which differs from two others and to generalize this principle whether the object differs in form or in colour; and finally, the development of a concept, that of a triangle regardless of its spatial disposition and colour. This last example is particularly striking when it is remembered that Kant specifically chose a triangle to illustrate conceptual thought in man: that is, a plane figure with three sides and three angles regardless of its other physical variables.

Mental representation, the establishment of relationships, the development of strategies based on probabilities, generalization and conceptualization are all thought processes which can be agreed to occur in the absence of language. Different learning situations have permitted their separation but in one, described by Köhler[5] more than 40 years ago, the solution of the problem included all these processes as well as others: a hungry chimpanzee named Sultan saw a banana hanging from the ceiling of his cage but he was too short to reach it; seeing boxes and canes lying on the floor he climbed on a box but did not succeed; he then placed one box on

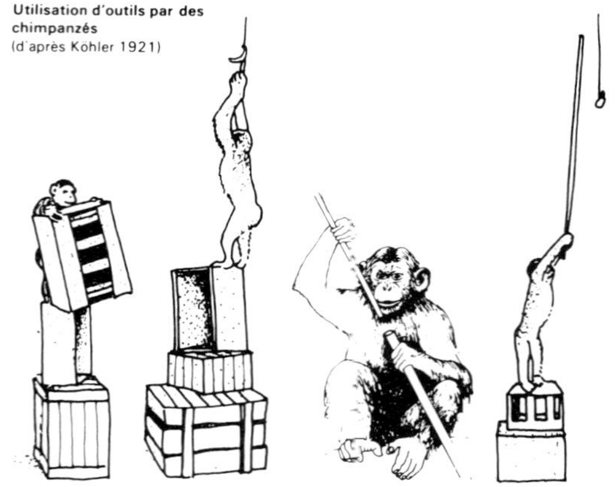

Fig. 19-1 *Use of tools by Köhler's chimpanzee. Adapted from Köhler (1951).*

top of another and climbed on this scaffold, but to no avail; he then used a cane to help but still could not reach; next, he joined two canes together—they were designed to permit this—and, perched on the boxes, he finally grasped the banana and ... ate it (Fig. 19-1). The unfolding of the successive steps in this performance provides more than analogies with what is called logical reasoning, even if this reasoning is applied to physical instruments. What the chimpanzee lacked in this feat was surely not the language to subtend his thinking but rather the language to tell us about it.

Let us now consider humans. Infants acquire the rudiments of language only after the age of 12 or 18 months (see Chapter 8-2). Nevertheless, who would dare to say that infants—and perhaps even newborns—do not think? Common sense suggests a germ of thought behind the baby's smile when he recognizes his mother, behind some of his tears or behind the attention which he focuses on his hands, on the objects which he manipulates, and somewhat later, on his games. Psychoanalytical theory accords even more importance to the infant's mental life in the affective domain than in that of the initial organization of his/her eventual personality. We shall not continue along this path too full of untestable hypotheses. On the other hand, Piaget's work[6–11] has renewed ideas about the development of intelligence in children. In one of his last works, he expressed himself as follows: 'About 40 years ago, at a time when I believed in close relations between language and thought, I scarcely studied anything but verbal thought. Since then, different studies have taught me that there is a logic of the coordination of actions [which is] more profound than the logic tied to language ... It is on these insufficiencies of language that I will mainly insist, because if everyone notices its contribution, and I believe I am sufficiently aware of its finally decisive importance, one too often forgets the part of actions and of operational intelligence itself'[11].

The first degrees of intelligence develop before a child has acquired any language. This development is based on actions which gradually acquire the value of a concept which can be generalized to a group of actions, hence Piaget[9] named them sensorimotor schemata. Through covert combinations of these schemata, the small child suddenly becomes able to understand a situation: e.g., s/he discovers how to get objects which an observer has hidden in different ways. At a later stage, the language which is being acquired or has been acquired is insufficient to allow the child to solve certain concrete problems. Among many others, the problem called the conservation of liquids clearly shows that the child's successful solution does not depend on language but on the attainment of an internal logic governing the development of his/her actions. Thus, before the age of seven or eight years, a child thinks that the amount of water contained in a glass increases or decreases depending on whether it is poured into a narrower or a wider glass. The child's judgement is based only on the exterior aspect, that is on the height of the liquid, even though s/he possesses the vocabulary necessary to understand the experiment. After the age of seven or eight, the child can say that the amount of liquid remains the same, not because vocabulary is richer but because the development of logical reasoning, contemporaneous with progressively greater biological cerebral maturation[12–16] (see Chapter 8-2), allows him/her to nullify the apparent change in the volume of water when poured into a container of a different shape. In such cases, it is useless to give verbal rules. The solution of such problems depends on the level of intelligence. The role of language later increases, it being a necessary but insufficient condition for the completion of logical structures. In the brain, there are innate anatomofunctional systems which, under pressure from the linguistic environment, will permit the acquisition of language; but there are also more generalized systems which, under pressure from the environment, will permit the development of cognitive activities. These systems are independent even if there are reciprocal influences between them.

Important information on this subject is provided by the congenitally deaf and the congenitally blind. Most deaf children do not begin to learn language before they begin school (i.e., around the age of five) and the language which is eventually acquired remains below normal levels. Intellectual development, however, is characterized only by a simple delay which is much less significant than that of language; moreover, it follows the same stages of elaboration as in hearing children. This is not the case for the congenitally blind, who acquire oral language normally but encounter serious difficulties on tests permitting the evaluation of their operational intellectual capacities. The explanation of this difference is that language is not the source of logic but is rather one of its products; as for visual information, it has a major role in the elaboration of schemata and the formation of logical structures.

What about those who are both deaf and blind since birth? The answer is not straightforward. Such cases are rare and generally the brain has also been the victim of a pathological process. The widely cited cases are those of Marie Heurtin and Helen Keller who surely did not suffer total auditory and visual deprivation. Nevertheless, these individuals' thought and their abilities to think had nothing to do with the delay and limits of their abilities in linguistic communication. In this regard we should mention a disconcerting pathological condition, namely *audi-mutité* (failure to acquire language as a consequence of congenital deafness). Here is the case of a child followed by Jean-Louis Signoret: at birth the child's brain had perhaps suffered a meningeal haemorrhage; this child, now 12 years old, developed normally with the exception of language. He uttered only a multitude of phonemes with some intonation and, occasionally, a word; he understood so little of the language of others that he could not point to pictures of objects named by the examiner; he was not deaf and could identify familiar noises and the sounds of musical instruments. Nevertheless his intelligence, as measured on non-verbal intelligence tests, was within the normal range. It is clear that this child thought; his emotions were lively and his personality was socially adapted. And this was true despite the absence of language mediation. Even if it is difficult to explain the 'how' of his thought mechanism, the fact remains that he did think. This must be accepted.

Lesions of adult brains provide other examples of a dissociation between language and thought. We have selected three illustrations. The most classical one is aphasia caused by a left hemisphere lesion in a right-hander. There is then a more or less severe disorganization of language. However, the loss of comprehension or of expression does not necessarily mean that what is appropriately called *inner language* has been destroyed, because these disturbances may be the result of a lesion which, in the former case, affects the decoding systems for auditory messages and, in the latter, the systems which ensure the organization and realization of articulatory movements. The same line of reasoning applies to written language. Nowadays, various tests allow these pitfalls to be avoided and the extent of properly linguistic impairments to be determined. What can then be said about the intellectual activities of those whose language, as a symbolic or semiotic function, is disorganized or lost? This is an old debate, lasting for more than a century, between those who maintain that there is a deterioration of intelligence in aphasics and those who defend its almost complete integrity. Obviously, no one claims that verbal thought is preserved and the question concerns only non-linguistic intellectual activities. In our opinion, it has received a scientific answer. Psychometric tests, Piaget's tests[7-11, 17] and various types of learning have shown that there is no correlation between aphasia and success or failure on these different tests: we have reported elsewhere an anatomoclinical study of a patient which clearly illustrates this fact (see Chapter 8-4, case of J. Com.). Aphasia does not entail, simply by its presence, a deterioration of general intelligence (Insertion 19.1). A fortiori, it is not the consequence of aphasia. If there are aphasics whose intelligence is generally impaired, it is because the cerebral lesion is not limited to the so-called language regions, but extends to other regions whose intactness is necessary for the performance of non-linguistic tasks. The behaviour of the great majority of aphasics remains adapted to the situations in which they find themselves; they are aware of their disability; they cope with their grief according to their personality—which remains unchanged—with their reactions ranging from resignation to despair. Certain mathematicians and physicists remain able to solve problems whose difficulty does not only impress the examining neurologist. The same is true of chemists.

Artistic creation merits particular mention. After becoming aphasic, Maurice Ravel was always able to pick out the smallest errors in musical selections which he heard, but was never able to create new works[23-25]. Perhaps this deficit was due to the extent of the cerebral lesions. The Soviet psychologist Luria[26] cited the case of a musician who continued to compose despite his aphasia, his music apparently being better than before his cerebral accident. Let us now consider the case of a painter, Gernez, who had a well-earned reputation during the post-impressionist era. At the age of 52, he was suddenly deprived of language and paralysed on the right side of his body. After a certain period of illness, and despite his hemiplegia and aphasia, he began to paint again: his stylistic characteristics had not changed; they were, perhaps, even stronger. Théophile Alajouanine[23] remained a close friend throughout these years. Here are some of the artist's reflections which Alajouanine gathered, retranscribed according to the rules of French (and then of English): 'There are two men in me; one who paints who is normal when he paints; the other who is in a haze, who is lost, who does not connect with life ... I say very badly what I want to say ... There is in me one who grasps reality, life; there is another one who is lost in the abstract ... When I paint, I am outside my existence, my vision of things is even more intense than before: I connect; I find everything again. There are two men in me: one who is connected by reality in order to paint; the other, the imbecile who no longer knows how to shift for himself with words ... it's strange, I painted again, some

Insertion 19.1

Cerebral lesions may sometimes cause both aphasia and [as can readily be demonstrated through the use of different psychometric tests (see Chapter 16)] a decrease in general intelligence. However, aphasia itself is not, as was claimed by Marie[18] and is still claimed by Bay[19] (see Chapter 1), a form of intellectual deterioration. This becomes obvious when considering the history of a patient who has been followed for some years by one of us (A.R.L.) and Joanette[20].

Brother J. was born in 1930. He is right-handed, as are all members of his family. He completed only ten years of school but has since continued his education through self-instruction. He has worked for several years on the staff of a religious periodical, his main responsibility being to answer letters from the readers.

Brother J. may have presented a first episode of *grand mal* at about the age of 15 and certainly presented another at the age of 20. He then received treatment in the form of different anticonvulsant drugs. Although *grand mal* has since recurred only once or twice, Brother J. has presented several episodes of paroxysmal aphasia without alteration of consciousness. Neurological and psychometric examinations carried out between these episodes were generally normal; electroencephalograms obtained during sleep nevertheless revealed the presence of left temporal epileptic activity and computerized tomography scans showed mild enlargement of the left lateral ventricle. An electroencephalogram obtained at the beginning of a spell (critical phase[21]) showed that the abnormal electrical activity then extended from the temporal region to the left frontal, central and parietal regions.

Brother J.'s episodes of paroxysmal aphasia have been of two types, some being long and others short. The short episodes may occur several times per day and weeks may go by without any occurring. They last from a few seconds to a maximum of a few minutes and, during this time, language is globally affected (impaired comprehension and production of written language was documented many times, since these episodes often occurred while the patient was at work, reading and answering letters related to the periodical). The long episodes have occurred from 10 to 15 times per year and have lasted between 2 and 11 hours (as a general rule, around four hours). Their progression is remarkable in the sense that they successively recapitulate, within a number of hours, the picture of several clinical forms of aphasia. The following sequence is observed in the most characteristic of these episodes (Fig. 19–2):

1. The episode begins with *global aphasia*, that is, with the suppression of oral and written expression and maximal impairment of oral and written comprehension.
2. This initial phase is short and soon followed by a qualitative and quantitative reduction which is at first massive and then gradually becomes less severe. An articulatory disturbance may then become evident and last for approximately half an hour. With its disappearance and decreased severity of the reduction, an increasing number of neologisms and all types of paraphasias can be distinguished in the patient's discourse; written expression is then very reduced, with or without a disturbance of graphism proper, and includes all types of paragraphias. At this time, the patient usually prints in block letters. The severity of the comprehension disturbance begins to decrease. The clinical picture can then be termed *mixed aphasia*; others would speak of reduced Wernicke's aphasia (see Insertion 4.1).
3. The quantitative reduction disappears when the patient's discourse still includes many deviant segments: jargonaphasia is then observed, with unequivocal logorrhoea during certain moments. Repetition and oral reading give rise to many phonemic paraphasias. Word-finding difficulty is still evident during naming. In written expression, the patient returns to the use of cursives and his production still includes deviations, especially literal paragraphias. Although improved, oral language comprehension remains impaired. Recovery of written language comprehension is somewhat more rapid. The clinical picture observed during this phase is clearly that of *Wernicke's aphasia proper*.
4. There may then be a period in which the patient's language is characterized by the (decreasing) production of paraphasias and by word-finding difficulty. Since the comprehension disturbance is then very slight, the clinical picture resembles that of *conduction aphasia*.
5. Word-finding difficulty and dysorthographia are the last anomalies to disappear. Thus the episode ends with the clinical picture of *amnesic aphasia*[22] which gradually disappears (Fig. 19–2).

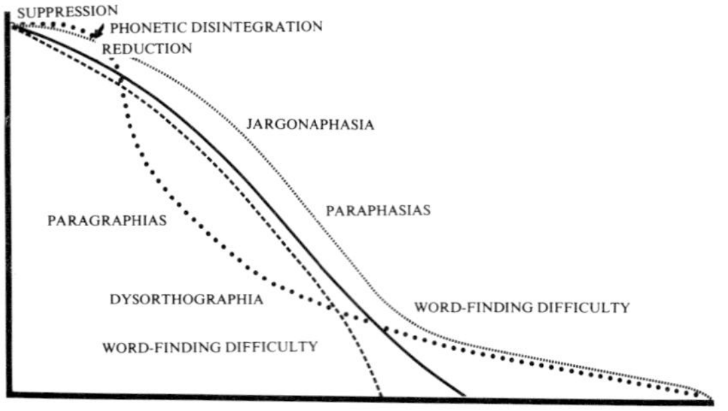

Fig. 19–2 *Evolution of the clinical manifestations of aphasia in Brother J's case. The severity of the different signs of aphasia is represented along the ordinate and time along the abscissa. .... Oral expression; .... written expression; ——— oral comprehension; - - - - - written comprehension.*

Other characteristics of Brother J.'s aphasic episodes are also noteworthy:

1. There is almost no change in his state of consciousness, even during the initial phases of the episode. At most, the beginning of a spell is accompanied by a desire to sleep, a desire which the patient can deliberately overcome if he so wishes and which an eventual examiner could easily overcome through his interventions. This characteristic obviously favours the diachronic description of the linguistic disturbance.
2. Throughout each episode, the patient remains aware of his aphasia (and often feels a profound sadness): thus, on one occasion when he could not avoid answering the telephone while his expressive ability was reduced, Brother J. repeated the word '*Allo*' more and more loudly, deliberately modifying his prosody to make his caller believe, before hanging up, that he could not be heard because of some defect in the telephone or transmission line. Brother J. nevertheless presents a form of anosognosia,* particularly during the jargonaphasic phase. He remains unaware of the deviant nature of the paraphasias and neologisms which he produces. Furthermore, he cannot remember having uttered certain words rather than others once his aphasic episode has ended, and would be astonished to learn that his discourse includes, as in the case of J. Com. (see Chapter 8–4), a preferred neologism (which remains the same from one episode to another: /twaʀe/, /fwaʀe/).
3. With the exception of this disturbance which may reflect some impairment of linguistic recall, the aphasic episodes do not affect Brother J's memory. During the course of an episode, he is therefore quite capable of following instructions given a long time ago (e.g., the instruction to tape-record a sample of his speech or to find a third party who would alert us by telephone). He also remembers personal and other events which occur during his spells and willingly discusses them once they have ended. If one gives credit to introspective data, Brother J's case is thus exceptional since, between episodes, he uses standard language to describe his repeated, conscious experience of aphasia.
4. Brother J's aphasic episodes affect his inner language (if it is defined as a person's ability to talk to himself, in words and sentences, without obvious peripheral manifestations). The patient definitely considers that this disturbance is proportional to that of overt expression, that is, any segment which is available for private use is also available, with or without deviations, for communication with others.
5. The aphasic episodes do not include an associated apraxia (apparently not even buccofacial apraxia although this has not been verified at the beginning of a spell). In this regard, Brother J. performs normally on different tests and, especially, carries out, during his aphasic episodes, various complex activities requiring praxic control (using an elevator, making a tape-recording, using scissors to cut up cigarette boxes and assembling the pieces to form an elaborate montage of predetermined design).
6. Testing also indicates that the aphasic episodes do not include the presence of an associated *visual* or *auditory agnosia*. Here again, certain observations gathered in the course of a spell are of obvious interest. While he is aphasic, Brother J. sometimes listens to music. He recognizes familiar people, whom he generally cannot name, by sight or, if they are unseen, by voice or other sounds (e.g. that of a colleague walking along the corridor with a cane). In addition, Brother J. sometimes tunes his radio to an all-talk programme in order to verify whether his comprehension is improving (i.e., to determine if his spell is ending).

* Probably the same as that observed in many aphasics.

Many of the facts pointed out—the deliberate feigning on the telephone, tape-recording a speech sample in accordance with previous instructions, using a radio station to verify the status of oral comprehension, etc.—clearly show that Brother J.'s general intelligence is not impaired during his aphasic episodes. The following anecdote is possibly even more demonstrative in this regard. One day while travelling by train from Italy to Switzerland, Brother J. experienced the onset of an aphasic episode a short time before arriving at the station in the city where he was to disembark, a fact which he had probably recognized before the beginning of his spell. In any case, when the train pulled into the station, his aphasia did not prevent him from collecting his luggage, disembarking from the train, presenting his tickets to the proper agent, leaving the station and setting out in search of a hotel. Having identified one from non-linguistic cues (since his alexia was then very severe), he entered, recognized the reception desk, and showed the attendant his *medic-alert* bracelet which he always wore. Understanding the receptionist's gestured response ('no room'), he left and continued his search. Finding a second hotel, the same initial scene was repeated but this time he recognized that a room was available. Brother J. then gave the receptionist his passport and pointed out the information which she needed to fill in his registration card. He correctly interpreted her gestured question ('Do you want to lie down now?') and nodded affirmatively. He then rested for about half an hour but, being unable to sleep because of anxiety and hunger, he left his room and found the hotel's restaurant (with no more difficulty than anyone who finds himself in an unfamiliar hotel in a foreign-language country). He sat at a table and, when the waiter came to take his order, Brother J. pointed to a line in that part of the menu which seemed most likely to be the list of main courses. He then waited, hoping that his finger had fallen on something he liked. He remembers feeling very disappointed when the waiter returned with a fish dish, a food which he particularly dislikes. After eating a little, nevertheless, he returned to his room by himself, unlocked the door without any difficulty, lay down and slept for several hours. By the time he awoke, his aphasia had disappeared.

It is clear that even when Brother J. is severely aphasic, he is able to carry out (relatively) complex activities and that his behaviour is coherent and completely adapted, that is, based on thought having the same characteristics. In this case, thought undoubtedly involves conceptual patterns established during times when Brother J.'s linguistic functioning was normal, but it can obviously occur when linguistic functioning is impaired. Just like Sultan[5], the aphasic Brother J. is unable to explain his thoughts by means of articulated language but, to a certain extent and in certain circumstances, language is not essential for adaptive and effective thought.

large pastels which are more alive than real life.' Subirana[27] also spoke of a patient whose pictorial talent was *heightened* after the *liberation* of right hemisphere activities, the liberation being related to the onset of a left hemisphere lesion (with right hemiplegia and aphasia). There is a fascinating duality in these two cases, between verbal thought and another activity, visual and emotional, which it will be generally agreed, is nevertheless part of human thought.

There is a pathological condition opposite to that just discussed, namely a disorganization of thought in the presence of normal language. It results from lesions affecting the frontal lobes (see Chapter 6). Their role is to exert a regulating and controlling function over all behaviours of a certain degree of complexity. Consider the example of an arithmetic problem, even a simple one. The task requires the gathering of information, the formation of a strategy or programme, and control over every stage of its execution. This is what these patients have lost. If the examiner is willing to guide the patient step by step (we were going to say 'lend him his own fontal lobes'), he will then be able to solve the problem[28]. These facts do not illustrate the existence of thought without language but the inefficacy of language without organization of thought.

The last example offered by cerebral pathology is truly fascinating. It is widely known that the brain is composed of two hemispheres which are linked together by associative fasciculi, the most important forming the corpus callosum[29] which, in man, is composed of more than two million fibres. Their role is to transfer information from one hemisphere to the other, in such a way that these reciprocal exchanges allow the two hemispheres to function as a whole. In animals, learning which, through different technical procedures would a priori occur in only a single hemisphere, also occurs in the other hemisphere because all information received and each of the animal's responses are transmitted by the corpus callosum to the other hemisphere. Sectioning of the corpus callosum is sufficient to confine all learning to the single hemisphere which receives information.

Twenty years ago, in the United States, a neurosurgeon, Bogen[30], and a psychologist, Sperry[31, 32], thought of treating patients with severe epilepsy by sectioning their corpus callosum and other commissures having a more accessory role. These cases were called *split-brain* patients, a term which has since been widely adopted. Following the surgical intervention, the two hemispheres are disconnected from each other so that their activities are henceforth independent. The functions of each hemisphere can therefore be studied individually (see Insertion 11.2). The question is truly captivating. The left hemisphere, in right-handers, is known to include the systems subtending language, gestures, and analytical and conceptual thought but what are the functions of the right hemisphere whose adjective 'minor' clearly expresses the small part which has been attributed to it in higher cerebral activities? It is first necessary to understand the experimental situation: when an object is placed in the right hand, the central neural pathways cross the midline so that information is transmitted to and processed in the left hemisphere; when an object is placed in the left hand, it is the right hemisphere which receives the information. The same is true of visual information (Fig. 19-3) although the situation is more complex because of scanning movements of the eyes which permit both hemispheres to receive all visual information. However only a few technical procedures—fixation of gaze on a central point and stimulus presentation in a quarter of a second flash—are necessary to ensure that each stimulus is projected to only one half of the visual field and therefore reaches only one hemisphere.

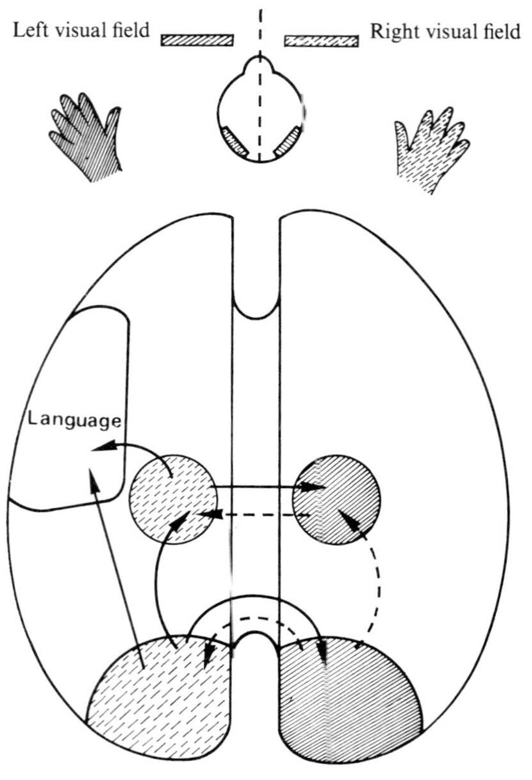

Fig. 19-3 *Anatomical pathways underlying naming of a stimulus presented in the left visual field (extramacular vision).*

When split-brain patients are tested under these conditions, all tactile or visual stimuli addressed to the left hemisphere are recognized and named. When addressed to the right hemisphere, however, they elicit no verbal response; the subject even denies having palpated an object or having seen a picture, but he speaks with his left hemisphere which did not receive this information. Nevertheless, the objects and pictures are accurately identified by the right hemisphere, the proof being that, when using his left hand (i.e., right hemisphere), the subject can find the object which had already been palpated and can point out, on a card showing many pictures, those which had been projected to his right hemisphere. This information is memorized because the subject can easily perform the same identification procedures after a long delay. Furthermore, in the absence of any language, the right hemisphere is able to form concepts. Consider, for example, that of a key: a picture of a small flat key is projected to the left visual field and thus to the right hemisphere and the subject must use his left hand to find it among other objects belonging to the same category; in this case, his hand does not grasp the small objects which resemble the small key in terms of size, but instead selects a very large key of the type used in wine cellars. Thus the subject's action was guided by a concept[32, 33].

An even more striking finding is the relative superiority of right hemisphere performance

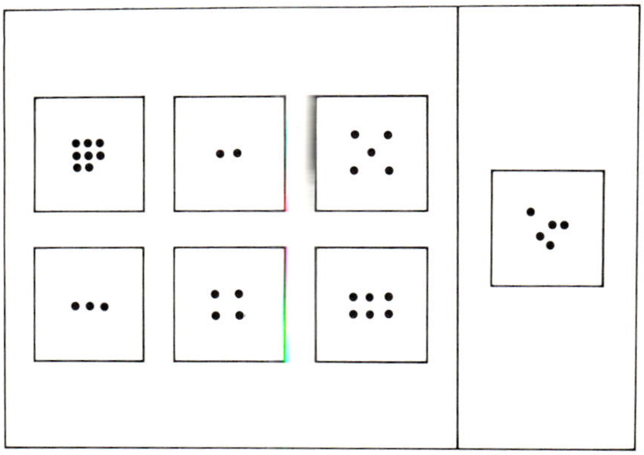

Fig. 19-4 *An example of stimuli used in the tachistoscopic dot-number test. Commentary in the text.*

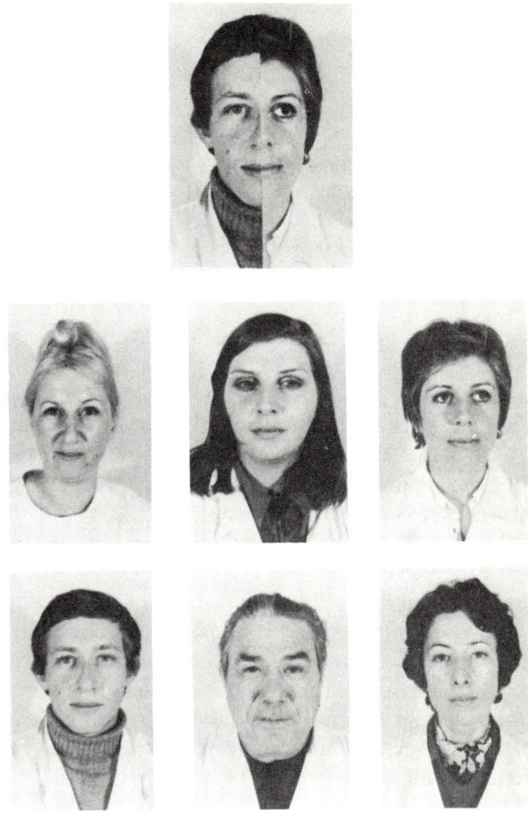

Fig. 19-5 *A stimulus used in an adaptation of the test by Levy, Trevarthen and Sperry*[35]*. Commentary in the text.*

over that of the left during many tasks which require visual discrimination and the construction, in space, of different two- or three-dimensional forms. When cards displaying a random array of dots are presented by flash projection and the subject is then asked to find the same number of dots among cards showing an aligned array, a normal subject is able to do so on trials which include up to six or seven dots, that is, his brain is able to apprehend the number, without counting, and to modify its spatial disposition in order to relocate it in a new configuration. If split-brain patients are tested on this task, as was done by one of us (F.L.) and collaborators[34] (Fig. 19-4), the left hemisphere does not exceed three dots while right hemisphere performance is the same as in normal subjects. The left hemisphere undoubtedly tries to count—verbally—the number of dots (which is impossible given the brevity of stimulus exposure) and this verbal constraint leads to failure; the right hemisphere does not need to count; it includes other mechanisms for spatial perception, mechanisms which enter into play in normal subjects although no one is subjectively aware of their intervention.

Another task merits attention here, namely face recognition. Using chimeric images composed of two different half-faces (Fig. 19-5) and projected for a quarter of a second, Levy, Trevarthen and Sperry[35], as well as one of us (F.L.) and collaborators[3[illegible]], were able to place the two hemispheres in competition, each one receiving only a half-face. If a split-brain patient is asked to describe verbally which face s/he saw, s/he responds, often in a rather confused fashion, by describing in every case the half-face which was seen by the left hemisphere; if the patient is then asked not to speak, but to identify the face which s/he saw by pointing it out in an array of faces, s/he immediately points to one which includes the half-face perceived only by the right hemisphere. In the competition between the hemispheres during this last task, it is the right one, that is, the hemisphere without language, which is dominant.

If these results are to be more fully understood, another fact of cerebral pathology should be considered: the loss of the ability to recognize faces, a syndrome whose origin is almost always related to a lesion of the occipital lobe of the minor hemisphere[36-38]. The deficit is so severe that the patient does not even recognize himself in pictures nor on a television screen directly transmitting images of his own face. In this case, only the left hemisphere functions normally. All information which it receives tends to be analysed and formulated in terms of language but this type of processing is ineffective in matters of physiognomy. It is usually very difficult, or impossible, for a normal individual to recognize a human face, an animal's appearance or the make of a car purely on the basis of someone's verbal description, that is, from information which is specifically addressed to the left hemisphere. In contrast, this operation is performed by the right hemisphere in only 1/125 of a second of visual information[34]. A final comment on this point: certain occipital lesions of the left hemisphere lead to the non-recognition of pictures of objects which have a name in the language. What can then be thought about a patient, observed by one of us (F.L.) and Chédru[39], who had such a lesion and who therefore processed visual information in the right hemisphere? When faced with reproductions of six famous paintings, she did not recognize either the church, the field, the meadow, or Pierrot but quickly said *'Tiens! Voici deux Van Gogh!'* ('Oh! Here are two Van Goghs.') The style of a painting leads to countless verbal comments but its intrinsic nature is not easily verbalized. It is the right hemisphere which, to a large extent, elaborates the assemblies which allow style to be distinguished, to be recognized and, who knows? to be more or less appreciated.

These facts suggest a general explanation of the functional organization of the brain which can be summarized as follows: until the age of about two years, the two hemispheres are equipotential; then the genetic factor of hemispheric dominance intervenes, fixing the logic of language so firmly in the left hemisphere of right-handers that all information tends to be processed according to its terms (see Chapter 11). This is an advantage in respect of certain forms of analytical and conceptual thought but a constraint on other activities, notably artistic ones, which are obviously linked to thought but which develop in a natural fashion in the hemisphere devoid of language. It might even be that, in certain cases, language stifles other potential cognitive modalities[27].

So many other questions can also be raised! Can the right hemisphere subtend affective reactions? A photograph of a naked woman was projected to the right hemisphere of a split-brain patient, a young American woman. She smiled but, when questioned, replied that she had not seen anything: she had spoken using her left hemisphere. When the photograph was presented several times, she laughed and covered her face with her hands in embarrassment but still said that she had not seen anything: she finally blamed the 'funny machine', namely the projection and recording equipment which were in front of her[40].

Our personality is neither simple nor homogeneous. While this is obvious, could it nevertheless have distinct traits depending on the hemisphere considered? Gazzaniga[40] followed the first split-brain patient, universally known as W.J., over a long time and reported the following anecdotes. W.J. once tried to strike his wife with his left arm while his right arm tried to oppose this and protect her. Another day, when walking with W.J., Gazzaniga saw him seize an axe with his left hand in a very threatening way. Gazzaniga rapidly slipped away, humorously reporting that he thus hoped to spare American courts the problem of determining which of the two hemispheres could be held responsible for a crime. One could also add which of the two hemispheres would deserve a medal.

It is clear that our two hemispheres have different modes of activity. But in what ways do they cooperate or, on the contrary, oppose each other? In a surely unconscious and probably natural way, we probably use them in alternation, depending on the task to be carried out. Will it some day be possible to overdevelop the functional capacities of each of the hemispheres? The question is of evident interest but actually belongs to the domain of futurology.

If we have stressed this subject, it is because it offers new insights into the organization of the cerebral systems which subtend the functions of our psychic individuality. But let us make no mistake about it. Thought exists without language, thought which precedes and exceeds language. It is clearly not supported by the left hemisphere alone; this would be too simple. It is the entire brain which participates. We wish to speak of creativity, be it in the form of a novel idea, the imaginary, an artistic creation, the emotional force of memory, or mathematical thought. Language must surely have been required by Archimedes in order to specify the nature of the problem but his discovery emerged suddenly with no arousal of verbal thought. It burst forth without his conscious awareness of the permanent action of his thought mechanisms and verbal formulation occurred only afterwards. Was it a question of language when Jules Verne imagined his worlds or Picasso jostled forms? 'I don't seek, I find' stated the latter. In the field of physics, Einstein stressed the non-verbal nature of his thought processes: his concepts initially arose in the form of psysic entities, signs and images of varying clarity which he strived to associate. These elements had 'a visual and sometimes muscular characteristic. It is only at the next stage that I must laboriously search for conventional terms and signs' to express them.

And is the same not also true of countless literary productions? Our reference on this topic has been so often quoted that we hesitate to repeat it again. It is Marcel Proust's[41] description of the slow and difficult resurgence of a given period of one's past. We will cite only small fragments of Proust's text (thereby diminishing its impact): 'And as soon as I had recognized the taste of a piece of sponge cake soaked in lime-blossom tea which my aunt gave me ... immediately the old grey house on the street, where my room was, came ... to give one's full attention to the small pavilion in the garden ...; and with the house, the city, from morning till night and in all weather, the place where I was sent before lunch, the streets where I used to shop, the paths that one took if the weather was nice'. And after comparing his thinking process to a Japanese game in which verbal messages are delivered by the blossoming of a flower, Proust continues: 'in the same way now all the flowers of our garden and those of Mr Swann's grounds, and the water lilies of the Vivonne, and the good people of the village and their small dwellings and the church and all of Combray and its surroundings, all that which takes form and solidity, came out, city and gardens, from my cup of tea'. The reader's emotions are partly attributable to Proust's literary genius, but who can minimize this world of thoughts which entered into his mind before any language to describe it to himself or to others?

Having begun with a quotation from Paul Valéry[3], extolling language, we shall close with other, highly critical ones taken from his Notebooks[42]: 'the pre-existence of words ... confines, in the germ itself, the production of our mind ... moulds this thought more than it expresses it and even develops it in a sense other than the initial one'; further on, Valéry insists that it is our nature to believe that 'what cannot be said and well said, does not exist'; finally, according to Robinson's abridgement[43], 'men have infinitely more trust in notions consecrated by language than in those often much more important which remain to be discovered in every direction and beyond all familiar words.'

REFERENCES

1. Lhermitte, F. (1973) Le cerveau et la pensée. *La revue des deux mondes*, 524, Paris.
2. Lhermitte, F. (1976) Peut-on penser sans langage? *Réalités*, **363,** 40.
3. Valéry, P. (1960) *Cahiers*. Paris: Gallimard.
4. Buyssens, E. (1967) *La communication et l'articulation linguistique*. Paris: Presses Universitaires de France.
5. Köhler, W. (1951) *Mentality of Apes*. New York: The Humanities Press.
6. Piaget, J. (1923) *Le langage et la pensée chez l'enfant*. Paris: Delachaux and Niestlé.
7. Piaget, J. (1949) *La psychologie de l'intelligence*. Paris: Colin.
8. Piaget, J. (1954) Le langage et la pensée du point de vue génétique. *Acta Psychologica*, **10,** 51.
9. Piaget, J. (1959) *La formation du symbole chez l'enfant*. Paris: Delachaux and Niestlé.
10. Piaget, J. (1965) Langage et pensée. *Revue pratique* (Paris), **15,** 2253.
11. Piaget, J. (1967) *Biologie et connaissance*. Paris: Gallimard.
12. Kaes, T. (1907) *Die Grosshirnrinde des Menschen in ihrem Massen und in ihrem Fasengehalt*. Iéna: Fischer.
13. Yakovlev, P.I. (1962) Morphological criteria of growth and maturation of the nervous system in man. *Research Publications, Association for Research in Nervous and Mental Diseases*, **39,** 3.
14. Yakovlev, P.I. & Lecours, A.R. (1967) The myelogenetic cycles of regional maturation of the brain. In *Regional Development of the Brain in Early Life* (Ed.) Minkowski, A. p. 3. Oxford: Blackwell.
15. Lecours, A.R. (1975) Myelinogenetic correlates of the development of speech and language. In *Foundations of Language Development: a Multidisciplinary Approach* (Ed.) Lenneberg, E. & Lenneberg, E. Vol. 1, p. 121. New York: Academic Press.
16. Lecours, A.R. (1982) Correlates of developmental behavior in brain maturation. In *Regression in Development* (Ed.) Bever, T. Hillsdale, NJ: LEA Press.
17. Tissot, R., Lhermitte, F. & Ducarne, B. (1963) Etat intellectuel des aphasiques. *Encéphale*, **52,** 285.
18. Marie, P. (1926) *Travaux et mémoires*. Tome I Paris: Masson.
19. Bay, E. (1964) Aphasia and intelligence. *International Journal of Neurology*, **4,** 252.
20. Lecours, A.R. & Joanette, Y. (1980) Linguistic and other

psychological aspects of paroxysmal aphasia. *Brain and Language*, **10,** 1. (Case presented to the XV Annual Congress of the Academy of Aphasia, Montreal, October, 1977.)
21. Alajouanine, Th. & Sabouraud, O. (1960) Les perturbations paroxystiques du langage dans l'épilepsie. *Encéphale*, **49,** 95.
22. Lhermitte, F. & Derouesné, J. (1976) L'aphasie amnésique; étude de 25 cas. *Revue neurologique*, **132,** 669.
23. Alajouanine, Th. (1948) Aphasia and artistic realization. *Brain*, **71,** 229.
24. Alajouanine, Th. (1965) Sur l'état intellectuel des aphasiques. *Revue pratique* (Paris), **5,** 2325.
25. Alajouanine, Th. (1968) *L'aphasie et le langage pathologique*. Paris: Baillière.
26. Luria, A.R., Tsvetkova, L.S. & Futer, D.S. (1965) Aphasia in a composer. *Journal of the Neurological Sciences*, **2,** 288.
27. Subirana, A. (1953) Sur les bienfaits éventuels de certaines maladies neurologiques. In *Livre jubilaire du Professeur Roger*. p. 117. Marseille: Faculté de Médecine.
28. Lhermitte, F., Derouesné, J. & Signoret, J.L. (1972) Analyse neuropsychologique du syndrome frontal. *Revue neurologique*, **127,** 415.
29. Selnes, O.A. (1974) The corpus callosum: some anatomical and functional considerations with special reference to language. *Brain and Language*, **1,** 111.
30. Bogen, J.E. & Vogel, P.J. (1962) Cerebral commissurotomy in man; preliminary report. *Bulletin of the Los Angeles Neurological Sciences*, **27,** 169.
31. Sperry, R.W. (1962) Some general aspects of interhemispheric integration. In *Interhemispheric Relations and Cerebral Dominance* (Ed.) Mountcastle, V.B. p. 43. Baltimore, MA: Johns Hopkins.
32. Sperry, R.W. (1964) The great cerebral commissure. *Scientific American*, **210,** 42.
33. Lecours, A.R. & Poncet, M. (1975) Syndrome calleux. *Encyclopédie médico-chirurgicale*, *17036 C^{10}*, 1.
34. Lhermitte, F., Chain, F., Chedru, F. & Penet, C. (1974) Syndrome de déconnexion interhémisphérique. *Revue neurologique*, **130,** 247.
35. Levy, J., Trevarthen, C. & Sperry, R.W. (1972) Perception of bilateral chimeric figures following hemispheric deconnexion. *Brain*, **95,** 61.
36. Hécaen, H. & Angerlergues, R. (1962) Agnosia for faces. *Archives of Neurology* (Chicago), **7,** 92.
37. Hécaen, H. & Angelergues, R. (1963) *La cécité psychique*. Paris: Masson.
38. Lhermitte, F., Chain, F., Escourolle, R., Ducarne, B. & Pillon, B. (1972) Etude anatomoclinique d'un cas de prosopagnosie. *Revue neurologique*, **126,** 329.
39. Lhermitte, F., Chédru, F. & Chain, F. (1973) A propos d'un cas d'agnosie visuelle. *Revue neurologique*, **128,** 301.
40. Gazzaniga, M.S. (1973) The split brain in man. *Scientific American*, **228,** 24.
41. Proust, M. (1954) *Du côté de chez Swan*. Paris: La Pléiade, Gallimard.
42. Valéry, P. (1960) *Cahiers de Paul Valéry (XXIII)*. Paris: La Pléiade, Gallimard.
43. Robinson, J. (1963) *L'analyse de l'esprit dans les cahiers de Valéry*. Paris: José Corti.

BIBLIOGRAPHY

Alajouanine, Th. & Lhermitte, F. (1964) Essai d'introspection de l'aphasie; l'aphasie vue par les aphasiques *Revue neurologie*, **110,** 609.

Alajouanine, Th. & Lhermitte, F. (1964) Non-verbal communication in aphasia. In *Disorders of Language* (Ed.) de Reuck, A.V.S. & O'Connor, M. p. 168. London: Churchill.

Alford, L.B. (1933) Localization of consciousness and emotion. *American Journal of Psychiatry*, **89** (*new series 12*), 789.

Alford, L.B. (1943) Mental state associated with cerebral lesions. *Psychosomatic Medicine*, **5,** 15.

Ballet, G. (1886) *Le langage intérieur*. Paris: Ancienne librairie Germer Baillière.

Bay, E. (1973) Afasia, pensamiento conceptual e inteligencia. *Acta Audiologica y Foniatrica Hispano-americana*, **10,** 137.

Benvéniste, E. (1958) Catégories de pensée et catégories de langue. *Les Etudes philosophiques*, **4,** 419.

Bergson, H. (1912) *Matière et mémoire*. Paris: Alcan.

Beyn, E.S. (1958) Peculiarities of thought in patients with sensory aphasia. *Language and Speech*, **1,** 233.

Blum, G.S. (1961) *A Model of the Mind*. New York: Wiley.

Bogen, J.E. (1969) The other side of the brain II: an appositional mind. *Bulletin of the Los Angeles Neurological Society*, **34,** 135.

Bogen, J.E. (1969) The other side of the brain III: the corpus callosum and creativity. *Bulletin of the Los Angeles Neurological Society*, **34,** 191.

Brain, R. (1951) *Mind, Perception and Science*. Oxford: Blackwell.

Broadbent, W.H. (1872) On the cerebral mechanism of speech and thought. *Medico-chirurgical Transactions*, **55,** 145.

Brown, J.W. (1976) Consciousness and pathology of language. In *The Neuropsychology of Language: Essays in Honor of Eric Lenneberg* (Ed.) Rieber, R.W. New York: Plenum Press.

Brown, J.W. (1977) *Mind, Brain, and Consciousness: the Neuropsychology of Cognition*. New York: Academic Press.

Buyssens, E. (1954) Speaking and thinking from the linguistic standpoint. *Acta Psychologica*, **10,** 136.

Cassirer, E. (1929) La pathologie de la conscience symbolique. *Journal de Psychologie*, **26,** 289.

Chomsky, N. (1968) *Language and Mind*. New York: Harcourt Brace Jovanovich.

Doehring, D.G. & Reitan, R.M. (1962) Concept attainment of human adults with lateralized cerebral lesions. *Perceptual and Motor Skills*, **14,** 27.

Egger, V. (1881) *La parole intérieure.* Paris: Librairie Germer Baillière.

Ford, A. (1929) Attention-automatization: an investigation of the transitional nature of mind. *American Journal of Psychology*, **41,** 1.

Fraisse, P. & Piaget, J. (1963) *Traité de psychologie expérimentale.* Vol. VIII: *Langage, communication et décision.* Paris: Presses Universitaires de France.

Furth, H.G. (1966) *Thinking without Language. Psychological Implications of Deafness.* New York: Free Press.

Gazzaniga, M.S. & Sperry, R.W. (1965) Language in human patients after brain bisection. *Federation Proceedings*, **24,** 522.

Gazzaniga, M.S. & Sperry, R.W. (1967) Language after section of the cerebral commissures. *Brain*, **90,** 131.

Geets, W. (1972) Le langage perdu ou l'histoire d'un aphasique. *Le langage et l'homme*, **18,** 36.

Gelb, A. (1933) Remarques générales sur l'utilisation des données pathologiques pour la psychologie et la philosophie du langage. *Journal de Psychologie*, **30,** 403.

Goodglass, H., Denes, G. & Calderon, M. (1974) The absence of covert verbal mediation in aphasia. *Cortex*, **10,** 264.

Griffith, J.S. (1967) Neural organization underlying conscious thought. *Nature*, **214,** 345.

Hall, W.A. (1961) Return from silence—a personal experience. *Journal of Speech Disorders*, **26,** 174.

Harl, J.M. (1954) *Contribution à l'étude de l'intelligence non verbale chez les aphasiques.* Medical thesis, Paris.

Jakobson, E. (1911) On meaning and understanding. *American Journal of Psychology*, **22.**

Jørgensen, J. (1954) Some remarks concerning thinking and talking. *Acta Psychologica* (Amsterdam), **10,** 125.

Karlin, I.W. & Hirscherfang, S. (1963) Evaluation of language and intellectual disturbances in patients with space occupying brain lesions. *Logos*, **6,** 33.

Kertesz, A. & McCabe, P. (1975) Intelligence and aphasia: performance of aphasics on Raven's coloured progressive matrices (RCPM). *Brain and Language*, **2,** 387.

Kennedy, F. & Wolf, A. (1936) Relationship of intellect to speech defect in aphasic patients, with illustrative cases. *Journal of Nervous and Mental Diseases*, **84,** 125 and 293.

Köhler, W. (1951) *Mentality of Apes.* New York: The Humanities Press.

Kornyey, E. (1977) Aphasie et création artistique. *Encéphale*, **3,** 71.

Lashley, K.S. (1963) *Brain Mechanisms and Intelligence: a Quantitative Study of Injuries to the Brain.* New York: Dover.

Lebrun, Y. & Hoops, R. (1974) *Intelligence and Aphasia.* Amsterdam: Swets and Zeitlinger.

Lhermitte, J. (1957) *Le cerveau et la pensée.* Paris: Bloud and Gay.

Liublinskaya, A.A. (1957) The development of children's speech and thought. In *Psychology in the Soviet Union* (Ed.) Simon, B. p. 197. Stanford: Stanford University Press.

Lordat, J. (1843) Analyse de la parole pour servir à la théorie de divers cas d'alalie et de palilalie (de mutisme et d'imperfection de parler) que les neurologistes ont mal connus. *Journal de la Société pratique de Montpellier*, **7,** 333, 417 and **8,** 1.

Luria, A.R. (1957) The role of language in the formation of temporary connections. In *Psychology in the Soviet Union* (Ed.) Simon, B. p. 115. Stanford: Stanford University Press.

Meyers, R. (1948) The relation between 'thinking' and language: an experimental approach using dysphasic patients. *Archives of Neurology and Psychiatry* (Chicago), **9,** 119.

Ombredane, A. (1951) *L'aphasie et l'élaboration de la pensée explicite.* Paris: Presses Universitaires de France.

Orgass, B., Hartje, W., Kerschensteiner, M. & Poeck, K. (1972) Aphasie und nichtsprachliche Intelligenz. *Nervenarzt*, **43,** 623.

Piaget, J. (1954) Le langage et la pensée du point de vue génétique. *Acta Psychologica* (Amsterdam), **10,** 51.

Premack, D. (1971) Language in chimpanzee. *Science*, **172,** 808.

Premack, D. (1971) *Intelligence in Ape and Man.* Hillsdale, NJ: Lawrence Erlbaum.

Shank, R.C. & Colby, K.M. (1973) *Computer Models of Thought and Language.* San Francisco: Freeman.

Sinclair-de Zwart, H. (1967) *Acquisition du langage et développement de la pensée.* Paris: Dunod.

Sokolov, A.N. (1969) Studies of the speech mechanisms of thinking. In *A Handbook of Contemporary Soviet Psychology* (Ed.) Cole, M. & Maltzman, J. p. 531. New York: Basic Books.

Sokolov, A.N. (1972) *Inner Speech and Thought.* New York: Plenum-Rosetta Press.

Teleki, G. (1974) Chimpanzee subsistence technology: materials and skills. *Journal of Human Evolution*, **3,** 575.

Tilney, F. (1936) Discussion of Kennedy, F. and Wolf, A. Relationship of intellect to speech in patients with aphasia, with illustrative cases. *Archives of Neurology and Psychiatry* (Chicago), **36,** 897.

Vigotsky, L.S. (1939) Thought and speech. *Psychiatry*, **2,** 29.

Whorf, B. (1956) *Language, Thought, Reality.* New York: Wiley.

Woerkom, W. (van) (1923) Sur l'état psychique des aphasiques. *Encéphale*, **18,** 286.

Woodworth, R.S. (1915) A revision of imageless thought. *Psychological Review*, **22.**

Zangwill, O.L. (1964) Intelligence in aphasia. In *Disorders of Language* (Ed.) de Reuck, A.V.S. & O'Connor, M. p. 261. London: Churchill.

Zaslow, R.W. (1961) A study of concept formation in normals, mental defectives, and brain-damaged adults. *Genetic Psychology Monographs*, **63,** 279.

Index

Note: Page numbers of chapter titles are in **bold face** type

15

£21·50